THE PLANT BASED Diet Cookbook

800 Foolproof Recipes to Lose Weight by Cooking Wholesome Green Foods | **28-Day Meal Plan** Included to Detox Your Body and Feel Great Again

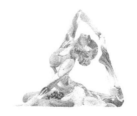

by
EMMA J. GUIDE

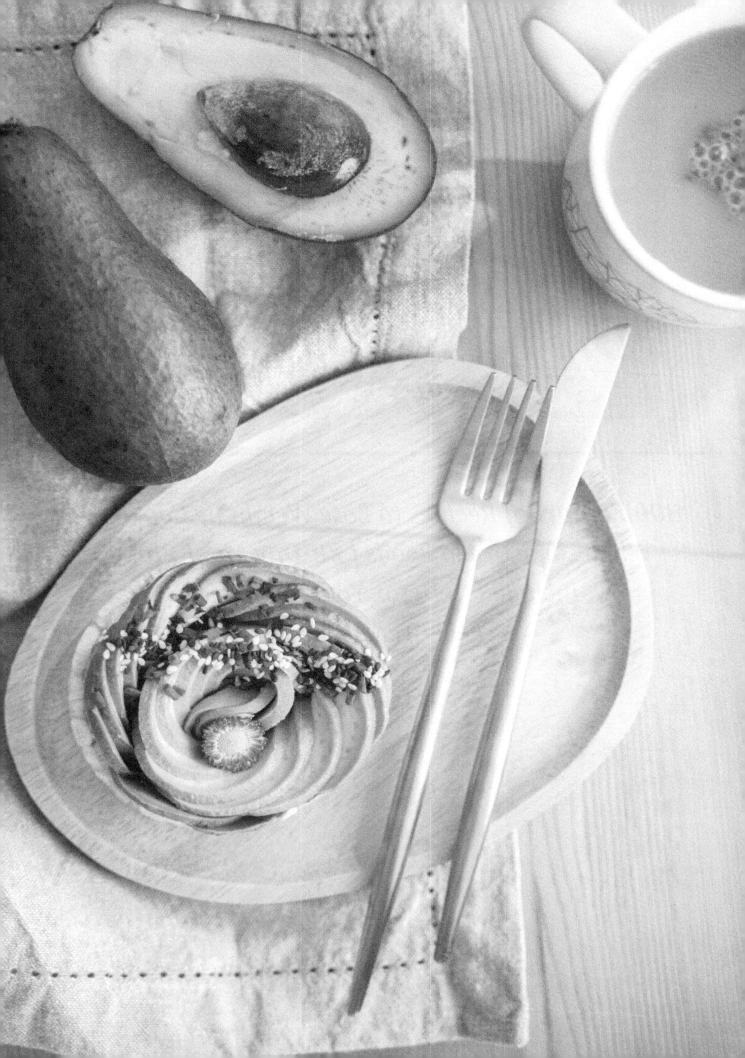

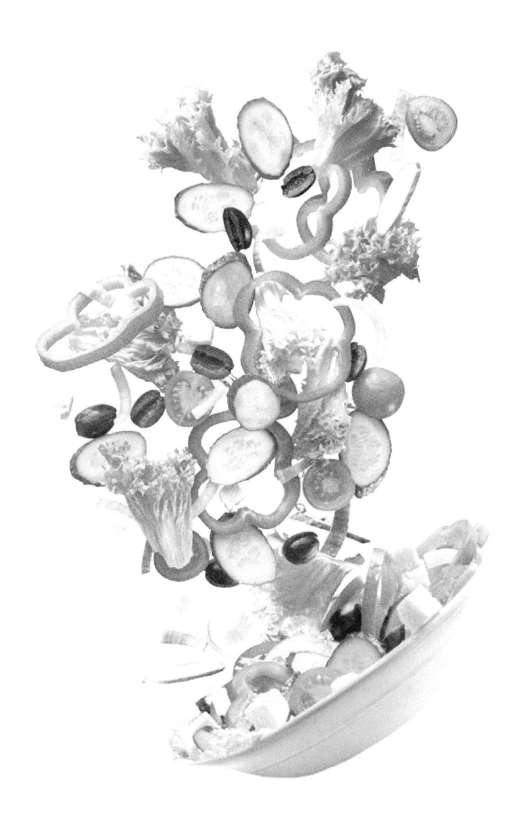

About the Author

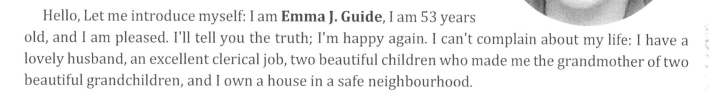

One day, without knowing how, I lost myself. Compared to any other period in my life, my body has changed too quickly: I have gained weight, I can't recognize myself in the mirror, I have been tired all the time, my mood is low, and I have entered an alienated one.

The negative spiral comes from everyone, including my husband. He always said that I am beautiful, but his words do not match the facts; our intimacy is getting less and less, and I am afraid of losing him.

Hello, Let me introduce myself: I am **Emma J. Guide**, I am 53 years old, and I am pleased. I'll tell you the truth; I'm happy again. I can't complain about my life: I have a lovely husband, an excellent clerical job, two beautiful children who made me the grandmother of two beautiful grandchildren, and I own a house in a safe neighbourhood.

All this sounds great, but there was a dark period after 41 years. As I wrote before, I feel bad and close to depression. After menopause, I gained 45 pounds; I changed my whole wardrobe and no longer liked myself. I locked myself at home and never went out again because I always felt exhausted and uncomfortable. I am afraid of the expression on other people's faces. My husband also walked away, and to overcome the sadness, I continued to eat. I tried to react by testing any diet available on the market, Keto, Dukan, and Paleo, but I couldn't return to my original self.

Yes, I lost weight immediately, and I can see some effects, but between the side effects of these ultra-protein diets and dietary restrictions, I gave up quickly. Then I started to know the Plant-Based Diet, and my life changed drastically. All of this seems unbelievable. According to the letter, I have to reduce the excess weight by dividing the time between eating and fasting. Don't give up any food dreams. Soon, I will be able to wear my favourite clothes back; I will feel more energetic and confident. I went back in the evening to go out with friends. I was relieved or disappeared from the pain, and I found my husband again. He is even jealous of my young colleague now.

Given my success using a **Plant-Based Diet**, I decided to research and explore this topic with some nutritionists to achieve my goal: to help all women like me encounter the problems I have encountered. I don't want any woman to have my recent feelings. So I am here to help you find your best self and regain the fun of beauty and sexiness.

In this book, you will find all the topics I have explored that have helped me on my journey:

- ✅ A brief introduction to **Plant-Based Diet** and its basic principles.
- ✅ Follow all the best protocols to get results in the shortest possible time.
- ✅ 8 easy ways to get started with a **Plant-Based Diet**.
- ✅ Tips and tricks to cook plant-based and its anti-aging effects.
- ✅ The correlation between **Plant-Based Diet** and exercise.
- ✅ Foods to avoid or limit on the Plant-Based Diet.
- ✅ A complete **28-Day Meal Plan** with exercises to activate the metabolism, burn fat and lose weight by eating more food

...and much more!

I Can Already Feel Your Satisfaction!

☆ **Here Is the First Tips:** <u>Start Now</u>!
It's time for you to decide and plan for a healthier life for yourself and your family.
Then, with a straightforward purchase that you can set up in your kitchen, you can begin cooking delicious meals suitable for your body and soul. It's time to take control of your culinary fate, so come on in and learn about what a wood pellet smoker has to offer.

So, What Are You Waiting For? It's Time for You to Take Charge!

Good Luck!

Table of Contents

ABOUT THE AUTHOR 5
INTRODUCTION 15
CHAPTER 1. THE PLANT-BASED EXPLAINED 19
How To Build A New Flavor? 19
An Alternative Food Concept 21
8 Ways To Get Started With A Plant-Based Diet..........22
Some Plant-Based Substitutes 22
Plant-Based Diet Using A Meal Plan.....................24

CHAPTER 2. UNDERSTANDING PLANT-BASED DIET 27
What Is a Plant-Based Diet? 27
Foods To Eat On The Plant-Based-Diet...................29
Cooking Equipment Used To Prepare Plant-Based Diet....30
Knife Types For Cutting Plant-Based Diet 33
Cutting Techniques According To Food...................34
Things to keep in your mind while cutting..............35

CHAPTER 3. TYPES OF A PLANT-BASED DIET 37
Types Of Plant-Based Diets 38
Understanding Plants....................................39
Essential Plant-Based Pantry 40
Tips And Tricks For Going Plant-Based 41

CHAPTER 4. PLANT-BASED DIET 43
Macrobiotic Plant-Based Diet 43
Vegan Lifestyle 44
Pros And Cons Of Plant-Based Diet 44
Difference Between Vegan And Vegetarian Diet............45
Benefits 45
Daily Exercise: 15 Minutes For Day 46

CHAPTER 5. 28-DAY MEAL PLAN 47
Week 1 48
Week 2 49
Week 3 50
Week 4 51

CHAPTER 6. BREAKFAST RECIPES...........................53
1.   Banana-Amaranth Porridge..........................54
2.   Jalapeño Cornbread.................................54
3.   Japanese-Pumpkin Rice..............................54
4.   Polenta With Herbs.................................54
5.   Blueberry Pancakes.................................55
6.   Baked Apples.......................................55
7.   Maple Cashew Apple Toast...........................56
8.   Mango Ginger Oats Recipe...........................56
9.   Acai-Bowl Recipe...................................56
10. Plant-Based Burrito Breakfast......................56
11. Crunchy-Egg-Salad..................................57
12. No-Bake Cookies....................................57
13. No-Bake-Energy-Balls...............................57

14. Breakfast-Veggie-Burger Recipe 58
15. Banana-Buckwheat Porridge 58
16. Black Bean Plus Sweet Potato Hash.................58
17. Blueberry Muffins 59
18. Breakfast Burritos 59
19. Breakfast Scramble................................60
20. Breakfast Tofu Scramble...........................60
21. Chai-Spiced Oatmeal With Mango 61
22. Coconut-Almond Risotto 61
23. Cranberry-Walnut Quinoa 61
24. Nutty Granola 61
25. Pear Oats With Walnuts 62
26. Pumpkin Spice Oatmeal With Brown Sugar
     Topping 62
27. Soy Yogurt 62
28. Strawberry Muffins 63
29. Whole-Wheat Banana Pecan Pancakes 63
30. Bowl With Amaranth Granola 64
31. Portobello Mushroom Burger 64
32. Toast With Radishes & Dandelion Greens 65
33. Wild Rice Soup 65
34. Roasted Brussels Sprouts 66
35. Easiest Chia Pudding 66
36. Roasted Chickpeas 66
37. Verde Avocado Salsa 67
38. Lemon Thyme Oil & Burrata 67
39. Miso Soup 67
40. Carrot Smorrebrod Crisps 68
41. Cream Of Mushroom Soup 68
42. Sweet & Spicy Popcorn.............................69
43. Vegetarian Tacos With Avocado Sauce 69
44. Blistered Shishito Peppers 70
45. Burrata 70
46. Mango Coconut Muffins.............................70
47. Vegan Pasta Salad.................................71
48. Matcha Milkshakes.................................71
49. Chocolate Cups 71
50. The Best Guacamole 72
51. Vegan Pimento Dip 72
52. Cilantro Lime Rice 72
53. Vegan Cashews Dip 73
54. Sheet Pan Nachos 73
55. Vegan 7 Layer Dip 73
56. Kale Pesto 74
57. Original Baba Ganoush 74
58. Edible Cookie Dough...............................75
59. Sweet Vegan Nachos 75
60. Vegan Bacon 75
61. Tzatziki Sauce 76

62.	Pomegranate Potato Crostini	76
63.	Strawberry Basil Avocado Toast	76
64.	Vegan-Pumpkin Bars	77
65.	Strawberry Rhubarb Bars	77
66.	Rhubarb Chia Strawberry Overnight Oat Parfaits	78
67.	Almond Butter Brown Rice Crispy Treats	78
68.	Pumpkin Spiced Corn Muffins	79
69.	Falafel	79
70.	Best Lentil Soup	80
71.	Vegan Lemon Muffins	80
72.	Chocolate Avocado Pudding Pops	81
73.	Healthy Loaded Vegan Nachos	81
74.	Jamaican Jerk Vegan Tacos	82
75.	Marinated Baked Tempeh	82
76.	Many-Veggie Vegetable Soup	83
77.	Yellow Split Pea Soup	83
78.	Twice Baked Sweet Potatoes	84
79.	Grilled Tartines	84
80.	Corn "Ceviche" Crostini	85

CHAPTER 7. SNACKS, SIDES DISHES & WRAPS 86

81.	Alanna's Pumpkin Cranberry Nut & Seed Loaf	87
82.	Cashew Cream For 2	87
83.	Almost-Raw Carrot Balls	87
84.	Fresh Spring Rolls	88
85.	Fried Green Tomatoes	88
86.	Herb Compound Butter	89
87.	Deviled-Potato Sandwiches	89
88.	Sweet-Potato & Veggie-Roll-Ups	90
89.	Spicy-Tempeh-Mango-Spring Rolls	90
90.	California Burritos	91
91.	Blueberry-Banana-Wraps	91
92.	Tortilla-Roll-Ups & Lentils-Spinach	92
93.	Rainbow-Veggie-Slaw Wrap	92
94.	Spanish-Rice & Black-Beans With Burrito	92
95.	Spinach-Tomatillo-Wraps With Hearty-Tahini-Spread	93
96.	Avocado And White-Bean-Salad Wraps	93
97.	Vegan-Spring-Rolls	94
98.	Vegan-Snack-Wrap	95
99.	Summer Rolls	95
100.	Fresh Spring-Rolls	95
101.	Nori Wraps	96
102.	Chickpea-Salad-Wraps With Avocado-Dill-Sauce	96
103.	Steamed Dumplings	97
104.	Steamed Bao-Buns	97
105.	Homemade Soft-Pretzels	98
106.	Rosemary-Focaccia-Bread	99
107.	Vegan-Pecan-Apple-Chickpea-Salad Wraps	99
108.	Green Pea, Lettuce And Tomato Sandwich	100
109.	Chickpea-Salad-Sandwiches	100
110.	Puffed Rice Balls	101
111.	Roasted Cauliflower Hummus	101
112.	Thai Chickpeas	101
113.	Sweet Potato Appetizer Bites	102
114.	Roasted Corn With Poblano-Cilantro Butter	102
115.	Porcini Mushroom Pate	103
116.	Red Pepper Hummus In Cucumber Cups	103
117.	Stir-Fried Chinese Cress With Fermented Black Beans	103
118.	Stuffed Artichokes	104
119.	Stuffed Mushrooms	104

120.	Latkes	105
121.	Curry Roasted Cauliflower	105
122.	Easy Garlic-Roasted Potatoes	106
123.	Almond And Breadcrumb–Stuffed Piquillo Peppers	106
124.	Roasted Radishes And Carrots With A Lemon Butter Dill Sauce	106
125.	Warm Caper With Beet Salad	107
126.	Braised Brussels Sprouts With Chestnuts	107
127.	Imam Bayildi- Turkish Stuffed Eggplant	108
128.	Sweet-Potato-Appetizer-Bites	108
129.	Orange-Scented Green Beans With Toasted Almond	109
130.	Roasted Root Vegetable Medley	109
131.	Spinach And Rice–Stuffed Tomatoes	109
132.	Turmeric Ginger Spiced Cauliflower	110
133.	Vegan Stuffed Eggplant Provençal	110
134.	Asparagus Avocado Soup	111
135.	Chicken- Less Soup	112
136.	Classic Vegetable Soup	112
137.	Cold Tomato Summer Vegetable Soup	113
138.	Cream Of Mushroom Soup	113
139.	Cream Of Thyme Tomato Soup	113
140.	Creamy Cauliflower Soup	114
141.	Creamy Corn Chowder	114
142.	Curried Cauliflower Coconut Soup	115
143.	Giambotta- Italian Summer Vegetable Stew	115
144.	Ginger Kale Soup	116
145.	Grandma's Chicken Noodle Soup	116
146.	Green Curry Vegetable Stew	117
147.	Guacamole Soup	117
148.	Gumbo Filé	118
149.	Lime-Mint Soup	118
150.	Meaty Mushroom Stew	119
151.	Vegan-Miso Soup	119
152.	Miso Udon Bowl	120
153.	Mushroom And Cabbage Borscht	120
154.	Mushroom Barley Soup	121
155.	Roasted Tomato Soup	121
156.	Smoky White Bean And Tomato Soup	122
157.	Tom Yum Soup	122
158.	Rosemary Garlic Popcorn	123
159.	Classic Hummus	123
160.	Herbed Zucchini	123
161.	Homemade Marinated Mushrooms	124
162.	Mushroom Bun Sliders	124
163.	Banh-Mi-Sandwich	125
164.	Chickpea-Salad Sandwich	125
165.	Carrot-Smorrebrod-Crisps	126
166.	Blt Sandwich	126
167.	Jackfruit-Bbq-Sandwiches	126
168.	No-Tuna-Salad-Sandwich	127
169.	Greens & Things Sandwiches	127
170.	Jackfruit-Barbecue-Sandwiches And Broccoli-Slaw	128
171.	Stacked-Vegetable-Sandwiches & Cilantro Chutney	128
172.	Buffalo-Cauliflower-Pita-Pockets	129
173.	Super-Sloppy-Joes	129
174.	Sautéed Brussels-Sprouts	130
175.	Baba Ganoush	130
176.	Tomato Bruschetta	130

177. Grilled-Ratatouille-Tartines 131
178. Socca Recipe 131
179. Loaded-Potato-Skins 131
180. Vegan Portobello-Pizzas 132
181. Vegan-Lemon-Muffins 132
182. Healthy Banana-Muffins 133
183. Mango-Coconut-Muffins 133
184. Portobello-Mushroom-Burger 134
185. Maki-Sushi-Recipe 134
186. Vegan-7-Layer-Dip 135
187. 2-Mins, Steamed Asparagus 135
188. Sun-Dried-Tomato & Chickpea Sliders 136
189. Mexican Cauliflower Rice 136
190. Minted Peas And Baby Potatoes 136
191. Mushroom Risotto 137
192. Red Cabbage With Apples And Pecans 137
193. Fragrant Cauliflower Rice 138
194. Garlic Sautéed Spinach 138
195. Roasted Tomatoes 139
196. Sautéed Broccoli Rabe 139
197. Sautéed Zucchini And Cherry Tomatoes 139
198. Sesame Asparagus 140
199. Sesame Ginger Broccoli 140
200. Smoky Lima Beans 140
201. Southern Sweet Potatoes With Pecan Streusel 141
202. Southern-Style Braised Greens 141
203. Steamed Artichokes 142
204. Sweet Thai Coconut Rice 142
205. Vegan-Welsh-Rarebit & Mushrooms 142
206. Air-Fryer Onion-Rings 143
207. Wasabi-Ginger-Beet & Avocado With Tartines 143
208. Roasted-Kabocha Squash 144
209. Roasted Pumpkin-Seeds 144
210. Avocado Fries 144
211. Baked Potato-Wedges 145
212. Instant-Pot Mashed-Potatoes 145
213. Homemade Granola 145
214. Homemade Taquitos 146
215. Sheet-Pan-Nachos 146
216. Crispy-Roasted-Chickpeas 146
217. Roasted Cauliflower & Lemon Zest 147
218. Homemade Salsa 147
219. Mango Salsa 147
220. French-Onion-Dip 148
221. Tomatillo-Salsa-Verde 148
222. Cowboy Caviar 148
223. Air Fryer-French- Fries 149
224. Baked-Sweet-Potato-Fries 149

CHAPTER 8. SUPPER & SAVORY BOWLS **151**
225. Instant-Pot-Black-Beans 152
226. Black-Bean-Chili 152
227. Roasted-Golden-Beets 152
228. Butternut-Squash-Risotto 153
229. Arugula-Salad With Lemon-Vinaigrette 153
230. Brown Rice 154
231. Kimchi-Brown-Rice-Bliss-Bowls 154
232. Box-Buddha-Bowls 154
233. Curried-Lentil-Salad 154
234. Cinnamon-Roasted-Sweet-Potato-Salad With
       Wild-Rice 155
235. Shiitake Bacon 155

236. Coconut Bacon 156
237. Avocado-Sweet-Potato-Tacos 156
238. Macro-Veggie-Bowl 156
239. Falafel Flatbread 157
240. Vegan-Egg-Salad 157
241. Adzuki-Bean-Bowls 158
242. Roasted-Veggie-Grain-Bowl 158
243. Sweet-Potato-Quinoa-Bowl 159
244. Mango-Ginger-Rice-Bowl 159
245. Sesame-Soba-Noodles 159
246. Vegan-Burrito-Bowl 160
247. Cauliflower-Rice-Kimchi-Bowls 160
248. Spaghetti Squash 161
249. Stuffed-Acorn Squash 161
250. Stuffed-Poblano-Peppers 162
251. Avocado-Cucumber-Sushi-Roll 162
252. Spicy-Mango & Avocado-Rice-Bowl 163
253. Quinoa-Pilaf-Recipe 163
254. Radish-Salad W/Radish-Top-Pesto 164
255. Kale-Salad W/Carrot-Ginger-Dressing 164
256. Roasted-Cauliflower-Salad 165
257. Taco Salad 165
258. Coconut Curry 166
259. Bibim-Bap 166
260. Tamago-Kake-Gohan 167
261. Vegan-Poke-Bowl 167
262. Avocado-Crispbreads W/Everything-Bagel-
       Seasoning 167
263. Mixed-Greens-Salad W/Pumpkin-Vinaigrette 168
264. Veggie-Rice-Bowl Recipe 168
265. Grilled-Vegetable-Wrap W/Balsamic-Mayo 168
266. Mushroom-Cheesesteak Recipe 169
267. Nutrient Packed-Simmered-Lentils Recipe 169

CHAPTER 9. SOUPS & STEWS RECIPES **171**
268. Butternut-Squash-Soup 172
269. Vegan-Broccoli-Soup 172
270. Tomato- Basil Soup 173
271. Creamy-Mushroom-Soup 173
272. Wild Rice 174
273. Potato-Leek-Soup 174
274. Pumpkin-Tortilla-Soup 174
275. Tomato-Basil-Soup 175
276. Carrot-Soup-Recipe W/Ginger 176
277. Roasted-Red-Pepper-Soup 176
278. Cauliflower Soup 176
279. Red-Curry-Lemongrass-Soup 177
280. Carrot-Coconut-Soup 177
281. French-Onion-Soup 178
282. Oyster-Mushroom-Soup 178
283. Tortellini Soup 179
284. Vegetarian Pho 179
285. Spiralized-Zucchini-Vegetable-Noodle Soup 180
286. Ginger-Miso-Soup 180
287. Cabbage Soup 181
288. Ribollita Tuscan Bean Soup 181
289. Veggie Soup 181
290. Vegetable Stock 182
291. Creamy-Potato-Soup 182
292. Sweet-Potato-Soup 183
293. Instant-Pot-Lentil-Soup 183
294. Barley With Winter Vegetable Soup 184

295. Black Bean Soup 184
296. Vegan Chili Soup 184
297. Creamy Broccoli Soup With "Chicken" And Rice.185
298. Lentil And Vegetable Dal 185
299. Lentil Soup With Cumin And Coriander 186
300. Meaty Seitan Stew 187
301. Mexican Baked Potato Soup 187
302. Minestrone...187
303. Mushroom & Jalapeño Stew 188
304. Red Curry-Coconut Milk Soup 188
305. Root Veggie Soup 189
306. Spicy Chili With Red Lentils 189
307. Split-Pea Soup 189
308. Tofu Stir Fry With Asparagus Stew 190
309. Tomato Rice Soup 190
310. Turkish Soup 190
311. Veggie-Quinoa Soup 191
312. Weeknight 3-Bean Chili 191
313. Vegetable Detox Soup 192
314. Mean Green Detox Vegetable Soup 192
315. Cleansing Detox Soup 193
316. Vegan Turmeric Cauliflower Chickpea Stew ...193
317. Chicken Detox Soup 194
318. Slimming Detox Soup 194
319. Cleansing Carrot Autumn Squash Soup ...195
320. Tomato Basil Soup 195
321. Lentil And Kale Soup 196
322. Roasted Cauliflower Soup 196
323. Creamy Butternut Squash Soup 196
324. Raw Red Pepper Soup 197
325. Broccoli Basil Cream Soup 197
326. Cremini Mushroom Soup 198
327. Protein Packed Black Bean And Lentil Soup ...198
328. Thai Roasted Sweet Potato Soup 198
329. Slow Cooker Savory Superfood Soup......199
330. Flush The Fat Away Vegetable Soup.......199
331. Slow Cooker Butternut Squash & Kale Stew....200
332. Slow Cooker Chicken Enchilada Stew........200
333. Slow Cooker Black Bean & Veggie Soup....200
334. Pesto White Bean Soup 201
335. Skinny Detox Soup 201
336. Weight Loss Soup 202
337. Superfoods Detox Soup 202
338. Creamy Nutmeg Broccoli Soup 202
339. Broccoli And Arugula Soup 203
340. Detox Deliciously: Ginger-Carrot Soup ...203
341. Spring Detox Soup 204
342. Vegan Black Bean Soup 204
343. Tuscan Portobello Stew 205
344. Braised Pork Stew 205
345. Pork And Green Chile Stew....................205
346. Moroccan Vegetarian Stew 206
347. Wintertime Braised Beef Stew 206
348. Beefy Cabbage Bean Stew 207
349. Chicken Mushroom Stew 207
350. 1-Pot Beef & Pepper Stew 208
351. Manchester Stew 208
352. Teriyaki Beef Stew 208
353. West African Chicken Stew....................209
354. Slow-Cooked Lentil Stew 209
355. Root Stew 210
356. Curried Beef Stew 210

357. Sweet Potato Lentil Stew 210
358. Spicy Chicken Stew 211
359. Spicy Beef Vegetable Stew 211
360. Sweet Potato Stew 211
361. Apple Chicken Stew 212
362. Beefless Stew 212

CHAPTER 10. LUNCH & DINNER RECIPES........... 213
363. Arancini- Risotto Balls 214
364. Bisteeya- Moroccan Phyllo Pie 214
365. Butternut Squash Tagine 215
366. Cassoulet 215
367. Clean Vegan Pad Thai 216
368. Creamy Pasta With Swiss Chard And Tomatoes... 216
369. Crispy Quinoa Cakes 217
370. Eggplant And Roasted Tomato Polenta Lasagna.. 217
371. Farro Risotto With Roasted Fennel And Mushrooms 218
372. Grilled Tofu Caprese 219
373. Hearty Seitan Roast 219
374. Mixed Vegetable Cottage Pie 220
375. Moroccan Couscous 221
376. Mushroom Lasagna 221
377. 1-Pan Pasta Primavera 222
378. Quinoa Vegetable Salad 222
379. Risotto Milanese 223
380. Savory Stuffed Cabbage 223
381. Seitan And Dumplings 224
382. Seitan Satay 225
383. Sesame Noodles 225
384. Sesame Tofu Cutlets 226
385. Summer Squash And Onion Bake...........226
386. Swiss Chard Ravioli 227
387. Tamale Casserole 227
388. Tempeh Milanese 228
389. Tofu And Veggie Stir-Fry 229
390. Tofu Summer Rolls 229
391. Vegetable Enchiladas With Roasted Tomato Sauce 230
392. Whole-Wheat Pasta & Ceci- Pasta With Chickpeas 230
393. Winter Vegetable Pot Pie.......................231
394. Tofu Stir-Fry 232
395. Spinach & Chickpeas With 5 Ingredient Ziti Baked.............................232

CHAPTER 11. NOODLES & PASTA RECIPES 233
396. Spinach Parmesan Zucchini Noodles 234
397. No-Boil Vegetable Lasagna 234
398. Blt Pasta Salad 234
399. Pesto Pasta Salad..................................235
400. How To Make Veggie Noodles 235
401. Spaghetti And Meatballs 236
402. Sesame Soba Noodles 236
403. Zucchini Noodles & Lemon /Ricotta 236
404. Easy Peanut Noodles 237
405. Cold Cucumber Soba 237
406. Zucchini Noodles & Avocado-Miso Sauce ...238
407. Cashew Broccoli Soba Noodles 238
408. Ginger Noodles With Kale & Shiitakes....238
409. Cucumber Mango Miso Noodle Bowl 239
410. Tahini Noodle Salad With Roasted Carrots & Chickpeas 239

411. Roasted Cauliflower Pasta 240
412. Tahini Zucchini Noodles 241
413. Roasted Tomato Brown Rice Pasta.........241
414. Creamy Butternut Squash Pasta............242
415. Zucchini Noodles 242
416. Spiralized Daikon "Rice Noodle" Bowl......243
417. Soba Noodles With Shishitos & Avocado 243
418. Spicy Kohlrabi Noodles 244
419. Cold Sesame Noodles With Kale & Shiitakes....244
420. Butternut Squash Noodle Pasta 245
421. Zucchini Coconut Noodles 245
422. Ginger Miso Noodles With Eggplant 246
423. Sesame Noodle Bowl 246
424. Golden Turmeric Noodle Miso Soup 247
425. Creamy Vegan Shiitake & Kale Pasta........247
426. Creamy Pumpkin Pasta Sauce 248
427. Broccoli Tahini Pasta Salad 248
428. Creamy Vegan Pasta 249
429. Rosemary Lemon Pasta 249
430. Slow Roasted Tomato Pasta 250
431. Vegan Sweet Potato..........................250
432. Cauliflower Mac & Cheese 251
433. Hazelnut Tahini Pasta 252
434. Anna's Avocado & Lemon Zest Spaghetti.....252
435. Shells & Roasted Cauliflower 253
436. Tagliatelle With Tomatoes And Greens 253
437. Spaghetti Bolognese 254
438. Spring Green Lemon & Basil Pasta...........254
439. Fettuccine & Sweet Corn Cream 255
440. Sweet Potato Surprise 256
441. Creamy Pasta Pomodoro 256
442. Orecchiette With Broccoli Rabe 257
443. Summer Squash & Corn Orzo................258
444. 1 Pot Vegetable Penne Pasta 258
445. Easy Pesto Pasta 258
446. Creamy Vegan Pasta Bake With Brussels Sprouts .259
447. Spaghetti Aglio E Olio........................259

CHAPTER 12. LEGUME RECIPES............... 261
448. Smokey Tempeh Bacon 262
449. Burrito With Tofu Scramble 262
450. Huevos Rancheros Casserole 263
451. Burrito 263
452. Vegan Collard Greens.......................264
453. Chipotle Black Bean Avocado Toast 264
454. Baked Bean Toast- 3-Ingredient............264
455. Black Bean Breakfast Burritos 265
456. Tofu Scramble Stuffed Breakfast Sweet Potatoes ..265
457. Butternut Squash Black Bean Enchiladas With Jalapeño Cashew Crema......................266
458. Vegetarian Chili.............................267
459. Black Bean Chili.............................267
460. Instant Pot Black Beans 268
461. Creamy Potato Soup.........................268
462. Smoky-Sweet Potatoes With Black Beans & Corn 268
463. Santa Fe Black Bean Burger 269
464. Caesar Salad 269
465. Curried Chickpea Salad 270
466. Greek Quinoa Salad 270
467. Black Bean, Corn & Avocado Salad..........270
468. Pozole- Posole Verde 271
469. Lemon Rosemary White Bean Soup 271

470. Green Beans Almondine- Amandine 271
471. Hearty Lentil Soup 272
472. Chickpea Tikka Masala 272
473. 1 Pot Chili Mac 273
474. Bean Chili 273
475. Collard Greens..............................274
476. Rustic Cabbage, Potato & White Bean Soup 274
477. Barley Bowl..................................274
478. Kale + Black Bean Burrito Bowl 275
479. Roasted Poblano Tacos 276
480. Creamy Dill Potato Salad 276
481. Balela Salad.................................277
482. Black Bean + Quinoa Burritos..............277
483. Refried Beans...............................278
484. Healthy Baked Beans 278
485. Chickpea Noodle Soup 279
486. Crispy Chickpeas 279
487. Black Beans 279
488. Red Beans & Rice 280
489. Peanut Butter Plus Rice Crispy Cacao Nibs Treats 280
490. Teriyaki Tofu-Tempeh Casserole 281
491. Spanish Vegan Paella 281
492. Lemon Chickpea Orzo Soup................282
493. Rosemary Bread 283
494. Vegetable Chili..............................283

CHAPTER 13. GRAINS RECIPES 285
495. Ingredients Mexican Quinoa 286
496. Healthy Huevos Rancheros Tacos...........286
497. Vanilla Vegan Buckwheat Pancakes 286
498. Chocolate Chip, Apricot, And Orange Scones ..287
499. Enchilada Rice 287
500. Healthy Carrot Cake Cookies 288
501. Carrot Muffins 288
502. Pumpkin Spice Overnight Oats Recipe 288
503. Healthy Chai-Spiced Carrot Banana Bread With Cream Cheese Frosting 289
504. Peanut Butter Cinnamon Toast 289
505. Quinoa & Chia Oatmeal Mix 290
506. Savory Vegan Breakfast Bowl 290
507. Easy Oil-Free Granola- With Lots Of Crunchy Clusters! 290
508. Instant Pot Buckwheat Porridge 291
509. Creamy Tomato, Basil & Rice Soup.........291
510. Vegan Coconut Rice Pudding 291
511. Easy Low Fodmap Shakshuka 292
512. Pina Colada Granola- Vegan & Can Be Gf ..292
513. Cauliflower Rice Kimchi Bowls 293
514. Stuffed Yellow Peppers......................293
515. Roasted Veggie Brown Rice Buddha Bowl ..294
516. Spinach, Feta & Rice Casserole 294
517. Cooked Brown Rice 294
518. Chana Masala 295
519. Kimchi Brown Rice Bliss Bowls 295
520. Pomegranate Rice Salad 295
521. Stuffed Poblano Peppers....................296
522. Vegan Sushi.................................296
523. Vegan Burrito Bowl 297
524. Mango Ginger Rice Bowl....................298
525. Avocado Cucumber Sushi Roll 298
526. Butternut Squash Burrito Bowls 299

527. Toasted Oats Cereal- Camping Breakfast 299
528. Chia Overnight Oats 2 Ways! 300

Chapter 14. Salad Recipes 301

529. Autumn Wheat Berry Salad 302
530. Baby Bok Choy Salad With Sesame Dressing 302
531. Baby Lima Bean And Quinoa Salad 302
532. Bulgur, Cucumber, And Tomato Salad 303
533. Buttery Garlic Green Beans 303
534. Citrus Green Beans With Pine Nuts 303
535. Curried Rice Salad 304
536. Fruited Millet Salad 304
537. Greek Broccoli Salad 305
538. Israeli Quinoa Salad 305
539. Quinoa Arugula Salad 305
540. Quinoa Tabbouleh 306
541. Quinoa, Corn, And Black Bean Salad 306
542. Rice Salad With Fennel, Chickpeas, And Orange ..306
543. Spicy Asian Quinoa Salad 307
544. Spring Asparagus Salad With Lemon Vinaigrette ..307
545. Warm Rice And Bean Salad 307
546. Winter Greens Salad With Pomegranate &
     Kumquats 308
547. Zucchini And Avocado Salad With Garlic
     Herb Dressing 308

Chapter 15. Vegan Recipes 311

548. Slow-Cooker Chicken & Chickpea Soup 312
549. Butternut Squash Soup With Apple Grilled
     Cheese Sandwiches 312
550. Wheat Berry Salad With Roasted Beets & Curry
     Cashew Dressing 313
551. Carrot And Ginger Soup Recipe 313
552. Warm Broccoli And Chicken Salad Recipe 314
553. Cheesy Ground Beef & Cauliflower Casserole 314
554. Easy Italian Wedding Soup 315
555. Slow-Cooker Chicken & White Bean Stew 315
556. Spinach & Artichoke Casserole With Chicken
     And Cauliflower Rice 315
557. Spicy Weight-Loss Cabbage Soup 316
558. Chicken Cutlets With Sun-Dried Tomato Cream
     Sauce 316
559. American Goulash 317
560. 1-Pot Chicken & Cabbage Soup 317
561. Cabbage Roll Casserole 318
562. Vegan Almond Flour Shortbread Cookies 318
563. Vegan Carrot Almond Breakfast Pudding 319
564. Wild Rice Mason Jar Salad With Basil Pesto 319
565. Thai Salad With Ginger Peanut Sauce 320
566. The Ultimate Detox Salad With Lemon Ginger
     Dressing 320
567. Zucchini Noodles With Pesto 320
568. Vegan Quinoa Salad 321
569. Vegan Taco Salad 321
570. Southwest Quinoa Salad 322
571. Mediterranean Quinoa Salad 322
572. Vegan Spring Rolls With Sweet Potato Noodles ...323
573. Easy Guacamole 323
574. Vegan Cheddar Cheese With Jalapeño 323
575. 4 Ingredient Cookies 324
576. Roasted Garlic Hummus 324
577. Vegan Queso 324
578. Mexican-Style Stuffed Zucchini Boats 325

579. Vegan Enchiladas Skillet 326
580. Eggplant Chickpea Curry 326
581. Vegan Bolognese Sauce With Mushrooms 327
582. Portobello Steaks 327
583. Vegan Zucchini Noodle Lasagna 327
584. Vegan Sushi Bowl 328
585. Lemon Pepper Cauliflower Steaks 329
586. Tofu Stir Fry With Broccoli And Bell Peppers 329
587. Black Beans And Rice 330
588. Raw Chocolate Chia Pudding 330
589. Vegan Chocolate Cheesecake Bars 330
590. Raw Carrot Cake Bites 331
591. Raw Chunky Monkey Ice Cream 332
592. Vegan Chocolate Banana Cream Pie 332
593. Raw Chocolate Peanut Butter Cups 333
594. Blueberry Overnight Oats 333
595. Protein Packed Chia Pudding 333
596. Matcha Chia Pudding 334
597. Gluten-Free, Vegan Breakfast Cookies 334
598. Chocolate Peanut Butter Oatmeal 335

Chapter 16. Vegetable Recipes 337

599. Best Roasted Vegetables- Perfectly Seasoned! 338
600. Dipping Sauce 338
601. Ultimate Sauteed Vegetables 338
602. Fat Free Crock Pot Chili 339
603. Vegan Apple Cinnamon Oatmeal 339
604. Curried Tempeh Quinoa Breakfast Hash 339
605. Detox Turmeric Ginger Miso Soup 340
606. Smoky Roasted Eggplant Soup With Za'atar-
     Fat Free 340
607. Mixed Beans Bowl With Sweet Potatoes &
     Turmeric Rice 341
608. Sweet Potato & Black Bean Chili 342
609. Corn Pakora, Baked, No Oil 342
610. Slow Cooker Butternut Squash Dal 342
611. Slow Cooker Chana Masala 343
612. Vegan Lentil Tacos 343
613. Vegan Gumbo 344
614. Quick Sauteed Peppers And Onions 344
615. Simple Sauteed Broccoli 345
616. Sauteed Spinach- That Tastes Amazing 345
617. Perfect Sauteed Carrots 346
618. Sauteed Rainbow Chard 346
619. Easy Sauteed Cabbage 346
620. Perfect Sauteed Zucchini 346
621. Sauteed Mushrooms 347
622. Best Ever Sauteed Kale 347
623. Perfect Sauteed Green Beans 348
624. Simple Sauteed Onions 348
625. Quinoa Salad 348
626. Super Crunch Salad 348
627. Turmeric Noodle Soup 349
628. Millet Medley Nourish Bowl 349
629. Root Bowl With Meyer Garlic Sauce Recipe 350
630. Coconut Lemongrass Noodle Soup 350
631. Mixed Spice Muesli Recipe 350
632. Cucumber And Prawn Stir-Fry Recipe 351
633. Soy-Cured Tuna Noodles Recipe 351
634. Roast Tomato And Orange Soup Recipe 352
635. Avocado Couscous Salad Recipe 352
636. Chunky English Garden Salad Recipe 352

637. Thai Quinoa Salad 353
638. Creamy Pea And Watercress Soup Recipe 353
639. Anthony Worrall Thompson's Herby Fruit
Salad Recipe 354
640. 7-Veg Stir-Fry Recipe 354
641. Quinoa And Butternut Squash Salad Recipe 354
642. Roasted Minty Beetroot And Goat's
Cheese Recipe 355
643. Granola Recipe 355
644. Beetroot, Pomegranate, And Parsnip Soup
Recipe 355
645. Stir-Fry Prawns With Mushroom And Broccoli
Recipe 356
646. Sea Bass With Squash And Stir-Fry Recipe 356
647. Quinoa Lentil Salad 357

CHAPTER 17. SWEET DISHES RECIPES 359
648. Apricot-Pear Cake 360
649. Applesauce Cake 360
650. Homemade Brownies 360
651. Paleo-Blackberry-Cashew-Chia Pudding 361
652. Apple-Oatmeal-Cookies 361
653. Jessica's-Pistachio-Oat-Squares 361
654. Oatmeal Cookies 362
655. Vegan-Ice Cream 362
656. Tahini Cookies 362
657. Oatmeal-With-Peanut Butter & Banana Recipe 363
658. Honey Pecan Granola With Cherry Recipe 363
659. Chocolate-Avocado-Pudding-Pops 363
660. Vegan-Butternut-Squash-Pudding 364
661. Raspberry-Cheesecake 364
662. Tart-Cherry And Mint-Sorbet 364
663. Pumpkin Pudding 365
664. Oatmeal-Pancakes With Apples-Cinnamon
Recipe 365
665. Peach Cobbler 365
666. Summer-Strawberry-Crumble 366
667. Peach Crisp 366
668. Best-Zucchini-Bread 366
669. Pumpkin Bars 367
670. Healthy-Banana-Bread 367
671. Black Rice Pudding With Coconut 367
672. Buckwheat Apple Cobbler 368
673. Chocolate Cheesecake 368
674. Chocolate Fondue With Coconut Cream 369
675. Cinnamon-Poached Pears With Chocolate Sauce 369
676. Orange-Glazed Poached Pears 369
677. Pineapple Upside-Down Cake 370
678. Pumpkin-Spice Brown Rice Pudding With Dates ..370
679. Stuffed Pears With Salted Caramel Sauce 371
680. Tapioca Pudding 371
681. Vegan Cheesecake With Raspberries 371

CHAPTER 18. STAPLES & SEASONINGS 373
682. Honey Butter 374
683. Apple-Pie-Spice 374
684. Chili Powder 374
685. Homemade Applesauce 374
686. Chipotle-Ranch-Dressing 374
687. Oat Milk 375
688. Lentils 375
689. Cashew Cream 375
690. Cheese Sauce 375

691. Pico-De-Gallo......................................376
692. Almond Flour 376
693. Creamy-Chipotle-Sauce 376
694. Oat Flour 376
695. Vegan Mayo 377
696. Radish-Greens-Pesto 377
697. Easy-Vegan-Chili 377
698. Ranch Dressing 377
699. Best Hummus 378

CHAPTER 19. SAUCES, DRESSING & DIPS 379
700. Béchamel Sauce 380
701. White-Bean-Dip 380
702. Vegan-Pimento-Cheese-Dip 380
703. Carrot-Tomato Sauce 380
704. Cashew Ricotta 381
705. Endo Guacamole 381
706. Fava Bean Dip 381
707. Homemade Ketchup 382
708. Lemon And Thyme Sauce 382
709. Lentil Bolognese 383
710. Mango Chutney 383
711. Raspberry Vinaigrette 383
712. Mixed-Veggie Sauce 384
713. Sage-Butternut Squash Sauce 384
714. Tangy Honey Mustard Dressing 384
715. White Wine Sherry Sauce 385
716. Vinegar Honey Sauce 385
717. Teriyaki Sauce -Asian Inspired 385
718. Vegan "Cheese" Sauce 385
719. Vegan Alfredo Sauce 386
720. Vinaigrette 386

CHAPTER 20. SMOOTHIES & FRESH JUICES 387
721. Anti-Inflammatory Juice Recipe 388
722. Apple Berry Detox Smoothie 388
723. Apple-Strawberry Smoothie 388
724. Apricot-Mango Madness 388
725. Avocado Detox Smoothie 388
726. Banana Ginger Smoothie 389
727. Banana-Blueberry-Soy Smoothie 389
728. Beet Greens Smoothie 389
729. Blackberry Soda Syrup 389
730. Blueberry Detox Smoothie 390
731. Broccoli Apple Smoothie 390
732. Carrot And Apple Juice 390
733. Carrot And Orange Juice 390
734. Celery Cucumber Green Juice 390
735. Cherry Beet Smoothie 391
736. Cherry Mango Anti-Inflammatory Smoothie 391
737. Coconut-Water-Smoothie 391
738. Cranberry Simple Syrup 391
739. Dairy, Sugar & Gluten-Free Smoothie 392
740. Detox Green Smoothie With Grapes 392
741. Detox Smoothie 392
742. Digestive Aid Green Juice 392
743. Easy Detox Smoothie 393
744. Elderberry Syrup 393
745. Glowing Green Detox Smoothie 393
746. Golden Detox Smoothie 393
747. Grapefruit Smoothie 394
748. Green Detox Smoothie 394
749. Green Dragon Veggie Juice 394

750.	Green Juice For Beginners	394
751.	Green Protein Detox Smoothie	395
752.	Green Tea, Blueberry, And Banana Smoothie	395
753.	Healthy Green Juice	395
754.	Healthy Green Juice With Lemon	396
755.	Homemade Ginger-Lemon Cough Syrup	396
756.	Homemade Vanilla Extract	396
757.	Jumping Jack Smoothie Recipe	396
758.	Just Peachy Smoothie	397
759.	Kale And Apple Green Detox Smoothie	397
760.	Kale Banana Strawberry Detox Smoothie	397
761.	Kale Coconut Pineapple Detox Smoothie	397
762.	Keto Avocado Smoothie	398
763.	Mango-Kale Smoothie	398
764.	Mint Chip Smoothie	398
765.	Mixed-Fruit-Smoothie	398
766.	My Favorite Green Juice	399
767.	Orange And Spinach Juice	399
768.	Orange Dream Creamsicle	399
769.	Peach Simple Syrup	399
770.	Peaches And Cream Oatmeal Green Smoothie	399
771.	Peppermint Crio Bru	400
772.	Pineapple And Avocado Detox Smoothie	400
773.	Pineapple Banana Detox Smoothie	400
774.	Pineapple Passion	400
775.	Pineapple Sunrise	401
776.	Pomegranate, Raspberry, And Banana Smoothie	401
777.	Pomegranate Smoothie	401
778.	Pressure-Cooker Chai Tea	401
779.	Raspberry & Blueberry Smoothie	401
780.	Strawberry-Banana Smoothie	402
781.	Strawberry-Kiwi Smoothie	402
782.	Sunrise Detox Smoothie	402
783.	Sunrise Smoothie	402
784.	Tomato-Kale Gazpacho Smoothie	402
785.	Tropical Papaya Perfection	403
786.	Turmeric Ginger C Boost Life Juice	403
787.	Vanilla-Ginger Syrup	403
788.	Very Berry Breakfast	403
789.	Wassail- Hot Mulled Cider	404
790.	Watermelon Wonder	404
791.	World's Best Smoothie	404
792.	Yummy Mango Citrus Drink	404
793.	Avocado Pesto Pasta Salad	405
794.	Endo Parm Asparagus	405
795.	Green Quinoa Salad	405
796.	Vegetable Fried Rice	405
797.	Tofu Stir-Fry	406
798.	Almonds & Blueberries Smoothie	406
799.	Almonds And Zucchini Smoothie	406
800.	Avocado With Walnut Butter Smoothie	407
801.	Baby Spinach And Dill Smoothie	407
802.	Blueberries And Coconut Smoothie	407

CHAPTER 21. MEASUREMENT CONVERSION CHART 409

Weights	410
Common Ingredient Measures	411
Baking Measurements	412
Volume Measurements	413
Weight Measurements	413
Temperature Conversions	414
Temperatures	414

CONCLUSION 417

RECIPES INDEX 422

Introduction

If you're on a vegan diet or just want to change things up, it's a good idea to consume more natural foods and veggies. Rather than relying on animal protein, we rely on beans, legumes, whole grains, and nuts in this healthy eating plan, which emphasizes a plant-based diet. You don't have to worry about not getting enough protein if you eat meat if you plan out your meals correctly. Plant-based meals are also high in fiber, another satiating element, making them ideal for weight loss. Additionally, fiber keeps us full, ensuring that we remain satisfied all day long.

On a whole-food, plant-based diet, we recommend 1,500 calories per day, which most people lose weight at, with the option of 1,200 or 2,000 calories per day for those who need more calories. As far as I can tell, all of these interpretations are correct. The term "plant-based diet" may be used as a synonym for the vegan diet, according to Summer Yule, RDN, a nutritionist in Hartford, Connecticut. The phrase "plant-based" may describe diets mostly made up of plant foods, but not entirely.

"Other people may use the word in a broader meaning to apply to all vegetarian diets, and I've also seen persons use the term 'plant-based."

GRUPPO

"A plant-based diet promotes the consumption of fruits, vegetables, and legumes while avoiding meat, dairy, and eggs," says Manaker. If you wish to go any further, additional restrictions may be applied. According to Manaker, animal products may either be banned entirely or restricted depending on the individual's viewpoint.

So, meat and fish don't have to be off-limits, but you may limit how frequently you eat them. Think of the term "plant-based" as an umbrella term for a wide range of more specific diets. A plant-based diet emphasizes foods derived from plants, such as vegetables, whole grains, fruits, nuts, beans, seeds, and legumes, while avoiding foods derived from animals, such as dairy, meat, eggs, and food components such as honey and gelatin.

However, there are still excellent and unhealthy options in the world of plant-based diets. Eating a plant-based diet makes it possible to make poor decisions. However, whole foods in their original state are far superior to processed meals from a supermarket freezer or a fast-food restaurant, so choose thoughtfully and mindfully.

WHY CHOOSE PLANTS?

People switch to a plant-based diet for various reasons, including improved health, increased energy, disease treatment and prevention, and weight loss, to mention a few. The list below may give you the motivation you need to switch to a plant-based diet.

A PLANT-BASED DIET KEEPS YOU LOOKING YOUNG.

A 2013 study by the University of California, San Francisco, and the Preventive Medicine Research Institute cited the plant-based diet as a crucial element in reversing the aging process. Participants in the study who ate a plant-based diet (and exercised consistently) had their telomeres (the protecting ends of DNA strands) lengthened by 10%, resulting in extended cell life. On the other hand, participants who continued to eat an animal-based diet had their telomeres shortened by 3%. "Shortened telomeres have been proven to play a role in colon cancer, dementia, heart disease, stroke, and early death," says Dr. Dean Ornish, the study's lead author.

A PLANT-BASED DIET IS BENEFICIAL TO ONE'S HEALTH.

Many cardiologists recommend a plant-based diet to prevent and even treat heart disease. Cancer prevention, keeping healthy intestinal flora, weight loss, treating diseases like Parkinson's and multiple sclerosis, eye problems, diabetes, and various other ailments have all been related to a plant-based diet. It's lovely to eat a plant-based diet. Who doesn't want clearer skin, a smaller waistline, and more energy? You'll look and feel great if you switch to a healthy, plant-based diet that emphasizes fresh, complete foods.

IT IS HEALTHY TO EAT A PLANT-BASED DIET.

In addition to the use of antibiotics, the meat business is plagued with disease. Food recalls are becoming more common due to meat contamination, resulting in illness outbreaks from potentially dangerous food-borne germs.

A PLANT-BASED DIET IS LONG-TERM.

Agriculture, particularly dairy and meat products, accounts for 70% of worldwide freshwater use, 38% of total land usage, and 19% of global greenhouse gas emissions, according to the United Nations' Millennium Ecosystem Assessment from 2005. Antibiotic resistance, water pollution, and many other environmental disasters are all tied to livestock farming. This book emphasizes that plant-based recipes and easy to make to lead a healthy life and lose weight. This book also contains a simple plant-based meal plan for losing weight while avoiding dairy and meat products. Switching to a plant-based diet enhances your health, increases energy, and prevents chronic illnesses. According to scientific data, many chronic diseases can be avoided, treated, or even reversed with a plant-based diet. According to findings published in the classic book

The China Study, a plant-based diet can lower the risk of type 2 diabetes, cardiovascular disease, some forms of cancer, and other serious ailments. A whole-food, plant-based diet is based on the following concepts. First, it allows you to achieve your nutritional requirements by focusing on organic, minimally processed plant foods: Natural, less processed foods are referred to as "whole foods." Second, it refers to entire, unprocessed, or lightly processed substances. Third, plant-based food is defined as food made entirely of plants and does not include animal products such as meat, eggs, milk, or honey.

FOOD GROUPS

Here's a rundown of the primary food groups you'll find on a plant-based diet, along with some examples:

- **Fruits**: Any fruit, such as bananas, apples, grapes, citrus fruits, strawberries, etc.
- **Vegetables**: Peppers, maize, spinach, lettuce, kale, collards, peas, and other vegetables are plentiful.
- **Tubers**: Potatoes, parsnips, carrots, beets, sweet potatoes, and other root vegetables are examples of tubers.
- **Whole grains**: Entire grains are cereals, whole grains, quinoa, millet, brown rice, oats, whole wheat, and barley. Popcorn, too, is a whole grain.
- **Legumes**: Beans of all kinds, as well as pulses, lentils, and other legumes.

Nuts, avocados, seeds, tempeh, whole-grain flour and bread, tofu, and plant-based milk are just a few of the items you can eat. However, these foods are higher in calories and might lead to weight gain.

BENEFITS OF A WHOLE-FOOD, PLANT-BASED DIET

Easy weight loss and maintenance: People who consume a plant-based diet are slimmer than those who don't, and the diet makes it simple to lose weight & keep it off, even if you don't monitor calories. Chronic illnesses, such as heart disease & type 2 diabetes, may be prevented, halted, or even reversed with a whole-food, plant-based diet.

ENVIRONMENTALLY FRIENDLY: A PLANT-BASED DIET HAS A FAR LOWER ENVIRONMENTAL IMPACT.

There is no precise description of a plant-based, whole-food diet. WFPB diet is much more of a way of life than a specific diet. It's because plants' diets may vary substantially depending on how many animal items are included in an individual diet. Nonetheless, the essential concept of a plant-based, whole-food diet is: Animal products are limited or avoided. Whole, less processed meals are emphasized. Plants, such as vegetables, whole grains, fruits, seeds, legumes, and nuts, should account for the bulk of your diet. Food quality is prioritized, with several supporters of the WFPB diet advocating for locally produced, organic foods wherever feasible. Refined foods like white flour, added sugars, and processed oils are excluded. This menu is often mistaken for vegetarian or vegan due to these factors. Although comparable in some aspects, these diets are different and not the same.

Vegans avoid all animal products, especially dairy, eggs, poultry, meat, fish, and honey. Vegetarians avoid all meat & poultry. However, some vegetarians consume eggs, fish, or dairy products. But on the other side, the WFPB diet is more adaptable. Animal items are not forbidden to followers who consume vegetables essentially. While a WFPB dieter may avoid all animal foods, another may have limited quantities of poultry, eggs, fish, meat, or milk. Changing your diet to a diet based on plants is not only good for your health, but it's also good for the environment. People who eat plant-based food have a reduced environmental impact. Applying sustainable dietary habits may help decrease carbon dioxide emissions, water use, and industrial farming land usage, all of which contribute to global warming & environmental damage.

Compared to non-vegetarians, those who follow plant-based food have a reduced chance of suffering from heart disease. Plant-based meals have been shown to decrease improved cholesterol and blood pressure and treat and prevent cardiac disease. In addition, eliminating animal and high-fat diets in favor of plant-based diets may help reduce the risk of some cancers. Also, without workouts or calorie tracking, plant-based meals help people lose weight. Consumption of calories is decreased automatically when high-fat meals are replaced with vegetables, fruits, legumes, and healthy grains.

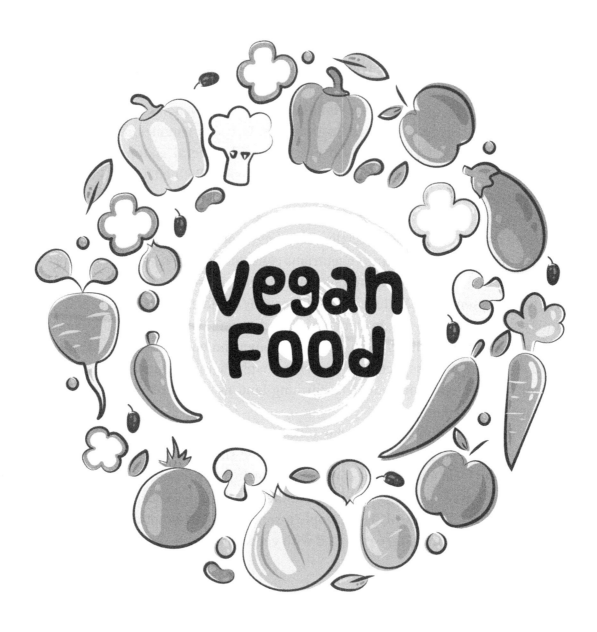

Chapter 1.

The Plant-Based Explained

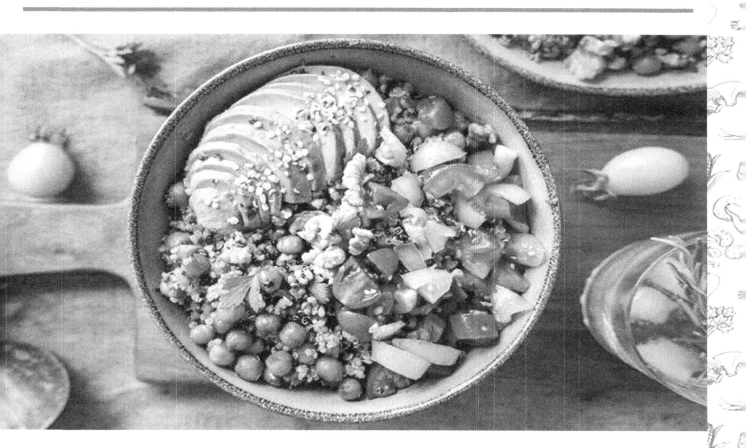

A plant-based food consists primarily of meals derived from plants, including very few or even no animal products. Vegetables, nuts, seeds, legumes, whole grains, and fruits all fall within this category. A plant-based meal may be the right choice for you for several reasons. Concerns regarding health benefits, animal welfare, the environment, or even a personal choice may fall under this category. Every age or stage of life may benefit from a plant-based lifestyle. In the same way as any other diet, you must plan a daily plant-based diet to achieve your nutritional requirements.

How To Build A New Flavor?

When individuals switch to a plant-based diet, one of the most common complaints is that their meals lack flavor. They think this is undoubtedly true, but it's not because plants are plants - it's simply that people don't often realize how big of difference spices can make! You can't understand why individuals say meatless dishes are bland or tasteless.

From sausage to vegetarian burgers, consumers are more likely to notice the flavor than the food in every cuisine. Some of the most common ingredients in most recipes are herbs, spices, vegetables, and other fruits. When vegans cook using grains or beans, it is believed that they end up with tasteless food. You hardly ever eat a meal consisting only of grains or beans, and you never prepare such a meal for yourself. Grains or beans are bland when eaten according to their own.

To get the most out of chickpeas, you'll need to cook them. Hummus, on the other hand, is a very tasty spread. Add the right spices and tastes, and your dish will be delicious. Chickpeas are a terrific source of protein and fiber, but they're also tasty and healthful when you add garlic, cumin, lemon juice, and a pinch of paprika.

Fresh herbs, ginger, garlic, or other herbs and spices, whether fresh or dried, may enhance the nutritional value of your food, so don't be afraid to use them liberally. Marinating cooked beans and grains in a dressing or sauce for at least an hour before serving is a good idea since this will enhance their taste.

Beans & grains may be jazzed up in several ways. You may if you wish:

- You may serve them with a variety of veggies or fruits.
- Mix herbs and spices into the water when they are cooking.
- When cooking, use a few vegetables, juice, or broth.
- A tasty sauce may be used to dress them up.
- Then blend them into a sauce or dip them in seasonings.
- Adding grains, beans, & bean dips may transform a lightweight salad into a full dinner.
- Add these to a vegetable-based dish such as vegetable soup.
- Toss cooked whole-grain pasta with your favorite spaghetti sauce.
- Add spices to beans or lentils to create a taco filler or burrito filling.

USING SALT

Don't be frightened of using salt in your cooking. Vegetables will taste more affable, and you'll need to eat much of the nutritious meal you're creating, thanks to the softening of their harshness. Likewise, good hummus doesn't just taste like hummus; it tastes like all its ingredients come together.

USING SPICES

Adding spices to the food is a great way to get more nutrients, antioxidants, & protein into your diet. Spices come in a broad range of flavors and nutritional advantages, so it's best to stock up on as many as possible. Try different spices like cardamom, cloves, or paprika instead of the customary few. When you're unsure, start a little and build from there. You can still add more, yet you can't withdraw.

An unpleasant bitterness, particularly if you overuse spices, may feel a tingling sensation on the tongue.

1. Make a dish out of them (try to utilize whole food fat like seeds, avocados, and nuts, most often)
2. Simmering them with beans or veggies like squash in a thick sauce
3. Cooking water for soup, grains, or beans with entire spices (cinnamon stick, cumin seeds, etc.)
4. Before using spices, dry taste them (whether ground or whole)

USING HERBS

Use herbs since they're packed with nutrients, including vitamins, minerals, & antioxidants! When possible, utilize fresh herbs rather than dried ones since they have added nutrients and taste. When it comes to food, fresh veggies are an excellent addition. They may be used in salads, bean dips, smoothies, and more. Fresh herbs rapidly lose their taste when heated, so use them as a garnish or add them only at the end of the cooking.

When fresh herbs are scarce in the winter, dried herbs may still provide a shocking number of nutritional values. However, if they don't have their flavor released, they won't taste delicious. As you put them into your meal, rub them on your fingers, or infuse these in Fat based sauces to transmit their flavor. Dried herbs may be used to flavor soups, sauces, & whole-grain cooking water.

SEASONING COMBINATIONS

To get you started, here are a few tried-and-true taste pairings:

- You may use sesame oil, soy sauce, and ginger to enhance the taste of vegetables such as dark and kale green leafy greens such as broccoli.
- The typical herbs for seasoning tomato sauce include basil, oregano, & marjoram.
- Adding a creamy sauce made of onion powder, dill, & nutritional yeast over brown rice & steamed vegetables makes this dish even better.
- Mushroom gravy and squash risotto may be enhanced by adding thyme, parsley, & bay leaves.
- It's easy to prepare a basic curry powder by combining spices, ginger, turmeric, cumin, coriander, & cayenne.
- Cayenne, cumin, & allspice form the foundation of a delicious chili that includes tomatoes, mushrooms, kidney beans, and zucchini.
- If you're making gingerbread or even porridge, molasses & cinnamon are the right additions.

Then, once you've honed your seasoning skills, you can add a pinch of spice, like cinnamon or cardamom, with powdered curry. Don't ever be afraid to add a little salt and pepper to your food! If you want to prepare a fantastic vegan meal, you need to pay attention to the details. You can impress anyone's palate with the right seasonings.

AN ALTERNATIVE FOOD CONCEPT

Plant-based diets emphasize consuming primarily plant-based foods like oils, nuts, seeds, legumes, whole grains, beans, fruits, and veggies. The term "vegan" or "vegetarian" does not imply complete abstinence from animal products. Instead, you're choosing to eat more plant-based meals in proportion to your overall calorie intake.

MEDITERRANEAN & VEGETARIAN DIETS

In what ways are plant-based diets shown to be beneficial? Nutrition Facts Per Servings studies have extensively studied plant-based dietary patterns like Mediterranean or vegetarian diets. Foods such as fish, chicken, eggs, yogurt, and cheese are included in the Mediterranean diet weekly, but meat or sweets are consumed less often. This meal has reduced heart disease risk, diabetes, metabolic syndrome, certain cancers (especially breast and colon cancer), depression, or frailty risk in older individuals. It has also been found to improve physical and mental function in older adults on the Dietary pattern. Lowering the heart disease risk, diabetes, and obesity has also benefited vegan diets.

Plant-based diets include all the essential components for maximum health, including protein, lipids, carbs, vitamins, & minerals, as well as fiber plus phytonutrients. But some vegans might have to take a supplement (particularly vitamin B-12) to guarantee they get all the necessary elements to be healthy and strong.

VEGETARIAN DIET VARIETY

Choose the vegetarian diet that works most for you based on your preferences. Eggs, dairy products, and sometimes meat, poultry, fish, and shellfish are included in a semi-vegetarian and flexitarian diet.

There is no meat and poultry in the diet of a pescatarian. Lacto-Ovo vegetarians consume dairy products and eggs but no meat, poultry, fish, or seafood.

No animal products are allowed in vegan diets.

8 Ways To Get Started With A Plant-Based Diet

Here are a few suggestions to consider to assist you in getting started on the plant-based lifestyle.

1) **Eat lots of vegetables.**
   Vegetables should make up most of your meal at both lunch and supper time. Make sure to incorporate a wide variety of veggies into your meal. With salsa, hummus, or guacamole, serve veggies as a snack.
2) **Make a shift in your thinking regarding meat.**
   Utilize lesser portions. Instead of a centerpiece, use it as a garnish.
3) **Fats that are excellent for you should be your priority.**
   Olive, olives oil, nuts & nut butter, avocados, and seeds are all excellent sources of healthful fats.
4) **At least once a week, prepare a vegetarian dish.**
   These meals are based on a combination of whole grains, beans, and veggies.
   Breakfast should contain whole grain products.
   You may start with oats, buckwheat, quinoa, or barley, but don't be afraid to experiment. Then, in addition to fresh fruit, include some seeds or nuts.
5) **Veggies are the way to go.**
   Explore a range of leafy green vegetables, including kale, collards, spinach, Swiss chard, & other greens, every day to stabilize your blood sugar. Preserve the Nutrition Facts Per Serving and taste your food by steaming, grilling, braising, or stir-frying.
6) **Salad as the centerpiece of your dinner.**
   Toss the greens into a large salad dish with spinach, romaine, or Bibb lettuce. Fresh herbs, peas, beans, or tofu may also be added to this dish.
7) **Eat a piece of fruit as a sweet treat.**
   Fresh peaches, juicy watermelon slices, or crisp apples can satisfy your post-meal sweet need.

Some Plant-Based Substitutes

A few of your favorite and most comfortable items may be substituted with plant-based alternatives. It's understandable if you're perplexed about how a plant-based substitute for particular items may be found. The following is a list of some of the most often-used ingredients in vegetarian cuisine.

MILK SUBSTITUTES FOR PLANT-BASED EATING

Fortunately, many non-dairy milk substitutes may either be purchased at a shop or made at home. Coconut, rice, almond, & hempseed milk are just some of the many options available. If a recipe asks for milk, you may simply swap one of these (in equal proportion) for it. Calcium isn't lost when you drink non-dairy milk. Many plant-based meals, such as kale, almonds, or bok choy, are rich in these vitamins and minerals. Milk isn't the only place you'll find them!

SUBSTITUTES FOR EGGS IN A PLANT-BASED DIET

Many people are unsure about what to use in place of an egg. When making the muffin's "stock," the absence of an egg is an obvious problem. Concerns may be justified. The truth is, you've got many more possibilities than you realize!

Try the following: each one yields one egg's worth of product:

- Water, flax seeds, chia seeds, and three tbsp of the combination are all you need to get started
- A quarter cup of mashed banana
- ¼ cup of apple juice

MEAT SUBSTITUTES IN A PLANT-BASED DIET

In a plant-based diet, meat isn't an option. Tempeh, beans, tofu, & portobello mushrooms are the key plant-based products to start stocking up on for a robust, rich texture & something which fills you up. Marinating any of these ingredients in almost any flavorful sauce is possible. It's also possible to cut or cut them up and utilize them in any manner you would use meat: like burgers, into stews & chili, or even baked on the plate.

CHEESE SUBSTITUTES FOR PLANT-BASED EATING

Most individuals find it quite tricky to surrender something as deeply ingrained in their being as this. Cheese is a food that most people can't resist. You may get creamy, velvety textures from luscious and indulgent plants instead of cheese. Avocado, soaked & blended cashews, organic tofu sprouted soft, plus nutritional yeast is just a few of my favorites. There are many ways to include these ingredients in your favorite pizza, tacos, sandwiches, quesadilla, and more.

Most non-dairy cheeses on the market are made from highly processed soy, which may harm your health. Maintain a moderate intake of this product since it is still packaged food. Make sure to steer clear of products made from either soy or rice that are too processed and do not satisfy your cheese cravings. There may also be traces of dairy in these alternatives. If you're having difficulty letting go of cow's milk cheese, know that sheep or goat's milk cheeses are an alternative. As a result, they are simpler to digest and less lactose-heavy than cows, and their treatment within the food business is much more humane than that of cows.

PLANT-BASED THICKENERS

What is the secret ingredient that keeps your beef gravy around each other?? You may not want to find out. It doesn't matter if cornstarch is plant-based since it's probably genetically engineered. It's best to use tapioca and arrowroot powder instead. Each of these ingredients adds natural gooeyness to your sauces and puddings. You may find these ingredients in the baking area throughout many health foods shops or supermarkets.

MOCK MEATS

Soybean oil waste product is utilized as a meat substitute. There are a variety of "meatless meats" on the market nowadays. Even though they don't include any animal products, plant-based meals aren't something you should rely on if you require a meaty fix. Stick to the meat substitutes that have previously been suggested.

MYTHS AND MISCONCEPTIONS ABOUT A PLANT-BASED DIET

It's difficult to understand what to trust when this comes to diet. Several misconceptions about plant-based eating stem from a total lack of knowledge about the topic. In addition, it's tough to keep up with the newest events because of the rapid spread of false or contradicting information. Plant-based eating has a bad rap when it comes to people's perceptions of its benefits in terms of health, taste, and safety, but experts are here to debunk those myths on Monday with the help of solid evidence from reputable sources. Our collection of plant-based eating misconceptions will help you conquer your anxiety about incorporating more variety into your diet without hesitation.

MYTH: EATING A PLANT-BASED DIET DOESN'T PROVIDE ENOUGH PROTEIN

As long as you're consuming enough calories to maintain weight & eating a diverse diet, you're practically assured of obtaining enough protein. Most Americans consume one and a half times extra protein than they need per day, & protein shortage is rare in the United States. Even though many plant-based meals are high in protein, you may need to consume enough of them to equal the protein levels found in dairy sources.

For example, a 3-ounce serving of meat has the same amount of protein as cooked beans. A spoonful of plant-based whey protein may be added to your smoothie for an additional protein boost if you're anxious about having enough of it.

MYTH: PLANT-BASED MEALS DON'T HAVE TO BE EATEN IN PRECISE COMBINATIONS TO PROVIDE A COMPLETE PROTEIN.

Plant-based nutrients are naturally combined in your body to create a complete protein. It isn't required to combine meals to make "complete proteins" since most vegetable protein sources contain just a small quantity of several important amino acids. A varied diet will ensure that your body has all the amino acids this needs to produce new proteins. It doesn't matter where you consume your protein since your metabolism "completes" this for you.

MYTH: PEOPLE WHO EAT A PLANT-BASED DIET ARE ILL (IRON DEFICIENT)

Fact: A wide range of plant-based foods contain various quantities of iron. These include lentils & chickpeas as well as leafy greens. Many people have been misinformed about the difference between iron contained in meat and that found in plant-based foods (non-heme iron). Foods rich in vitamin C and even other sources of bioavailable iron may boost the absorption of the plant protein's iron. Tofu alongside broccoli and a dish of beans containing diced red peppers are just two examples.

MYTH: NO KIDS LIKE VEGETABLES, ACCORDING TO POPULAR BELIEF.

Many children appreciate veggies and healthful dishes, particularly if they are involved in the cooking process. It's easy to get youngsters excited about veggies like broccoli, cauliflower, & asparagus if they're cooked correctly. Kids are more likely to eat their vegetables if they have a hand in picking and preparing them. To get youngsters excited about eating more plant-based meals, consider creating familiar recipes like Buffalo nuggets like eggplant & onion "meatballs."

MYTH: PLANT DIETS ARE LACKING IN NUTRIENTS.

Is it possible to have a meat-free diet? The answer is yes! It's rare for anyone's nutrient to be lacking in the population. When it comes to vitamin & mineral intake, several foods consumed are either supplied or fortified with these nutrients. Vegans may have to supplement their diets with vitamin B12 and iron, although these elements may also be found in fortified plant-based meals, including milk, cereal, and other types of fortified food.

PLANT-BASED DIET USING A MEAL PLAN

Here's a sample of a **One-Week Meal Plan** for the plant-based diet.

MONDAY

- **Breakfast:** Carrot Muffins
- **Lunch:** Instant Pot Black Beans
- **Snack:** Herb Compound Butter
- **Dinner:** Pina Colada Granola

TUESDAY

- **Breakfast:** Easy low fodmap shakshuka
- **Lunch:** Butternut Squash Black Bean Enchiladas with Jalapeño Cashew Crema
- **Snack:** Blistered Shishito Peppers
- **Dinner:** Chana Masala

WEDNESDAY

- **Breakfast:** Roasted Veggie Brown Rice Buddha Bowl
- **Lunch:** Curried Chickpea Salad
- **Snack:** Cashew Cream
- **Dinner:** Mango Ginger Rice Bowl

THURSDAY

- **Breakfast:** Stuffed Poblano Peppers
- **Lunch:** Pozole (Posole Verde)
- **Snack:** Vegan Pimento Dip
- **Dinner:** Burrito

FRIDAY

- **Breakfast:** Avocado Cucumber Sushi Roll
- **Lunch:** Lemon Rosemary White Bean Soup
- **Snack:** Vegan Seven Layer Dip
- **Dinner:** Vegetarian Chili

SATURDAY

- **Breakfast:** Toasted Oats Cereal (Camping Breakfast)
- **Lunch:** Collard Greens
- **Snack:** Edible Cookie Dough
- **Dinner:** Green Beans Almondine (Amandine)

SUNDAY

- **Breakfast:** Tofu Scramble Stuffed Breakfast, Sweet Potatoes
- **Lunch:** Crispy Roasted Chickpeas
- **Snack:** Golden Turmeric Noodle Miso Soup
- **Dinner:** Teriyaki Tofu-Tempeh Casserole

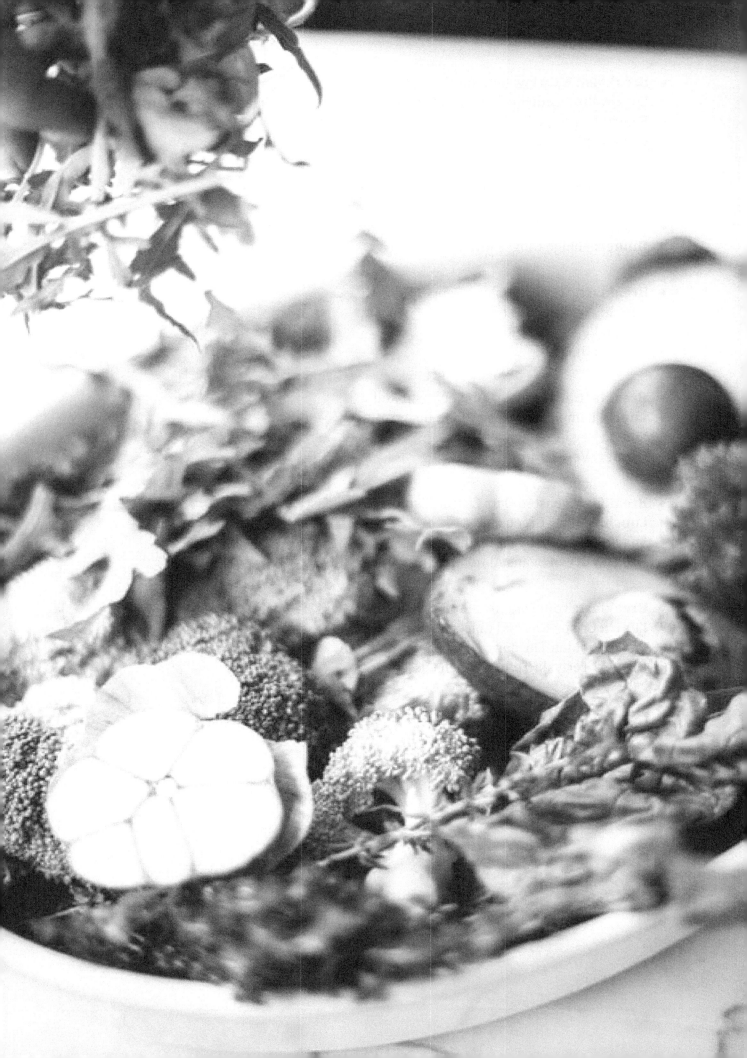

Chapter 2.

Understanding Plant-Based Diet

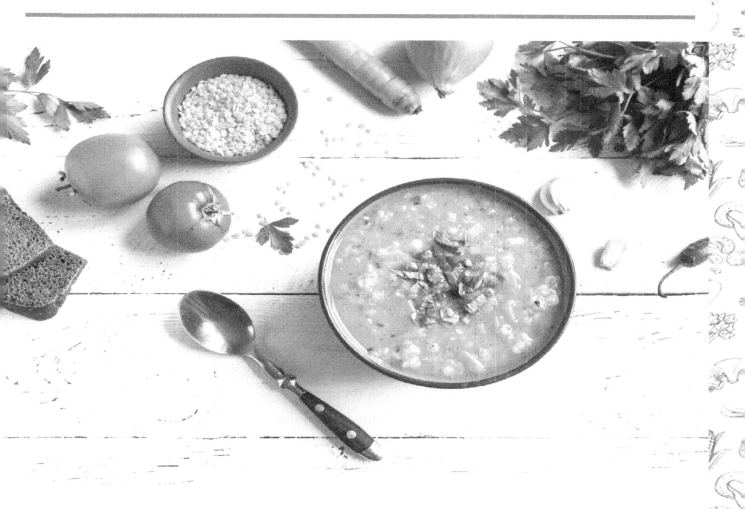

This chapter gives detail about the plant-based diet. What is it, which foods you can eat in a plant-based diet, and what to avoid or limit while following a plant-based diet is included in the chapter? How cooking equipment works for this diet and its work are also discussed in detail and depth. This chapter also includes the knife types used for cutting plant-based diets, how they work, and food-cutting techniques.

WHAT IS A PLANT-BASED DIET?

Plant-forward or plant-based eating patterns emphasize foods that come from plants. This comprises nuts, oils, seeds, legumes, whole grains, beans, and fruits & vegetables. It does not imply that you are a vegan or vegetarian, so you can never consume meat or dairy products. Rather, you are consuming a more significant amount of your diet from sources of plants.

Plant-based diets have indeed been linked to improved health, including a reduced risk of coronary heart disease, diabetes, high bp, and longer life. This is because plant-based diets are rich in fiber and phytonutrients and include all of the required protein, fats, carbs, minerals & vitamins for optimum health. However, some vegans may need to take a supplement (particularly vitamin B12) to get all the necessary nutrients they need.

VARIETY OF PLANT-BASED DIET

Vegetarian diets exist in various sizes and forms, and you must choose the one that best suits your needs.

- Vegan excludes all animal products.
- A pescatarian diet consists of eggs, dairy products, fish, & seafood but excludes meat and poultry.
- Eggs, dairy products, and sometimes meat, fish, poultry, & seafood are included in a flexitarian or semi-vegetarian diet.
- Vegetarian foods contain eggs and dairy products but exclude meat, fish, poultry, and seafood.

WFPB DIET HELPS TO IMPROVE A VARIETY OF HEALTH CONSEQUENCES

Adopting a WFPB whole-foods & plant-based diet may help you lose weight while also lowering your risk of chronic illness and alleviating symptoms.

CANCER

According to research, eating a plant-based diet may lower your risk of some cancers. For example, in research, vegetarian diets were linked to a decreased incidence of gastrointestinal cancer, particularly for those who adopted a Lacto-Ovo vegan lifestyle (vegetarians who take dairy and eggs). In addition, when compared to non-vegs, Pescatarians (vegetarians who consume fish) exhibited the best protection against colorectal cancer, with a 43 percent lower risk.

HEART DISEASE

The most famous and useful advantage of the WFPB diet is that it is heart-healthy. On the other hand, both the quality and kinds of foods consumed in the diet are important. According to a study, those who ate a healthy diet based on plant food rich in fruits, vegetables, whole grains, nuts, and legumes had a decreased risk of heart disease as compared to those who ate non-veg diets.

On the other hand, unhealthy diets based on plant food containing sugary beverages, refined grains, and fruit juices were linked to a slightly higher risk of cardiovascular disease.

COGNITIVE DECLINE

According to research, eating a diet rich in fruits and vegetables may assist older persons in reducing or avoiding cognitive loss and Alzheimer's disease. Diets based on plant foods include more antioxidants and plant compounds, which have been demonstrated to reduce Alzheimer's disease development and cognitive repair impairments.

BRAIN HEALTH

Saturated and trans fats, which are present in meat, dairy products, and fried meals, have been linked to an increased risk of Alzheimer's disease as well as other cognitive disorders. These items are avoided in a plant-based lifestyle, which is high in folate, antioxidants, and vitamin E, all of which may have a protective impact.

DIABETES

Adopting a diet based on plant food may help you manage your current diabetes and lower your chances of acquiring it. According to research, those who ate a healthy veg diet had a 34% reduced chance of contracting diabetes compared to others who ate unhealthily, non-veg diets.

FOODS TO EAT ON THE PLANT-BASED-DIET

For many individuals, animal foods emphasize most meals, from bacon and eggs in the morning to steak in the evening. Meals should revolve around foods sourced from plants while transitioning to a plant-based lifestyle. If animal products are consumed, they should be consumed in lower amounts and with special care given to the item's quality. Dairy, poultry, eggs, meat, & fish should be served as a side dish to a diet based on plant food rather than as the main course.

A WFPB - DIET LIST

- Vegetables: Spinach, kale, tomatoes, cauliflower, broccoli, carrots, peppers, asparagus & many more.
- Fruits: Citrus fruits, berries, pears, pineapple, peaches, bananas &many more.
- Starchy vegetables: Sweet potatoes, potatoes, butternut squash & many more.
- Healthy fats: Olive oil, avocados, unsweetened coconut & many more.
- Whole grains: Rolled oats, brown rice, farro, pasta made from brown rice, quinoa, barley & many more.
- Legumes: Chickpeas, peas, lentils, black beans, peanuts & many more.
- Beverages: Tea, coffee, sparkling water & many more.
- Unsweetened milk based on plant diet: Almond milk, coconut milk, cashew milk, & many more.
- Nuts, seeds & nut butter: Cashews, almonds, macadamia nuts, tahini, sunflower seeds, pumpkin seeds, natural peanut butter & many more.
- Herbs, spices & seasonings: Rosemary, Basil, turmeric, black pepper, curry, salt & many more.
- Protein based on plant food: Tempeh, Tofu, powders, or protein sources based on plant food with no artificial ingredients or added sugar.
- Condiments: Mustard, Salsa, nutritional yeast, vinegar, soy sauce, lemon juice & many more.

If you want to include animal products in your diet based on plant food, look for high-quality foods at grocery shops or, even better, buy them from nearby farms.

- Poultry: Organic & free-range.
- Eggs: Pastured.
- Pork and beef: Grass-fed or Pastured.
- Dairy: Pastured and organic.
- Seafood: If feasible, source from reliable fisheries.

FOODS TO AVOID OR LIMIT ON THE PLANT BASED-DIET

The Whole Foods Plant-Based Diet (WFPB) is a manner of eating that emphasizes eating products in their very natural state. This implies that items that have been excessively processed are not allowed. Focus on freshly prepared foods while shopping for groceries, and when buying products with a label, go for those with the fewest ingredients possible.

FOODS THAT YOU SHOULD AVOID

- Added sweets & sugars: Soda, Table sugar, juice, cookies, pastries, candy, sugary cereals, sweet tea & many more.
- Fast food: Chicken nuggets, cheeseburgers, French fries, hot dogs & many more.

- Refined grains: Bagels, white pasta, White rice, white bread & many more.
- Processed animal foods: Beef jerky, lunch meats, bacon, sausage & many more.
- Vegan-friendly processed foods: Meats based on plant diet like Faux cheeses, Tofurkey, vegan butter & many more.
- Convenience & packaged foods: Frozen dinners, crackers, chips, cereal bars & many more.
- Artificial sweeteners: Splenda, Equal, Sweet'N Low.

FOODS YOU SHOULD CONTACT LIMITATE.

While it is possible to incorporate healthful animal foods in a diet based on plant food, the following items should be avoided.

- Pork
- Beef
- Sheep
- Poultry
- Game meats
- Eggs
- Seafood
- Dairy

COOKING EQUIPMENT USED TO PREPARE PLANT-BASED DIET

You've probably already begun gathering some essential kitchen items and appliances to cook your own nutritious meals.

Even with only these instruments, you can make beautiful and enjoyable foods.

CUTTING BOARD

Cutting boards come in helpful when it comes to cutting and slicing your items before cooking. Wood or plastic may be used to make them. It's often a great idea to keep aromatic vegetables like garlic and onions on a separate chopping board so they don't contaminate the taste of other vegetables & fruits.

SHARP KNIFE

Investing in an excellent chef's knife is a smart place to start since it will be your frequently used kitchen utensils. Because prices vary, you may select a sharp knife for cutting that fits your budget. In addition, preparing ingredients with a decent knife is fast, simple, and considerably safer.

LARGE & SMALL POT

To cook sauces, soups, cereals, curries, stews, and other meals, may benefit at minimum 1 small and 1 big pot. Large pots are ideal for cooking in bulk or for feeding a large household. In addition, it makes sense to have many pots since you may have to cook some grains as well as sauce or vegetables simultaneously.

MIXING BOWL

A mixing bowl made of metal is ideal for making delicious baked items, stirring salads, and mixing pancakes. Metal bowls are less heavy than glass and take up less space. We suggest obtaining ones with lids so they may be used as food storage boxes.

NON-STICK FRYING PANS

When making vegan omelets or pancakes without oil, water-sautéing your veggies, or dry-frying your tofu, a non-stick skillet or a frying pan is essential. We wouldn't recommend spending much money on this since non-stick frying pans seldom survive more than just a few years. As a result, they are highly cost-friendly, although useful kitchen addition. We utilize ours on a daily basis.

WHISK

When it comes to preparing pancake batter, blending up a sauce, or obtaining a light, fluffy mixture of cake, whisks are essential. Choose a balloon stainless steel design to avoid flavor transfer in acidic dishes.

MEASURING SPOONS & CUPS

Get some purposeful measuring spoons and cups & stop working with guesses. They're essential if you really want to go with baking Directions and always obtain the greatest results. Measurement cups are also useful for determining how much quantity of water to add to the cooking oats or grains.

BAKING SHEETS

Friendly not only for baking bread or cookies, as well as for roasting potatoes and vegetables but also for making beanballs from home and burgers. Line it with parchment paper or place a silicone-baking mat on the top to minimize sticking.

DINNER BOWLS

We like a delicious supper bowl brimming with spaghetti, noodles, or a lovely Buddha bowl dish. Bowls are actually more multipurpose than plates since they may be used to handle a variety of foods.

PEELER

A peeler, which comes in various designs and shapes, is necessary for peeling sweet potatoes, potatoes, carrots, & some other veggies. A peeler may also be used to prepare veggie spaghetti.

SPATULA

Spatulas are particularly handy for flipping foods such as burgers, pancakes, and waffles and serving meals from casserole dishes or baking pans. Ours are often used to keep veggies from sticking together when sautéing.

WOODEN SPOONS

This vintage kitchenware is ideal for stirring gravies & sauces as they simmer and mix batter for cake and preparing oatmeal. The handle will not get hot when cooking and will not leave a mark on your ceramic pans and pots.

FOOD PROCESSOR

Food processors are better at breaking down and mixing items than blenders to purify them into a fine liquid form. For example, suppose you want to create homemade vegetarian burgers, brownies, or energy balls using chickpeas or beans. In that case, a food processor may help you achieve the exact consistency you desire while mixing the flavors throughout. You can even use this appliance to prepare your homemade nut butter and flour from oats or almonds for nutritious baked products.

BLENDER

High-powered blenders are a lifesaver when it comes to making healthful and fresh soups or smoothies that retain all of the fiber. For a smoother consistency, some brands may even be used to blend sauces, gravies, and dressings.

TONGS

When presenting challenging foods like spaghetti or noodles or scooping up hot products like vegan sausages, burgers, falafels, hot dumplings, or veggies, some firm tongs might come in very handy.

CAST-IRON-SKILLET

A cast-iron skillet is a heavier-duty pan that maintains heat so well, making it ideal for frittatas, sautéed vegetables, cornbread, and even gooey desserts. It'll also survive for years, ensuring that you receive your money's payback. Furthermore, research has revealed that food cooked in a cast-iron pan has more iron, making it ideal for plant-eaters.

WOK

Woks are great pieces of equipment with a wide range of applications. You may use woks for curries, stir-fries, stews, stir-frying veggies, and even as a different frying pan. They are also reasonably priced and come in a variety of sizes.

STEAMER BASKET

Steaming potatoes, vegetables, and other items is an excellent preparation technique since nutrients are not wasted in the water as they are when they are boiled. Consequently, the vegetables are firm yet tender, fast to cook, and flavorful.

MANDOLINE

A mandoline reduces the time it takes to slice, cut, chop and shred vegetables by almost half. So, if you dislike the preparation phase of cooking food, this one can be a good option. This instrument also allows you to obtain uniformly sized pieces, which benefits processing times and makes your meal appear nice.

GRATER

Most graters have a box-like shape and many sides, allowing them to be used for more than simply grating vegan cheese. They may also be used for shredding and slicing vegetables and zesting out citrus fruits.

SILICONE-BAKING-MATS

Baking mats made up of silicone are an excellent low-waste substitute for parchment paper or tin foil. They may be used to roast veggies and potatoes and bake biscuits and cookies in an oven without using any oil when spread over a baking pan. They may simply be cleaned in warm water with soap and dried after use.

FOOD CONTAINERS

Having food storage containers on hand to keep any remains for another day is among the easiest ways to decrease waste in your kitchen. Glass, followed by metal, is the safest choice to keep food and preserve freshness. If you have the option, choose these. If you just have plastic containers, you may put them to good use first. If at all possible, make sure they're airtight.

MASON JARS

Mason jars are quite multifunctional, in addition to being extremely attractive. They're fantastic for preserving leftover sauces & dressings in your fridge, bringing a stacked salad to work for lunch, keeping prepared vegetables in water, freezing bulk-cooked meals, and even bringing a self-made smoothie.

FOOD WRAPS

These kitchen wares have been renowned in the zero waste sector for a time as plant-based wraps and beeswax wraps. You may wash and then reuse these wraps made of organic cotton, coconut oil & soy wax to wrap your self-prepared meals again and again.

NUT-MILK-BAG

Are you concerned about the cost of plant-based replacements for milk, or do you wish to decrease your disposal? Nut milk bags lets you prepare your homemade milk by using any seed or nut, including cashews, almonds, macadamia nuts, rice, and sesame seeds. Of course, we used to prepare our homemade soy milk as well.

This little cost-friendly piece of cotton is quite multipurpose and may have been used as a tea bag or to prep your homemade juice while using a blender, so this milk bag. Definitely one of our favorite little shenanigans.

CASSEROLE DISH OR BAKING PAN

Pasta bakes, stews, lasagnas, vegetable casseroles, and other set-and-forget dinners benefit greatly from casserole dishes & baking pans. They can also be used to make baked foods like oatmeal or risotto, which aren't your typical baked foods.

SLOW COOKER OR CROCK POT

Make huge amounts of curries, spaghetti sauces, risotto, stews, or even oatmeal in a slow cooker or crock pot. Simply add your ingredients, spices, and liquids, then close the lid, and adjust the temperature to your requirement. The slow cooker performs all the job for you, whether you keep it while you are at work or overnight, so you can arrive back to a great dinner with very little effort.

TOFU PRESS

A tofu press, which is made up of two parts, will strain all of the liquid from your tofu in mins without even using paper towels. Consequently, you'll have delightfully firm tofu ready to absorb all of your fav sauces. But, of course, if you do not want to spend the money on one, a dry towel and several weighty books will do.

AIR FRYER

An air-fryer is such an amazing appliance whether you're looking for a healthy substitute for fries or want to prepare the tastiest crispy tofu. The air fryer enables you to cook a variety of your favorite recipes more healthily by using just a little or no oil. For example, a fryer may be used to prepare tacos, sushi, cauliflower wings, falafel, potato chips, roasted chickpeas, and sometimes even toast, in addition to potato wedges or fries. The possibilities are limitless.

SPIRALIZER

Spiralizing is an excellent method to get more vegetables into your own meals and into the meals of your kids as well. Spiralizers come in a variety of sizes and shapes, but they all accomplish the same stuff, they transform zucchini, sweet potatoes, carrots, as well as other vegetables into long, delicious spaghetti or noodles.

Toss them into Thai meals, salads, or pasta sauces for a tasty alternative.

KNIFE TYPES FOR CUTTING PLANT-BASED DIET

GRANTON EDGE

The Granton edge appears as evenly distributed dimples around a centimeter through from the cutting edge. This knife was originally created for cutting meat, but then it has since been adopted by other knife kinds to allow air as well as water to release, making it simpler to cut both vegetables and fruit. These really are entertaining to practice with, but we've not discovered any big benefits.

SERRATED

Serrated or scalloped knives are almost a must for tomatoes, bread, pineapple, or something more challenging outside than an insider. In particular, Tomatoes may be sliced with an extremely sharp, well-maintained flat blade. So getting at least a serrated knife on hand is a smart idea among soft fruit.

HOLLOW GROUND

These knives are useful for delicate jobs like peeling because the tip of the knife is worn down from the depth of the knife. However, they are fragile and should not be used for something hard, and they require more regular sharpening. The paring knife seems to be more versatile and may do the same duties as a chef's knife.

PARING KNIFE

Paring knives come in a variety of shapes and sizes. The first is a spike-tip paring knife that is ideal for most fruits, tiny vegetables, or peeling by hand. The other is a stylet, sometimes known as a sheep's feet paring blade, which has a curved tip and a plain cutting edge and is useful for tiny jobs such as slicing garlic. Depending on your customary applications, this knife is less of a day-to-day knife than a regular paring knife.

Finally, a bird's mouth-paring blade, which curls in from the tip, can help you make your masterpieces if you want to get into food artistry, transforming apples into the swan and melons into flowers.

STRAIGHT & CURVED KNIVES

Plain blades are choppers that work well with hard fruits and veggies like squash and sweet potatoes. For almost everything else, the curved or chef's knife is preferred. On the other hand, a sufficiently sturdy and sharp chef's knife will operate very well on hard veggies.

CUTTING TECHNIQUES ACCORDING TO FOOD

WATERMELON

A particular watermelon knife appears like a green and pink bread blade but doesn't have a hollow ground. As a result, a chef's blade or bread knife can readily cut through watermelon unless you eat it twice a day. The problem is that watermelons are bigger than the tools we use to cut them, resulting in uneven slices.

LEAFY GREENS

Serrated knives work well with leafy greens, particularly ones with tough stems such as Swiss chard or certain types of cut kale. Flat blades tend to etch lines onto greens rather than completely slice them through them.

ROOT VEGETABLES & HARD SQUASH

A sharp, sleek chef's knife is ideal for cutting tough vegetables. However, a sharpened knife will need to be hacked or pressed harder, and it is possibly deadly.

ONIONS

While cutting with a non-serrated knife is feasible, a serrated knife cuts through more readily and without slipping. Also, once you've become accustomed to cutting onions, they're really rather simple.

SOFT FRUIT

Use a serrated knife for anything soft, particularly with a harder hide like tomatoes, a keen paring blade, or a chef's knife for more accurate slices. Most people, particularly amateur cooks, prefer a serrated knife for tomatoes, figs, and other similar fruits. If you like non-serrated knives or don't have one, use a chef's knife for bigger fruits and vegetables and a paring blade for smaller ones, but this isn't a hard and fast rule.

GARLIC

Garlic is easy to cut with almost any knife. A pairing blade or chef's knife can suffice, but a specialist knife such as a sheep's feet paring blade or a similar flat-edged knife will make mincing simpler. Use a paring blade for complete slices, such as those seen in classic Chinese broccoli & garlic dishes.

THINGS TO KEEP IN YOUR MIND WHILE CUTTING

The best sort of knife is determined by how a person cooks, cuts, as well as maintains their knives. Carbon steel blades are often pricey and regarded as good quality, although they need some maintenance. If exposed to moisture, the carbon steel, as well as iron-carbon alloys, may rust. Nevertheless, these are popular among professional cooks because they can withstand a great deal of usage and damage, so they're a favorite for hard labor. Knives should be sharpened twice a year at home or more often when used regularly. Dull knives take more force to wield and are potentially hazardous, making prep work very difficult.

Ceramic blades are intended to hold their sharpness for far longer than that of the ordinary blade without honing. However, they are difficult to polish by a non-professional when worn out or when you need a special knife stone made of a harder substance than ceramic.

Stainless steel seems to be a widely used material for cookware since it's simple to clean and doesn't trust easily. In addition, stainless steel blades are easy to break and hone than carbon steel knives, although they are less costly, needless sharpening, and more suitable for the home cook.

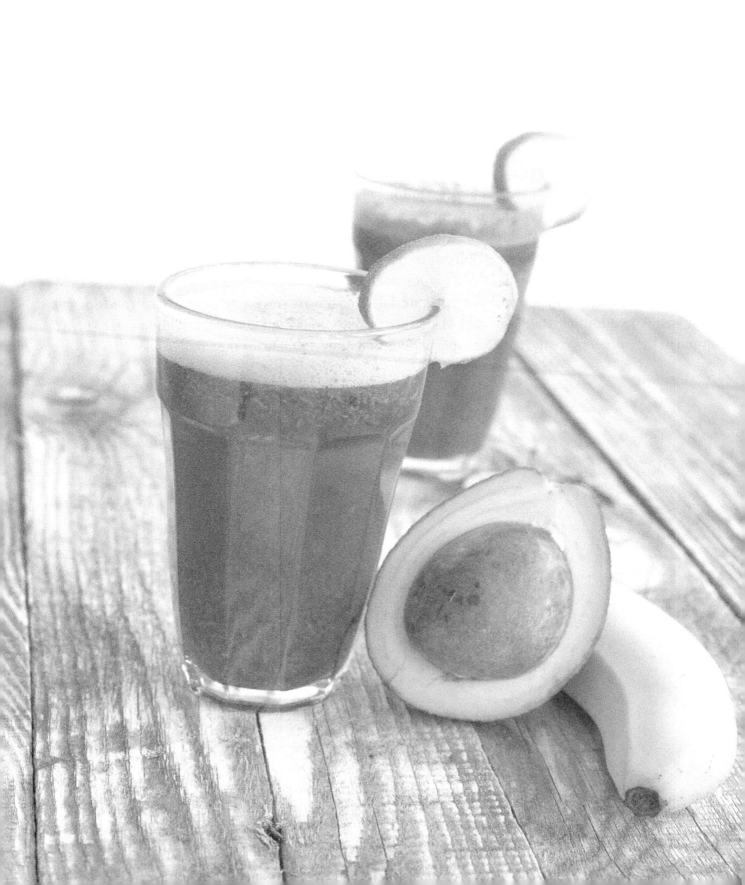

Chapter 3.

Types of a Plant-Based Diet

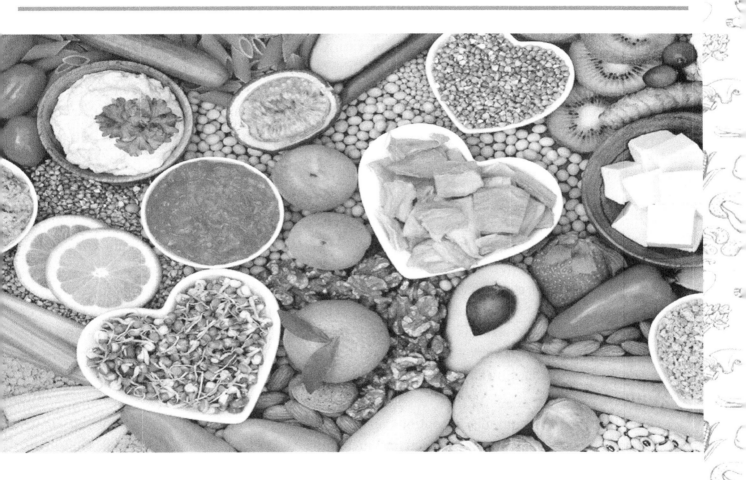

Plant-based diets have no conventional definition. However, the most popular definition of a plant-based diet is an eating pattern centered on plant-based foods (as contrasted to animal products/ingredients).

A wide variety of plant foods comprise legumes, grains, nuts, seeds, vegetables, fruits, and herbs or spices. To say that a diet is "plant-based" usually indicates that animal items are avoided to some extent as well. However, you don't have to eliminate all animal-based items; just cut down on their intake. Anywhere along this line is where a plant-based diet may be found. There are no hard and fast rules for a plant-based diet. What your plant-based diet looks like after that is entirely up to every individual.

As a result, there are several plant-based diets to choose from.

TYPES OF PLANT-BASED DIETS

Plant-based diets come in a variety of forms, including:

- Mediterranean
- Flexitarian
- Vegan & Vegetarian
- Whole diet plant-based

As well as anything else you can think of. Of course, plenty of vegans and vegetarians don't follow any of these rules, and it's ok!

THE DIET OF THE MEDITERRANEAN

As a result of extensive scientific study, a Mediterranean diet is good for health. The Mediterranean diet, particularly, has been linked to improved cardiovascular health1. Vegetables, fruits, seeds, legumes, nuts, or whole grains make up the bulk of the Mediterranean diet. Fish, shellfish, olive oil, & a small quantity of red wine are also included in this diet. A few times a month is all that is allowed for red meats, processed meats, or sweets, such as cookies. Smaller servings are less frequent than in normal Western diets; maybe one serves eggs, poultry, and dairy products daily.

The Mediterranean meal also promotes socializing or having a happy dining environment in addition to these food-specific guidelines. There's also a suggestion to engage in some kind of physical activity every day.

THE FLEXITARIAN DIET

Increasingly popular & for a good cause is the phrase "Flexitarian." People seek methods to enhance their health & lessen the environmental effect of their dietary choices but would not need to wipe out animal products fully. In comparison to vegetarianism, the flexitarian diet is more flexible. People may still consume some meat & other animal products, but they should do so less frequently and in smaller portions. It is also characterized as a semi-vegetarian meal or a flexitarian meal. Several studies have shown that reducing one's intake of animal-based meals may enhance one's health. Some of these benefits of healthy eating may be achieved with a flexitarian diet.

THE VEGAN AND VEGETARIAN DIET

One of the most common misconceptions about the phrase "plant-based diet" is that this means something similar to a vegan meal. There is no such thing as a vegan diet in and of itself. Those who are vegan abstain from using any animal foods (including food); hence their diet is entirely composed of plant-based foods (hence the term "plant-based food"). Plant-based food isn't just about a vegan diet and veganism since one may still incorporate certain animal foods into a plant-based meal.

THE WHOLE FOOD PLANT-BASED DIET

A whole cuisine plant-based diet restricts plant-based eating since not a single processed food is permitted. This diet is based on eating solely whole foods and avoiding items that have been processed in any manner. Some advocates of whole foods plant-based diet advocate for an unprocessed diet, while others advocate for a diet that includes no packaged foods at all. Many individuals might benefit from more plant foods in their diets, demonstrated to be a health-boosting dietary strategy 3. However, a meal with such stringent guidelines may raise concerns about sustainability & may contribute to problematic eating patterns or bad food-related relationships.

UNDERSTANDING PLANTS

WHY GO PLANT-BASED?

It boosts your body's natural defenses. Plants are rich in nutrients that can't be found in other foods, such as vitamins and minerals. Antioxidants within plants help maintain your cells healthy such that your immunity can perform at its peak. Andrea Murray, a health promotion expert at MD Anderson, adds that "plants provide your body the nutrients that this needs to assist fight illness." You can protect yourself against germs & microbes by eating a plant-based meal. A robust immune system is vital to minimizing your cancer risk as it can identify and combat cell abnormalities before they may lead to illness. In addition, inflammation is reduced by eating plant-based meals. Inflammation within your body may be alleviated by consuming plants' important elements. Immune system-supporting phytochemicals & antioxidants also work to neutralize toxins in the body, such as pollution, processed foods, germs, and viruses. To counteract these free radicals, Murray believes "antioxidants within plants" are the answer. Eat a plant-based diet & listen to the body's cues on what foods work best for you to prevent inflammation.

Cancer & other inflammatory disorders, such as arthritis, have been related to chronic inflammation. These illnesses can be prevented by eating a plant-based diet that eliminates some of the causes. With a plant-based meal, you can keep your weight stable. An essential thing you could do to lower your cancer risk is to maintain a healthy weight. Not smoking seems to be the only factor more essential than a healthy weight for cancer prevention. Inflammation and hormone imbalance are caused by excess weight. In addition, 12 distinct forms of cancer, comprising postmenopausal breast, colorectal, or esophageal, kidney, uterine, & pancreatic cancers, are more likely if you are obese or overweight. Plant-based diets exclude several of the dietary items that contribute to weight gain. You're now on the road to weight reduction if you add a workout to your diet.

Fiber is abundant in plants. Every non-processed plant food has fiber. If you consume a lot of it, you'll get the advantages of the plant's structure, which is made up of it. To effectively absorb the macronutrients that strengthen your immunity and decrease inflammation, the plant-based diet is essential; in addition to lowering cholesterol & stabilizing blood sugar, fiber aids in proper bowel control. In addition, fiber is essential to lowering your risk of cancer. Colorectal cancer is the 3rd most frequent cancer in the United States. There are several health benefits to a plant-based meal. The health advantages of eating a plant-based diet are not confined to cancer prevention. Additionally, a plant-based meal has been found to lessen your risk of heart disease, diabetes, stroke, and several mental health issues.

MAKE SURE YOUR PLANT-BASED MEALS ARE HEALTHY

Plant-based meals need you to eliminate the most common dietary hazards, such as fat and sugar, even if you're eating them. You could get the full advantages of the plant-based meal if you use appropriate cooking techniques & understand how to maximize the nutritional value of your veggies. There are no more deep-fried veggies. Crackers and cookies are also high-processed meals. In addition to limiting sugary treats, be sure to choose entire grains. White rice, white pasta, and white bread are all plant goods, but they're not whole-grain goods. Choose 100 percent wheat bread and pasta & eat rice (brown) instead of white rice.

The body's systems will run more efficiently if you eat more vegetables. Eating plants is all that's required. As Murray puts it, "They have become so crucial to your long-term health."

WHAT DOES EATING PLANT-BASED MEAN?

You're likely to have considered your nutrition when it comes to preventing cancer. Weekly, a new health food fad is making headlines. It may be almost hard to plan what to consume and what to avoid when it comes to food. However, a diet has repeatedly been shown to lessen cancer risk for more than 2 decades. Plant-based food is the primary source of nutrition.

A plant-based diet does not imply that you cannot consume animal products. Instead, it indicates that your diet consists mostly of plant-based foods, such as vegetables, grains, & fruits. There are also a variety of legumes, seeds, & nuts. These plant-based items should make up 2/3 of your diet. The remaining 1/3 of the meal should be a protein such as fish, chicken, or beans.

ESSENTIAL PLANT-BASED PANTRY

Building a better diet requires having a well-stocked pantry. A pantry full of nutritious, complete foods will keep you cooking and eating well all week. While everyone's pantry needs are different, here are some general guidelines to help you get your plant-based pantry fully stocked. But, first and foremost, don't be intimidated by the list! Don't stress about stocking the entire cupboard at once if you're just starting to incorporate more whole foods into your diet and more plant-based items into your meals.

That can be intimidating and costly and may rapidly turn you away from the project. Instead, consider adding a few new products each week to gradually expand your pantry depending on the meals you believe are the greatest fit. Focus on healthful, whole foods in their original, unadulterated state while stocking your plant-based pantry.

Additionally, experiment with some of the specialty foods and ingredients that can make cooking more enjoyable and delicious.

VEGETABLES

Salad greens, leafy greens like collards or kale, mushrooms, cruciferous veggies like cauliflower and cabbage, and aromatics like onions, carrots, and celery are among the many fresh and frozen vegetables to choose from. Frozen veggies are a healthy alternative to fresh vegetables, and in-season vegetables from a local farm are more cost-effective and tasty. In addition, the pantry should include broccoli, peas, greens, and maize from the farmers' market.

FRUITS

Fresh fruits like bananas, cherries, apples, and pears are delicious on their own or in baked goods. Frozen fruits are great in smoothies and pies and peeled; ripe bananas should always be kept on hand in the freezer for baking emergencies.

BEANS AND LEGUMES

To give an affordable, easy-to-cook protein supply, use a variety of dry and canned beans and legumes. In a pantry, store lentils, chickpeas, black beans, kidney beans, and cannellini beans. Because most busy cooks rely on canned beans to get dinner on the table, many of the recipes in this book call for them. However, don't be frightened to cook dried beans from scratch; it's simple and cost-effective.

GRAINS

Brown rice, basmati rice, cornmeal, whole-wheat pastry flour, all-purpose flour, wholewheat and semolina pasta, rolled oats, barley, millet, farro, couscous, rice noodles, and quinoa are some of the grains and grain-like seeds to keep on hand. In addition, if you follow a gluten-free diet, almond flour, gluten-free flour mix, and oat flour are excellent pantry additions.

VINEGAR AND OILS

Begin with a high-quality extra-virgin olive oil and a neutral-flavored oil like grapeseed. Curries and baked dishes benefit greatly from the use of coconut oil. Baked products and salad dressings benefit from nut oils, and toasted sesame oil has a smokey, nutty flavor. Oils that aren't used every day should be kept refrigerated. The flexibility of apple cider vinegar, red wine vinegar, and balsamic vinegar is unrivaled. Rice vinegar is great in Asian foods, while umeboshi plum vinegar adds a particular salty, sour, spicy flavor.

NUTS AND SEEDS

Raw almonds and cashews can be kept in the cupboard for baking, "cheese" fillings, nut milk, and just plain munching. Everything tastes better with walnuts and pecans, especially when they're roasted. Salads, fruit dishes, bread, and oats can benefit from adding chia and flaxseeds to the plant-based baking cabinet. Pumpkin seeds (pepitas) that have been roasted and salted are very delicious. Nuts and seeds should be stored in tightly-sealed glass jars, and rarely-used items should be frozen.

PRODUCTS MADE FROM SOY

Tofu, tempeh, edamame, and miso are essential ingredients in any plant-based pantry. Because tofu absorbs the taste of whatever it's cooked with, it's perfect for curries and stews. Tempeh is a fermented soy product with a meaty texture and umami flavor that's great for grilling, sandwiches, and casseroles. Edamame is whole soybeans that can be used in soups, stews, and salads, just like beans. When it comes to creating umami flavor, miso is a must-have ingredient.

CONDIMENTS

Keep a range of homemade and store-bought condiments on hand in recipes or topping for cooked foods. Ketchup, spicy sauce, whole-grain Dijon mustard, and vegan mayo are all must-haves.

SPICES, HERBS, AND SEASONINGS

Fresh basil, chervil, cilantro, dill, parsley, and tarragon; herbes de Provence; Himalayan black sea salt; kosher salt; nutritional yeast; sea salt (normal and smoked); smoked paprika; turmeric; and more!

SUGAR AND SWEETENERS

Raw Sugar/Turbinado Sugar, Sucanat/Evaporated Cane Juice, Coconut Sugar, Agave nectar, Maple Syrup, Honey, and Stevia.

FLOUR

Whole wheat pastry flour, Buckwheat flour, Chickpea Flour, Spelt, einkorn, Kamut, Amaranth flour, Quinoa flour, Millet flour, Sorghum Coconut Flour, and Almond flour.

TIPS AND TRICKS FOR GOING PLANT-BASED

It doesn't have to be tough to switch to a plant-based diet. On the contrary, it's simple to acquire all the nutrients you need from plant sources without relying on processed, refined foods—and without feeling like you're missing out on anything—with a bit of planning.

BEGIN WITH TINY ADJUSTMENTS

For many people, switching to a plant-based diet is a gradual process. It's a good idea to start with a "meatless Monday." Start with one plant-based meal per day and gradually increase to two. Begin by removing the worst offenders from your diet, such as bacon and cheese, and replacing them with a fresh vegetable dish or two at each meal.

HAVE A PLAN

You'll want to plan your meals if you're new to the plant-based lifestyle. Planning your meals and perhaps doing some cooking on your day off will help you avoid the temptation to revert to harmful eating habits. For example, suppose you've bought healthy ingredients and have a vegetarian casserole in the freezer. In that case, you'll be less likely to give in and order that sausage and pepperoni pizza when you're hungry but don't have much time.

EAT YOUR VEGGIES

For individuals accustomed to harmful processed foods, huge amounts of meat, and few, if any, fresh fruits, vegetables, and whole grains, the additional fiber in a plant-based diet might be a shock to the system. However, gradually increasing your fiber intake can help if you're prone to digestive problems. Begin by consuming a large, raw salad on a daily basis. Then, reduce or eliminate meat, dairy, and eggs while increasing the number of beans, fruits, legumes, and vegetables you consume. Tomatoes, zucchini, black beans, onions, corn, and peppers combine with plant-based cheese in this zesty comfort food.

SEEK INSPIRATION

Inspiration can be found in various places, including websites, publications, blogs, and cookbooks. Don't be scared to branch out and try new things. The worst that can happen is that you will dislike a certain dish or meal. So instead, try something new, add your favorite meals to your repertoire a few times a week, and forget about the rest.

NEW FRONTIERS SHOULD BE EXPLORED

The plant-based diet is a fantastic way to branch out and try something new. Whether you go to an Indian vegetarian restaurant or make a Middle Eastern meze with your friends, you'll notice that many cuisines around the world use very little (or no) meat, with vegetables and whole grains making up the majority of the meal. Recipes based on that tradition and ones that explore cuisines you may not be familiar with can be found throughout this book. So take a chance and dive right in!

FAUX IT!

Do you crave some meat? From Tofurky to "veggie" pepperoni, there's a whole universe of meat substitutes out there ready for you to try. Eating these processed meals on a daily basis is not recommended, but they can help satisfy the desire for comfort foods. Who doesn't enjoy a little soy chorizo or a grilled veggie dog every now and then?

MOVE AT YOUR OWN PACE

Finally, following a plant-based diet is all about the journey, and every one of us has a unique experience along the way. Open your mind and heart, and commit to eating for health and happiness. Challenges will arise when you're traveling, staying in someone else's house, or simply tired, hungry, and enticed by the familiar. When you fall, pick yourself up and try again. Any improvement is a positive thing. Give yourself a break and try your hardest.

Chapter 4.

Plant-Based Diet

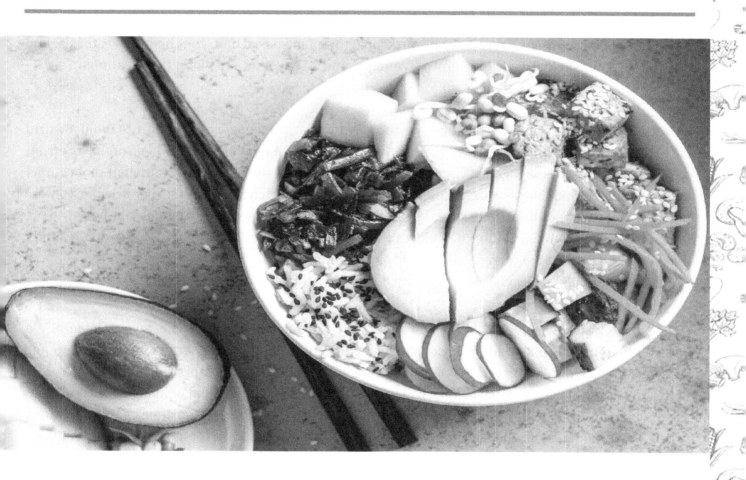

MACROBIOTIC PLANT-BASED DIET

George, a Japanese philosopher, was the first to invent the term macrobiotically. However, macrobiotics did not become popular in the United States until the 1960s. Macrobiotics is a lifestyle that emphasizes balance and stability.

Macrobiotics is based on the habits and practices of long-established global civilizations that have avoided chronic sickness for millennia. Its goal is to achieve a healthy balance of physical and mental well-being.

Whole grains, legumes, vegetables, nuts, seeds, fruits, and naturally pickled & fermented foods are all part of the macrobiotic plant-based diet. In addition, meat, dairy, artificial components, and processed foods are eliminated or reduced.

MACROBIOTIC DIET BENEFITS

A macrobiotic diet has several health advantages. Fiber, nutrients, and minerals are abundant in plant-based diets. As a result, a nutritious plant-based diet helps in bodily balance, improved stomach and digestion, immunity, and toxin elimination.

High blood pressure, diabetes, & hypoglycemia may all be prevented by eating a diet rich in vegetables and whole grains. These meals are well-balanced and consistent. As a result, they aid in the maintenance of your blood pressure. In addition, plant-based meals help with weight control and enhance body functioning; therefore, the macrobiotic diet lowers the risk of cardiovascular disease.

Compared to a diet heavy in processed foods, your heart doesn't have to work as hard. Fatigue - Today's diet is excessively acidic and unbalanced. As a result, it becomes more difficult for the body to provide oxygen to important organs. Furthermore, the digestive tract has difficulty absorbing nutrients and minerals. As a result, when you switch to a plant-based diet, your body starts to heal and rejuvenate. You will feel more invigorated, younger, and stronger as a result of this treatment.

VEGAN LIFESTYLE

Vegans take charge with purpose. No matter how modest, they make every effort to build a world without human service hurting animals. And it's not just about food. Vegans have been at the forefront of several demonstrations against circus performances and other forms of entertainment that compel animals to act for human pleasure. A circus has nothing to do with Nutrition Facts Per Servings(unless popcorn and cotton candy are included) but all to do with animal welfare. Animals compelled to act for human pleasure often exhibit no evidence of enjoyment or desire to do so. As a result, trainers must use pain to elicit the correct behavior from the animal.

Veganism entails consciously avoiding any behavior that harms animal welfare.

VEGANISM

Veganism is a belief and way of life that rejects the existence of other animals for our benefit. We were all here on this planet for a reason, and species other than humans serve just as much to our ecosystem as we do. Vegans think that rather than living as "apex predators," mankind can coexist with animals. Rather than imposing our will on animals, we may assist them in living as natural a life as possible. Diet is an important part of the vegan lifestyle. Vegans refuse to consume eggs, dairy, meat, or any other animal byproduct, even honey produced by bees. But it's a lot more than that. Animals are employed in producing a wide range of consumer goods and cosmetics, including soaps and apparel. Vegans, for example, use synthetic textiles rather than wool from llamas, alpacas, sheep, and other animals. True, these animals aren't slaughtered for their fur. They are, however, terrified throughout the shearing process that they do not comprehend and are left without their natural shelter from the outdoors. The vegan way of life is all about intention, but it's also about awareness. Before purchasing anything from the shop, a vegan evaluates if it negatively influences animals.

PROS AND CONS OF PLANT-BASED DIET

PROS

- Protection from certain types of cancer
- Improved glycemic control (reduction of Hemoglobin A1C in people with Diabetes Type II)
- Weight management
- Lower total cholesterol and LDL levels

- Improved neurocognitive function, prevention, and management of dementia and Alzheimer's Disease
- Reduced carbon footprint
- Lower risk of developing diabetes type II
- Improved cardiovascular health (decreased blood pressure, lowered heart rate, reduced risk for cardiovascular events)

Cons

There are several methods to consume a plant-based diet that are harmful. In addition to boosting plant products, the research on the advantages of a plant-based diet stresses fresh, complete components and reducing processed meals. Changing to a plant-based diet or just adding more fresh food to one's diet can undoubtedly enhance one's health.

Plant-based diets, on the other hand, may entail the following health risks if they are not properly planned and educated about foods:

- Low calcium and vitamin D consumption leads to decreased bone mineralization and an increased risk of fractures.
- Lower essential fatty acid intake
- Iron deficiency
- Low protein intake
- Vitamin B12 deficiency

DIFFERENCE BETWEEN VEGAN AND VEGETARIAN DIET

WHAT IS A VEGAN DIET?

A vegan diet forbids the use of both animal protein and animal products. Meat, shellfish, dairy, milk, eggs, cheese, and honey are all examples. A vegan diet may also be tailored to the individual.

For example, someone may abstain from using animal-tested cosmetics due to animal welfare and rights concerns. Instead, choose a raw vegan diet and eat largely uncooked and unprocessed foods for health reasons.

WHAT IS A VEGETARIAN DIET?

A vegetarian diet avoids animal protein and meat, which is comparable to a vegan diet. The difference between a vegan and a vegetarian diet is that a vegetarian diet may include animal products such as milk, dairy, cheese, eggs, and honey.

WHAT IS A MACROBIOTIC DIET AND LIFESTYLE?

A macrobiotic definition is a concept of holistic principles & dynamic practices that direct nutritional, physical, mental, social, & environmental health through choices in diet, exercise, and lifestyle. As a result, you may be a macrobiotic vegan or vegetarian, but being vegetarian or vegan does not imply you are macrobiotic.

BENEFITS

WHY PLANT-BASED?

Maintaining a healthy weight is easier with a plant-based diet. One of the essential things you can do to lower your cancer risk is to maintain a healthy weight. The only thing more essential than keeping a healthy weight for cancer prevention is not smoking. It is because being overweight induces inflammation as well as hormone imbalances. If you're overweight or obese, you're more likely to get colorectal, postmenopausal breast, uterine, esophageal, kidney, and pancreatic cancers, to name a few.

Many things that cause weight gain are eliminated when you largely eat vegetables. When you add exercise to the mix, you're on your way to losing weight.

Fiber is abundant in plants. All raw plant foods include fiber. It's what gives the plant its structure, and eating more of it gives you access to a slew of advantages. A plant-based diet enhances gut health, allowing you to absorb more nutrients from the food that help your immune system and decrease inflammation. Fiber may help decrease cholesterol and blood sugar levels, and it's also beneficial for intestinal health.

Fiber is crucial in lowering your cancer risk. It is particularly true if you're at risk for colorectal cancer, the third most prevalent cancer. A plant-based diet also lowers your chances of contracting other ailments. However, the advantages of eating primarily vegetables go beyond lowering your cancer risk. A plant-based diet has also been demonstrated to lower the risk of heart disease, stroke, diabetes, and some mental diseases.

DAILY EXERCISE: 15 MINUTES FOR DAY

1) **Walk-Out Push-Up**

   This technique, according to Watkins, engages numerous muscle groups and includes different planes of movement, increasing heart rate. Begin by standing with the feet about hip-width apart. Next, bend forward at the hips and slowly bring the hands to the floor. Next, slowly move your hands forward after touching the bottom until the spine is straight and you're in the push-up beginning position. Complete a push-up, then walk the hands back to the feet and carefully roll the spine up 1 vertebra at a time to return to standing.

2) **Standard Squat**

   Squats compel the brain to participate actively. For example, to concentrate on equal weight distribution between the left and right leg; to maintain the chest-high & back straight; to activate the glutes; to halt at the change of direction to prevent momentum from accumulating; and to stand with full extension of the hips.

3) **Jumping Jacks**

   The age-old jumping jack causes a lot of folks to roll their eyes. However, a sprinkle of plyometrics is quite advantageous when it comes to functional fitness. Due to living in shoes and being sedentary, neurotransmitters in the feet become drowsy. The light impact is a terrific way to get those wacky animals to wake up. When done correctly, the jacks, like the walk-outs, activate various muscular groups and raise the heart rate.

4) **Hip Bridge**

   A degree of happiness for everybody. Furthermore, like with the squat, your brain is actively involved in this movement. Foot positioning, weight distribution, and breathing are crucial. Another aspect of this regulated proprioception is maintaining the toes on the floor. When your heels take all body weight, the lower back is under extra strain. On the other hand, the hamstrings and glutes engage and help extend the hips when the body shifts direction while the toes remain down.

Chapter 5.

28-Day Meal Plan

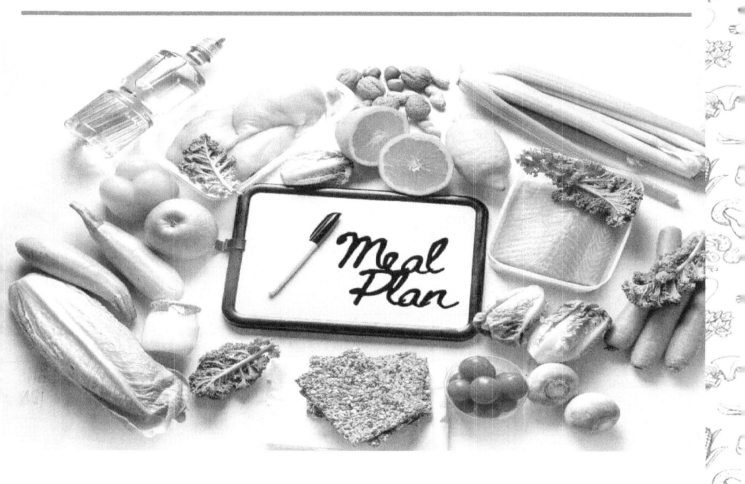

Consider your time, tastes, and nutritional value of your eating items while making meal plans. Do as much cooking and prep work as you can ahead of time—a little work on your day off makes the rest of the week go more smoothly. Chop the onions, celery, and carrots ahead of time; store in 1 cup pieces in zipper-lock plastic freezer bags or containers; and use straight from the freezer—no need to thaw. Make a batch of granola on the weekend and store it in an airtight jar for convenient grab-and-go snacks. Soups and stews are great to prepare ahead of time and store in the refrigerator or freezer.

Prepare and chill pizza dough up to 2 days ahead of time. Next, make a double batch of vinaigrette, chill for up to 5 days, mix well, then drizzle over daily salads. When you can, double a soup or casserole recipe and freeze half of it in individual or family-size quantities. You'll soon have a freezer full of meals that you can defrost if you're short on time.

WEEK 1

DAYS/MEALS	DAY 1	DAY 2	DAY 3	DAY 4	DAY 5	DAY 6	DAY 7
BREAK-FAST	Banana-Amarnath Porridge	Pear Oats with walnuts	Breakfast Tofu Scramble	Beet Greens Smoothie	Coconut-Almond Risotto	Broccoli Apple Smoothie	Breakfast Burritos
SNACK	An apple	Easy garlic-roasted potatoes	Stuffed mushroom	One ounce of water	Latkes	An orange	Classic Hummus
LUNCH	Curried Rice Salad	Grilled tofu Caprese	Clean Vegan Pad Thai	Seitan Satay	Warm rice and Bean Salad	Mushroom Lasagna	Spicy Asian Quinoa Salad
SNACK	Soy yogurt	Mushroom bun Sliders	One cup of frozen and dried berries	An apple	Classic Hummus	Rosemary Garlic Popcorn	An orange
DINNER	Tofu Stir-Fry	Zucchini and Avocado Salad with garlic herb dressing	Swiss Chard Ravioli	Quinoa Vegetable Salad	Summer squash and onion bake	Autumn Wheat Berry Salad	Winter vegetable pot pie

WEEK 2

DAYS/ MEALS	DAY 1	DAY 2	DAY 3	DAY 4	DAY 5	DAY 6	DAY 7
BREAK-FAST	Banana-Amarnath Porridge	Coconut-Almond Risotto	Breakfast Tofu Scramble	Beet Greens Smoothie	Pear Oats with walnuts	Breakfast Tofu Scramble	Beet Greens Smoothie
SNACK	Classic Hummus	Roasted Corn with poblano-cilantro butter	Mushroom bun sliders	Roasted Cauliflower Hummus	Puffed Rice Balls	Latkes	Red cabbage with apples and pecans
LUNCH	Tofu Stir-Fry	Zucchini and Avocado Salad with garlic herb dressing	Tofu summer rolls	Quinoa Vegetable Salad	Tamale Casserole	Autumn Wheat Berry Salad	Moroccan Lasagna
SNACK	An apple	Easy garlic-roasted potatoes	Stuffed mushroom	One ounce of water	Latkes	An orange	Classic Hummus
DINNER	Curried Rice Salad	Grilled tofu Caprese	Clean Vegan Pad Thai	Seitan Satay	Warm rice and Bean Salad	Mushroom Lasagna	Spicy Asian Quinoa Salad

WEEK 3

DAYS/ MEALS	DAY 1	DAY 2	DAY 3	DAY 4	DAY 5	DAY 6	DAY 7
BREAK-FAST	Banana-Amarnath Porridge	Pear Oats with walnuts	Breakfast Tofu Scramble	Beet Greens Smoothie	Coconut-Almond Risotto	Broccoli Apple Smoothie	Breakfast Burritos
SNACK	Soy yogurt	Mushroom bun Sliders	One cup of frozen and dried berries	An apple	Classic Hummus	Rosemary Garlic Popcorn	An orange
LUNCH	Farro risotto with roasted fennel and mushroom	Winter vegetable pot pie	Mixed vegetable cottage pie	Rice Salad with Fennel, Chickpeas, and orange	Cassoulet	Fruited Millet Salad	One-pan Pasta primavera
SNACK	Classic Hummus	Roasted Corn with poblano-cilantro butter	Mushroom bun sliders	Roasted Cauliflower Hummus	Puffed Rice Balls	Latkes	Red cabbage with apples and pecans
DINNER	Tofu Stir-Fry	Zucchini and Avocado Salad with garlic herb dressing	Swiss Chard Ravioli	Quinoa Vegetable Salad	Summer squash and onion bake	Autumn Wheat Berry Salad	Winter vegetable pot pie

WEEK 4

DAYS/ MEALS	DAY 1	DAY 2	DAY 3	DAY 4	DAY 5	DAY 6	DAY 7
BREAK-FAST	Banana-Amarnath Porridge	Coconut-Almond Risotto	Breakfast Tofu Scramble	Beet Greens Smoothie	Pear Oats with walnuts	Breakfast Tofu Scramble	Beet Greens Smoothie
SNACK	An apple	Easy garlic-roasted potatoes	Stuffed mushroom	One ounce of water	Latkes	An orange	Classic Hummus
LUNCH	Tofu Stir-Fry	Zucchini and Avocado Salad with garlic herb dressing	Swiss Chard Ravioli	Quinoa Vegetable Salad	Summer squash and onion bake	Autumn Wheat Berry Salad	Winter vegetable pot pie
SNACK	Soy yogurt	Mushroom bun Sliders	One cup of frozen and dried berries	An apple	Classic Hummus	Rosemary Garlic Popcorn	An orange
DINNER	Farro risotto with roasted fennel and mushroom	Winter vegetable pot pie	Mixed vegetable cottage pie	Rice Salad with Fennel, Chickpeas, and orange	Cassoulet	Fruited Millet Salad	One-pan Pasta primavera

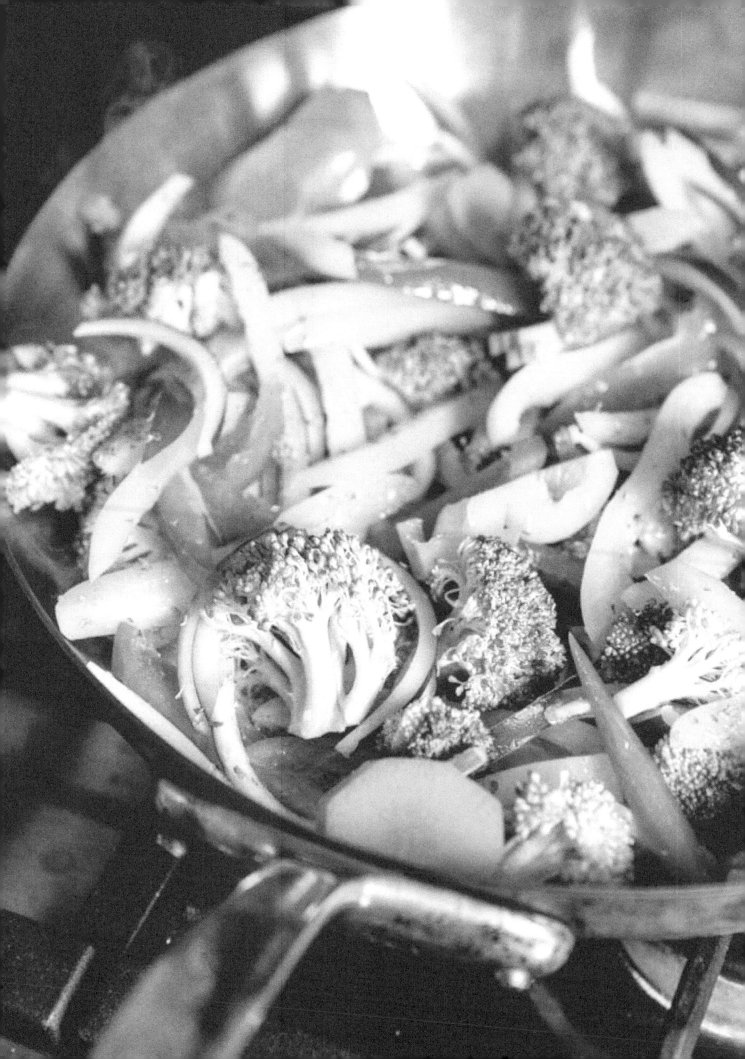

Chapter 6.

Breakfast Recipes

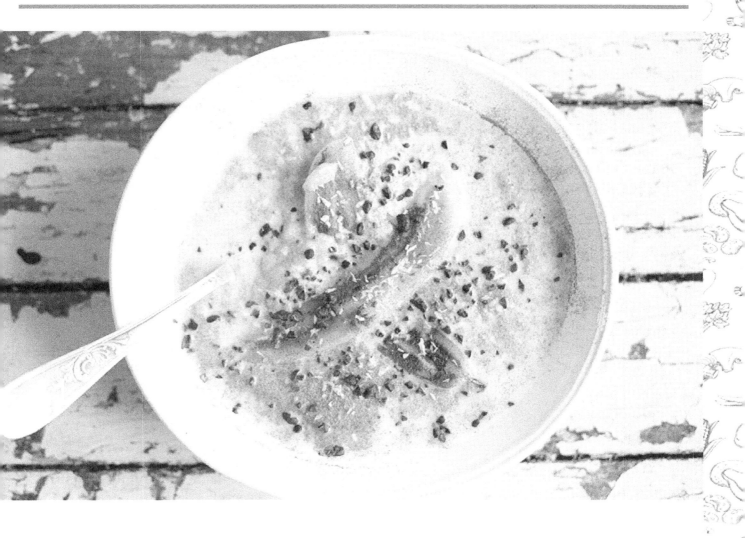

1. BANANA-AMARANTH PORRIDGE

- Breakfast - Prep time: 10 mins, Cook time: 10 mins, Total time: 20 mins, Servings: 4, Grill temp: 350°F

Ingredients

- 2 ½ cups of unsweetened almond milk
- 1 cup of amaranth
- 2 sliced bananas
- Dash of cinnamon

Directions

1. Mix the amaranth, milk, and bananas in your pressure cooker or a deep pan.
2. Close the lid.
3. Cook on high pressure/heat for about 5 mins.
4. When the time is up, wait for the pressure to come down on its own.
5. You can serve the porridge with cinnamon when all the pressure is gone.

Nutritional Values

Calories 271, Fat 6g, Chol 0mg, Sodium 71.4mg, Potassium 67.7mg, Carbs 47g, Protein 8g

2. JALAPEÑO CORNBREAD

- Breakfast - Prep time: 10 mins, Cook time: Ready in about: 40 mins, Servings: 12, Grill temp: Medium

Ingredients

- 1 cup flour, all-purpose
- 1 cup of cornmeal
- 2 tsp baking powder
- ¼ tsp baking soda
- ½ tsp sea salt
- 1 cup of almond milk
- ¼ cup of maple syrup
- 1 egg
- ¼ cup of olive oil, extra-virgin
- ¾ cup of jalapeño peppers, diced
- 4 chopped scallions, chopped
- ¾ cup of cheddar cheese
- - For serving Honey Butter
- 1 tbsp butter

Directions

1. Preheat your oven to around 350°F.
2. Add cornmeal, baking powder, flour, salt, & baking soda in it.
3. Take another bowl, add egg, almond milk, maple syrup, & oil, and whisk well.
4. Combine wet ingredients with the dry ingredients & stir well. Also, add jalapeños, scallions, and cheese to it.
5. Put your batter into a pre-oiled pan, sprinkle some leftover jalapeños & scallions, then bake for around 20-24 mins.
6. Serve it with some honey butter.

Nutritional Values

Calories 222, Carbs 30g, Protein 8.9g, Fat 15g, Sodium 886mg, Potassium 734mg, Chol 0mg

3. JAPANESE-PUMPKIN RICE

- Breakfast - Prep time: 5 mins, Cook time: 10 mins, Total time: 15 mins, Servings: 4, Grill temp: 300°F

Ingredients

- 2 cups of cubed Kabocha squash
- 2 cups of rice
- 1 ½ cups of water
- 4 drops of sesame oil
- 1 tbsp of cooking sake
- 1 tsp of salt

Directions

1. Mix rice, water, sake, sesame oil, and salt in a deep-bottomed saucepan with a lid and keep it on medium flame.
2. Add the squash.
3. Close and seal the lid.
4. Cook on high flame for 7 mins.
5. Turn off the flame and wait for 10 mins.
6. Stir and serve!

Nutritional Values

Calories 355, Fat 4g, Chol 0mg, Sodium 71.4mg, Potassium 67.7mg, Carbs 82g, Protein 9g

4. POLENTA WITH HERBS

- Breakfast - Prep time: 10 mins, Cook time: 5 mins, Total time: 10 mins, Servings: 4, Grill temp: 300°F

Ingredients

- 3 cups of vegetable broth

- 1 cup of water
- 1 cup of coarse-ground polenta
- 1 large minced onion
- 3 tbsp of fresh, chopped thyme
- 2 tbsp of fresh, chopped Italian parsley
- 1 tbsp of minced garlic
- 1 tsp of fresh, chopped sage
- Salt and pepper to taste

Directions

1. Put a deep-bottomed saucepan/pot with a lid on heat and sauté the onion for about a minute.
2. Add the minced garlic and cook for 1 more minute.
3. Pour in the broth with the thyme, parsley, and sage. Stir.
4. Sprinkle the polenta in the pot, but don't stir it in.
5. Close and seal the lid.
6. Cook on high flame for 5 mins.
7. Turn off the flame and let it stand for 10 mins.
8. Pick out the bay leaf.
9. Using a whisk, stir the polenta to smooth it.
10. Season to taste with salt and pepper before serving.

Nutritional Values

Calories 103kcal, Fat 0g, Chol 0mg, Sodium 71.4mg, Potassium 67.7mg, Carbs 3g, Protein 0g

5. BLUEBERRY PANCAKES

- Breakfast - Prep time: 10 mins, Cook time: ready in about 20 mins, Servings: 2, Grill temp: Medium

Ingredients

- 2 tbsp cane sugar
- 1½ cups of flour, all-purpose
- 2 tsp baking powder
- ½ tsp cinnamon
- ½ tsp baking soda
- ¼ tsp sea salt
- 1 cup of almond milk
- 1 egg
- ½ cup of whole milk- Greek yogurt
- Maple syrup
- 1½ tsp of vanilla extract
- 2 tbsp avocado oil

- 2 cups of blueberries

Directions

1. Take a bowl, add sugar, flour, baking powder, cinnamon, baking soda, and salt, and stir well.
2. Take another bowl, add egg, yogurt, almond milk, avocado oil, & vanilla in it, and whisk well.
3. Combine your wet ingredients with your dry ingredients fully.
4. Take a non-stick pan, place it on medium flame and spray with little oil.
5. Pour the mixture into the pan, place blueberries over each pancake, and cook for around 1-2 mins.
6. Turn around & again cook for 1-2 mins.
7. Serve them hot with some maple syrup.

Nutritional Values

Calories 272kcal, Carbs 30g, Protein 8g, Fat 15g, Sodium 686mg, Potassium 734mg, Chol 0mg

6. BAKED APPLES

- Breakfast - Prep time: ready in about: 30 mins, Servings: 4, Grill temp: Medium

Ingredients

- ½ cup of almond flour
- ½ cup of rolled oats, whole
- ⅓ cup of brown sugar
- ½ tsp Apple-Pie-Spice
- ¼ cup of crushed walnuts
- ¼ tsp sea salt
- 4 halved apples
- Ice cream - for serving
- ¼ cup of coconut oil

Directions

1. Preheat your oven to around 375°F.
2. Take a medium bowl, add oats, brown sugar, almond flour, walnuts, salt, coconut oil & apple spice in it, and make your mixture with a thick consistency.
3. Next, scoop out each ½ apple from the center.
4. Put them in a baking pan and drizzle with some coconut oil, spreading all over your apples.
5. Cover using foil & bake for around 10 mins.

6. Uncover and top each piece with a spoonful of your prepared topping.
7. Add some more coconut oil & bake for around 20 mins.
8. Let them cool for a while & serve them with some ice cream.

Nutritional Values

Calories 222kcal, Carbs 30g, Protein 8g, Fat 15g, Sodium 886mg, Potassium 734mg, Chol 0mg

7. MAPLE CASHEW APPLE TOAST

- Breakfast - Prep time: ready in about: 10 mins, Servings: 4, Grill temp: Medium

Ingredients

- 4 tsp of maple syrup
- 1/4 cup of cashew butter
- 4 slices of toasted wheat bread
- 1/8 tsp of ground cinnamon
- ½ apple, sliced thinly

Directions

1. Take a medium bowl, add cashew butter & syrup, and stir well.
2. Pour over toasted bread.
3. Sprinkle with some cinnamon & top with some apple wedges.

Nutritional Values

Calories 227kcal, Carbs 30g, Protein 5g, Fat 10g, Sodium 208mg, Potassium 734mg, Chol 0mg

8. MANGO GINGER OATS RECIPE

- Breakfast - Prep time: ready in about: 40 mins, Servings: 4, Grill temp: Medium

Ingredients

- 1 to 1/3 cups of water
- 2 cups of oats
- 2/3 cup of coconut milk, unsweetened
- ½ tsp ginger, grated
- seeds of Pomegranate
- 2 Tbsp of honey
- 2 cups of mango

Directions

1. Divide oats in Mason jars equally.
2. Mix water, honey, coconut milk, & ginger, then pour this mixture over oats in each

jar. Also, put some mango into your jars, cover them, and let them chill overnight.
3. Then add some pomegranate seeds on the top, if required, and serve.

Nutritional Values

Calories 264kcal, Carbs 30g, Protein 6g, Fat 6g, Sodium 38mg, Potassium 734mg, Chol 0mg

9. ACAI-BOWL RECIPE

- Breakfast - Prep time: ready in about: 40 mins, Servings: 2, Grill temp: Medium

Ingredients

- 2 bananas, ripped & frozen
- 3.5-ounce acai pulp, frozen
- 1 Tbsp of honey
- 1 cup blueberries
- 4 to 5 Tbsp of water
- 1 sliced kiwi
- 2 Tbsp of unsweetened toasted coconut
- 2 Tbsp toasted almonds
- 2 Tbsp of cocoa nibs

Directions

1. Take a blender, put acai pulp, banana chunks, & honey in it, and blend well.
2. Divide into 2 bowls and top each with your leftover ingredients
3. Serve.

Nutritional Values

Calories 388 kcal, Carbs 30g, Protein 5g, Fat 15g, Sodium 16mg, Potassium 89mg, Chol 0mg

10. PLANT-BASED BURRITO BREAKFAST

- Breakfast - Prep time: ready in about: 40 mins, Servings: 6, Grill temp: Medium

Ingredients

- ½ diced onion
- 1 tsp of canola oil
- ½ bell pepper, red and diced
- 1 container of Lightlife Ground- Plant-Based
- 1 packet of taco seasoning
- 3 eggs
- 6 Cassava Wraps
- Black beans
- ¼ cup of shredded cheese

- Cilantro- fresh
- Hot sauce

1. Take a skillet, add oil & sauté bell pepper and onion over medium flame.
2. Cook for around 3 mins while occasionally stirring, then put seasoning & Light-life ground to your frying pan.
3. Cook for around 5-7 mins, until browned.
4. Place another pan over the flame, coat it with your cooking spray, put eggs & whisk to form a scramble.
5. Toast your wraps for a while. Then assemble your burrito, first layer your prepared ground mixture, & then black beans, scrambled eggs, & cheese.
6. Top them with fresh cilantro & hot sauce. Serve hot.

Nutritional Values

Calories 322kcal, Carbs 30g, Protein 8g, Fat 15g, Sodium 586mg, Potassium 734mg, Chol 0mg

11. CRUNCHY-EGG-SALAD

- Breakfast - Prep time: ready in about: 30 mins, Servings: 2, Grill temp: 0

Ingredients

- 2 cups of butter lettuce
- 2 eggs
- 4 sliced radishes
- 1 small cucumber
- ¼ cup of snap peas
- 2 Tbsp walnuts, chopped
- 2 Tbsp of balsamic vinegar
- Fresh dill
- 1 tsp of Dijon mustard
- Salt & pepper
- ¼ cup of olive oil, extra-virgin

Directions

1. Take your eggs & boil for around 10 mins, then slice them into halves.
2. While taking a bowl, add all of your dressing ingredients to it and toss them well.
3. Take another bowl, put radishes, butter lettuce, snap peas, walnuts, and cucumber in it, and mix with dressing.

4. Transfer to a bowl & top with egg halves and some fresh dill.

Nutritional Values

Calories 222kcal, Carbs 30g, Protein 8g, Fat 15.5g, Sodium 886mg, Potassium 734mg, Chol 0mg

12. NO-BAKE COOKIES

- Breakfast - Prep time: ready in about: 35 mins, Servings: 12, Grill temp: 0

Ingredients

- ½ cup of maple syrup
- ¼ cup of coconut oil
- 1½ cups of rolled oats
- ¼ cup of almond milk
- ¼ cup of peanut butter, creamy
- 2 tbsp of cocoa powder
- ½ tsp vanilla

Directions

1. Take a baking sheet lined with baking paper.
2. Take a pan, add coconut oil, maple syrup, cocoa, almond milk, peanut butter, & vanilla in it, and cook over medium flame for around 2 mins while stirring.
3. Then stir your prepared sauce in oats.
4. Scoop this batter on your baking sheet, let them chill for around 30 mins, and then serve.

Nutritional Values

Calories 165kcal, Carbs 14g, Protein 7g, Fat 10g, Sodium 627mg, Potassium 834mg, Chol 0mg

13. NO-BAKE-ENERGY-BALLS

- Breakfast - Prep time: ready in about: 10 mins, Servings: 12 balls, Grill temp: 0

Ingredients

- 1 tbsp flaxseed & 3 tbsp warm water
- 1 cup of rolled oats
- ¼ cup of almond butter, roasted
- 3 pitted Medjool dates
- 2 tbsp maple syrup
- 2 tbsp coconut oil
- ¼ tsp cinnamon
- ½ tsp vanilla extract
- ¼ tsp sea salt

- ½ cup of shredded coconut
- ¼ cup walnuts, chopped
- ⅓ cup of chocolate chips

Directions

1. Slightly toast your oats over medium-low flame for around 2 mins.
2. Take a food processor, add almond butter, dates, maple syrup, coconut oil, cinnamon, salt, vanilla, and thickened flaxseed in it, and blend well.
3. Then put walnuts, coconut, oats, & chocolate chips in it and mix fully.
4. Make balls using this mixture and let them chill for around 30 mins.
5. Then serve and enjoy your food.

Nutritional Values

Calories 253kcal, Carbs 33g, Protein 10g, Fat 9g, Sodium 680mg, Potassium 834mg, Chol 0mg

14. BREAKFAST-VEGGIE-BURGER RECIPE

- Breakfast - Prep time: ready in about: 40 mins, Servings: 1, Grill temp: Medium-high

Ingredients

- 1 thick tomato
- 1 burger patty should be veggie
- 3 slices of red onion
- 1 tsp of canola oil
- ¼ sliced avocado
- 1 egg
- Fresh parsley
- Black pepper

Directions

1. Take a pan, place it over medium flame, and cook patty from both sides for around 3 mins each.
2. Put tomato slice on your plate, then add sliced onion & veggie patty on it.
3. Cook egg in a frying pan for around 3-5 mins, then place it on your burger's top.
4. Sprinkle some parsley & black pepper, and serve.

Nutritional Values

Calories 265kcal, Carbs 14g, Protein 7g, Fat 11g, Sodium 627mg, Potassium 834mg, Chol 0mg

15. BANANA-BUCKWHEAT PORRIDGE

- Breakfast - Prep time: 10 mins, Cook time: 10 mins, Total time: 20 mins, Servings: 3 to 4, Grill temp: 350°F

Ingredients

- 3 cups of almond- or rice milk
- 1 cup of buckwheat groats
- 1 sliced banana
- ¼ cup of raisins
- 1 tsp of cinnamon
- ½ tsp of pure vanilla extract

Directions

1. Rinse off the buckwheat and put it right in the pressure cooker or a deep pan with a lid.
2. Pour in the milk, and add the rest of the ingredients.
3. Close the lid.
4. Cook for 6 mins on high pressure/heat.
5. When time is up, wait 20 minutes or so for the pressure to go down.
6. Open the lid and stir well. Add more milk if it's too thick for you.
7. Serve!

Nutritional Values

Calories 240, Fat 4g, Chol 0mg, Sodium 21.4mg, Potassium 77.2mg, Carbs 46g, Protein 6g

16. BLACK BEAN PLUS SWEET POTATO HASH

- Breakfast - Prep time: 5 mins, Cook time: 10 mins, Total time: 15 mins, Servings: 4, Grill temp: 350°F

Ingredients

- 2 cups of peeled, chopped sweet potatoes
- 1 cup of chopped onion
- 1 cup of cooked and drained black beans
- 1 minced garlic clove
- ⅓ cup of vegetable broth
- ¼ cup of chopped scallions
- 2 tsps of hot chili powder

Directions

1. Prepare your vegetables.
2. In a deep saucepan with a lid, saute and cook the chopped onion for 2-3 mins, stirring so it doesn't burn.

3. Add the garlic and stir until fragrant.
4. Add the sweet potatoes and chili powder and stir.
5. Pour in the broth and give 1 last stir before locking the lid.
6. Cook on high pressure for 3 mins.
7. When time is up, quick release the pressure carefully.
8. Add the black beans and scallions and stir to heat everything up.
9. Season with salt and more chili powder if desired.

Nutritional Values

Calories 133, Fat 1g, Chol 0mg, Sodium 32.4mg, Potassium 57.7mg, Carbs 28g, Protein 5g

17. BLUEBERRY MUFFINS

- Breakfast - Prep time: 15 mins, Cook time: 25 mins, Total time: 40 mins, Servings: 12, Grill temp: 350°F

Ingredients

- 1 and ¾ cups of all-purpose flour
- ½ tsp of baking soda
- ½ cup of sugar
- ½ tsp of baking powder
- ¼ tsp of kosher salt
- ¼ tsp of ground cinnamon
- 3 tsps of egg replacer, such as Ener-G
- ¼ cup of warm water
- ½ cup of nondairy vanilla yogurt
- ¼ cup of grapeseed oil
- 2 tbsp of non-dairy milk
- 1 tsp of lemon zest
- 1 tsp of freshly squeezed lemon juice
- 1 and ¼ cups of roughly chopped fresh or frozen blueberries

Directions

1. Preheat the oven to 350°F - 180°C. Lightly coat the cups of a 12-cup muffin tin with nonstick baking spray.
2. Whisk together baking soda, all-purpose flour, kosher salt, sugar, baking powder, and cinnamon in a medium bowl.
3. Whisk egg replacer with warm water in a small bowl until well blended. Whisk in vanilla nondairy yogurt, grapeseed oil, lemon zest, and lemon juice.

4. Quickly stir wet ingredients into the flour mixture until ingredients are just combined, taking care not to overmix. Fold in blueberries.
5. Using an ice cream scoop or a large spoon, evenly divide the batter among muffin cups. The batter will be thick, like biscuit dough.
6. Bake on the bottom rack of the oven for 22 to 25 mins or until muffins spring back when lightly pressed in the center. Cool in the pan for 5 mins before turning out on a wire rack to cool. Serve warm or at room temperature.

Nutritional Values

Calories 113, Fat 1.8g, Chol 5mg, Sodium 71.4mg, Potassium 67.7mg, Carbs 22g, Protein 2.3g

18. BREAKFAST BURRITOS

- Breakfast - Prep time: 10 mins, Cook time: 10 mins, Total time: 20 mins, Servings: 2, Grill temp: 300°F

Ingredients

- 2 tbsp of olive oil
- ½ small red onion, thinly sliced- ¼ cup
- 2 cups of sliced button mushrooms
- 1 tsp of crumbled dried sage
- ½ tsp of kosher salt
- ½ tsp of freshly ground black pepper
- 1 cup of cooked black beans
- 2- 10-in. whole-wheat tortillas
- 1 large tomato, diced- 1 cup
- 1 medium Hass avocado halved, seeded, and sliced
- ¼ cup of prepared salsa

Directions

1. Heat olive oil in a medium sautés pan over medium-high heat. Cook, stirring once or twice, for 2 to 3 mins, with button mushrooms and red onion.
2. Cook for 2 mins or more after adding the kosher salt, sage, and black pepper.
3. Cook, stirring a few times and pressing to break up the beans and brown them a little, for approximately 5 mins, turning a few times and pushing to break them up and

brown them a little. Remove the pan from the heat and set it aside.

4. Place ½ of the mushroom filling in the center of each tortilla, then divide the avocado, tomato, and salsa among the burritos. Fold the 2 short ends first, then fold 1 long end inside to form a burrito.

Nutritional Values

Calories 113, Fat 1.8g, Chol 0mg, Sodium 61.4mg, Potassium 37.7mg, Carbs 22g, Protein 2.3g

19. BREAKFAST SCRAMBLE

- Breakfast - Prep time: 10 mins, Cook time: 10 mins, Total time: 20 mins, Servings: 2, Grill temp: 300°F

Ingredients

- 2 tbsp of olive oil
- ½ cup of silken tofu
- ½ small red onion, thinly sliced- ¼ cup
- 1 tbsp of nutritional yeast
- 2 cups of sliced button mushrooms
- 1 tsp of crumbled dried sage
- ½ tsp of kosher salt
- ½ tsp of freshly ground black pepper
- 1 cup of cooked black beans
- 2- 10-in., 25cm whole-wheat tortillas
- 1 large tomato, diced- 1 cup
- 1 medium Hass avocado halved, seeded, and sliced
- ¼ cup of plant-based sour cream
- A handful of chopped cilantro
- Chopped fruits and vegetables of your choice
- ¼ cup of prepared salsa

Directions

1. Heat olive oil in a medium sautés pan over medium-high heat. Cook, stirring once or twice, for 2 to 3 mins, with button mushrooms and red onion.
2. Cook for 2 mins or more after adding the kosher salt, sage, and black pepper.
3. Cook, stirring a few times and pressing to break up the beans and brown them a little, for approximately 5 mins, turning a few times and pushing to break them up and brown them a little.

4. Toss ½ a cup of crumbled silken tofu and 1 tbsp of nutritional yeast into the pan with black beans. Remove the pan from the heat and set it aside.
5. Place ½ of the mushroom filling in the center of each tortilla, then divide the avocado, tomato, and salsa among the burritos.
6. Add plant-based sour cream, chopped cilantro, or chopped fresh fruits or veggies to your burrito.
7. Fold the 2 short ends first, then fold 1 long end inside to form a breakfast scramble.

Nutritional Values

Calories 113, Fat 1.8g, Chol 3mg, Sodium 31.4mg, Potassium 87.7mg, Carbs 22g, Protein 2.3g

20. BREAKFAST TOFU SCRAMBLE

- Breakfast - Prep time: 5 mins, Cook time: 5 mins, Total time: 10 mins, Servings: 4, Grill temp: 350°F

Ingredients

- 1 block of extra-firm, crumbled tofu
- 1 cup of cherry tomatoes
- 1 onion
- 1 diced potato
- 1 diced apple
- ¼ cup of veggie broth
- 2 minced garlic cloves
- 1 tsp of dry dill
- ½ tsp of ground turmeric
- Salt and pepper to taste

Directions

1. Sauté and dry-cook the garlic and onion until the onion begins to soften in a deep saucepan with a lid.
2. Add a bit of water if it starts to stick.
3. Pour broth and add the rest of the ingredients.
4. Close the lid.
5. Cook on high pressure for 4 mins.
6. Stir, season to taste, and enjoy!

Nutritional Values

Calories 139, Fat 5g, Chol 5mg, Sodium 61.4mg, Potassium 57.7mg, Carbs 15g, Protein 12g

21. CHAI-SPICED OATMEAL WITH MANGO

- Breakfast - Prep time: 10 mins, Cook time: 10 mins, Total time: 20 mins, Servings: 2 to 3, Grill temp: 350°F

Ingredients
- 3 cups of water
- 1 cup of steel-cut oats
- ½ tsp of vanilla
- Dash of cinnamon
- Dash of ginger
- Dash of cloves
- Dash of cardamom
- Dash of salt
- ½ mango, cut into pieces

Directions
1. Mix water and oats in a deep saucepan with a lid.
2. Close the lid.
3. Cook for 5 mins on high flame.
4. Turn off the flame and let it rest.
5. Open the lid and stir well.
6. Season and taste.
7. Divide into even servings and add chopped mango.

Nutritional Values
Calories 236, Fat 4g, Chol 0mg, Sodium 74mg, Potassium 67mg, Carbs 44g, Protein 6g

22. COCONUT-ALMOND RISOTTO

- Breakfast - Prep time: 10 mins, Cook time: 10 mins, Total time: 20 mins, Servings: 4, Grill temp: 350°F

Ingredients
- 2 cups of vanilla almond milk
- 1 cup of coconut milk
- 1 cup of Arborio rice
- ⅓ cup of sugar
- 2 tsps of pure vanilla
- ¼ cup of sliced almonds and coconut flakes

Directions
1. Pour the milk into a deep-bottomed saucepan with a lid.
2. Stir until it boils.
3. Add the rice and stir before closing the lid.
4. Cook for 5 mins on high pressure.
5. Turn off the flame and wait 10 mins.
6. Add the sugar and vanilla.

7. Divide up oats and top with almonds and coconut.

Nutritional Values
Calories 337, Fat 7g, Chol 4mg, Sodium 41.4mg, Potassium 87.7mg, Carbs 66g, Protein 6g

23. CRANBERRY-WALNUT QUINOA

- Breakfast - Prep time: 10 mins, Cook time: 10 mins, Total time: 20 mins, Servings: 4, Grill temp: 350°F

Ingredients
- 2 cups of water
- 2 cups of dried cranberries
- 1 cup of quinoa
- 1 cup of chopped walnuts
- 1 cup of sunflower seeds
- ½ tbsp of cinnamon

Directions
1. Rinse quinoa.
2. Put quinoa, water, and salt in a deep-bottomed saucepan with a lid.
3. Lock the lid.
4. Cook for 10 mins, on high pressure.
5. Turn off the flame.
6. When the pressure is gone, open the lid.
7. Mix dried cranberries, nuts, seeds, sweeteners, and cinnamon.
8. Serve and enjoy!

Nutritional Values
Calories 611, Fat 29g, Chol 11mg, Sodium 73mg, Potassium 65mg, Carbs 85g, Protein 13g

24. NUTTY GRANOLA

- Breakfast - Prep time: 5 mins, Cook time: 25 mins, Total time: 30 mins, Servings: 10, Grill temp: 300°F

Ingredients
- 4 cups of rolled oats- not instant
- 2 tbsp of lightly packed brown sugar
- 1 tsp of ground cinnamon
- ½ tsp of kosher salt
- ½ cup of grapeseed oil
- ½ cup of maple syrup
- ½ cup of chopped pecans, walnuts, or your favorite nut

- ½ cup of raisins
- ¼ cup of roasted, salted, shelled pumpkin seeds- pepitas

Directions

1. Preheat the oven to 300°F - 150°C.
2. Combine cinnamon, brown sugar, rolled oats, and kosher salt in a large mixing bowl.
3. Whisk maple syrup and grapeseed oil together in a small basin, then pour over the oat mixture. Fold the ingredients together with a big spatula until well combined.
4. Spread the granola out on a big baking sheet and toast it for 20 to 25 mins, stirring twice, until golden brown.
5. Allow to cool completely in a clean basin, stirring in raisins, pecans, and pumpkin seeds.
6. For up to a week, store in a firmly sealed glass jar.

Nutritional Values

Calories 113, Fat 1.8g, Chol 0mg, Sodium 54mg, Potassium 77mg, Carbs 22g, Protein 2.3g

25. PEAR OATS WITH WALNUTS

- Breakfast - Prep time: 10 mins, Cook time: 10 mins, Total time: 20 mins, Servings: 4, Grill temp: 350°F

Ingredients

- 2 cups of almond milk
- 2 cups of peeled and cut pears
- 1 cup of rolled oats
- ½ cup of chopped walnuts
- ¼ cup of sugar
- 1 tbsp of melted coconut oil
- ¼ tsp of salt
- Dash of cinnamon

Directions

1. Mix everything except the walnuts and cinnamon in an oven-safe bowl.
2. Preheat the oven to 350°F.
3. Put the bowl in the oven.
4. Set the timer for 10 mins.
5. When time is up, carefully remove the bowl, divide it into 4 servings, and season with salt and cinnamon.

Nutritional Values

Calories 288, Fat 13g, Chol 2mg, Sodium 67mg, Potassium 57.7mg, Carbs 39g, Protein 5g

26. PUMPKIN SPICE OATMEAL WITH BROWN SUGAR TOPPING

- Breakfast - Prep time: 10 mins, Cook time: 10 mins, Total time: 20 mins, Servings: 6 to 8, Grill temp: 350°F

Ingredients

- 4 ½ cups of water
- 1 ½ cups of steel-cut oats
- 1 ½ cups of pumpkin puree
- 2 tsps of cinnamon
- 1 tsp of vanilla
- 1 tsp of allspice
- ½ cup of brown sugar
- ¼ cup of chopped pecans
- 1 tbsp of cinnamon

Directions

1. Pour 1 cup of water into a deep-bottomed saucepan.
2. Add everything from the first ingredient list- including the rest of the water, into an oven-safe bowl and set it in the steamer basket.
3. Lower the basket into the saucepan and lock the lid.
4. Cook on high pressure for 3 mins.
5. Turn off the flame.
6. Mix the topping ingredients in a small bowl.
7. When you serve, sprinkle on top. If necessary, add a little almond milk to the oats.

Nutritional Values

Calories 207, Fat 4g, Chol 0mg, Sodium 71.4mg, Potassium 67.7mg, Carbs 38g, Protein 4g

27. SOY YOGURT

- Breakfast - Prep time: Midnight, Cook time: 0 mins, Total time: Midnight, Servings: 8, Grill temp: 125°F

Ingredients

- 2 quarts of soy milk
- 1 packet of vegan yogurt culture

Directions

1. Mix milk and yogurt cultures together.
2. Pour into a container.
3. Close the lid.
4. Store in a dry place.
5. After 12 to 13 hours, take out the yogurt.
6. Put the lids on the containers and store them in the fridge for at least 6 hours.
7. The yogurt will be very tangy and sweetened with vanilla, sugar, jam, fruit, and so on!

Nutritional Values

Calories 55, Fat 2g, Chol 2mg, Sodium 67mg, Potassium 57.7mg, Carbs 5g, Protein 4g

28. STRAWBERRY MUFFINS

- Breakfast - Prep time: 15 mins, Cook time: 25 mins, Total time: 40 mins, Servings: 12, Grill temp: 350°F

Ingredients

- 1 and ¾ cups of all-purpose flour
- ½ cup of sugar
- ½ tsp of baking powder
- ½ tsp of baking soda
- ¼ tsp of kosher salt
- ¼ tsp of ground nutmeg
- 3 tsps of egg replacer, such as Ener-G
- ¼ cup of warm water
- ½ cup of nondairy vanilla yogurt
- ¼ cup of grapeseed oil
- 2 tbsp of non-dairy milk
- 1 tsp of lemon zest
- 1 tsp of freshly squeezed lemon juice
- 1 and ¼ cups of roughly chopped fresh or frozen strawberries

Directions

1. Preheat the oven to 350°F - 180°C. Lightly coat the cups of a 12-cup muffin tin with nonstick baking spray.
2. Whisk together sugar, kosher salt, all-purpose flour, baking powder, baking soda, and nutmeg in a medium bowl.
3. Whisk egg replacer with warm water in a small bowl until well blended. Whisk in vanilla nondairy yogurt, grapeseed oil, lemon zest, and lemon juice.
4. Quickly stir wet ingredients into the flour mixture until ingredients are just combined, taking care not to overmix. Fold in strawberries.
5. Using an ice cream scoop or a large spoon, evenly divide the batter among muffin cups. The batter will be thick, like biscuit dough.
6. Bake on the bottom rack of the oven for 22 to 25 mins or until muffins spring back when lightly pressed in the center. Cool in the pan for 5 mins before turning out on a wire rack to cool. Serve warm or at room temperature.

Nutritional Values

Calories 113, Fat 1.8g, Chol 0mg, Sodium 71.4mg, Potassium 67.7mg, Carbs 22g, Protein 2.3g

29. WHOLE-WHEAT BANANA PECAN PANCAKES

- Breakfast - Prep time: 15 mins, Cook time: 15 mins, Total time: 30 mins, Servings: 4, Grill temp: 300°F

Ingredients

- 1 and ¼ cups of soy milk or coconut milk beverage, plus ¼ cup if needed
- 1 tbsp of flax meal- ground flaxseeds
- 1 tsp of apple cider vinegar
- 1 large ripe banana, peeled and mashed well
- 1 tbsp of brown sugar
- 1 tbsp of maple syrup, plus more for serving- optional
- 1 tsp of vanilla extract
- 1 cup of white whole-wheat flour or whole-wheat pastry flour
- 1 /3 cup of buckwheat flour
- 2 tsps of baking powder
- ½ tsp of kosher salt
- ½ tsp of ground cinnamon
- ¼ tsp of ground nutmeg
- ½ cup of finely chopped toasted pecans
- 1 cup of fresh mixed raspberries, blueberries, and/or strawberries- optional

Directions

1. In a small saucepan, warm ¼ cup of soy milk over medium-high heat.
2. Place flax meal in a small bowl, add warm milk, stir well, and set aside.

3. Whisk apple cider vinegar into the remaining soy milk in a small bowl and set aside to thicken and curdle.
4. In another small bowl, mash the banana with brown sugar, maple syrup, and vanilla extract. Whisk in the flax mixture, followed by curdled soy milk, and blend well.
5. Heat a cast-iron skillet or frying pan over medium heat until a drop of water sizzles and evaporates immediately.
6. Meanwhile, in a medium bowl, whisk together white whole-wheat flour, buckwheat flour, baking powder, kosher salt, cinnamon, and nutmeg. Stir in wet ingredients until just combined, and quickly fold in chopped pecans. Stir in more soy milk as needed to make a thick batter, the consistency of a heavy-pound cake batter.
7. Lightly oil or butter the griddle, and drop 3 tbsp-size scoops of batter into the pan, spreading with a small spatula if necessary. Cook for 2 mins, without disturbing or until bubbles form on the surface of the pancakes; carefully flip over pancakes and cook for 1 ½ more mins. Grease the pan a little between each batch, as these pancakes will want to stick to the pan otherwise.
8. Serve hot with mixed fruit- if using and more maple syrup- if using. The success of this recipe depends on using nondairy milk that will curdle. Instead, choose a soy or coconut milk beverage, as both will thicken and sour nicely when the apple cider vinegar is introduced.

Nutritional Values

Calories 113, Fat 1.8g, Chol 0mg, Sodium 31.4mg, Potassium 97.7mg, Carbs 22g, Protein 2.3g

30. BOWL WITH AMARANTH GRANOLA

- Breakfast - Prep time: 10 mins, Cook time: 30, Total time: 40 mins, Grill temp: 300°F, Servings: 8

Ingredients

- 1 cup oats rolled
- ½ cup of amaranth
- ½ cup almonds chopped
- ½ tsp salt
- 2 tbsp coconut oil melted
- 2 tsp cinnamon
- 2 tbsp butter almond
- 4 tbsp syrup maple
- Fresh fruit, dried or frozen
- Original Almond milk

Directions

1. In the oven, set the temp to 300°F and line the baking sheet with parchment paper.
2. A mixing bowl is an ideal size for combining all of the components. Then whisk in the maple syrup, coconut oil, and almond butter until everything is well combined.
3. Bake for 15 mins, then spread out on a baking pan to cool. After moving the pan into the oven, bake for another 15 mins or until golden brown. Allow the dish to cool for at least 15 mins before serving.
4. In bowls, combine the granola, fruit, and almond milk and serve immediately.
5. Extra granola may be stored for up to a week in an airtight container.

Nutritional Values

Fat 7.2g, Chol 6mg, Sodium 9mg, Potassium 76mg, Carbs 56g, Calories 423, Protein 12g

31. PORTOBELLO MUSHROOM BURGER

- Breakfast - Prep time: 5 mins, Cook time: 13 mins, Total time: 18 mins, Grill temp: 0, Servings: 4

Ingredients

- 4 portobello mushrooms
- Olive oil or drizzling
- Balsamic vinegar
- Tamari
- Sea salt & black pepper freshly ground

For serving
- 4 toasted hamburger buns
- Lettuce
- Tomato finely sliced
- Red onion finely sliced
- pickle
- Ketchup, mustard, mayonnaise
- Pesto

1. Clean the caps of the mushrooms by removing the stems and wiping them clean with a paper towel. Drizzle olive oil, tamari, balsamic vinegar, salt, and pepper over the mushrooms on a rimmed plate. Cover all sides of the mushrooms with your hands.
2. Preheat a grill pan over medium heat. Arrange the mushrooms on top of the grill pan. Cook for 5 to 7 mins each side or until the mushrooms are tender.
3. Place the mushrooms on top of the buns and add your preferred toppings.

Nutritional Values

Fat 9g, Chol 3mg, Sodium 5mg, Potassium 12mg, Carbs 54g, Calories 289, Protein 13g

32. TOAST WITH RADISHES & DANDELION GREENS

- Breakfast - Prep time: 10 mins, Cook time: 10 mins, Total time: 20 mins, Grill temp: 0, Servings: 3-4

Ingredients

- olive oil
- ¼ cup spring onions chopped
- sliced radishes
- ½ bunch of greens dandelion
- ¼ cup thawed & chopped frozen edamame
- 4-6 slices of grainy toasted bread
- pepper flakes red
- salt & pepper

Directions

1. In a food processor or blender, combine all of the seed spread ingredients and process until smooth. 1 more time, blend in the herbs. Place it in the refrigerator whenever you're ready to use it.
2. Sauté the onion until translucent, then add it to the radishes with pepper and salt. Cover and cook for 5 mins, or until the radishes are fork-tender.
3. Add the dandelion greens and a hefty lemon squeeze when the radishes are nearly done. Cook until the greens are just starting to wilt. Season with kosher salt and freshly cracked black pepper to taste.

4. Before serving, garnish with radishes, seed spread, chopped greens, and a pinch of chili flakes.
5. Store the sunflower spread in the refrigerator for up to 4 days.

Nutritional Values

Fat 6.4g, Chol 9mg, Sodium 12mg, Potassium 70mg, Carbs 57g, Calories 426, Protein 14g

33. WILD RICE SOUP

- Breakfast - Prep time: 10 mins, Cook time: 35 mins, Total time: 45 mins, Grill temp: 0, Servings: 4

Ingredients

Creamy base
- 1 cup almond milk
- ⅓ cup cashews
- ¼ cup drained cannellini beans
- white miso paste tbsp
- Dijon mustard 2 tsp

Soup
- 2 tbsp olive oil
- 1 bunch of chopped scallions
- 1 chopped celery stalk
- 1 chopped carrot
- 8 oz. sliced cremini mushrooms
- 1 tsp of sea salt
- 4 minced garlic cloves
- 2 tbsp of minced rosemary
- 1 thyme bunch
- 1¼ cup drained cannellini beans
- ½ tsp black pepper freshly ground
- 4 cups of water
- 1 cup of wild rice cooked
- 1-2 tbsp of lemon juice fresh
- 4 cups of chopped kale
- Chopped parsley
- Red chili flakes

Directions

1. To make the cream base, start by following these steps: Combine the almond milk, white beans, cashews, miso paste, and Dijon mustard in a blender and blend until smooth. Then, remove the item from the table.
2. Follow these directions: Heat the oil over medium heat in a medium-sized Dutch large pot to make the soup. Stir in the

celery, scallions, carrots, and mushrooms, followed by the salt, until well incorporated. Cook for 8-10 mins, occasionally stirring, or until the mushrooms are tender. Combine the rosemary, garlic, and thyme, as well as the pepper, cannellini beans, and water, in a large mixing bowl. Cook with the lid on for at least 20 mins.

3. In a large mixing bowl, combine the rice, cashew mixture, 1 tbsp fresh lemon juice, and kale, discarding the thyme. Cook for 5 mins, stirring regularly unless the kale is done. Season to taste and serve with extra parsley, lemon juice, and red chili flakes if desired.

Nutritional Values

Fat 9.7g, Chol 6mg, Sodium 14mg, Potassium 76mg, Carbs 59g, Calories 485, Protein 14g

34. ROASTED BRUSSELS SPROUTS

- Breakfast - Prep time: 5 mins, Cook time: 30 mins, Total time: 35 mins, Grill temp: 425°F, Servings: 3-4

Ingredients

- 1 pound of Brussels sprouts
- Olive oil for drizzling
- Sea salt & black pepper freshly ground
- Lemon Parmesan for seasoning
- 1 tbsp lemon juice
- 1 tbsp lemon zest
- 1 tbsp of grated Parmesan cheese
- 1 tbsp thyme leaves fresh
- parsley leaves
- pinch of red chili flakes

Directions

1. Preheat the oven to 425°F and prepare a baking pan with parchment paper. Cut the Brussels stems in ½ and place them on a baking dish with oil, salt, and pepper drizzle. Roast for 20-30 mins or until the veggies are tender and golden. You'll need to modify the time based on the size of the sprouts.
2. Toss roasted Brussels sprouts with lemon zest, Parmesan cheese, and fresh thyme leaves, if desired.

3. Serve garnished with parsley and red chili flakes.

Nutritional Values

Fat 7g, Chol 12mg, Sodium 19mg, Potassium 78mg, Carbs 56g, Calories 314, Protein 18g

35. EASIEST CHIA PUDDING

- Breakfast - Prep time: 10 mins, Cook time: 15 mins, Total time: 25 mins, Grill temp: 0, Servings: 4

Ingredients

- ¼ cup seeds chia
- 1 & ½ cups milk cashew
- 1 tbsp maple syrup
- ¼ tsp of cinnamon
- sea salt pinch
- ½ tbsp lemon juice Meyer
- zest lemon
- fruit seasonal

Directions

1. Combine the cinnamon, salt, milk, chia seeds, maple syrup, and any extra lemon juice and zest in a jar or plate.
2. After cooling covered for 30 mins, stir in the chia seeds collected to the bottom of the basin. Depending on how thick you want your chia pudding, refrigerate for at least 6 hr or overnight. If it gets too thick, thin it with a tiny bit of milk.
3. Scoop pudding onto serving plates and sprinkle with desired toppings such as berries, nuts, and maple syrup.

Nutritional Values

Fat 6.3g, Chol 9mg, Sodium 12mg, Potassium 79mg, Carbs 54g, Calories 379, Protein 13g

36. ROASTED CHICKPEAS

- Breakfast - Prep time: 5 mins, Cook time: 20 mins, Total time: 25 mins, Grill temp: 425°F, Servings: 1.5

Ingredients

- 1-½ cups chickpeas drained
- Olive oil for drizzling
- Sea salt
- paprika

Directions

1. Preheat the oven to 425°F and line a baking sheet with parchment paper.
2. Spread the chickpeas out on the cloth to drain. Any skins that have come free should be discarded.
3. Combine the dry chickpeas with a splash of oil and a few pinches of salt on a baking pan.
4. Roast for 20-30 mins, or until roasted and crispy, depending on your oven; if your beans aren't crispy, keep cooking them until they are.
5. Remove the chickpeas from the oven and season them with your choice of spices while they are still warm.
6. Store toasted chickpeas in an airtight jar at 25°C. It is suggested that you use them within 2 days.

Nutritional Values
Fat 4.6g, Chol 9mg, Sodium 16mg, Potassium 74mg, Carbs 53g, Calories 348, Protein 14g

37. VERDE AVOCADO SALSA

- Breakfast - Prep time: 20 mins, Cook time: 10 mins, Total time: 30 mins, Grill temp: 0, Servings: 2

Ingredients
- 2 chopped scallions
- 1 diced avocado
- ½ cup chopped cilantro
- ¼ cup red onion chopped
- 1-2 limes juice & zest
- sea salt
- 1 minced garlic clove
- 1 thinly sliced jalapeño pepper

Directions
1. In a small bowl, combine the kiwi, onions, and avocado. If using, add the garlic, jalapenos, lime zest, and juice.
2. To taste, add more sea salt and lime juice.
3. Serve.

Nutritional Values
Fat 4.7g, Chol 17mg, Sodium 8mg, Potassium 76mg, Carbs 45g, Calories 327, Protein 11g

38. LEMON THYME OIL & BURRATA

- Breakfast - Prep time: 5 mins, Cook time: 15 mins, Total time: 20 mins, Grill temp: 0, Servings: 4

Ingredients
Lemon-thyme oil
- ½ cup of olive oil
- 1 crushed garlic clove
- 1 small lemon peel
- 4 thyme sprigs

Burrata platter
- 4 tomatoes
- 1 ripe sliced peach
- 1- 8 oz. burrata
- ½ cup fresh mint leaves
- 1 tbsp of toasted pistachios
- Sea salt & black pepper freshly ground
- Fresh cherries
- Toasted bread

Directions
1. Combine the oil, lemon peel, garlic, and thyme in a small stovetop saucepan.
2. After slowly warming the mixture, remove it from the fire.
3. Allow for 20 mins of steeping time before straining.
4. Arrange the tomatoes, peach segments, and burrata on a serving platter. Season with salt after sprinkling the lemon thyme oil on top. Pistachios should be sprinkled on top of the basil and mint.
5. Garnish with cherry and currants if preferred. Season with salt and pepper to taste, and serve with buttered bread.

Nutritional Values
Fat 4.8g, Chol 6mg, Sodium 9mg, Potassium 72mg, Carbs 40g, Calories 310, Protein 13g

39. MISO SOUP

- Breakfast - Prep time: 15 mins, Cook time: 15 mins, Total time: 30 mins, Grill temp: 0, Servings: 4

Ingredients
- 1 kombu piece
- 4 cups of water
- 4 tbsp dried seaweed wakame
- ¼ cup miso paste white
- ⅓ cup scallions chopped

- 6 oz. cubed silken tofu
- Tamari

Directions

1. Rinse each kombu piece carefully under running water to remove any remaining grit. Cook the Kombu in a saucepan with water for 10 mins to soften the texture. It will become bitter if you boil the Kombu for an extended period.
2. Rehydrate your wakame by soaking it in a bowl of hot water for about 5 mins.
3. Strain the broth and set the Kombu aside to chill. Return a portion of the hot broth to the soup after stirring it into miso paste in a separate dish until smooth.
4. Place the scallions, wakame, and tofu in a soup pot after draining them. Allow 1 to 2 mins of low heat simmering time. Use tamari for the seasoning.

Nutritional Values

Fat 4.9g, Chol 9mg, Sodium 13mg, Potassium 82mg, Carbs 52g, Calories 376, Protein 13g

40. CARROT SMORREBROD CRISPS

- Breakfast - Prep time: 5 mins, Cook time: 10 mins, Total time: 15 mins, Grill temp: 475°F, Servings: 4

Ingredients

- 4 carrots
- Sea salt

Marinade
- 3 tbsp of olive oil
- 1 tbsp of rice vinegar
- ½ tsp of smoked paprika
- Fresh lemon juice
- Black pepper freshly ground

For assembly
- Rye Crispbreads
- Vegan cheese creamy
- Finely sliced Persian cucumbers
- Finely sliced Radishes
- Capers
- Chives Chopped
- Dill chopped

Directions

1. Bake for 30 mins at 475°F, then remove from the oven and cool for 15 mins on a baking sheet lined with parchment paper. Place the whole carrots in the dish, then season liberally with salt after a 14-inch-thick layer of salt is applied on the base. I guarantee you that salt will not be consumed in the completed product. Make sure your carrots are soft by roasting them long enough. The freshness and size of the carrots will influence when they should be cooked. After around 40 mins, start keeping an eye on them.
2. Put your items in a bowl and prepare a marinade: In a small bowl, combine the oil, rice vinegar, lemon juice, paprika, and black pepper.
3. Remove the veggies from the oven and set them aside to cool. Rub any excess salt off with your hands to get rid of it. Next, tear the carrot into strips by slicing a horizontal layer and then using a peeler to remove the remaining carrot skin. To make the marinade, whisk together all of the ingredients in a large mixing basin.
4. When ready to serve, make sandwiches with crispbread, cucumber, cream cheese, and sliced radish. Before serving, toss in the capers, chives, carrot ribbons, and dill.
5. You may keep the rest of the carrots in the marinade for up to 4 days in the refrigerator. After that, these may be added to salads or other dishes.

Nutritional Values

Fat 4.2g, Chol 9mg, Sodium 13mg, Potassium 85mg, Carbs 42g, Calories 388, Protein 14g

41. CREAM OF MUSHROOM SOUP

- Breakfast - Prep time: 15 mins, Cook time: 15 mins, Total time: 30 mins, Grill temp: 0, Servings: 4-6

Ingredients

- 2 tbsp olive oil extra-virgin
- 2 white & light green medium leeks
- 2 diced celery stalks
- 16 oz. chopped cremini mushrooms
- 2 tbsp of tamari
- ½ cup white wine dry
- 2 large, chopped garlic cloves
- 2 tbsp thyme leaves fresh
- 4 cups broth vegetable

- 1 lb broken cauliflower
- 1 tsp mustard Dijon
- 1 tbsp vinegar balsamic
- Sea salt & black pepper

Directions

1. In a large saucepan, heat some oil over medium heat. Cook for 5 mins with the leeks and celery before adding the salt. After adding the mushrooms, simmer for another 8-10 mins.
2. Cook garlic and thyme for 30 seconds to 1 min, depending on your tamari's strength. In a large saucepan, combine the cauliflower and the stock.
3. Cover and cook the cauliflower for about 20 mins or until very soft. In a blender, combine the mustard and vinegar and mix until smooth. Allow for a few mins of resting time before serving, and then top with desired toppings.

Nutritional Values

Fat 6.3g, Chol 13mg, Sodium 15mg, Potassium 77mg, Carbs 51g, Calories 365, Protein 12g

42. SWEET & SPICY POPCORN

- Breakfast - Prep time: 10 mins, Cook time: 15 mins, Total time: 25 mins, Grill temp: 300°F, Servings: 4

Ingredients

- 8-10 cups of popcorn
- 3 tbsp of sunflower oil
- 3 tbsp of maple syrup
- ½ tsp of cinnamon
- 1 pinch of Cayenne pepper
- ¼ tsp of sea salt

Directions

1. Before you start cooking, preheat your oven to 300°F.
2. In a small saucepan, combine the cinnamon, maple syrup, sunflower oil, and cayenne pepper. Cook, stirring periodically, for 1–2 mins over low heat.
3. On a baking sheet, spread the seasoned mixture over the popcorn. Mix in the salt well. Stir the ingredients halfway through the baking period of 30 mins. Allow cooling before transferring to airtight containers.

Nutritional Values

Fat 2.7g, Chol 4mg, Sodium 12mg, Potassium 67mg, Carbs 32, Calories 265, Protein 13g

43. VEGETARIAN TACOS WITH AVOCADO SAUCE

- Breakfast - Prep time: 15 mins, Cook time: 20 mins, Total time: 35 mins, Grill temp: 400°F, Servings: 2-3

Ingredients

- 1 chopped Japanese eggplant
- 1 cup summer squash chopped
- 1 chopped bell pepper
- 1 cup sliced cherry tomatoes
- olive oil extra-virgin
- 6 of tortillas
- 2 cups drained & rinsed black beans cooked
- 1 diced avocado
- 1 sliced serrano pepper
- 2 cotija cheese crumbled
- sea salt & black pepper
- 1/3 cup salsa tomatillo
- ¼ cup of pepitas
- ½ avocado
- Spinach
- 2 tbsp olive oil extra-virgin
- Lime juice
- Sea salt and black pepper

Directions

1. Line a baking sheet with parchment paper and preheat the oven to 400°F. On a baking sheet, spread out the chopped vegetables: red pepper, eggplant, squash, and tomatoes. Roast for 25-30 mins, often baste with olive oil and season with pepper and salt.
2. In the meanwhile, make your sauce. Mix all ingredients except the lime juice, salt, and pepper in a food processor. Keep refrigerated until ready to serve.
3. If using, top tacos with cotija or serrano cheese and generous portions of the sauce. Serve right away. If desired, the extra sauce may be utilized as a dipping sauce.

Nutritional Values

Fat 7.2g, Chol 3mg, Sodium 5mg, Potassium 12mg, Carbs 58g, Calories 467, Protein 14g

44. BLISTERED SHISHITO PEPPERS

- Breakfast - Prep time: 5 mins, Cook time: 8 mins, Total time: 15 mins, Grill temp: 0, Servings: 4

Ingredients

- 8 oz. of shishito peppers
- Sesame oil
- Sea salt
- Sesame seeds
- Tamari
- Peanut Sauce

Directions

1. A big iron pan should be heated to high heat. Cook, turning periodically, unless the peppers are tender & scorching, for approximately 6-8 mins in a dry pan. Place the chilies in a thin layer as you work to make sure regular contact is well with a hot skillet.
2. Sprinkle sesame oil over the peppers, then season with sesame seeds and sea salt. To dip, sprinkle with tamari & peanut sauce.

Nutritional Values

Fat 12.6g, Chol 19mg, Sodium 7mg, Potassium 88mg, Carbs 32g, Calories 258, Protein 13 g

45. BURRATA

- Breakfast - Prep time: 5 mins, Cook time: 15 mins, Total time: 20 mins, Grill temp: 0, Servings: 4

Ingredients

- ½ cup olive oil
- 1 garlic clove
- 1 small lemon
- Thyme springs 4

Directions

1. Combine the thyme, oil, garlic, and lemon peel in a small saucepan over low heat. After slowly warming the mixture, turn off the heat. Allow 20 mins for steeping before straining.
2. To serve, place the tomatoes, peach, and burrata on a dish, sliced. Drizzle liberally with salt and lemon oil. Garnish with mint and basil once the nuts have been sprinkled on top. Garnish with cherries and

currants if desired. Serve with toast, then season to taste with salt and pepper.

Nutritional Values

Fat 14g, Chol 7mg, Sodium 12mg, Potassium 75mg, Carbs 39g, Calories 345, Protein 14g

46. MANGO COCONUT MUFFINS

- Breakfast - Prep time: 15 mins, Cook time: 10 mins, Total time: 25 mins, Grill temp: 350°F, Servings: 12

Ingredients

- 1 tbsp flaxseed ground
- 3 tbsp of water
- 2 tsp lime juice fresh
- ¾ cup milk almond
- ½ tsp salt
- 2 cups of spelled flour
- 2 tsp baking powder
- ½ tsp cinnamon
- ½ cup of cane sugar
- ¼ cup coconut oil melted unrefined
- 1 tsp of vanilla
- 1 cup ripe mango finely diced
- ½-¾ cup coconut flakes unsweetened

Directions

1. Preheat the oven to 350°F and line a muffin pan with paper liners.
2. Remove from heat and set aside to thicken ground flaxseed with water. After whisking in the lime juice, set aside your almond milk.
3. Combine the sugar, cinnamon, and baking powder in a mixing dish. In a mixing bowl, whisk the flaxseed mixture, almond milk or lime juice, coconut oil, and vanilla until smooth.
4. After putting the liquid components into the dry ingredients dish, stir them in until barely combined. Make sure you don't overmix the components. Next, mix in the diced mango well.
5. Fill about 3-quarters full of batter in each muffin cup, then equally distribute in the pan. The amount of time it takes to bake depends on how thick your coconut milk is, but it should take between 15 and 20 mins. If using, add a light sprinkling of the remaining sugar. After 10 mins of chili ng

on the counter, transfer to the metal rack to finish cooling.

Fat 4.3g, Chol 10mg, Sodium 9mg, Potassium 94mg, Carbs 48g, Calories 387, Protein 12g

47. VEGAN PASTA SALAD

- Breakfast - Prep time: 15 mins, Cook time: 15 mins, Total time: 30 mins, Grill temp: 0, Servings: 8

Ingredients

- 1 cup sliced haricots verts
- 8 oz. curly pasta short
- 2 medium spiralized yellow squash
- 1 can drain artichoke hearts
- ¾ cup drained navy beans cooked
- 1 cup cherry tomatoes halved
- ¼ cup red onion thinly sliced
- ¼ cup sliced Kalamata olives
- ½ cup chopped parsley
- ½ cup chopped basil
- 2 tbsp seeds of sunflower
- ½ tsp of sea salt

Directions

1. On the burner should be a medium saucepan of salted water and an ice-water basin at the same time. After 1 min of blanching, toss the haricots verts with the ice water. Once you've emptied the water, pat yourself dry.
2. In a large saucepan, boil salted water. Follow the package guidelines for cooking the pasta until it is just tender-crisp. Drain and rinse with cold water.
3. Follow these directions to make the dressing: In a mixing bowl, combine the milk, tahini, apple cider vinegar, and other ingredients.
4. Combine the pasta, red onion, haricots verts, artichoke hearts, yellow squash, cherry tomatoes, navy beans, and olives in a mixing bowl. Toss the salad in the dressing to coat it completely. Then, add the sunflower seeds and mix thoroughly with the parsley, basil, and oregano. If required, season with more salt to taste.

5. Refrigerate for roughly 2 days before serving at room temp. Season with salt and pepper before serving.

Nutritional Values

Fat 3.8g, Chol 13mg, Sodium 18mg, Potassium 70mg, Carbs 52g, Calories 420, Protein 13g

48. MATCHA MILKSHAKES

- Breakfast - Prep time: 5 mins, Cook time: 5 mins, Total time: 10 mins, Grill temp: 0, Servings: 1

Ingredients

- ¼ cup Almond milk
- 1 tsp matcha
- 1-2 scoops of ice cream

Directions

1. Combine the almond milk and matcha powders in a mixing dish. To blend, whisk everything together well. If the matcha isn't smooth, use a tea filter to remove the lumps.
2. Shake the ice cream in a container thoroughly. Shake. Allow some room for thinning. In a mixing dish, combine all of the ingredients and whisk well.

Nutritional Values

Fat 3g, Chol 9mg, Sodium 4mg, Potassium 73mg, Carbs 31g, Calories 285, Protein 11g

49. CHOCOLATE CUPS

- Breakfast - Prep time: 10 mins, Cook time: 20 mins, Total time: 30 mins, Grill temp: 0, Servings: 2

Ingredients:

- 9 oz. baked chocolate
- 2 tbsp of coconut oil
- ⅓ cup of peanut butter
- 1-2 tbsp of sugar
- Strawberry jelly

Directions

1. Melt chocolate chips and oil in a boiler to make a mixture.
2. Fill cupcake liners with a little quantity of chocolate to cover the base pulse corners of the cupcakes and place them in a muffin tray. This recipe makes 16 small cupcakes.

Use a little brush to carefully press the cocoa up the liners' edges. Refrigerate until the chocolate is solid.

3. Add the butter and icing sugar to a mixing dish and whisk until completely blended. Place a little amount of butter and jelly in each cup.

4. To get a cake-like finish, add more chocolate to the top. To expedite the procedure, place it in the freezer. Add the sea salt when the chocolate begins to solidify on top. Return to the freezer- or refrigerator and set aside until completely frozen.

5. These mugs may be kept at room temp or kept in the fridge.

Nutritional Values

Fat 4.7g, Chol 12.9mg, Sodium 18mg, Potassium 69.8mg, Carbs 49g, Calories 382Kcal, Protein 13.2g

50. THE BEST GUACAMOLE

- Breakfast - Prep time: 10 mins, Cook time: 10 mins, Total time: 20 mins, Grill temp: 0, Servings: 4-6

Ingredients

- 3 avocados ripe
- ¼ cup red onion diced
- ¼ cup chopped cilantro finely
- 2 limes, zest & juice
- 1 diced jalapeño small
- ½ tsp sea salt coarse
- ½ tsp cumin
- Tortilla chips

Directions

1. In a mixing dish, combine all of the ingredients. Toss in the jalapenos, cumin, and season with salt and pepper to taste. Using the ingredients, make a smooth but lumpy mash. Season with salt and pepper to taste.

2. If desired, serve with corn or flour tortilla chips.

Nutritional Values

Fat 5g, Chol 7mg, Sodium 9.5mg, Potassium 84.3mg, Carbs 49g, Calories 346, Protein 11.98 g

51. VEGAN PIMENTO DIP

- Breakfast - Prep time: 5 mins, Cook time: 5 mins, Total time: 10 mins, Grill temp: 0, Servings: 2

Ingredients

- 1 & ½ cups raw cashews
- ½ cup of water
- 3 tbsp lemon juice fresh
- 2 tsp mustard Dijon
- 1 tsp of sriracha
- 2 tbsp pimento peppers jarred
- 1 clove garlic
- ½ tsp paprika smoked
- ½ tsp of salt
- Black pepper
- 1 tbsp chopped chives

Directions

1. Combine the salt, lemon juice, cashews, water, Dijon mustard, pimento peppers, sriracha, smoked paprika, garlic, and plenty of pepper in a blender. Blend until smooth, using the mixer baton to keep the blades moving. If required, gradually add more water until the mixture is smooth. Keep refrigerated until ready to serve.

2. Serve with celery, crackers, and radishes, then garnish with minced chives.

Nutritional Values

Fat 6.7g, Chol 9mg, Sodium 5.6mg, Potassium 65mg, Carbs 56g, Calories 387, Protein 13.42g

52. CILANTRO LIME RICE

- Breakfast - Prep time: 3 mins, Cook time: 25 mins, Total time: 30 mins, Grill temp: 0, Servings: 4

Ingredients

- 1 cup of long-grain rinsed well & drained jasmine rice
- 1 & ½ cups of water
- 3 tsp olive oil extra-virgin
- 1 small finely minced garlic clove
- 2 finely chopped scallions
- 1 tsp zest lime
- ¼-½ tsp sea salt
- 1 & ½ tbsp juice lime
- ½ cup chopped cilantro finely

- ¼ jalapeño diced

Directions

1. Combine the water, rice, and olive oil in a saucepan. Bring to a boil, then reduce to low heat and cook for 20 mins. Cook on low heat for 20 mins.
2. Mash the avocado with a fork until smooth. Mix in the lime juice and zest until everything is well combined. Set aside for 1 min, then add lime juice, cilantro, and any more pepper flakes or jalapenos to taste. Season with salt and pepper and toss everything together.

Nutritional Values

Fat 4.4g, Chol 4.5mg, Sodium 9.5mg, Potassium 99mg, Carbs 55g, Calories 397, Protein 12 g

53. VEGAN CASHEWS DIP

- Breakfast - Prep time: 10 mins, Cook time: 5 mins, Total time: 15 mins, Servings: 2, Grill temp: 0

Ingredients

- 1 & ½ cups raw cashews
- ½ cup of water
- 3 tbsp lemon juice fresh
- 2 tsp mustard Dijon
- 1 tsp of sriracha
- 2 tbsp pimento peppers jarred
- 1 clove garlic
- ½ tsp paprika smoked
- ½ tsp of salt
- black pepper
- 1 tbsp chopped chives

Directions

1. Puree the cashews with the other ingredients- excluding pepper and salt, until smooth and creamy using a food processor or blender. Serve right away or keep refrigerated in an airtight container. To make blending easier, use your blender baton to keep the blades moving while blending until smooth. Slowly drizzle in more water to thin down the thick mixture. Place it in the refrigerator whenever you're ready to use it.

2. Decorate the dip with chopped chives and serve it with celery, crackers, and radishes as a dip accompaniment.

Nutritional Values

Fat 5.9g, Chol 9mg, Sodium 15mg, Potassium 67mg, Carbs 54g, Calories 367, Protein 13 g

54. SHEET PAN NACHOS

- Breakfast - Prep time: 15 mins, Cook time: 15 mins, Total time: 30 mins, Grill temp: 0, Servings: 4

Ingredients

- Chips of Tortilla
- Cheese of Vegan
- tomato Chopped
- 2 tbsp scallions chopped
- 1 thinly sliced serrano
- Sliced avocado
- sliced radishes or Pickled Onions
- 1 tbsp chopped cilantro finely
- Lime wedges

Directions

1. Place your tortilla chips on a dish and put them on top of it. Arrange the tacos on the dish. Drizzle some cheese sauce on top.
2. Serve with scallions on top. Toss in the avocado and radishes. Coriander should be included, as well as lime wedges for squeezing.

Nutritional Values

Fat 5.8g, Chol 12mg, Sodium 19mg, Potassium 74mg, Carbs 49g, Calories 386, Protein 13 g

55. VEGAN 7-LAYER DIP

- Breakfast - Prep time: 12 mins, Cook time: 15 mins, Total time: 27 mins, Grill temp: 0, Servings: 6-8

Ingredients

- 1 can bean refried
- 1 classic guacamole or Kale Guacamole
- 1 cup cherry tomatoes halved
- ½ diced bunch of scallions
- ½ cup chopped cilantro
- 1 diced or thinly sliced jalapeño
- Cashew Cream
- Tortilla Chips
- 1 cup raw cashews

- ½ cup of water
- 2 tbsp olive oil extra-virgin
- 2 tbsp juice of the lemon
- ½ tsp sea salt
- 1 & ½ cups red quinoa cooked
- 1 minced garlic clove
- 1 tsp powdered chili
- 1 tsp paprika smoked
- ½ tsp of cumin
- ½ tbsp lime juice fresh
- 1 tsp olive oil extra-virgin
- ¼ tsp maple syrup
- ½ tsp sea salt

Directions

1. Cashew Cream: In a blender, combine all ingredients and mix until smooth and creamy- about 30 seconds. Place it in the refrigerator whenever you're ready to use it.
2. Spiced Quinoa Preparation: Stir the quinoa into the remaining ingredients until everything is completely blended. Place it in the refrigerator whenever you're ready to use it.
3. On the serving plate, layer the refried beans, cashew cream, kale guacamole, spicy quinoa- or something similar. If using jalapenos, sprinkle them over the top after adding the scallions, tomatoes, and cilantro.
4. Serve with tortilla chips on the side.

Nutritional Values

Fat 5.3g, Chol 13mg, Sodium 19mg, Potassium 65mg, Carbs 48g, Calories 345, Protein 11g

56. KALE PESTO

- Breakfast - Prep time: 10 mins, Cook time: 15 mins, Total time: 25 mins, Grill temp: 0, Servings: 8

Ingredients

- 1 cup of pepitas
- 1 garlic clove small
- ¼ cup Parmesan cheese grated
- ¼ tsp sea salt
- black pepper
- 2 cups curly kale chopped
- 2 tbsp juice of the lemon
- ½ cup olive oil extra-virgin

Directions

1. In a food processor, pulse the pepitas and garlic until the pepitas are finely crushed. Then, pulse in the nutritional yeast, cheese, pepper, and salt to taste.
2. Stir together the greens and lemon juice in a mixing dish. While the food processor is running, drizzle in some olive oil and pulse until well combined. Season with salt and pepper to taste.

Nutritional Values

Fat 5g, Chol 8mg, Sodium 14mg, Potassium 67mg, Carbs 46g, Calories 363, Protein 12g

57. ORIGINAL BABA GANOUSH

- Appetizer - Prep time: 20 mins, Cook time: 50 mins, Total time: 1 hr 10 mins, Grill temp: 425°F, Servings: 2 cups

Ingredients

- 2 eggplants medium or 1 large
- ¼ cup of tahini
- 3 tbsp lemon juice fresh
- 2 tbsp olive oil extra-virgin
- 2 cloves garlic
- ½ tsp of sea salt
- 1 tbsp plain Greek yogurt, optional
- chopped parsley
- smoked paprika Pinch
- pepper flakes Pinch
- Toasted pine nuts for garnish, optional
- Pita and Veggies

Directions

1. Wrap your eggplant in Al foil and bake it at 425°F for 30 mins. Depending on how tender you want your eggplant, it should be roasted for 20-30 mins. Remove the dish from the oven and set it on a serving platter.
2. When the eggplant is cool enough to handle, peel off the skin and remove any big clusters of seeds.
3. Combine the eggplant and all other ingredients in a blender, except the olive oil and garlic, and pulse until smooth.
4. Place in a serving dish and season with parsley and additional ingredients as desired. Pita bread and steamed or grilled veggies are good accompaniments.

58. EDIBLE COOKIE DOUGH

- Breakfast - Prep time: 15 mins, Cook time: 10, Total time: 25 mins, Grill temp: 0, Servings: 8

Ingredients

- ¾ cups peanut butter, very smooth
- 1/3 cup coconut oil melted
- 1/3 cup syrup maple
- 2 tsp vanilla
- ½ tsp sea salt
- 3 cups flour almond
- ½ cup chocolate chips mini

Directions

1. In a mixing basin, whisk together all ingredients until thoroughly blended- about 3 mins.
2. Make a well in the middle of the mixture and add the almond flour. To integrate, stir everything together. Adding 1 tbsp of water at a time may make the crumbly mix smooth and cohesive.
3. Mix in the chocolate chips well.
4. Serve with a cookie scoop after baking-on-baking sheets. To keep the food fresh, place it in the refrigerator or freezer.

Nutritional Values

Fat 4.8g, Chol 9mg, Sodium 15mg, Potassium 22mg, Carbs 59g, Calories 425, Protein 9g

59. SWEET VEGAN NACHOS

- Breakfast - Prep time: 10 mins, Cook time: 20, Total time: 30 mins, Grill temp: 0, Servings: 4

Ingredients

- 2 tbsp scallions chopped
- 1 thinly sliced serrano
- Sliced avocado
- Vegan Cheese
- Tortilla Chips
- Taco
- tomato Chopped
- Onions Pickled
- 1 tbsp cilantro finely chopped
- Lime wedges

Directions

1. Set a platter on the table and top it with fresh tortilla chips. Next, arrange the tacos on a platter. Drizzle some cheese sauce on top.
2. Serve with scallions on top. Toss in the avocado and radishes. Coriander should be included, as well as lime wedges for squeezing.

Nutritional Values

Fat 9.6g, Chol 3.5mg, Sodium 18mg, Potassium 25mg, Carbs 49g, Calories 485, Protein 20g

60. VEGAN BACON

- Breakfast - Prep time: 10 mins, Cook time: 20, Total time: 30 mins, Grill temp: 425°F, Servings: 5

Ingredients

- Tempeh Bacon
- 8 oz. sliced crosswise tempeh
- ¼ cup of tamari
- 2 tbsp vinegar rice
- 2 tbsp syrup maple
- 1 tbsp olive oil extra-virgin
- ½ tsp of cumin
- ½ tsp paprika smoked
- Shiitake Bacon
- black pepper
- 8 oz. mushrooms shiitake
- 2 tbsp olive oil extra-virgin
- Coconut Bacon
- 1 tbsp of tamari
- ¾ cup coconut flakes unsweetened
- ¾ tbsp of tamari
- ½ tbsp syrup maple
- ¼ tsp paprika smoked

Directions

1. Preheat the oven to 425°F and line a baking sheet with parchment paper for the tempeh bacon. Steamed tempeh should be placed in a baking dish. Before adding the soy sauce to the pan, combine it with the other ingredients. After you've done mixing the mixture, sprinkle some pepper on top and serve. Set aside 15 mins to marinate your tempeh. Bake for 8-10 mins, or until

the tempeh strips are crisp and browned on the exterior. Remove the pan from the oven and set it aside to cool for 10 mins. Crush some crispy tempeh with your hands to make "bacon bits" if desired.

2. Preheat the oven to 300°F and prepare a baking sheet for the shiitake bacon. Using a damp cloth, wipe the mushrooms down. Drizzle the olive oil and tamari over the cut mushrooms on a baking sheet and toss to mix. Depending on how crispy you want your mushrooms, bake for 30-40 mins, flipping halfway through or until wilted and crispy.

3. Preheat the oven to 350°F and prepare a baking pan for the coconut bacon. Pour in the maple syrup, tamari, and smoked paprika, then stir in the coconut flakes. Bake on a baking sheet for 6-10 mins or until golden brown and crispy. Because oven temps may vary and coconut flakes can burn quickly, keep an eye on them.

Nutritional Values

Fat 5.9g, Chol 7mg, Sodium 11mg, Potassium 22.5mg, Carbs 53g, Calories 420, Protein 14g

61. TZATZIKI SAUCE

- Breakfast - Prep time: 10 mins, Cook time: 10, Total time: 20 mins, Grill temp: 0, Servings: 4-6

Ingredients

- ½ cup cucumber finely grated
- 1 cup Greek yogurt thick whole
- 1 tbsp juice of the lemon
- ½ tbsp olive oil extra-virgin
- 1 grated garlic clove
- ¼ tsp of sea salt
- 1 tbsp chopped dill
- 1 tbsp chopped mint

Directions

1. Using a towel, squeeze out some of the excess water from the cucumber.
2. In a mixing basin, whisk together all of the ingredients until smooth. If desired, garnish with fresh herbs. Place it in the refrigerator whenever you're ready to use it.

Nutritional Values

Fat 0.8g, Chol 2mg, Sodium 26mg, Potassium 27mg, Carbs 32g, Calories 210, Protein 7g

62. POMEGRANATE POTATO CROSTINI

- Breakfast - Prep time: 10 mins, Cook time: 15, Total time: 25 mins, Grill temp: 400°F, Servings: 16-20

Ingredients

- 1 medium chopped sweet potato
- olive oil Extra-virgin
- 1 sliced baguette
- ½ clove garlic
- Sunflower spread
- ½ cup seeds pomegranate

Directions

1. Before making the sunflower spread, drain and rinse all of the sunflower seeds. Then, combine sunflower seeds, garlic, lemon juice, water, vinegar, and salt until smooth in a food processor or blender. Place it in the refrigerator whenever you're ready to use it.
2. Preheat the oven to 400°F and parchment paper 2 baking pans. Before serving, drizzle olive oil over the potato cubes and baguette slices. Toss the potatoes with a pinch of salt and a few grinds of black pepper. Roast sweet potatoes for about 35 mins or until golden brown. Place the bread in the oven for 10-12 mins at 350°F for a crisp baguette. Garlic should be smeared on the heated baguette slices while still warm. Take a step back from the situation.
3. Before serving, top the crostini with pomegranate seeds, potato cubes, and cilantro leaves if used. Finish with a drizzle of olive oil and salt and pepper to taste.

Nutritional Values

Fat 7.3g, Chol 3.5mg, Sodium 19mg, Potassium 15mg, Carbs 58g, Calories 387, Protein 13g

63. STRAWBERRY BASIL AVOCADO TOAST

- Breakfast - Prep time: 5 mins, Cook time: 5, Total time: 10 mins, Grill temp: 0, Servings: 4

Ingredients

- Strawberry slices
- balsamic vinegar
- ripe avocado
- fresh lime juice
- sea salt
- toasted bread
- fresh basil
- hemp seeds

Directions

1. In a small dish, toss the strawberries with a splash of balsamic vinegar. Allow 5 mins to pass.
2. Cut the avocado into cubes using a knife. Combine the avocado, lemon juice, and a pinch of salt in a mixing bowl. Remove it from the oven and mash it into the bread with a fork.
3. To serve, top the toast with sliced strawberries, basil, hemp seeds if preferred, and salt and pepper to taste.

Nutritional Values

Fat 5.6g, Chol 6.7mg, Sodium 17mg, Potassium 45mg, Carbs 45g, Calories 376, Protein 10.34g

64. VEGAN-PUMPKIN BARS

- Breakfast - Prep time: 20 mins, Cook time: 20, Total time: 40 mins, Grill temp: 350°F, Servings: 16

Ingredients

- ¼ cup crushed flaxseed
- ¼ cup+ 2 tbsp warm water
- ¾ cup all-purpose flour
- ¾ cup almond flour
- 1 tbsp pumpkin pie spice
- 2 tsp baking powder
- ½ tsp baking soda
- ½ tsp sea salt
- 1 cup pumpkin puree, canned
- 2 tbsp coconut oil
- ⅓ cup maple syrup
- 1 tsp vanilla extract
- vegan chocolate chips
- Vegan Cream Cheese Frosting

Directions

1. Preheat the oven to 350°F and lightly oil the baking pan- by 8X8 inches.
2. In a small bowl, combine the flaxseed and water and set aside for 5 mins to thicken.
3. In a large mixing bowl, combine the almond flour, all-purpose flour, baking powder and soda, pumpkin, and salt.
4. Combine the coconut oil, pumpkin, vanilla, maple syrup, and flaxseed combination in a medium mixing bowl.
5. Whisk together the wet and dry ingredients in a mixing bowl until well combined. Preheat oven to 350°F and bake for 25-30 mins. Allow the cake to cool completely before frosting or slicing it.
6. While the cake is cooling, make the cake icing. Whip the butter and cream cheese together with an electric mixer until smooth. Combine the sugar and vanilla essence in a blender until smooth. Enjoy the cake once it has been frosted.

Nutritional Values

Fat 6.9g, Chol 5mg, Sodium 28.5mg, Potassium 27.4mg, Carbs 56g, Calories 425, Protein 12.98g

65. STRAWBERRY RHUBARB BARS

- Breakfast - Prep time: 15 mins, Cook time: 1 hr., Total time: 1 hr. 15 mins, Grill temp: 350°F, Servings: 16 bars

Ingredients

Fruit filling
- 1 cup strawberries, diced
- 1 cup rhubarb, diced
- 1 tsp cornstarch
- ½ tsp lime juice
- ½ tsp maple syrup
- ¼ tsp vanilla

Crumble crust & topping
- ⅔ cup whole rolled oats
- ⅔ cup walnuts, chopped
- ½ cup almond flour
- ½ cup brown sugar
- ¼ cup crushed flaxseed
- 1 tsp cinnamon
- heaping ¼ tsp sea salt
- 2 tbsp firm coconut oil
- 1½ tbsp water

Directions

1. Preheat the oven to 350°F and line an 8x8 inch baking sheet with parchment paper. Coat the pan's edges lightly with cooking spray.
2. Combine the strawberries, cornstarch, rhubarb, maple syrup, lemon juice, and vanilla in a basin to form the fruit filling.
3. In a food processor, combine the almond flour, oats, almonds, flaxseed, brown sugar, salt, and cinnamon to produce the crumble. Pulse the coconut oil in a food processor. After adding the water, pulse 1 more. 2/3 of the crumbles should be pressed into the baking sheet to produce a crust. Bake for 20-25 mins or until gently browned and firm around the edges. After removing from the oven, set aside for 15 mins to cool.
4. Extra fruit filling crumbles and rolled oats may be sprinkled on top. Bake for another 20 mins or until the fruit is soft and the crushed topping is lightly crispy. Allow it to cool completely before slicing and serving.

Nutritional Values

Fat 8.4g, Chol 4.1mg, Sodium 29mg, Potassium 31mg, Carbs 58g, Calories 465, Protein 13g

66. RHUBARB CHIA STRAWBERRY OVERNIGHT OAT PARFAITS

- Breakfast - Prep time: 6.5 hr., Cook time: 11 min, Total time: 6.5 hr. 11 min, Grill temp: 0, Servings: 2

Ingredients

Oats overnight
- 1 cup rolled oats whole
- 1 cup almond milk
- Pinch of salt
- 1 tbsp maple syrup

Strawberry rhubarb chia jam
- 2 cups strawberries, chopped
- 1 cup rhubarb, chopped
- ½ tsp lime juice
- Pinch of salt
- 1 ½-2 tbsp maple syrup
- 2 tbsp chia seeds

Directions

1. In a medium saucepan over medium-low heat, sauté the rhubarb, strawberries, salt, and lemon juice for 10 mins- to prevent the fruit from burning, stir it constantly. After removing the skillet from the heat, stir in the chia seeds and maple syrup. Allow 20-30 mins to cool to room temp. After transferring to a jar, let it cool for at least 1 hr.
2. Combine the oats, almond milk, maple syrup, and a pinch of salt in 2 glass jars. Combine the ingredients in a mixing basin, cover, and chill overnight.
3. In the morning, spoon a generous dollop of chia jam into oat containers.
4. Top with granola- if desired, the crunch contrasts well with the mushy oats, coconut cream, and maple syrup.

Nutritional Values

Fat 8.4g, Chol 5.4mg, Sodium 28mg, Potassium 19mg, Carbs 58g, Calories 398, Protein 13.76g

67. ALMOND BUTTER BROWN RICE CRISPY TREATS

- Breakfast - Prep time: 10 mins, Cook time: 30, Total time: 40 mins, Grill temp: 350°F, Servings: 12 bars

Ingredients

- 2 cups brown rice cereal
- ⅓ cup almonds, chopped and toasted
- ⅓ cup hemp seeds
- ⅓ cup coconut, shredded
- pinch of sea salt
- ½ cup almond butter
- ⅓ to ½ cup brown rice syrup
- 2 tbsp melted coconut oil

Chocolate topping
- ½ cup semi-sweet vegan chocolate chips
- 1 tsp coconut oil

Directions

1. Preheat the oven to 350°F and line a pan- 8X8 inch or similar size with parchment paper before baking.
2. Combine the almonds, brown rice cereal, hemp seeds, salt, and coconut in a large mixing bowl.

3. Mix the almond butter, coconut oil, and 1/3 cup brown rice syrup in a bowl.
4. In a large mixing bowl, combine the almond and butter mixture with the dry ingredients. To ensure that the components are evenly distributed, carefully combine them. If the batter is too dry, add a little browner rice syrup. To prevent sticking with your hands, press the mixture firmly into the pan's bottom with another piece of parchment paper and bake for 20 mins.
5. In a double boiler or a glass dish set over a small pot of boiling water, melt the chocolate with the coconut oil, then pour over the crispy treats. Place in the freezer for about 30 mins to solidify.
6. Remove the cake from the pan using the parchment paper's edges and place it on a cutting board after it has been set. Using a sharp knife, cut it into 12 bars. Cover and store at room temp.

Nutritional Values

Fat 7.8g, Chol 2.9mg, Sodium 20mg, Potassium 21.5mg, Carbs 58g, Calories 415, Protein 14 g

68. PUMPKIN SPICED CORN MUFFINS

- Breakfast - Prep time: 10 mins, Cook time: 25, Total time: 35 mins, Grill temp: 350°F, Servings: 10-12 muffins

Ingredients

- 1 cup cornmeal
- 1 cup spelled or whole wheat flour
- 2 tsp baking powder
- ¼ tsp baking soda
- 1 tsp cinnamon
- ½ tsp nutmeg
- ½ tsp salt
- 1 cup almond milk
- ½ cup canned pumpkin puree
- ⅓ cup maple syrup
- ¼ cup extra-virgin olive oil
- 1 tsp apple cider vinegar

Directions

1. Preheat the oven to 350°F. Line a 12-cup muffin tray with paper liners or nonstick cooking spray.

2. Combine the spelled flour, cornmeal, baking powder, soda, nutmeg, cinnamon, and salt in a large mixing bowl.
3. In a medium mixing bowl, combine the pumpkin puree, almond milk, olive oil, maple syrup, and apple cider vinegar.
4. In a mixing bowl, pour the puree over the dry ingredients and whisk until just combined. Make sure the ingredients aren't overmixed.
5. Fill each muffin tray halfway with batter and bake for 16–20 mins, or until a toothpick inserted in the center comes out clean. Remove the pan from the rack and leave it aside to cool for 5-10 mins.

Nutritional Values

Fat 6.3g, Chol 12mg, Sodium 17mg, Potassium 67mg, Carbs 50g, Calories 432, Protein 13g

69. FALAFEL

- Breakfast - Prep time: 15 mins, Cook time: 25, Total time: 35 mins, Grill temp: 400°F, Servings: 4

Ingredients

- 1 cup chickpeas, uncooked, soaked, rinsed, & patted dry
- ½ cup shallot/yellow onion, chopped
- 3 garlic cloves
- 1 tsp lime zest
- 1 tsp crushed cumin
- 1 tsp crushed coriander
- ¾ tsp sea salt
- ¼ tsp cayenne pepper
- ¼ tsp baking powder
- 1 cup fresh cilantro, chopped
- 1 cup fresh parsley, chopped
- 1 tbsp extra-virgin olive oil

Directions

1. Preheat the oven to 400°F. Line a large baking sheet with parchment paper. 2. Combine chickpeas, garlic, cumin, shallot, cayenne pepper, lemon zest, salt, coriander, baking powder, parsley, cilantro, and olive oil in a food processor. Pulse until everything is combined but not pureed. If necessary, scrape the basin's edges using a spatula.

2. Form the mixture into 12-15 thick patties-if they don't stay together, process the mixture a few more times.
3. Place the patties on the baking pan after they've been made. Drizzle some olive oil over them and bake for 14 mins. Bake for another 10-12 mins on the other side or until well browned and crispy on the exterior. Fold the pita in foil and finish baking it in the oven for the last few mins.
4. Hummus, diced veggies, pickled onions, herbs, falafel, and tahini sauce go into pitas.

Nutritional Values

Fat 6.3g, Chol 18mg, Sodium 22mg, Potassium 67mg, Carbs 57g, Calories 423, Protein 14g

70. BEST LENTIL SOUP

- Breakfast - Prep time: 10 mins, Cook time: 35, Total time: 45 mins, Grill temp: 0, Servings: 4-6

Ingredients

- 2 tbsp coconut oil
- 1 medium chopped onion
- 4 minced garlic cloves
- 3 tbsp ginger, minced
- 1 tbsp mild curry powder
- ¼ tsp red pepper flakes
- 1 can fire-roasted tomatoes, diced
- 1 cup French green lentils, dried
- 2½ cups water
- 1 can of full-Fat coconut milk
- ½ tsp sea salt
- Freshly crushed black pepper
- ½ cup cilantro, diced
- 2 tbsp fresh lemon juice

Directions

1. Heat the oil over medium heat in a large saucepan and mix the onions with a pinch of salt. Cook for 8-10 mins, or until the onions are soft and lightly caramelized around the edges.
2. Reduce the heat to low and stir in the ginger, garlic, red pepper flakes, and curry powder. Simmer for 2 mins or until fragrant.
3. In a large mixing bowl, combine the lentils, tomatoes, water, salt, coconut milk, and black pepper. Reduce the heat to low and

simmer for another 25-35 mins or until the lentils are tender. Then, to thin it out, add 1 to 2 cups more water or until it achieves the desired consistency.
4. Mix in the chopped cilantro and lemon juice well. Serve with a pinch of salt and black pepper.

Nutritional Values

Fat 6.5g, Chol 15mg, Sodium 19mg, Potassium 87mg, Carbs 57g, Calories 427, Protein 13g

71. VEGAN LEMON MUFFINS

- Breakfast - Prep time: 10 mins, Cook time: 15, Total time: 25 mins, Grill temp: 375°F, Servings: 9-10

Ingredients

- 1 cup Farms Almond Milk
- 1 tsp Vinegar Apple Cider
- 1 & ¾ cups Flour All Purpose
- ½ cup flour almond
- 2½ tsp Powder Baking
- ¼ tsp Soda Baking
- ½ tsp Sea Salt Stone mill
- ½ cup Sugar Coconut
- ⅓ cup Olive Oil Extra-Virgin
- 2 tbsp lemon zest Meyer
- glaze
- 3 tbsp lemon juice Meyer
- 1 tsp Vanilla Extract stone mill Pure
- 1 tbsp Chia Seeds Simply Nature
- ½ cup Vegan Cheese Earth Grown
- 2 tbsp lemon juice Meyer
- 2 tbsp Maple Syrup Selected Pure
- 1 tsp lemon zest Meyer

Directions

1. Preheat the oven to 375°F and lightly oil a nonstick muffin tray before baking.
2. In a mixing dish, combine the almond milk and apple vinegar.
3. Whisk the flours, baking soda, baking powder, and salt in a mixing basin until thoroughly blended.
4. Combine the sugar, lemon juice, lemon zest, olive oil, and vanilla in a mixing dish. Mix in the almond milk well. Combine the wet and dry ingredients in a mixing bowl and whisk just until combined. Fold the chia seeds, then use a 1/3 cup measuring

cup to pour the batter into muffin cups. After 16-17 mins of baking, check if a toothpick inserted in the middle comes out clean. After cooling for 10 mins in the pan, finish cooling on a wire rack.

5. Of course, you'll need to produce a glaze. Combine the maple syrup, lemon juice, cream cheese, and lemon zest in a food processor until smooth. Once the muffins have cooled, sprinkle them with chia seeds and lemon zest.

Nutritional Values

Fat 7.4g, Chol 8mg, Sodium 16mg, Potassium 97mg, Carbs 54g, Calories 423, Protein 14g

72. CHOCOLATE AVOCADO PUDDING POPS

- Breakfast - Prep time: 7 hr. 5 mins, Cook time: 2 hr., Total time: 9 hr. 5 mins, Grill temp: 0, Servings: 10

Ingredients

- 2 medium avocados ripe
- ¼ cup melted chocolate chips
- 3 tbsp powdered cacao
- 3 tbsp syrup maple
- 3 tbsp butter almond
- 1 tsp vanilla extract pure
- 2 cups Vanilla Almond milk
- ¼ tsp pure sea salt

Directions

1. In a food processor or blender, combine the avocados, vanilla, cacao powder, chocolate chips, almond butter, maple syrup, and sea salt until smooth. In a blender, puree the ingredients until perfectly smooth. Pour into ice pop molds after freezing overnight or for about 9 hr.
2. The pops will be loose enough to remove after a few mins of resting at room temp.
3. Topping option: Before adding the remaining chocolate chips to the cake, melt them with coconut oil. Place crushed nuts on top of the pops. Drizzle the syrup over the top.
4. If you choose, you may consume it as pudding. If you're using individual serving bowls, keep them in the fridge for roughly 4 hr after combining.

Nutritional Values

Fat 7.2g, Chol 8mg, Sodium 15mg, Potassium 90mg, Carbs 58g, Calories 487, Protein 13g

73. HEALTHY LOADED VEGAN NACHOS

- Breakfast - Prep time: 15 mins, Cook time: 15, Total time: 30 mins, Grill temp: 0, Servings: 4

Ingredients

- taco Mushroom-walnut
- 1 tbsp olive oil extra-virgin
- 1 & ½ cups shiitake mushrooms de-stemmed & diced
- 1 tsp cumin
- 1 cup raw walnuts chopped
- ½-1 tbsp tamari
- ¼ tsp powdered garlic
- ¼ tsp powdered onion
- 1 tsp coriander
- smoked paprika pinch
- ½ tsp vinegar balsamic
- ½ cup drained & rinsed black beans

For nachos
- chips tortilla
- 1 thinly sliced kale leaf
- 2 tbsp scallions chopped
- ½ cup cashew cream pumpkin
- 1 thinly sliced radish
- 1 diced small avocado
- 2 tbsp red onion diced
- ¼ cup chopped cilantro
- 1 sliced lime
- hot sauce

Directions

1. Heat some olive oil in a skillet over medium-high heat to prepare a mushroom-walnut taco. Pour in the mushrooms and cook, occasionally stirring, for 3-4 mins or until they begin to brown and soften. Toss in the walnuts and toast for 1-2 mins, swirling often. Along with the paprika and tamari, garlic powder and onion powder are added. 1 more time, stir in the balsamic vinegar. After the heat has been removed from the pan, add the black beans. After tasting and adjusting spices, add more tamari if necessary.
2. On a large dish, arrange ½ tortilla chips, taco, kale, scallions, and pumpkin cream to

make nachos. Toss with tortilla chips and serve. Sprinkle the remaining taco, radish, cashew cream, and avocado slices over the second layer of chips. Serve with lime slices that haven't been used and lime juice poured over the top.

3. Top with salsa sauce if desired. Prepare the dish and serve it as soon as possible.

Nutritional Values

Fat 7.3g, Chol 3.9mg, Sodium 5.7mg, Potassium 83mg, Carbs 56g, Calories 438, Protein 14g

74. JAMAICAN JERK VEGAN TACOS

- Breakfast - Prep time: 16 mins, Cook time: 26, Total time: 42 mins, Grill temp: 0, Servings: 4

Ingredients

- Salsa Mango Avocado
- 2 cups mango peeled diced
- 1 medium diced ripe avocado
- ¾ cup red onion diced
- ½ cup cucumber diced
- Sea salt
- 3 tbsp orange juice fresh
- 3 tbsp lime juice fresh
- ½ cup finely chopped cilantro

Jamaican jerk seasoning
- 1 & ½ tsp powdered onion
- 1 tsp paprika sweet/hot
- 1 tsp black pepper freshly ground
- 1 tsp thyme dried
- ½ tsp allspice ground
- ½ tsp cumin ground
- ¼ tsp pepper cayenne
- Jackfruit
- ¼ tsp cinnamon ground
- ¼ tsp of nutmeg
- 2 cans brine jackfruit
- 2 tbsp olive oil extra-virgin
- 6 sliced scallions
- 4 minced garlic cloves
- 1 & ½-inch grated ginger
- 1 minced habanero serrano
- 2 tbsp sugar coconut
- 2 tbsp paste tomato
- ¼ cup of tamari
- 3 tbsp lime juice fresh
- 12 charred corn tortillas

Directions

1. Serve the tacos with the mango-avocado salsa you made earlier. Toss the mango with the other ingredients until thoroughly incorporated in a mixing basin. Season to taste with salt, depending on how salty you want it.

2. Use the Jamaica Jerk Seasoning you just produced to add some kick to your cuisine. Combine all spices in a mixing dish.

3. Follow these procedures to prepare fresh jackfruit: Drain and shake the canned jackfruit to remove excess liquid. Thick cores can be removed with your fingers, and then the pieces may be peeled off.

4. In a large saucepan over medium heat, heat the oil. Add the scallions and cook for 1-2 mins or until browned. Sauté for a min, often rotating to prevent the ginger, garlic, and chili peppers from burning. Cook for about 30 seconds, turning regularly, until very fragrant, then add all the Jamaica jerk spice and mix to coat.

5. Toss the shredded jackfruit with coconut sugar, tamari, tomato paste, and lime juice. Stir everything together well. Add another ½ cup of water and mix well. Cook for about 20 mins with the cover on, occasionally stirring.

6. Serve the jackfruit with tortillas and mango-avocado salsa as a garnish.

Nutritional Values

Fat 6.2g, Chol 14mg, Sodium 18mg, Potassium 98mg, Carbs 56g, Calories 443, Protein 15g

75. MARINATED BAKED TEMPEH

- Breakfast - Prep time: 35 mins, Cook time: 25, Total time: 65 mins, Grill temp: 425°F, Servings: 4

Ingredients

- 1 package tempeh
- ¼ cup of tamari
- 2 tbsp vinegar rice
- 2 tbsp syrup maple
- 1 tbsp olive oil extra-virgin
- 1 tsp of sriracha
- Black pepper

Directions

1. Make tempeh cubes, place them in a steamer basket over a pot of water, and steam for 1 min. Set a timer for 10 mins and bring the water to a low boil before covering it. It becomes more soft and ready to absorb the flavors of the marinade.
2. In a mixing bowl, combine the sriracha, tamari, vinegar, olive oil, maple syrup, and a couple of grinds of black pepper. Toss the tempeh in the marinade in a small dish to coat it. A minimum of 30 mins of marinating time is advised.
3. Preheat the oven to 425°F to begin.
4. Place the cubes on the baking pan and set away from any leftover marinade.
5. 10 mins in the oven should be enough. Brush the cubes with a little more of your marinade after removing them from the oven. Allow the cubes to baking for another 10 mins or until the edges are browned. Use in salads or grain bowls.

Fat 5.9g, Chol 5mg, Sodium 17mg, Potassium 60mg, Carbs 53g, Calories 447, Protein 12g

76. MANY-VEGGIE VEGETABLE SOUP

- Breakfast - Prep time: 20 mins, Cook time: 25, Total time: 45 mins, Grill temp: 0, Servings: 6

Ingredients

- 2 tbsp olive oil extra-virgin
- 1 medium diced yellow onion
- Sea salt & black pepper
- 1 medium diced carrot
- 1 small diced sweet potato
- ¼ cup white wine dry
- 1 can roasted tomatoes diced fire
- 4 chopped garlic cloves
- 2 tsp oregano dried
- ¼ tsp pepper flakes red
- 4 cups broth vegetable
- 2 leaves bay
- 1 cup cherry tomatoes halved
- 1 cup green beans chopped
- 1 diced zucchini
- 1 can drain & rinse chickpeas
- 2 tbsp wine vinegar white
- 1 & ½ cups chopped kale

Directions

1. Warm the oil in a large saucepan over medium heat. With the onion, salt, and pepper, cook for about 8 mins, occasionally stirring. Whisk in the nutmeg for 2 mins after adding the carrots and sweet potatoes.
2. Pour in the wine and reduce it by ½ for 30 seconds before adding the tomato paste, oregano, garlic, and cayenne pepper. At this stage, you should also add broth and bay leaves. To blend, stir everything together well. Then, with the cover on, reduce the heat to low and cook for about 20 mins.
3. Cover and continue to cook for another 10-15 mins, or until the green beans are fork-tender. Now is the time to add the cherry tomatoes and chickpeas.
4. Toss the sauce with vinegar, kale, and salt.

Nutritional Values

Fat 6.4g, Chol 9mg, Sodium 14mg, Potassium 79mg, Carbs 53g, Calories 428, Protein 13g

77. YELLOW SPLIT PEA SOUP

- Breakfast - Prep time: 10 mins, Cook time: 1 hr., Total time: 1 hr. 10 mins, Grill temp: 0, Servings: 5

Ingredients

- 1 tbsp olive oil extra-virgin
- 1 chopped yellow onion
- 2 stalks of diced celery
- 3 cloves minced garlic
- 6 cups broth vegetable
- 1 cup split peas yellow
- 1 medium peeled & chopped gold potato
- Kernels 4 corn ears
- 3 /4 tsp paprika smoked
- 1 tsp sea salt
- 3 /4 cup of Creamy Cashew
- 1 & ½ tbsp cider vinegar apple
- 3 /4 cup of raw-soaked cashews
- 2/3 cup of water
- ¼ tsp of salt

Directions

1. Blend the nuts until smooth in a food processor to make cashew cream. Combine the water, cashews, and salt in a blender

until completely smooth. Season with salt to taste. Set aside ¾ cup of the mixture.

2. Warm the oil in a large saucepan over medium heat. Cook occasionally turns until the onion and celery are tender and translucent, about 5-7 mins. After adding the garlic, cook for 1 min, constantly stirring.

3. After adding the stock with split peas, potato, and corn, bring to a boil over high heat with the paprika and salt. Reduce the fire to a low level, cover, and cook the split peas for 45 mins, occasionally stirring.

4. Use a blender to make a partial puree of the soup, or puree it in a regular blender and return ½ of it to the pot. Toss in the Cashew Cream and the vinegar.

5. Taste and adjust the spices as needed. Serve immediately while still hot, garnished with desired toppings.

Nutritional Values

Fat 7.4g, Chol 6mg, Sodium 16mg, Potassium 84mg, Carbs 48g, Calories 432, Protein 16g

78. TWICE BAKED SWEET POTATOES

- Breakfast - Prep time: 10 mins, Cook time: 55, Total time: 65 mins, Grill temp: 400°F, Servings: 8

Ingredients

- 4 sweet potatoes medium
- 4 cups broccoli florets small
- 1 tsp olive oil extra-virgin
- 1 small minced garlic clove
- ½ tsp mustard Dijon
- 1 tbsp lemon juice fresh
- ⅓ cup scallions chopped
- 1 cup cheese cheddar
- ¼ cup seeds hemp
- ½ cup microgreens & chopped parsley
- Sea salt & black pepper freshly ground

Directions

1. Remove from the oven and put on a parchment-lined baking sheet after 20 mins of baking at 400 degrees. Place your sweet potatoes on a baking pan and pierce them with a fork many times. Remove from the oven after 45 mins or until fork-tender. Cut the mash in ½ and scoop out a

spoonful from each side to make room for the filling.

2. The Cashew Cream should be prepared in the following manner: In a blender, combine the water, lemon, mashed sweet potato, cashews, salt, pepper, and purée until smooth.

3. Check for tenderness after cooking broccoli for about 5 mins.

4. Combine the lemon juice, olive oil, Dijon mustard, garlic, and scallions in a mixing bowl. Toss in the steamed broccoli and season with salt and pepper to taste.

5. Before baking, top each potato ½ with scallions, cashew cream, broccoli mixture, cheddar cheese, and hemp seeds. The cheese should soften and melt after more than 10 mins in the oven. Serve the remaining cashew sauce beside the dish for sprinkling.

Nutritional Values

Fat 8.9g, Chol 9mg, Sodium 6mg, Potassium 93mg, Carbs 60g, Calories 448, Protein 14.5g

79. GRILLED TARTINES

- Breakfast - Prep time: 5 mins, Cook time: 10, Total time: 15 mins, Grill temp: 0, Servings: 4

Ingredients

- 1 sliced zucchini
- 1 sliced medium eggplant
- 1 halved bell pepper red
- 3 whole scallions
- extra-virgin olive oil for drizzling
- sea salt
- 1 cup halved cherry tomatoes
- 1 garlic clove, minced
- 1 tsp sherry vinegar
- 1 tsp herbs de Provence

Directions

1. A grill with a medium-high burner should be ready to begin.

2. Drizzle olive oil and salt over the zucchini, red pepper, eggplant, and scallions. 3 mins on each side, or until browned

3. Once the vegetables have cooled somewhat off the grill, cut everything into 1" pieces.

Combine sherry vinegar, garlic, cherry tomatoes, herbs, and basil in a mixing dish. Mix thoroughly.

4. Serve with hummus and lightly seasoned toasted bread.

Fat 6.4g, Chol 18mg, Sodium 23mg, Potassium 91mg, Carbs 57g, Calories 443, Protein 13.9g

80. CORN "CEVICHE" CROSTINI

- Breakfast - Prep time: 25 mins, Cook time: 10, Total time: 35 mins, Grill temp: 0, Servings: 8

Ingredient

- ½ cup corn kernels sweet
- 2 tbsp red onion minced
- ½ tsp jalapeño minced
- 2 tsp cilantro minced
- 1 tbsp lime juice
- ¼ tsp sea salt
- Lime Hummus Deli Jalapeño

Directions

1. Combine corn, onion, lime juice, jalapeno, cilantro, and sea salt in a dish. Serve right away. Place it in the refrigerator whenever you're ready to use it.
2. To go with the hummus, set out crostini, hummus, and ceviche.

Nutritional Values

Fat 6.3g, Chol 10mg, Sodium 16mg, Potassium 64mg, Carbs 55g, Calories 373, Protein 11 g

Chapter 7.

Snacks, Sides Dishes & Wraps

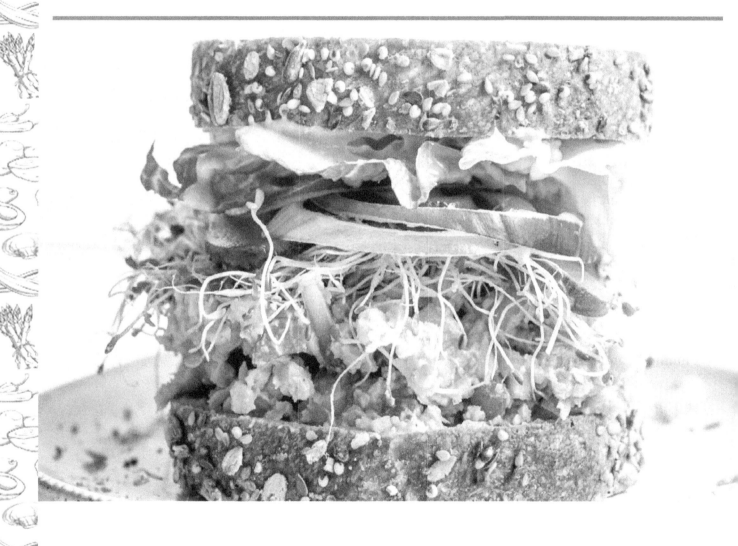

81. ALANNA'S PUMPKIN CRANBERRY NUT & SEED LOAF

- Snack - Prep time: 5 mins, Cook time: 15, Total time: 20 mins, Grill temp: 325°F, Servings: 1

Ingredients

- 1 & ½ cups walnut halves raw
- 1 cup pumpkin seeds raw
- 2 & ¾ cups rolled oats old-fashioned
- 1 cup cranberries dried
- ½ cup flaxseeds
- ½ cup husks psyllium
- ¼ cup seeds chia
- 2 tsp sea salt fine
- ¾ tsp cinnamon ground
- ½ tsp nutmeg freshly grated
- 1 can of pumpkin puree unsweetened
- 1 cup of water
- ¼ cup maple syrup
- ¼ cup oil of sunflower

Directions

1. Preheat the oven to 325°F - 165°C and place a rack in the center. Toast walnuts and pumpkin seeds on a rimmed baking sheet for 10-15 mins, turning the pan occasionally, until golden and fragrant. Remove the casserole from the oven.
2. Then, combine everything else in a large mixing bowl, including the salt and cinnamon. Stir everything together until it's completely smooth. With a wooden spoon, thoroughly mix the roasted walnuts and pumpkin seeds. Combine pumpkin puree, maple syrup, water, and sunflower oil in a mixing bowl using a sturdy wooden spoon, then stir until the "dough" is evenly soaked.
3. Set aside a parchment-lined loaf pan and scrape the dough into it. The dough should be packed in and slightly flattened over the top; it will not rise in the oven. Allow it to sit at room temp for 2-8 hr, covered with plastic wrap.
4. When you're ready to bake, preheat your oven to 400°F. Bake your loaf for 1 hr and 15 mins at 350°F to produce a rich brown crust and a sturdy texture. Even if the outside is black, let it cook for the whole time. Allow for chili ng for at least 2 hr before serving. For the best results, thinly slice your bread and toast it completely. If refrigerated airtight, it will last nearly 2 weeks.

Nutritional Values

Fat 7.5g, Chol 6mg, Sodium 10mg, Potassium 87.5mg, Carbs 58g, Calories 458, Protein 12g

82. CASHEW CREAM FOR 2

- Prep time: 5 mins, Cook time: 0 mins, Total time: 5 mins, Grill temp: 0, Servings: 2

Ingredients

- 1 cup raw cashews
- ½ cup of water
- 2 tbsp olive oil extra-virgin
- 2 tbsp juice of the lemon
- 1 peeled garlic clove
- ½ tsp salt
- ½ tsp mustard Dijon
- ¼ tsp powdered onion

Directions

1. Puree the cashews with water, garlic, lemon juice, olive oil, and salt in a blender until smooth and creamy.
2. When creating cashew cream using Cashew Sour Cream, replace 1 tbsp lemon juice with 1 tbsp wine vinegar. For added tang, add mustard and onion powder.

Nutritional Values

Fat 4.8g, Chol 10mg, Sodium 12mg, Potassium 82mg, Carbs 49g, Calories 378, Protein 13.65g

83. ALMOST-RAW CARROT BALLS

- Prep time: 15 mins, Cook time: 15 mins, Total time: 30 mins, Grill temp: 0, Servings: 16

Ingredients

- 1 cup sunflower seeds raw hulled
- 1 cup shredded coconut unsweetened
- ½ tsp of cinnamon
- ½ tsp of sea salt
- 12 soft pitted & soaked Medjool dates
- ⅔ cup carrots chopped
- 2 tsp syrup maple

Directions

1. To produce a finer meal, add cinnamon and salt to the food processor & sunflower seeds, and coconut.
2. Pulse in the dates and carrots until everything is well blended. Taste the bites and add more maple syrup as needed if you want them to be sweeter. If the mixture is too dry, additional maple syrup may be added. If it is too moist, more coconut can be added, or the mixture can be chilled for 20 mins.
3. Scoop a tbsp of the mixture onto your hands and shape it into 1" balls.
4. Use the remaining coconut to add a final layer of sweetness to the outside if desired. Keep refrigerated in an airtight container in the refrigerator for up to 5 days.

Nutritional Values

Fat 5.8g, Chol 9.8mg, Sodium 4.7mg, Potassium 76mg, Carbs 49g, Calories 424Kcal, Protein 12.54g

84. FRESH SPRING ROLLS

- Snack - Prep time: 5 mins, Cook time: 15 mins, Total time: 20 mins, Grill temp: 0, Servings: 2

Ingredients

for mushrooms
- ½ tsp olive oil extra-virgin
- 1 cup shiitake mushrooms or enoki
- ½ tsp of tamari

For spring rolls
- 4 oz. soba cooked
- 4 roll wrappers of Vietnamese rice
- Peanut Sauce
- 1 sliced avocado
- mint leaves & Fresh basil
- ¼ cup of microgreens
- Tamari

Directions

1. To make this recipe, all you need is a small skillet with oil on medium heat. Cook for about 5 mins or until the mushrooms are browned and soft. Remove the pan from the heat and add the tamari. Take a step back from the situation.

2. Before tossing the noodles, make sure they're well coated with peanut sauce.
3. Each rice paper wrap should be dipped in hot water for 5 seconds. Transfer to a clean towel to dry.
4. Arrange the avocado, herbs, noodles, mushrooms, and microgreens in the center of the rice paper. Wrap and tuck each wrapper's sides and bottom flaps, then gently roll it up to close.
5. More peanut sauce and tamari should be available for dunking.

Nutritional Values

Fat 4.9g, Chol 14mg, Sodium 20mg, Potassium 68mg, Carbs 47g, Calories 323, Protein 11g

85. FRIED GREEN TOMATOES

- Sides/Snacks; Prep time: 5 mins; Cook time: 10 mins; Total time: 15 mins; Servings: 4; Grill Temp: 300ºF

Ingredients

- 4 large, green beefsteak tomatoes
- ½ cup of unsweetened soy milk
- Juice of ½ lemon
- Kosher salt
- 1 and ¼ cups of fine cornmeal
- Grapeseed oil
- ½ tsp of kosher salt
- ½ tsp of freshly ground black pepper

Directions

1. Core each beefsteak tomato, trim and discard 1 /8 inch (3mm) from the top and bottom, and cut into 5 even slices. Set aside.
2. In a medium bowl, whisk together soy milk and lemon juice. Set aside to curdle for a few minutes.
3. Place cornmeal on a rimmed plate.
4. In a large frying pan over medium-high heat, heat 1 /2 inch (1.25cm) grapeseed oil until it's shimmering.
5. Working with just enough tomato slices to fit comfortably in the pan, dip each tomato slice in soy milk mixture and dredge in cornmeal. Add to the pan, and fry for about 2 minutes, adjusting heat as necessary to prevent burning. Turn carefully with a spatula, and fry the other side for 2 more minutes. Transfer to a plate lined with

several thicknesses of paper towels, season with a little kosher salt and black pepper, and keep warm. Continue until all tomato slices have been fried, replacing oil if cornmeal begins to burn. Serve hot.

6. For a Fried Green Tomato Sandwich, pile fried tomato slices on a crusty roll spread with a little plant-based mayo, hot sauce, and crispy lettuce.

Nutritional Values

Calories 223, Fat 3.8g, Chol 0mg, Sodium 71.4mg, Potassium 67.7mg, Carbohydrate-32g, Protein 2.3g

86. HERB COMPOUND BUTTER

- Snack - Prep time: 10 mins, Cook time: 10 mins, Total time: 20 mins, Servings: 8, Grill temp: 0

Ingredients

Garlic chive dill
- ½ cup butter
- 1 tbsp dill finely chopped
- 1 tbsp chives finely chopped
- ½ grated garlic clove
- ½ tsp of sea salt

Lemon thyme
- ½ cup of unsalted butter
- 2 tsp of thyme leaves fresh
- ¼ tsp of lemon zest
- ½ tsp of sea salt
- Pinch red chili flakes

Honey rosemary sage
- ½ cup butter
- 1 tsp rosemary finely chopped
- 1 tsp sage, finely chopped
- 1 tsp maple syrup or honey
- ½ tsp of sea salt

Sun-dried tomato basil
- ½ cup of butter
- 1 tbsp basil leaves finely chopped
- 1 tbsp dried tomatoes finely chopped
- ½ grated garlic clove
- ¼ tsp sea salt

Directions

1. Combine the softened butter and the ingredients from 1 of the herb combinations above in a small dish.

2. Scoop the herb butter onto parchment paper or plastic wrap, make it into a log, and twist the ends to seal it. Chill for at least an hour or until firm.

Nutritional Values

Fat 3.2g, Chol 9mg, Sodium 12mg, Potassium 93mg, Carbs 38g, Calories 323, Protein 13g

87. DEVILED-POTATO SANDWICHES

- Snack - Prep time: ready in about: 30 mins, Servings: 10, Grill temp: Medium

Ingredients

- ½ cup of unflavored, unsweetened plant milk, for example, cashew, almond, soy, water, or rice
- 1 large-sized Yukon Gold potato
- ¼ tsp of yellow mustard
- Black salt, Dash
- Ground turmeric, Dash
- 1 14-ounce can of palm heart, finely chopped and drained
- 1 thinly sliced scallion, green and white parts
- 1 finely chopped celery stalk
- Sea salt and white pepper
- 2 thinly sliced tomatoes
- 9 leaves of lettuce
- 18 slices of bread, whole-wheat

Directions

1. In a large skillet, place the potato chunks in a steamer basket.
2. Fill the saucepan halfway with water, slightly below the basket.
3. Bring the water to a boil. Steam 10 to 15 mins, covered, or until fairly tender.
4. Remove the potato and set it aside to chill.
5. Combine the milk, potato, turmeric, mustard, & black salt, if preferred, in a blender.
6. Cover with plastic wrap and process until smooth.
7. Place the ingredients in a medium mixing bowl.
8. Add the celery, palm hearts, & scallion and mix well. Season with kosher salt and freshly ground white pepper between bread pieces, layer potato filling, and, if preferred, tomatoes and lettuce.

9. Serve right away, or wrap tightly in waxed paper and keep refrigerated for up to 2 days.

Nutritional Values

Calories 225kcal, Carbs 18g, Protein 10.6g, Fat 10g, Sodium 627mg, Potassium 405mg, Chol 0mg

88. SWEET-POTATO & VEGGIE-ROLL-UPS

- Snack - Prep time: ready in about: 15 mins, Servings: 10, Grill temp: Medium

Ingredients

- ¼ cup of sliced scallions
- ⅔ cup of hummus, oil-free
- 4 6-inch tortillas, whole wheat
- 1 cup sweet potato, baked and chopped
- 2 tbsp of toasted sunflower kernels
- 1½ cups of baby spinach
- ¼ cup of red bell pepper, chopped

Directions

1. Combine the hummus & scallions in a small mixing basin.
2. Spread the mixture on the tortillas.
3. Add the sweet potato, spinach, bell pepper, & sunflower kernels to the hummus & gently press them in. To pack tortillas separately, roll them up and cover them in plastic wrap.
4. Refrigerate for at least 1 hour before serving.
5. Rolls should be cut into 1-inch sections.

Nutritional Values

Calories 155kcal, Carbs 14g, Protein 17g, Fat 10.1g, Sodium 427mg, Potassium 545mg, Chol 0mg

89. SPICY-TEMPEH-MANGO-SPRING ROLLS

- Snack - Prep time: ready in about: 1 hr 10 mins, Servings: 8-10, Grill temp: Medium

Ingredients

- 2 tbsp of tamari or soy sauce, reduced-sodium
- 8 oz. of tempeh
- 2 tbsp of vinegar, rice wine
- 2 tbsp of tamari or soy sauce reduced-sodium
- 1-2 tbsp of hot sauce
- 2 tbsp of lime juice
- 1½ tsp of maple syrup
- 1½ tsp of hot sauce
- ¾ tsp of ginger juice
- 1 head of Boston lettuce
- 8-10 wrappers of brown rice paper
- 1 mango
- 1 cucumber
- Fresh herbs like cilantro or mint
- 1 orange or red bell pepper
- 5 scallions

Directions

1. In a broad, shallow bowl, arrange tempeh in a thin layer.
2. In a small mixing dish, combine the rest of the marinade ingredients. Over tempeh, pour the mixture. Flip tempeh a couple of times until all of the pieces are well-coated.
3. Allow approximately 30 mins to marinate, turning and mixing tempeh 2 - 3 times. In the meantime, prepare a baking sheet by lining it using parchment paper.
4. Preheat your oven to 375°F and place the oven rack in the center. In a small dish, mix together all of the dipping sauce ingredients.
5. Place marinated tempeh on the parchment-lined pan in 1 layer. Any leftover marinade should be discarded.
6. Cook tempeh for 10 mins in the oven. Bake for 10 mins on the other side. Remove the pan from the oven and set it aside to cool. Set up an assembly station with rice paper, veggies, and tempeh. Fill a broad, shallow dish partly with lukewarm water and position it at the front of your assembly line, along with a cutting board. 1 rice paper completely in water for 5 seconds. Remove the paper & let any remaining water drain away.
7. On the cutting board, place the rice paper. Place 1 lettuce leaf or 1 to 2 big spinach leaves a bit off-center on the rice paper nearest side. 1 - 2 mango strips, 1 strip of tempeh, 2 strips of bell pepper, cucumber strips, 1 piece of onion, and a few sprigs of fresh herbs- if using.
8. On top of it, place 1 more lettuce leaf. To complete the roll, wrap the nearest edge of

rice paper over the filling, curling it under the roll and bringing it toward you.

9. Wrap the left & right edges of the wrapper over the filling to seal the sides, holding the fold in position with both thumbs on each side- like a burrito. Continue rolling the wrap away from the body until it is completely folded up. Using the leftover rice paper & filling ingredients, continue the cycle. Serve with dipping sauce on the side.

10. Refrigerate leftover rolls for up to 2 days in an airtight container.

Nutritional Values

Calories 195kcal, Carbs 14g, Protein 16g, Fat 12g, Sodium 547mg, Potassium 440mg, Chol 0mg

90. CALIFORNIA BURRITOS

- Snack - Prep time: ready in about: 20 mins, Servings: 4, Grill temp: Medium-low

Ingredients

- ¼ cup of vegetable broth, low-sodium
- ½ cup of chopped onion
- ¾ tsp of chili powder
- ⅛ tsp of ground turmeric
- ½ tsp of ground cumin
- ⅛ tsp of cayenne pepper
- ¾ cup of pinto beans, canned
- 1 cup of frozen corn
- 1 tbsp of nutritional yeast
- 4 7-8-inch of tortillas, whole grain
- Sea salt
- 2 cups of kale or lettuce, shredded
- ¼ -½ cup of salsa
- ½ avocado
- Hot sauce of pepper

Directions

1. Cook onion with vegetable broth in a big skillet over moderate heat for 5 mins, stirring often.
2. Cook & stir for another minute after adding the chili powder, turmeric, cumin, & cayenne pepper- if using.
3. Cook, turning periodically, for 5 mins. Remove the pan from the heat. Stir with nutritional yeast if preferred. Season with pepper and salt.

4. Heat tortillas in a nonstick pan over medium heat for 40 seconds, rotating once. To stay warm, cover with a moist towel. ¼ of the bean mixture should be spread slightly below the middle of each tortilla. 12 cup lettuce, 2 or 3 avocado slices, and 2 tbsp salsa atop.
5. Each tortilla's bottom border should be folded over the contents.
6. Fold in the opposite edges of the tortilla and wrap it up.
7. Place the burritos on a dish and seam sides down.
8. Warm the dish before serving. Pass spicy pepper sauce if requested.

Nutritional Values

Calories 265kcal, Carbs 11.2g, Protein 7.4g, Fat 10g, Sodium 437mg, Potassium 245mg, Chol 0mg

91. BLUEBERRY-BANANA-WRAPS

- Snack - Prep time: ready in about: 15 mins, Servings: 4, Grill temp: Medium-low

Ingredients

- ½ cup of chopped celery
- 1 cup of fresh blueberries
- 4 peeled ripe bananas
- ¼ cup of crushed peanuts or walnuts
- 4 8-inch of tortillas, whole wheat
- 4-5 finely chopped mint leaves
- 2 cups of baby spinach

Directions

1. Combine blueberries, walnuts, celery, and mint in a mixing dish.
2. Warm a tortilla in a pan over moderate heat for 30 seconds on each side for every wrap.
3. Place the tortilla on a chopping board while it is still warm. On a tortilla, spread 1 or 2 cups of spinach.
4. Add a banana on top and mash it with a fork. 1-4th of the blueberry mixture should be placed on top.
5. Fold in the sides of the tortilla as you roll it up.
6. Place the wrap on a dish with the curled sides down.
7. Make 4 wraps by repeating the process.

Calories 265kcal, Carbs 12g, Protein 14g, Fat 6g, Sodium 627mg, Potassium 845mg, Chol 0mg

92. TORTILLA-ROLL-UPS & LENTILS-SPINACH

- Snack - Prep time: ready in about: 20 mins, Servings: 15, Grill temp: Medium

Ingredients

- 6 minced cloves of garlic
- ½ onion
- 1 tsp of spice blend, ras el hanout
- 1 tbsp of lemon juice
- 1 15-ounce can of lentils
- Sea salt and black pepper
- 2 cups of fresh spinach
- 3 8-inch of tortillas, whole wheat
- 1 cup of hummus, oil-free

Directions

1. Combine garlic, onion, and ras-el-hanout in a pan. Add ¼ cup water and cook for 10 mins, pouring water 2 tbsp at a time to keep it from sticking.
2. Cook for 4 mins; further to build flavors with the lentils & lemon juice. Add Salt & pepper to taste. Remove the pan from the heat and set it aside to cool.
3. In the meantime, wrap the tortillas in a moist paper towel and cook for 30 seconds in the microwave. Place 1 hot tortilla on a level surface to create roll-ups. Pour 2 3 tbsp hummus equally on 1 side of the tortilla.
4. Over hummus, distribute an equal layer of spinach leaves, keeping 1 inch clean around the tortilla's borders. Spread 1/3 cup lentil mixture equally over spinach.
5. Roll the tortilla tightly and place it on a serving plate. Rep with the rest of the tortillas and toppings.
6. Trim all ends of every roll-up just before serving to create a neat log form. Each log should be cut into 5 sections that are approximately 1¼ inches thick.

Nutritional Values

Calories 365kcal, Carbs 14g, Protein 34g, Fat 10g, Sodium 627mg, Potassium 545mg, Chol 0mg

93. RAINBOW-VEGGIE-SLAW WRAP

- Snack - Prep time: ready in about: 20 mins, Servings: 8, Grill temp: Medium

Ingredients

- 3 cups of shredded zucchini
- 1 15 oz. can of garbanzo beans
- ½ cup of shredded carrot
- ½ cup of pods of snap pea
- ½ cup of shredded radishes
- ½ cup of shallots or red onion, chopped
- 2 tbsp of paste of white miso
- ¼ cup of fresh dill, finely snipped
- 16 leaves of lettuce
- 1½ tsp of yellow mustard
- Sea salt and black pepper
- 1 minced clove of garlic
- 8 7-8-inch of flour tortillas, whole wheat

Directions

1. In a large mixing basin, puree chickpeas for slaw.
2. Combine the following 9 ingredients in a mixing bowl- through garlic. Salt & pepper to taste.
3. Heat tortillas in a clean skillet until heated on both sides, each at a time. To keep warm, remove the pan & cover it with a cloth.
4. To prepare, place lettuce & slaw directly below the center of each tortilla.
5. Fold the tortilla's bottom edge over the contents. Fold in the opposite edges of the tortilla and wrap it up.

Nutritional Values

Calories 265kcal, Carbs 14g, Protein 17g, Fat 10g, Sodium 627mg, Potassium 445mg, Chol 0mg

94. SPANISH-RICE & BLACK-BEANS WITH BURRITO

- Snack - Prep time: ready in about: 35 mins, Servings: 8, Grill temp: Medium-low

Ingredients

- 1 yellow or green pepper
- 1 chopped onion

- ½ or 1 jalapeño chili
- 4 cups of brown rice, cooked
- 2 minced cloves of garlic
- 1½ cups of diced tomatoes
- 1 tsp of ground cumin
- 1½ cups of black beans
- 1 tsp of chili powder, ancho
- ½ tsp of smoked paprika
- ½ tsp of chili powder, chipotle
- 8 7-8-inch of tortillas
- Salt and black pepper

Directions

1. Over medium heat, place a deep nonstick skillet.
2. Cook onions, constantly stirring, until they start to brown.
3. Cook for another 2 mins with the pepper, jalapeno, & garlic.
4. Add the other ingredients, mix, and simmer for approximately 15 mins, constantly stirring. If it gets too dry, add a splash of vegetable broth or the tomato juice you set aside.
5. Taste & season with salt and other ingredients. Heat tortillas in a nonstick pan over medium heat for 40 seconds, rotating once. To keep it warm, top it with a moist towel. Just below the center of each tortilla, spread approximately 1 cup of the veggie mixture.
6. Each tortilla's bottom border should be folded over the contents.
7. Fold in the opposite edges of the tortilla and wrap it up.
8. Place the burritos on a dish and seam sides down.
9. Warm the dish before serving. Pass spicy pepper sauce if requested.

Nutritional Values

Calories 195kcal, Carbs 14g, Protein 17.8g, Fat 10g, Sodium 617mg, Potassium 445mg, Chol 0mg

95. SPINACH-TOMATILLO-WRAPS WITH HEARTY-TAHINI-SPREAD

- Snack - Prep time: ready in about: 20 mins, Servings: 4, Grill temp: Medium

Ingredients

- ½ cup packed fresh cilantro

- 1 cup of canned chickpeas
- 1 tbsp of tahini
- ¼ tsp of red pepper, crushed
- 1 tbsp of lime juice
- 4 7-8-inch of tortillas, whole wheat
- ½ cup of sweet onion, thinly sliced
- 2 tomatillos or/and green tomatoes
- 3 cups of baby spinach packed
- 1 cup of cucumber, thinly sliced

Directions

1. To make the bean spread, put the first 5 ingredients with 2 tbsp of water in a food processor.
2. Cover & process until it turns smooth, incorporating 1 tbsp of water at a time if necessary.
3. Cover tortillas with bean spread.
4. Add the rest of the ingredients on top.
5. Tortillas should be rolled up. To serve, split the wraps in ½ if desired.

Nutritional Values

Calories 212kcal, Carbs 14g, Protein 18.25g, Fat 10g, Sodium 627mg, Potassium 435mg, Chol 0mg

96. AVOCADO AND WHITE-BEAN-SALAD WRAPS

- Snack - Prep time: ready in about: 25 mins, Servings: 2, Grill temp: Medium-high

Ingredients

- 1 tbsp of liquid aminos
- 1½ cups of northern beans
- 1 tbsp balsamic vinegar
- 2 tbsp of lime juice
- 1-2 avocados
- 2 tbsp of cilantro or parsley
- 1 tsp of garlic powder
- 1 tbsp of green chilies, diced canned
- 1 tsp of smoked paprika
- Sea salt
- ½ tsp of onion powder
- Black pepper
- 1-2 Roma thinly sliced tomatoes
- 2 wheat tortillas or lavash wraps
- Baby spinach

Directions

1. In a frying pan over moderate heat, sauté the beans for 1 to 2 mins or until heated.

2. Cook, stirring periodically, until liquid aminos have completely evaporated.
3. Cook for a few mins, stirring once until the liquid has evaporated.
4. Take beans off the heated mash with a fork. Scoop avocado flesh into a mixing bowl & mash until smooth.
5. Combine mashed beans, parsley, lime juice, green chilies, paprika, garlic powder, and onion powder in a mixing bowl.
6. Mix until everything is well blended. Season to taste with salt & pepper. ½ of the avocado mixture should be spread on 1 wrap or tortilla.
7. Add a line of tomatoes across the wrap's shorter dimension, about an inch from 1 edge, followed by a row of spinach, the second row of tomatoes, and yet another line of spinach.
8. Keep rolling wrap over an initial row of tomatoes until it's all folded up.
9. Cut into 3 to 4 parts. Repeat with the rest of the ingredients for the second wrap.
10. Refrigerate for up to 3 days in an airtight container.

Nutritional Values

Calories 265kcal, Carbs 14g, Protein 18g, Fat 10g, Sodium 627mg, Potassium 245mg, Chol 0mg

97. VEGAN-SPRING-ROLLS

- Snack - Prep time: ready in about: 1 hr 15 mins, Servings: 12-16, Grill temp: Medium

Ingredients

- 4 ounces of sliced mushrooms
- 7 ounces of mung bean vermicelli
- 1 tbsp of fresh ginger, finely chopped
- 3 tbsp of tamari, low-sodium
- 1 cup of green onions, finely chopped
- ¼ tsp of black pepper
- 10 leaves of romaine lettuce
- 24-48 leaves of baby spinach
- 12-16 paper sheets of rice- 8½-inch
- 1 cucumber
- 2 carrots
- 1 cup of fresh cilantro, finely chopped
- Wasabi Orange Sauce
- 1 cup of mint leaves, finely chopped

Directions

1. Boil water in a moderately sized pan.
2. Take the pan off the heat, stir the vermicelli, & cover it. Allow 15 mins for the noodles to become transparent. Drain the noodles and slice them into smaller pieces using scissors- 2 - 3 inches long. Place aside.- If you leave the noodles out for too long, they will clump together.
3. Meanwhile, mix the ginger, mushrooms, and ¼ cup of water in a large pan with a lid, simmer, covered, on medium heat until water is bubbling, approximately 2 mins. Cook, covered, for 2 mins, or until the mushrooms are soft after adding the tamari, green onions, and pepper.
4. Stir in the prepared vermicelli, gently breaking up the noodles with a fork. Cook, uncovered, for 2 mins. Place the mixture in a mixing bowl and put it aside to cool.
5. Using cold water, scrub spinach leaves. To dry leaves, pat them dry with a towel. The leaves must be totally dry before being used. Rep with the remaining lettuce leaves.
6. Remove the lettuce leaves' central ribs and cut the remaining leaves into about 3-x 2-inch sections. ½-fill a medium bowl with water and place it near your work area.
7. Arrange a board, the rice paper, noodle mixture, carrots, cilantro, cucumber, and mint so that they are all easily accessible. To make the wraps, carefully dip a rice paper sheet in a water bowl for around 20 seconds to soak.
8. Place it on the chopping board after removing it from the water. Place 2 lettuce leaves on the side nearest to you. Add ½ cup of noodle mixture on top. Top with a few carrot & cucumber slices.
9. Serve with a garnish of cilantro and mint leaves. 3 spinach leaves should be placed on top of the filling. While bringing the package toward you, fold the edge of the rice paper nearest to you over the filling and fold it under on another side. Using 1 hand, maintain the fold in place, while with the other, tuck in the left & right edges of rice paper in the stuffing. Continue rolling the wrap backward until it is completely folded up.

10. Place aside the remaining rice paper & filling materials and proceed with the rest of the rice paper & filling ingredients.
11. Serve Wasabi Sauce in a dish with the halves on a large plate.

Nutritional Values

Calories 115kcal, Carbs 14g, Protein 7g, Fat 10g, Sodium 627mg, Potassium 445mg, Chol 0mg

98. VEGAN-SNACK-WRAP

- Snack - Prep time: ready in about: 5 mins, Servings: 1, Grill temp: Medium

Ingredients

- 1 tsp of lime juice
- ½ avocado
- ¼ tsp of salt
- 1 tsp of cilantro
- 1/8 tsp of pepper
- 1/10 inch of vegan tortilla
- ¼ bell pepper
- ½ carrot
- 2 slices of red onion
- 4 slices of cucumber
- 2 slices of tomato
- ¼ cup of mixed greens

Directions

1. Combine the avocado, salt, lime juice, pepper, & cilantro in a medium mixing bowl. Smash the avocado with a fork until it's nearly smooth.
2. Using 1-½ of the tortilla, spread the avocado mixture.
3. Combine the carrots, red onion, bell pepper, cucumber, tomato, and mixed greens in a large mixing bowl.
4. Wrap the tortilla in the shape of a sushi roll, with the bottom narrow and broad on top.
5. Serve right away.

Nutritional Values

Calories 272kcal, Carbs 30g, Protein 8g, Fat 15g, Sodium 886mg, Potassium 734mg, Chol 0mg

99. SUMMER ROLLS

- Snack - Prep time: ready in about: 30 mins, Servings: 3-8, Grill temp: Medium-low

Ingredients

- ¼ cup of basil
- ½ cup of coconut milk
- 1 tbsp cashew butter
- ¼ jalapeño
- 1 tbsp lime juice
- ½ clove of garlic
- ¼ tsp sea salt
- ½ tsp fresh ginger
- 6 roll-rice-wrappers
- 4 ounces of tofu- sliced
- 4-ounce rice noodles, cooked
- 1 avocado, sliced
- ½ watermelon-radish
- 2 peaches /1 mango- sliced
- Fresh herbs
- Tamari & sriracha, optional
- sesame seeds

Directions

1. To make basil sauce, mix the basil, coconut milk, cashew butter, chilies, lime juice, ginger, garlic, and salt in a blender.
2. Pulse until everything is properly blended. Season as per taste. Assemble your summer rolls in the following order: 1 inch of hot water in a glass baking dish. Soak 1 rice paper for 6 seconds in hot water, then place the loosened wrapper on a nice, moist kitchen towel.
3. Fill the wrapper with fillings of your choice. Tuck is filled beneath the wrapper by folding the base of the wrapper over it. Fold the edges of the envelope overfilling. Then, to make a summer roll, keep on rolling & tucking rice paper.
4. Continue with the rest of the rice sheets.
5. Serve with a dipping sauce made of basil and coconut. If preferred, serve some tamari & sriracha on the side.

Nutritional Values

Calories 272kcal, Carbs 30g, Protein 10g, Fat 15g, Sodium 886mg, Potassium 734mg, Chol 0mg

100. FRESH SPRING-ROLLS

- Snack - Prep time: ready in about: 15 mins, Servings: 2, Grill temp: Medium

Ingredients

- 1 cup of shiitake mushrooms
- ½ tsp of olive oil
- ½ tsp tamari
- Peanut Sauce
- 4 oz. cooked soba noodles
- 4 rice-spring-roll-wrappers
- basil and mint leaves
- Tamari
- 1 sliced avocado
- ¼ cup of microgreens

Directions

1. In a tiny pan, heat the oil on a moderate flame.
2. Cook mushrooms, occasionally stirring, until mushrooms are browned and tender, approximately 5 mins. Pan off the heat & mix in the tamari. Place aside. Toss noodles in peanut sauce until fully covered.
3. Dip rice paper in hot water for 5 seconds, 1 at a time.
4. Remove and set it on a clean cloth. In the middle of the rice paper, arrange noodles, avocado, herbs, & microgreens.
5. Wrap and tuck the sides, then the bottom flap, and roll the wrapper until it is completely closed. For dipping, serve with more peanut sauce plus tamari.

Nutritional Values

Calories 272kcal, Carbs 30g, Protein 8g, Fat 15g, Sodium 888mg, Potassium 734mg, Chol 0mg

101. NORI WRAPS

- Snack - Prep time: ready in about: 20 mins, Servings: 2, Grill temp: Medium

Ingredients

- rice vinegar
- 2 cups of white rice, cooked
- cane sugar
- 2 tbsp lime juice
- 2 tbsp tamari
- 2-3 nori sheets, slices form
- 1 mango, sliced
- ½ cucumber, sliced
- ½ sliced avocado
- sesame seeds
- pickled ginger
- spicy mayo

- 2 tsp sriracha
- ⅓ cup of mayo
- umeboshi paste
- basil leaves
- 3 oz. baked tofu
- microgreens

Directions

1. In a large mixing bowl, combine the sugar, rice vinegar, & salt.
2. Cover and set aside until primed to use. Mix the tamari & lime juice in a tiny bowl & put aside. To make spicy mayo, follow these steps:
3. Combine the mayonnaise & sriracha in a small mixing bowl.
4. Serve rice, nori squares, cucumber, avocado, mango, sesame seeds, pickled ginger, and any additions on a tray to compose as you eat.
5. Serve alongside spicy mayo & tamari dipping sauce.

Nutritional Values

Calories 242kcal, Carbs 30g, Protein 8.16g, Fat 15g, Sodium 886mg, Potassium 734mg, Chol 0mg

102. CHICKPEA-SALAD-WRAPS WITH AVOCADO-DILL-SAUCE

- Snack - Prep time: ready in about: 30 mins, Servings: 4-6, Grill temp: Medium

Ingredients

- ⅓ cup of chopped celery
- 1 14-ounce chickpea
- ¼ cup of chopped scallions
- 2 tbsp fresh dill
- 6 cornichons, chopped
- 2 tbsp lemon juice and a zest
- 1 tsp Dijon mustard
- 1 tbsp vegan mayo
- 1 tsp capers
- black pepper
- 1 clove garlic
- 1 avocado
- 2 tbsp lemon juice
- ½ cup of Almond milk- Unsweetened
- 2 tbsp fresh dill
- black pepper
- ¼ tsp salt
- 12 lettuce leaves

- ¼ cup red onions, pickled
- ¼ cup of radishes, sliced

Directions

1. Combine chickpeas, scallions, celery, cornichons, dill, garlic, lemon zest and juice, mayonnaise, capers, Dijon mustard, and a few pinches of pepper in a small mixing bowl.
2. Use a potato masher to mash the potatoes. If desired, season with a pinch of salt.
3. Refrigerate until set to use.
4. Blend the almond milk, avocado, lemon juice, salt, and dill, as well as several grinds of pepper to make avocado dill sauce. If required, add additional almond milk to make the mixture creamy.
5. Prepare lettuce wraps by layering chickpea salad, radishes, avocado dill sauce, and red onions on top.

Nutritional Values

Calories 272kcal, Carbs 33g, Protein 8g, Fat 15g, Sodium 686mg, Potassium 734mg, Chol 0mg

103. STEAMED DUMPLINGS

- Snack - Prep time: ready in about: 40 mins, Servings: 35, Grill temp: Medium

Ingredients

- 1 tbsp olive oil
- 4 oz. of tempeh
- 6 ox shiitake diced mushrooms
- ¼ cup of chopped scallions
- 1 tbsp tamari
- ⅓ cup chopped kimchi
- ½ tsp grated ginger
- 1 tsp toasted sesame oil
- ½ tsp sriracha
- Tamari/chili oil
- 35 dumpling-wrappers

Directions

1. Put the tempeh in a steamer basket & place it over 1-inch of water in a pot. Bring water to a low boil, cover, and set aside for 10 mins to steam.
2. Take the tempeh o, set it aside to cool, & crumble it with your hands in a wide skillet; heat oil over moderate flame.
3. Cook, occasionally stirring, until mushrooms are tender, approximately 5 mins. Cook for another 3 mins after adding the tempeh & tamari.
4. Add scallions, sesame oil, kimchi, ginger, & sriracha to a mixing bowl. To blend, stir everything together.
5. Scoop 1 heaping spoonful of filling onto every wrapper to make dumplings. Dab the sides of the wrapper using cold water with the fingertips, fold in part over the filling, then squeeze to seal. At the peak of the crescent, tuck 3 pleats into the wrapper.
6. Arrange dumplings in a bamboo steamer, making sure they don't touch, and top them with a lid. In a pan large enough for the steamer to hover over, bring 1 inch of water to a simmer.
7. Heat for around 10 mins, with the steamer on top.
8. Serve alongside dipping sauces such as tamari or chili oil.

Nutritional Values

Calories 222kcal, Carbs 30g, Protein 8.9g, Fat 15g, Sodium 886mg, Potassium 734mg, Chol 0mg

104. STEAMED BAO-BUNS

- Snack - Prep time: ready in about: 2 hr 25 mins, Servings: 4-6, Grill temp: Medium-high

Ingredients

- 2 tbsp sugar
- 2 tsp dry yeast
- ½ cup of hot water
- ½ tsp baking powder
- 2½ cups of flour, all-purpose
- ½ tsp baking soda
- ¼ cup of avocado oil
- 2 tsp sea salt
- 8 oz. tempeh, sliced
- 3 tbsp sriracha
- 6 tbsp hoisin sauce
- 1 tsp fresh ginger
- Avocado slices
- 1 tsp lime zest
- Sliced cucumber
- Thai chilies, diced
- Mint/cilantro

- For serving Lime wedges

Directions

1. To make bao buns, Stir together the sugar, yeast, and water in a bowl. Leave for around 5 mins.
2. Combine the baking powder, flour, baking soda, & salt in a large mixing bowl. Mix avocado oil & yeast in the mixture until the dough ball forms; if the dough is too dry, use 2 tbsp Additional water.
3. Move to a floured area, roll into a ball, & firmly knead for 5 mins.
4. Place dough into a bowl that has been brushed with some oil. Cover & put aside for 45 mins in a hot location. To make tempeh filling, preheat the oven to 425°F and place parchment paper on a baking pan.
5. Mix together the sriracha, hoisin sauce, ginger, & lime zest in a mixing bowl. ½ of the sauce should be saved away for serving, while the other ½ should be mixed with tempeh pieces and left to soak for 20 mins. Place tempeh on a baking sheet & bake for 12 mins.
6. Complete the buns. Using parchment paper, slice twelve 4-inch squares and arrange them on a baking sheet. Roll out dough to a thickness of ¼ inches on a clean surface. Cut into circles with a 3-inch glass and set them on squares. Brush tops with some oil, then flip every circle in ½ & carefully press down. Wrap in plastic wrap and set aside for 1 hour or until puffy. Place in a bamboo steamer over 1 inch of water in a pan. Bring water to a simmer, place lid, and steam for 11 min. Assemble.
7. Over cucumber, avocado, cucumber, & carrot, drizzle some lime juice. Stack each bun with avocado, tempeh, vegetables, herbs, & chilies, spooning some sauce over the tempeh pieces.
8. Serve with fresh lime slices and the leftover sauce on the side.

Nutritional Values

Calories 272kcal, Carbs 30g, Protein 8g, Fat 15g, Sodium 686mg, Potassium 734mg, Chol 0mg

105. HOMEMADE SOFT-PRETZELS

- Snack - Prep time: ready in about: 1 hr 15 mins, Servings: 4-8, Grill temp: Medium

Ingredients

- ¼ oz. of dry yeast
- 2 tbsp maple syrup
- 1½ cups of warm water
- 2 tsp sea salt
- 4½ cups of all-purpose flour
- ¼ cup of olive oil
- 6 cups of water
- sea salt
- 2 tbsp baking soda

Directions

1. To make pretzel dough, mix yeast, maple syrup, & water in a small basin and let sit for 5 mins or until frothy. Place the salt, flour, olive oil, & yeast mixture in the bowl of a mixer. Mix for 6 mins at moderate speed. After 3 mins, if the dough is still extremely dry, put 1 tbsp of water.
2. Place dough on a lightly floured surface & knead slightly to create a ball. Add a bit of extra flour if the dough is too gooey. Place dough in a big bowl that has been brushed with ½ tsps of olive oil. Wrap the dough in plastic wrap and place it in a warm place for 90 mins or until it has approximately doubled in size.
3. Preheat the oven to 450°F and line parchment paper on a baking sheet. Divide dough into 8 equal pieces & place it on a clean- non-floured work surface. Make an 18-inch rope out of 1 piece of dough. Make a U shape with the ends of the dough rope. Cross 1 of the ropes ends over the other, leaving a large dough loop beneath them. Then, to produce the pretzel's twist, wrap the ends of the dough around each other once more. To produce a pretzel shape, curl the twist into you and into the middle of the dough loop.
4. Continue with the leftover dough and put it on a baking sheet. Make poaching water as follows: Bring the baking soda 6 cups of water to a boil in a big saucepan. 1 by 1, add pretzels into the saucepan. Boil for thirty seconds, then transfer to a baking sheet with a slotted spoon. Scatter coarse

salt over the dough while it is still moist. Cut a 4-inch slice down the bottom of every pretzel using a sharp knife. Bake for around 14 mins.

106. ROSEMARY-FOCACCIA-BREAD

- Prep time: Snack, ready in about: 2 hrs, Servings: 10, Grill temp: Medium

Ingredients

- ¼ oz. of dry yeast
- 1¾ cup of warm water
- 1 tbsp cane sugar
- 1½ cups of wheat flour
- 3½ cups of all-purpose flour
- ½ tsp red-pepper-flakes
- 1 tbsp sea salt
- 1 bulb of Roasted Garlic
- ½ cup of olive oil, extra-virgin
- 2 tbsp chopped rosemary

Directions

1. Combine the yeast, water, and sugar in a medium mixing bowl. Allow it to sit for 5 mins.
2. Place the salt, flours, ¼ cup olive oil, & yeast mixture in the bowl of a stand mixer equipped with a dough hook connection and beat on moderate speed for 6 mins. Knead dough multiple times on a floured surface, sprinkle with extra flour as required, and shape it into a ball.
3. Place dough in a large mixing bowl that has been brushed with olive oil. Wrap with plastic wrap & leave aside to rise for 50 mins. Using the leftover ¼ cup olive oil, oil a 10 x 15-inch baking sheet. Punch down the dough & knead it several times on a lightly floured board.
4. Place dough in the pan and stretch it out to the pan's edges using your fingers. Turn the dough over and re-stretch it to the edges. Make markings with your fingertips all over the dough, spaced a few inches away. Cover the baking sheet using plastic wrap and let the dough rise for approximately 40 mins.

5. Preheat the oven to 425°F. Remove plastic wrap. Slice the garlic cloves into pieces and press them into the dough's surface.
6. Bake for twenty mins, with rosemary & red pepper flakes, sprinkled on top.

107. VEGAN-PECAN-APPLE-CHICKPEA-SALAD WRAPS

- Prep time: Snack, ready in about: 15 mins, Servings: 3, Grill temp: Medium

Ingredients

- 1 cup of diced Honey crisp-apple
- 1 can of chickpeas
- 1/3 cup of chopped toasted pecans
- 1 stalk celery
- 1/3 cup of tart cherries
- 2 tbsp parsley
- 3 tbsp tahini
- ¼ cup of green onions
- 2 tsp maple syrup
- 1 tsp of apple-cider-vinegar
- 1 tsp of Dijon mustard
- ¼ tsp of garlic powder
- black pepper
- ¼ tsp of salt
- 2 to 3 tbsp warm water
- 3 to 4 cups of organic spinach
- 3 spinach tortillas
- ¾ cup of shredded carrots

Directions

1. In a large mixing bowl, mash chickpeas with a masher after they have been washed & drained. Add chopped pecans, Diced apples, tart cherries, parsley, celery, and green onions.
2. Make the dressing in another bowl: Combine the tahini, honey, apple vinegar, Dijon mustard, salt, garlic powder, pepper, and warm water in a mixing bowl. If required, add extra water.
3. Toss chickpea salad with dressing. Toss everything together and coat everything with dressing. Taste and make any necessary adjustments. You may wish to season with a little extra pepper and salt.

4. Put 1 cup of spinach in the center of the spinach wraps, then top with ¼ cup of shredded carrots. 1/3 of the chickpea salad mixture should be on top.
5. Roll the wrap tightly, pinching in the ends as you go.

Calories 558 kcal, Carbs 76.3g, Protein 16.2g, Fat 23.5g, Sodium 607mg, Potassium 834mg, Chol 0mg

108. GREEN PEA, LETTUCE, AND TOMATO SANDWICH

- Prep time: Snack, ready in about: 20 mins, Servings: 4, Grill temp: Medium

Ingredients

- ¼ cup of fresh basil, packed
- 2½ cups of green peas
- 1 tbsp of nutritional yeast
- 1 tbsp of almond or sunflower butter
- 1 tbsp of lemon juice
- 2 minced garlic cloves
- Red pepper flakes
- Dijon mustard
- ½ tsp of salt
- 1–2 tbsp of water
- 4–6 romaine leaves of lettuce
- 1–2 thinly sliced tomatoes
- 8 slices of bread, whole grain, toasted

Directions

1. If adding fresh peas, blanch them for around 3 mins in boiling water, then rapidly move them to a dish of cold water to chill. Give or allow 5 mins. If you're adding frozen peas, make sure you defrost them first.
2. Drain peas and combine them with basil, lemon juice, nutritional yeast, sunflower butter, garlic, red pepper flakes, salt, & 1 tbsp water in a food processor. Pulse until the mixture is well blended but not totally smooth. If necessary, add additional water to get the required consistency. Season to taste and adjust spices as necessary.
3. Fill a glass dish halfway with the spread. Toast bread- 2 slices per for each sandwich. Spread 1 piece of bread with Dijon mustard & the other with ¼ cup of Pea Spread to form each sandwich.

Between the bread pieces, layer diced tomatoes & romaine lettuce.

Calories 265kcal, Carbs 14g, Protein 7.5g, Fat 10g, Sodium 527mg, Potassium 445mg, Chol 0mg

109. CHICKPEA-SALAD-SANDWICHES

- Prep time: Snack, ready in about: 30 mins, Servings: 10, Grill temp: Medium

Ingredients

- 2 tbsp of tahini
- ½ clove of garlic
- 1 tsp of Dijon mustard
- 1 tsp of capers
- 2 tbsp of chopped cilantro
- 1½ cups of cooked chickpeas
- 1 chopped green onion
- 2 tbsp of lemon juice
- sea salt and black pepper
- 1 soft baguette
- Green beans
- 8-10 Kalamata olives
- vegan mayo
- Red onion, thinly sliced
- ¼ thinly sliced English cucumber
- 6-8 basil leaves
- 1 thinly sliced radish
- Sea salt and black pepper

Directions

1. To prepare chickpea salad, put the chickpeas, Dijon mustard, tahini, garlic, green onions, capers, cilantro, lemon juice, and a bit of salt & pepper in a blender. Pulse until everything is incorporated, but don't purée it. Season as per taste. Green beans should be blanched.
2. Bring a small saucepan of salted water to a boil, and have an ice bath nearby. Put green beans in a pot of boiling water for 1½ mins, scoop them out and place them in cold water to halt the cooking. Rinse, pat dry, and slice into 1-inch chunks once cold.
3. Prepare the sandwiches as follows: On 1 side of the sandwich, distribute the chickpea salad.
4. Toss the green beans with the olives & red onion pieces in the chickpea salad. On the other ½ of the baguette, pour a layer of

mayo and cover it with radishes, cucumbers, and basil. To taste, season with pepper and salt.

110. PUFFED RICE BALLS

- Snacks - Prep time: 10 mins, Cook time: 15 mins, Total time: 25 mins, Servings: 6 to 8, Grill temp: 300°F

Ingredients

- 1/8 tsp of cardamom powder
- ½ cup of jaggery
- 1/8 cup of water
- 2 cups of puffed rice
- 1/8 tsp of ginger powder

Directions

1. Melt the jaggery in a pan using water.- jaggery should be immersed in water.
2. Remove impurities from jaggery, place the pan on a low flame, and heat it to form a thick jaggery syrup- you should be able to make a firm ball out of it.
3. Pour syrup over puffed rice.
4. Mix ginger powder and cardamom. Toss them.
5. Make bite-sized balls of your requirement.
6. Store in an airtight jar.

111. ROASTED CAULIFLOWER HUMMUS

- Sides/Snacks - Prep time: 10 mins, Cook time: 20 mins, Total time: 30 mins, Servings: 4, Grill temp: 400°F

Ingredients

- ¼ tsp of salt
- 1 garlic clove
- 1 large head of cauliflower
- 3 tbsp of olive oil
- ¼ cup of tahini
- Juice from 1 lemon
- pinch of ground coriander
- 2 tbsp of water
- Pepper to taste
- Olive oil for garnishing
- Chopped parsley for garnishing
- ¼ tsp of ground cumin
- Sunflower seeds for garnishing

Directions

1. Oven preheated to 200 degrees C.
2. Take the cauliflower head from the florets and put the florets on a cookie tray. Add 1 tbsp of olive oil & toss to mix. In the oven, put the cookie tray and bake for twenty mins.
3. Move the cauliflower to the food processor. Put the leftover 2 tbsp of olive oil, lemon juice, water, garlic cloves, cumin, salt, coriander & tahini. To taste, add pepper. Mix on high till creamy & smooth.
4. Move it to a bowl & season it with seeds of a sunflower & minced parsley.

112. THAI CHICKPEAS

- Snacks - Prep time: 10 mins, Cook time: 20 mins, Total time: 30 mins, Servings: 6 to 8, Grill temp: 300°F

Ingredients

- 1 ½ cups of soaked chickpeas
- 3 cups of coconut milk
- ¾ pound of peeled and chopped sweet potatoes
- 1 cup of chopped canned plum tomatoes
- 1 tbsp of mild curry powder
- ¼ cup of fresh, minced coriander
- ½ cup of fresh, minced basil
- 1 tbsp of tamari
- 1 tsp of minced garlic

Directions

1. The night before, soak the chickpeas in water on the counter. When ready, drain and rinse.
2. Add chickpeas to your pressure cooker, along with garlic, potatoes, tomatoes,

curry powder, coriander, and coconut milk.

3. Close and seal the lid. Cook on high pressure for 18 mins.
4. When time is up, turn it off and carefully quick-release.
5. If the chickpeas are not done, put the lid back on and simmer.
6. Add basil and tamari.
7. Break up the sweet potatoes with a wooden spoon and stir so you get a sauce.
8. Serve as is or with rice.

Calories 104, Fat 4g, Chol 0mg, Sodium 71.4mg, Potassium 67.7mg, Carbs 15g, Protein 2g

113. SWEET POTATO APPETIZER BITES

- Snacks/Appetizers - Prep time: 20 mins, Cook time: 30 mins, Total time: 50 mins, Grill temp: 0, Servings: 4

Ingredients

- 2 medium sweet potatoes
- olive oil Extra virgin
- Sea salt & black pepper, freshly ground
- 1 thinly sliced watermelon radish
- 2 tsp of white/black sesame seeds
- tartare Avocado
- 1 tsp oil sesame
- 2 tsp lemon juice fresh
- ¼ tsp mustard Dijon
- ¼ cup red onion diced
- 1 ripe avocado medium-large
- salt Sea

Directions

1. Remove from the oven after 30 mins and lay a large baking sheet with parchment paper on the bottom of the oven.
2. The thick cores of sweet potatoes should be cut into little rings.
3. Roast the sweet potatoes for 20 mins, spreading them out in a single layer on the baking sheet. Season with salt and pepper after drizzling with olive oil. Return to the oven for another 10-15 mins, or until the slices are fork-tender.

4. Follow these directions to make Avocado Tartare: In a mixing dish, combine the mustard, lemon juice, sesame oil, and salt. After adding the red onion, set it aside.
5. When the sweet potatoes are almost done cooking, toss in the avocado with a squeeze of lemon. Season with salt and pepper to taste.
6. To make a vivid appearance, toss roasted potato rounds with watermelon radish slices and avocado tartare. Toss in the sesame seeds and season with kosher salt to taste.

Nutritional Values

Fat 7.2g, Chol 3mg, Sodium 5mg, Potassium 12mg, Carbs 58g, Calories 467, Protein 14g

114. ROASTED CORN WITH POBLANO-CILANTRO BUTTER

- Appetizers/Snacks - Prep time: 5 mins, Cook time: 10 mins, Total time: 15 mins, Servings: 6, Grill temp: 425°F

Ingredients

- 1 poblano pepper
- 6 ears of fresh corn, shucked and trimmed
- 1 tbsp of extra-virgin olive oil
- ½ tsp of kosher salt
- ½ tsp of freshly ground black pepper
- ¼ cup of plant-based butter softened
- 2 tbsp of finely chopped fresh cilantro
- 1 tbsp of nutritional yeast

Directions

1. Preheat the oven to 425°F - 220°C.
2. Place poblano pepper directly over the flame on a gas stove, or roast under the broiler as it preheats before you cook corn, turning to char on all sides.
3. Transfer to a small bowl, cover with plastic wrap, and set aside to steam charred skin. After 5 mins, remove the plastic wrap. Core, seed, and peel poblano, and chop very finely- or pulse in the small bowl of a food processor until it's nearly smooth. Set aside.
4. Brush corn with extra-virgin olive oil, and sprinkle with kosher salt and black pepper. Place corn on a large rimmed

baking sheet and roast, turning once, for about 10 mins, or until tender and charred.

5. In a small bowl, stir chopped poblano into butter and cilantro, and nutritional yeast.
6. Spread hot corn with poblano butter, and serve. If fresh corn on the cob is out of season, look for frozen bags of roasted corn at your supermarket.
7. Heat and toss with poblano butter as directed. Leftover butter is fantastic with baked potatoes or steamed vegetables.

Nutritional Values

Calories 223Kcal, Fat 3.8g, Chol 0mg, Sodium 71.4mg, Potassium 67.7mg, Carbs 32g, Protein 2.3g

115. PORCINI MUSHROOM PATE

- Snacks/Appetizers - Prep time: 10 mins, Cook time: 11 min, Total time: 21 min, Servings: 6 to 8, Grill temp: 300°F

Ingredients

- 1 pound of sliced fresh cremini mushrooms
- 1 cup of rinsed dry porcini mushrooms
- 1 cup of boiling water
- ¼ cup of dry white wine
- 1 bay leaf
- 1 sliced shallot
- 2 tbsp of olive oil
- 1 ½ tsps of salt
- ½ tsp of white pepper

Directions

1. Place dry porcini mushrooms in a bowl and pour over boiling water.
2. Cover and set aside for now.
3. Heat 1 tbsp of oil in a deep pot.
4. When hot, cook the shallot until soft.
5. Add cremini mushrooms and cook until they've turned golden.
6. Deglaze with the wine, and let it evaporate.
7. Pour in the porcini mushrooms along with their water.
8. Toss in salt, pepper, and bay leaf.
9. Close and seal the lid.
10. Cook on high pressure for 10 mins.

11. Turn off the flame and let it rest for some time.
12. Pick out the bay leaf before adding the last tbsp of oil.
13. Puree the mixture until smooth.
14. Refrigerate in a closed container for at least 2 hours before eating.

Nutritional Values

Calories 70, Fat 4g, Chol 0mg, Sodium 71.4mg, Potassium 67.7mg, Carbs 6g, Protein 4g

116. RED PEPPER HUMMUS IN CUCUMBER CUPS

- Snacks/Appetizers - Prep time: 20 mins, Cook time: 20 mins, Total time: 40 mins, Servings: 20 pieces, Grill temp: 350°F

Ingredients

- 3 tbsp of Olive oil
- 1/3 cup of tahini
- 7 ounces of chopped cooked red pepper
- ¼ cup of lemon juice
- 2 cucumbers thick sliced
- Salt and pepper to taste
- 2 cups of chickpeas
- 1 chopped garlic
- ¼ tsp of powdered cumin

Directions

1. Blend tahini, red pepper, olive oil, salt, cumin, pepper, chickpeas, 1 tbsp of hot water, and lemon juice in a blender to get a smooth mixture.
2. Using a small spoon, scoop out the seeded portion from thick slices of cucumber.
3. Fill the center of the cucumbers with the blended mixture and serve.

Nutritional Values

Calories 54, Fat 5g, Chol 0mg, Sodium 71.4mg, Potassium 67.7mg, Carbs 6g, Protein 2g

117. STIR-FRIED CHINESE CRESS WITH FERMENTED BLACK BEANS

- Sides/Snacks/Appetizers - Prep time: 5 mins, Cook time: 5 mins, Total time: 10 mins, Servings: 4, Grill temp: 300°F

Ingredients

- 2 tbsp of grapeseed oil

- 8 cloves of garlic, very thinly sliced
- 1 tbsp of grated fresh ginger
- 4 bunches of Chinese watercress, washed well, bottom 1 in.- 2.5cm of stem removed
- ¼ cup of vegetable stock
- ½ cup of fermented black beans
- ½ tsp of crushed red pepper flakes

Directions

1. Heat a wok or large cast-iron skillet over medium heat until hot. Add grapeseed oil, garlic, and ginger, and stir for 30 seconds.
2. Add Chinese watercress, and stir for 30 seconds.
3. Stir in vegetable stock, fermented black beans, and crushed red pepper flakes. Stir for 1 or 2 more mins, or until beans are heated through and cress is tender, and serve immediately.

Nutritional Values

Calories 113, Fat 1.8g, Chol 0mg, Sodium 71.4mg, Potassium 67.7mg, Carbs 22g, Protein 2.3g

118. STUFFED ARTICHOKES

- Sides/Snacks/Appetizers - Prep time: 25 mins, Cook time: 50 mins, Total time: 1 hour 15 mins, Servings: 4, Grill temp: 375°F

Ingredients

- 4 large globe artichokes
- ½ cup of extra-virgin olive oil
- ¼ cup of green Spanish- Manzanilla olives, finely chopped
- 1 tbsp of salted capers, rinsed, drained, and finely chopped
- 6 cloves of garlic, minced
- 1 ½ cups of Italian-seasoned breadcrumbs
- ¼ cup of finely chopped fresh Italian flat-leaf parsley
- 1 tsp of grated lemon zest
- ½ tsp of freshly ground black pepper
- Boiling water

Directions

1. Preheat the oven to 375°F - 190°C. Lightly grease a baking dish large enough to hold artichokes.
2. Clean and prepare artichokes.

3. In a small sauté pan over medium heat, heat extra-virgin olive oil. Add Spanish olives, capers, and garlic, and cook, frequently stirring, for 3 mins or until garlic just begins to color. Remove from heat.
4. In a medium bowl, combine Italian-seasoned breadcrumbs, Italian flat-leaf parsley, lemon zest, black pepper, and olive oil mixture.
5. Pat artichokes dry. Spread apart the leaves of 1 artichoke, and spoon 1 /4 of the breadcrumb mixture between the leaves and into the center of the artichoke. Repeat with remaining artichokes, nestling them snugly in the baking dish after stuffing.
6. Pour 1 inch- 2.5cm boiling water around artichokes, taking care not to pour water directly over them- this will result in a soggy filling. Lightly grease a piece of aluminum foil, and cover the pan tightly.
7. Bake for 45 mins, uncover, and bake for 5 more mins. Serve hot or at room temperature.

Nutritional Values

Calories 223, Fat 3.8g, Chol 0mg, Sodium 61.4mg, Potassium 57.7mg, Carbs 32g, Protein 2.3g

119. STUFFED MUSHROOMS

- Sides/Snacks/Appetizers - Prep time: 10 mins, Cook time: 35 mins, Total time: 45 mins, Servings: 6, Grill temp: 400°F

Ingredients

- 5 tbsp of extra-virgin olive oil
- 2- 10 oz. pkg. of white button mushrooms
- ¼ of small red bell pepper, ribs, and seeds removed and finely chopped
- 2 small shallots, finely chopped
- 3 cloves of garlic, finely chopped
- 4 tbsp of dry white wine
- ½ cup of panko breadcrumbs
- 2 tbsp of finely chopped fresh Italian flat-leaf parsley
- 1 tsp of dried thyme
- ½ tsp of dried oregano
- 1 tsp of kosher salt

- ½ tsp of freshly ground black pepper

1. Preheat the oven to 400°F - 200°C. Brush a baking dish just large enough to hold mushroom caps with 1 tbsp of extra-virgin olive oil.
2. Gently remove stems from white button mushroom caps. Place mushrooms in the prepared baking dish. Chop mushroom stems finely.
3. In a medium sauté pan over medium-high heat, heat 2 tbsp of extra-virgin olive oil. Add mushroom stems, red bell pepper, shallots, and garlic, and cook for about 5 mins or until mushrooms begin to brown.
4. Deglaze the pan with 1 tbsp of white wine. Add panko breadcrumbs, Italian flat-leaf parsley, thyme, oregano, kosher salt, and black pepper, and remove from heat.
5. Pour the remaining 3 tbsp of white wine into the baking dish around the mushrooms. Evenly distribute filling among mushroom caps, lightly spooning a little filling into each. Drizzle the remaining 2 tbsp of extra-virgin olive oil over mushroom caps.
6. Bake for 20 mins, or until mushrooms are tender and the filling is golden. Serve hot, warm, or at room temperature.

Nutritional Values

Calories 113, Fat 1.8g, Chol 0mg, Sodium 71.4mg, Potassium 67.7mg, Carbs 22g, Protein 2.3g

120. LATKES

- Snacks/Appetizers - Prep time: 15 mins, Cook time: 10 mins, Total time: 25 mins, Servings: 4, Grill temp: 300°F

Ingredients

- 3 lb. of russet potatoes, peeled and grated
- 1 medium yellow onion, very finely chopped
- 2 tbsp of egg replacer, such as Ener-G
- 3 tbsp of warm water
- 2 tbsp of all-purpose flour

- 2 tbsp of potato starch or cornstarch
- 1 tsp of kosher salt
- ½ tsp of freshly ground black pepper
- ½ cup of grapeseed oil
- Applesauce or plant-based sour cream

Directions

1. Place grated potatoes in a large, fine-mesh strainer, and use a handful of paper towels to press down on them, removing as much liquid as possible.
2. In a large bowl, whisk yellow onion, egg replacer, warm water, all-purpose flour, potato starch, kosher salt, and black pepper until completely smooth.
3. Quickly stir the potatoes with the onion mixture when the potatoes are dry.
4. In a large, heavy frying pan over medium-high heat, heat ¼ cup of grapeseed oil.
5. Scoop ¼ cup of measures of potato mixture into the pan and press gently flat with a spatula. Fry for about 2 or 3 mins or until golden brown. Flip over and fry the other side until golden.
6. Remove to a metal cooling rack on a baking sheet and keep warm in the oven while you fry the remaining batches, adding additional oil and adjusting heat as necessary.
7. Serve hot with applesauce or plant-based sour cream.

Nutritional Values

Calories 193, Fat 1.8g, Chol 0mg, Sodium 71.4mg, Potassium 67.7mg, Carbs 28g, Protein 2.3g

121. CURRY ROASTED CAULIFLOWER

- Snacks/Sides/Appetizers - Prep time: 10 mins, Cook time: 15 mins, Total time: 25 mins, Servings: 4, Grill temp: 425°F

Ingredients

- 2 lb. of cauliflower
- 1 ½ tbsp of olive oil
- 1 ½ tsps of curry powder
- 1 tsp of kosher salt
- 1 tsp of lemon juice
- 1 tbsp of minced cilantro

Directions

1. Separate leaves of cauliflower and cut in into small pieces discarding the core.
2. Mix cauliflower, curry powder, oil, and salt in a bowl.
3. Place and spread the mixture over the baking sheet and bake in a preheated oven at 425°For 10 mins.
4. Change the side and bake for 7 more mins.
5. Combine cilantro and lemon juice and serve.

Nutritional Values

Calories 110, Fat 8g, Chol 0mg, Sodium 71.4mg, Potassium 67.7mg, Carbs 9g, Protein 3g

122. EASY GARLIC-ROASTED POTATOES

- Snacks/Sides/Appetizers - Prep time: 10 mins, Cook time: 7 mins, Total time: 17 mins, Servings: 4, Grill temp: 300°F

Ingredients

- 2 pounds of baby potatoes
- 4 tbsp of vegetable oil
- 3 garlic cloves
- ½ cup of vegetable stock
- 1 rosemary sprig
- Salt and pepper to taste

Directions

1. Take a deep-bottomed saucepan with a lid and let it heat.
2. When hot, add oil.
3. When the oil is hot, add potatoes, garlic, and rosemary.
4. Stir to coat the potatoes in oil and brown on all sides.
5. After 8-10 mins of browning, stop stirring, and pierce the middle of each potato with a knife.
6. Pour in the stock.
7. Close and seal the lid.
8. Cook on high for 7 mins. Then turn off the heat.
9. Let it stand for 10 mins.
10. Season before serving!

Nutritional Values

Calories 336, Fat 14g, Chol 0mg, Sodium 71.4mg, Potassium 67.7mg, Carbs 49g, Protein 5g

123. ALMOND AND BREADCRUMB–STUFFED PIQUILLO PEPPERS

- Snacks/Appetizers - Prep time: 10 mins, Cook time: 30 mins, Total time: 40 mins, Servings: 6 to 7, Grill temp: 350°F

Ingredients

- 3 tbsp of extra-virgin olive oil
- 2 cloves garlic, finely chopped
- 1 small shallot, finely chopped
- ½ tsp of crushed red pepper flakes
- 2 tbsp of finely chopped fresh Italian flat-leaf parsley
- 1 cup of fresh breadcrumbs
- ½ cup of finely chopped Marcona almonds
- 1 tbsp of salted capers, rinsed, drained, and finely chopped
- 1- 14 oz. can of piquillo peppers, drained

Directions

1. Preheat the oven to 350°F - 180°C.
2. In a small saucepan over medium-high heat, heat 1 tbsp of extra-virgin olive oil. Add garlic, shallot, and crushed red pepper flakes, and cook for 30 seconds. Stir in Italian flat-leaf parsley, and remove from heat.
3. In a small bowl, combine breadcrumbs, Marcona almonds, capers, and garlic mixture. Stir in 1 tbsp of extra-virgin olive oil.
4. Drizzle a medium baking dish with ½ of the remaining extra-virgin olive oil-about 1 tsp. Gently fill each piquillo pepper with about 1 tbsp of stuffing, and place the filled peppers in the baking dish.
5. Drizzle stuffed peppers with remaining extra-virgin olive oil, and bake for 20 mins.
6. Serve hot, warm, or at room temperature.

Nutritional Values

Calories 223, Fat 3.8g, Chol 0mg, Sodium 71.4mg, Potassium 67.7mg, Carbs 32g, Protein 2.3g

124. ROASTED RADISHES AND CARROTS WITH A LEMON BUTTER DILL SAUCE

- Appetizers/Snacks - Prep time: 10 mins, Cook time: 40 mins, Total time: 15 mins, Servings: 6, Grill temp: 400°F

Ingredients

- 1 pound of radishes trimmed and cut in ½
- 1 pound of baby carrots
- 2 tbsp of olive oil
- Salt to taste
- Pepper to taste

<u>Lemon butter dill sauce</u>

- 1 tbsp of butter
- 1 tbsp of lemon juice
- 1 tsp of fresh dill chopped

Directions

1. Preheat the oven to 400°F.
2. Toss the olive oil with the carrots and radishes.
3. On a baking sheet, spread the vegetables out in a thin layers.
4. Use salt and black pepper to sprinkle.
5. Cook for around 20 mins until it's soft with a fork.
6. Create the lemon butter dill sauce as the vegetable roast.
7. In a little pot or oven, heat the butter.
8. Stir in the dill and lemon juice.
9. Drizzle and eat the sauce over the vegetables.

Nutritional Values

Calories 97, Fat 6g, Chol 0mg, Sodium 71.4mg, Potassium 67.7mg, Carbs 9g, Protein 1g

125. WARM CAPER WITH BEET SALAD

- Appetizers/Sides/Snacks - Prep time: 5 mins, Cook time: 30 mins, Total time: 35 mins, Servings: 4 to 6, Grill temp: 300°F

Ingredients

- 4 medium-sized beets
- 1 cup of water
- 2 tbsp of rice wine vinegar
- 1 garlic clove
- 2 tbsp of capers
- 1 tbsp of chopped parsley
- 1 tbsp of olive oil
- ½ tsp of salt
- ½ tsp of black pepper

Directions

1. Pour 1 cup of water into a pressure cooker and lower it into the steamer basket.
2. Clean and trim the beets. Put beets in the steamer basket. Close and seal the lid.
3. Cook on high pressure for 25 mins.
4. While that cooks, make the dressing by shaking chopped garlic, parsley, oil, salt, pepper, and capers in a jar.
5. When the time is up, carefully quick-release the pressure.
6. Beets should be soft enough to pierce with a fork.
7. Run the beets under cold water and remove the skins.
8. Slice beets and serve with rice wine vinegar and jar dressing.

Nutritional Values

Calories 44, Fat 2.4g, Chol 0mg, Sodium 71.4mg, Potassium 67.7mg, Carbs 5.4g, Protein 7g

126. BRAISED BRUSSELS SPROUTS WITH CHESTNUTS

- Side/Appetizer - Prep time: 5 mins, Cook time: 15 mins, Total time: 20 mins, Servings: 8, Grill temp: 400°F

Ingredients

- 1 lb. of fresh brussels sprouts, trimmed and halved
- 1 tbsp of extra-virgin olive oil
- 1 tbsp of balsamic vinegar
- 1 tsp of kosher salt
- ½ tsp of freshly ground black pepper
- 2 tbsp of plant-based butter
- 1 tbsp of sugar
- 1 cup of roasted, peeled chestnuts, roughly chopped- about 18 chestnuts

Directions

1. Preheat the oven to 400°F - 200°C. Line a baking sheet with parchment paper.
2. In a large bowl, toss brussels sprouts with extra-virgin olive oil, balsamic vinegar, ½ tsp kosher salt, and black pepper. Spread sprouts on the prepared baking sheet, cut side down, and roast for 10 mins.

3. In a large sauté pan over medium-high heat, heat butter. Stir in sugar, remaining ½ tsp kosher salt, and chestnuts. Cook, stirring, for 2 mins.
4. Add brussels sprouts, and cook, stirring twice, for 2 mins. Serve immediately.
5. Look for firm chestnuts with a dark, glossy shell. To roast chestnuts, preheat the oven to 400°F - 200°C. Score each chestnut with an X and spread it on a baking sheet.
6. Roast for about 10 mins or until chestnuts split open. Let chestnuts cool until you can comfortably pick them up and peel them.
7. Eat out of hand or use in recipes.
8. Store roasted chestnuts in the refrigerator in a tightly sealed glass jar for up to 2 weeks.

Calories 113, Fat 1.8g, Chol 0mg, Sodium 71.4mg, Potassium 67.7mg, Carbs 22g, Protein 2.3g

127. IMAM BAYILDI- TURKISH STUFFED EGGPLANT

- Sides/Appetizers - Prep time: 10 mins, Cook time: 1 hour, Total time: 1 hour 10 mins, Servings: 6, Grill temp: 375°F

Ingredients

- 6 small eggplant stems removed
- ½ cup of extra-virgin olive oil, plus more to taste
- 3 large sweet onions, halved and thinly sliced
- 6 ripe plum tomatoes, peeled, julienne cut and juice reserved
- 6 cloves garlic, thinly sliced
- ¼ cup of fresh Italian flat-leaf parsley, finely chopped, plus more for garnish
- ¼ cup of toasted pine nuts- optional

Directions

1. Fill the kitchen sink or a large tub with well-salted water. Cut a small slit in each eggplant, add to the salt water bath, and soak for 1 hour. Drain, squeeze gently, and pat dry.

2. Heat extra-virgin olive oil in a wide, ovenproof sauté pan or a Dutch oven with a lid over medium heat. Add sweet onions, and cook, occasionally stirring, for about 5 to 10 mins or until golden.
3. Add eggplants, plum tomatoes, and garlic, reduce heat to medium-low- adjust as needed, cover, and cook, stirring onions once or twice without disturbing eggplants, for 10 mins. 4 Turn eggplants and cook for 10 mins.
4. Preheat the oven to 375°F - 190°C.
5. Remove the sauté pan from heat, and gently stuff some onion-tomato mixture into each eggplant. Pour reserved tomato juice over eggplants, sprinkle with Italian flat-leaf parsley, cover tightly with a lid or foil, and bake for 35 to 40 mins.
6. Remove from the oven, and cool slightly before garnishing with toasted pine nuts- if using and serving.

Nutritional Values

Calories 223, Fat 3.8g, Chol 0mg, Sodium 71.4mg, Potassium 67.7mg, Carbs 32g, Protein 2.3g

128. SWEET-POTATO-APPETIZER-BITES

- Snack - Prep time: ready in about: 35 mins, Servings: 4, Grill temp: Medium

Ingredients

- olive oil
- 2 sweet potatoes
- Sea salt & black pepper
- 2 tsp sesame seeds
- 1 watermelon-radish, sliced
- Avocado tartare
- 2 tsp lemon juice
- 1 tsp sesame oil
- ¼ tsp Dijon mustard
- Sea salt
- 1 ripe avocado
- ¼ cup of red onion, diced

Directions

1. Preheat your oven to 425°F and line parchment paper on a baking sheet.
2. From the thick center of potatoes, slice tiny rounds- tinier than ¼ inch, but not nearly as thin as 1/8 inch. This will give you 14–16 rounds.

3. Place potatoes in 1 layer on a baking sheet, sprinkle with olive oil, & season with pepper and salt before roasting for 20 mins.
4. Roast for another 15 mins after turning. To make avocado tartare, follow these steps: Whisk together lemon juice, sesame oil, mustard, and a couple salt pinches in a medium mixing bowl. Set aside after adding the red onion. When potatoes are nearly done, dice avocado and add it to tartare with a touch of lemon. Season as per taste.
5. Watermelon slices & avocado tartare go on top of sweet potato circles. Sesame seeds & coarse salt are sprinkled over the top.

Nutritional Values

Calories 272kcal, Carbs 30g, Protein 8g, Fat 15g, Sodium 186mg, Potassium 734mg, Chol 0mg

129. ORANGE-SCENTED GREEN BEANS WITH TOASTED ALMOND

- Appetizers/Sides - Prep time: 10 mins, Cook time: 15 mins, Total time: 25 mins, Servings: 4, Grill temp: 300°F

Ingredients

- 1 lb. of trimmed green beans
- ½ tsp of grated orange zest
- 1 tsp of olive oil
- ¼ cup of sliced almonds, toasted
- ¼ tsp of salt
- Freshly powdered pepper to taste

Directions

1. Place a basket steamer in a large saucepan, add water- 1 inch, and boil it. Put the green beans and steam in the basket for 6 mins, until tender.
2. Toss the green beans with the oil, almonds, orange zest, salt, and pepper in a large bowl.

Nutritional Values

Calories 83, Fat 4.3g, Chol 0mg, Sodium 71.4mg, Potassium 67.7mg, Carbs 10g, Protein 3.3g

130. ROASTED ROOT VEGETABLE MEDLEY

- Sides/Appetizers - Prep time: 20 mins, Cook time: 40 mins, Total time: 60 mins, Servings: 6, Grill temp: 400°F

Ingredients

- 6 cups of assorted root vegetables, peeled and cut into 1-in.- 2.5cm chunks
- ½ cup of extra-virgin olive oil
- 1 tsp of finely chopped fresh rosemary
- 1 tsp of fresh thyme leaves
- 1 tsp of fresh sage, finely chopped
- 1 tsp of kosher salt
- ½ tsp of freshly ground black pepper

Directions

1. Preheat the oven to 400°F - 200°C.
2. Place root vegetables in a 9×13-inch- 23×33cm glass baking pan, and drizzle extra-virgin olive oil evenly over the top. Season with rosemary, thyme, sage, kosher salt, and black pepper, and toss with your hands to mix well.
3. Bake, uncovered and stirring once or twice, for 35 to 40 mins, or until vegetables are tender and turning dark golden brown at the edges.
4. Serve hot or warm.

Nutritional Values

Calories 113, Fat 1.8g, Chol 0mg, Sodium 71.4mg, Potassium 67.7mg, Carbs 22g, Protein 2.3g

131. SPINACH AND RICE–STUFFED TOMATOES

- Sides/Appetizers - Prep time: 20 mins, Cook time: 60 mins, Total time: 1 hour 20 mins, Servings: 6, Grill temp: 400°F

Ingredients

- 2 ¾ cups of water
- ¾ cup of Arborio rice
- 1 ½ tsps of kosher salt
- 6 large beefsteak tomatoes
- 3 tbsp of olive oil
- 1 medium red onion, finely chopped
- 2 cloves garlic, thinly sliced
- 1 lb. of spinach washed in several changes of cold water, shaken dry in a colander, thick stems removed, thinly sliced

- 1 cup of shredded plant-based mozzarella-style cheese, preferably almond-based
- ½ cup of toasted pine nuts
- ¼ cup of nutritional yeast
- 2 tbsp of finely chopped fresh Italian flat-leaf parsley leaves
- 2 tbsp of torn or sliced fresh basil leaves
- ¼ tsp of freshly ground nutmeg
- ¼ tsp of freshly ground black pepper
- Juice of 1 lemon

Directions

1. Preheat the oven to 400°F - 200°C. Lightly grease a baking dish large enough to hold tomatoes snugly.
2. In a small saucepan over medium-high heat, bring water to a boil. Add Arborio rice and ½ tsp kosher salt, and cook for exactly 10 mins. Remove from heat, drain, and set aside.
3. Working over a colander set over a large bowl, core beefsteak tomatoes and scoop out insides, removing seeds and pulp while leaving outer flesh and skin intact. Press gently on the pulp to remove as much liquid as possible. Place hollowed tomatoes in a baking dish and set juice aside.
4. In a wide sauté pan over medium heat, heat olive oil. Add red onion, season with 1 /4 tsp kosher salt, and cook, frequently stirring, for about 5 to 7 mins, or until soft and beginning to color.
5. Add garlic, and cook for 1 minute.
6. Increase heat to high, add spinach, and cook for about 3 mins or until wilted.
7. In a large bowl, combine rice, spinach, mozzarella-style cheese, toasted pine nuts, nutritional yeast, Italian flat-leaf parsley, basil, nutmeg, black pepper, and the remaining ¾ tsp of salt.
8. Spoon rice mixture into tomatoes, filling each to the top. Pour tomato juice over and around stuffed tomatoes, cover pan tightly with aluminum foil, and bake for 25 mins, or until hot and bubbling.
9. Uncover, and cook for 5 more mins. Drizzle with lemon juice, and serve hot or warm.

Nutritional Values

Calories 223, Fat 3.8g, Chol 0mg, Sodium 61.4mg, Potassium 57.7mg, Carbs 32g, Protein 2.3g

132. TURMERIC GINGER SPICED CAULIFLOWER

- Sides/Appetizers - Prep time: 10 mins, Cook time: 20 mins, Total time: 30 mins, Servings: 4, Grill temp: 425°F

Ingredients

- 1 tbsp of Black mustard seeds
- 3 tbsp of Vegetable oil
- 1 head cauliflower- cut in florets
- 1 chopped jalapeno
- 1 tsp of Turmeric
- 1 tbsp of grated ginger
- Salt to taste

Directions

1. Heat oven up to 425°F.
2. Mix the oil, jalapeno, mustard seeds, turmeric, and ginger in a small container.
3. Put cauliflower in a baking dish of medium size, toss with the spiced oil and sprinkle with salt. Cook until just tender and light golden brown for about 20 - 25 mins. Enjoy hot.

Nutritional Values

Calories 139, Fat 11g, Chol 0mg, Sodium 71.4mg, Potassium 67.7mg, Carbs 9g, Protein 3g

133. VEGAN STUFFED EGGPLANT PROVENÇAL

- Sides/Appetizers - Prep time: 10 mins, Cook time: 30 mins, Total time: 40 mins, Servings: 4, Grill temp: 500°F

Ingredients

For the eggplants
- 3 eggplants
- Salt to taste
- 2 tsps of olive oil

For the sauce
- 1 tbsp of olive oil
- ½ chopped onion
- Salt to taste
- 1 chopped garlic clove
- 1 bay leaf

- 3 chopped tomatoes
- Pepper to taste
- 1/8 tsp of dried thyme
- 1 tsp of dried marjoram or ¾ tsp of dried oregano
- 1 tbsp of tomato paste

For the stuffing
- 1 tbsp of olive oil
- 1 chopped onion
- 2 minced garlic cloves
- 2 chopped carrots
- 1 diced red pepper
- 1 chopped zucchini
- 3 ½ ounces of chopped mushrooms
- 2 ½-ounce of pine nuts
- Black pepper to taste
- 2 tbsp of raisins
- 1 tsp of dried marjoram
- ½ tsps of dried thyme
- Salt to taste
- For the topping
- ½ cup of breadcrumbs

Directions

For the eggplants
1. Heat the oven to 260°C - or 500°F.
2. Slice the eggplants into halves and brush all cut sides with olive oil. Season with salt.
3. Put the eggplants on a greased baking tray, cut side down, and bake them until soft inside or around 20 mins. Eggplants should, however, be firm from the outside and be able to retain their form.
4. Take it out of the oven and put it aside.

For the sauce
1. In a medium-sized pan, heat the oil on medium heat. Sauté the onions until colorless.
2. Add in the bay leaf and garlic, and keep cooking for a couple of mins.
3. Add in the tomatoes and sprinkle salt, pepper, and herbs.
4. Cook on low heat for at least 15 mins or till the tomatoes have condensed and thickened. Lastly, include the paste of tomato and cook for an additional 10 mins.

For the stuffing
1. In a big pan, heat the oil on medium heat and sauté the onions until colorless.

2. Add in the garlic and carrots and keep cooking till the garlic is fragrant and soft.
3. Include the rest of the ingredients to be stuffed. Cook till all the veggies are tender or for up to 15 mins.

For the topping
1. On medium heat, heat a small pan and add the breadcrumbs to it., Stirring frequently, Toast until the color is golden brown.

For the stuffed eggplants
2. With the back of a spoon, push the eggplant's flesh to the sides to Stuff the eggplant halves.
3. Fill in the stuffing with the help of a spoon and cover the top with the toasted breadcrumbs.
4. Top with sauce and serve.

Nutritional Values

Calories 490, Fat 15g, Chol 0mg, Sodium 71.4mg, Potassium 67.7mg, Carbs 70g, Protein 11g

134. ASPARAGUS AVOCADO SOUP

- Appetizers - Prep time: 10 mins, Cook time: 20 mins, Total time: 30 mins, Servings: 4, Grill temp: 425°F

Ingredients
- 1 avocado, peeled, pitted, cubed
- Twelve ounces of asparagus
- ½ tsp of ground black pepper
- 1 tsp of garlic powder
- 1 tsp of sea salt
- 2 tbsp of olive oil, divided
- ½ of a lemon, juiced
- 2 cups of vegetable stock

Directions
1. Switch on the air fryer, insert the basket, grease it with olive oil, shut with its lid, set the fryer at 425°F, and preheat for 5 mins.
2. Meanwhile, place asparagus in a shallow dish, drizzle with 1 tbsp oil, sprinkle with garlic powder, salt, and black pepper, and toss until well mixed.
3. Add asparagus to the fryer, close with its lid, and cook for 10 mins until nicely golden and roasted, shaking halfway through the frying.

4. When the air fryer beeps, open its lid and transfer the asparagus to a food processor.
5. Add remaining ingredients into a food processor and pulse until well combined and smooth.
6. Tip the soup in a saucepan, pour in water if the soup is too thick, and heat it over medium-low heat for 5 mins until thoroughly heated.
7. Ladle soup into bowls and serve.

Nutritional Values

Calories 208, Fat 11g, Chol 0mg, Sodium 71.4mg, Potassium 67.7mg, Carbs 7g, Protein 4g

135. CHICKEN-LESS SOUP

- Main course/Appetizers - Prep time: 10 mins, Cook time: 15 mins, Total time: 25 mins, Servings: 4, Grill temp: 300°F

Ingredients

- 6 cups of hot water
- 1 cup of diced potatoes
- 2 diced carrots
- 1 minced onion
- 1 diced celery rib
- ¾ cup of cubed, extra-firm tofu
- 2 bay leaves
- 2 tbsp of seasoning blend
- 2 tsps of minced garlic
- 1 tsp of salt
- ⅛ tsp of dried thyme
- ¾ cup of nutritional yeast flakes
- 1 ½ tbsp of onion powder
- 1 tbsp of dried basil
- 1 tbsp of dried oregano
- 1 tbsp of dried parsley
- 1 tsp of salt
- ½ tsp of celery seed
- ¼ tsp of white pepper

Directions

1. To make your seasoning blend, put everything in a blender and process until it has become a fine powder. Don't breathe it in.
2. Mix 2 tbsp into your water and set aside.
3. Heat a deep-bottomed saucepan with a lid and saute the onion until brown.
4. Add garlic and cook for another minute.

5. Add the rest of the ingredients, including the seasoned water.
6. Close and seal the lid.
7. Let it boil for around 10 mins.
8. Turn off the heat and let it stand with a closed lid for about 5 mins.
9. Serve!

Nutritional Values

Calories 90, Fat 2g, Chol 0mg, Sodium 71.4mg, Potassium 67.7mg, Carbs 15g, Protein 6g

136. CLASSIC VEGETABLE SOUP

- Main course/Appetizers - Prep time: 10 mins, Cook time: 20 mins, Total time: 30 mins, Servings: 10, Grill temp: 300°F

Ingredients

- ¾ cup of alphabet pasta
- 1 tsp of grapeseed oil
- 1 medium yellow onion, finely chopped
- 2 large stalks of celery, finely chopped
- ¼ large red bell pepper, finely chopped
- 1 clove of garlic, minced
- 1 tsp of kosher salt
- ¼ tsp of ground allspice
- 4 cups of vegetable stock
- 2 cups of tomato-vegetable juice
- 2 cups of frozen mixed vegetables- green beans, peas, carrots, corn
- Juice of ½ a lemon

Directions

1. Bring a pot of water to a boil over medium heat, add alphabet pasta, and cook according to the package directions. Drain and set aside.
2. In a medium soup pot over medium heat, heat grapeseed oil. Add yellow onion, celery, red bell pepper, garlic, and kosher salt, and cook, frequently stirring, for about 5 mins, or until softened.
3. Add allspice, vegetable stock, tomato-vegetable juice, and frozen mixed vegetables, and bring to a boil. Reduce heat to medium, and cook, partially covered, for 10 mins.
4. Stir in cooked pasta and lemon juice, cook for 1 minute or until pasta is heated through, and serve.

Calories 113, Fat 1.8g, Chol 0mg, Sodium 71.4mg, Potassium 67.7mg, Carbs 22g, Protein 2.3g

137. COLD TOMATO SUMMER VEGETABLE SOUP

- Main Course/Appetizers - Prep time: 20 mins, Cook time: 0 mins, Total time: 20 mins, Servings: 6 to 8, Grill temp: 300°F

Ingredients

- ½ tsps of black pepper
- 2 minced zucchinis
- 2 chopped stalks of celery
- 2 tsps of sugar
- 2 chopped garlic cloves
- 2 tbsp of olive oil
- 1 chopped cucumber
- 6 chopped tomatoes
- ½ chopped onion
- 1 tsp of salt
- 1 chopped red bell pepper
- 1 tsp of chopped dry oregano
- 1 tsp of Vegan Worcestershire sauce
- ¼ cup of sherry vinegar
- 3 cups of tomato juice
- 1 ½ cups of vegetable broth
- 1 tbsp of chopped dill
- Hot sauce if needed

Directions

1. Take a big bowl.
2. Add all the ingredients and mix them all.
3. To adjust the consistency to the desired level, use extra tomato juice.
4. Add spices to the taste and serve the next day.

Nutritional Values

Calories 89, Fat 0.6g, Chol 0mg, Sodium 71.4mg, Potassium 67.7mg, Carbs 18.5g, Protein 4g

138. CREAM OF MUSHROOM SOUP

- Main Course/Appetizers - Prep time: 10 mins, Cook time: 6 hours, Total time: 15 mins, Servings: 5, Grill temp: 300°F

Ingredients

- 8 ounces of mushrooms, sliced
- ¼ cup of chopped onion
- 2 tbsp of plant-based butter
- 1 quart of vegetable broth
- ½ cup of vegan heavy cream
- ½ cup of vegan sour cream
- Salt and ground black pepper to taste
- Guar or xanthan- optional

Directions

1. In a big, heavy skillet, sauté the mushrooms and onion in the butter until the mushrooms soften and change color.
2. Transfer them to your slow cooker. Add the broth. Cover the slow cooker, set it to low, and let it cook for 5 to 6 hours.
3. When the time's up, scoop out the vegetables with a slotted spoon and put them in your blender or food processor. Add enough broth to help them process easily and purée them finely.
4. Pour the puréed vegetables back into the slow cooker, scraping out every last bit with a rubber scraper.
5. Now stir in the heavy cream and sour cream and season with salt and pepper to taste. Thicken a bit with guar or xanthan if you think it needs it. Serve immediately.

Nutritional Values

Calories 217, Fat 19g, Chol 0mg, Sodium 71.4mg, Potassium 67.7mg, Carbs 5g, Protein 6g

139. CREAM OF THYME TOMATO SOUP

- Main Course/Appetizers - Prep time: 10 mins, Cook time: 20 mins, Total time: 30 mins, Servings: 6, Grill temp: 300°F

Ingredients

- 2 tbsp of plant-based butter
- ½ cup of raw cashew nuts, diced
- 2- twenty-8 ounces cans of tomatoes
- 1 tsp of fresh thyme leaves plus extra to garnish
- 1 ½ cups of water
- Salt and black pepper to taste

Directions

1. Cook butter in a pot over medium heat and sauté the onions for 4 mins, until softened.

2. Stir in the tomatoes, thyme, water, cashews, and season with salt and black pepper.
3. Cover and bring to a simmer for 10 mins, until thoroughly cooked.
4. Open, turn the heat off, and puree the ingredients with an immersion blender.
5. Adjust to taste and stir in the heavy cream.
6. Spoon into soup bowls and serve.

Nutritional Values

Calories 310, Fat 27g, Chol 0mg, Sodium 71.4mg, Potassium 67.7mg, Carbs 5g, Protein 11g

140. CREAMY CAULIFLOWER SOUP

- Main Course/Appetizers - Prep time: 15 mins, Cook time: 30 mins, Total time: 45 mins, Servings: 6, Grill temp: 300°F

Ingredients

- 5 cups of cauliflower rice
- 8 ounces of vegan cheese, grated
- 2 cups of unsweetened almond milk
- 2 cups of vegetable stock
- 2 tbsp of water
- 2 garlic cloves, minced
- 1 tbsp of olive oil

Directions

1. Cook olive oil in a large stockpot over medium heat.
2. Add garlic and cook for 1-2 mins. Add cauliflower rice and water. Cover and cook for 5-7 mins.
3. Now add vegetable stock and almond milk and stir well. Bring to a boil.
4. Turn heat to low and simmer for 5 mins. Turn off the heat.
5. Slowly add cheddar cheese and stir until smooth.
6. Season soup with pepper and salt.
7. Stir well and serve hot.

Nutritional Values

Calories 214, Fat 17g, Chol 0mg, Sodium 71.4mg, Potassium 67.7mg, Carbs 9g, Protein 12g

141. CREAMY CORN CHOWDER

- Main Course/Appetizers - Prep time: 10 mins, Cook time: 20 mins, Total time: 30 mins, Servings: 4, Grill temp: 300°F

Ingredients

- 1 cup of blanched almonds
- 2 tbsp of extra-virgin olive oil
- 1 large yellow onion, finely chopped
- 2 small stalks of celery, finely chopped
- ½ medium red bell pepper, finely chopped
- 1 medium carrot, finely chopped
- 1 tsp of kosher salt
- 2 tbsp of all-purpose flour
- 6 cups of light vegetable stock
- 3 large Yukon gold potatoes, peeled and cut into 1 /4 -in.- .5cm dice
- 6 cups of corn kernels- shucked from about 4 ears of corn
- 1 tbsp of plant-based butter
- 1 tsp of freshly squeezed lemon juice
- ½ tsp of hot sauce, such as Sriracha
- ¼ tsp of freshly ground black pepper

Directions

1. Soak almonds in cold water overnight.
2. Discard water nuts soaked in, rinse nuts well, and drain. Set aside.
3. In a large soup pot over medium heat, heat extra-virgin olive oil. Add yellow onion, and cook, frequently stirring, for 5 mins.
4. Add celery, red bell pepper, carrot, and kosher salt, and cook for 3 more mins, or until vegetables are softened and just beginning to color.
5. Add all-purpose flour, and stir for 1 minute.
6. Add vegetable stock, stirring vigorously to combine. Bring to a boil, and reserve 1 cup of stock. Add Yukon gold potatoes and corn.
7. Combine almonds and reserved vegetable stock in a blender, and blend until smooth. Stir almond mixture into the soup, and simmer until potatoes are tender. 8 Add plant-based butter, lemon juice, hot sauce, and black pepper.
8. Serve immediately.

Nutritional Values

Calories 223, Fat 3.8g, Chol 0mg, Sodium 61.4mg, Potassium 57.7mg, Carbs 32g, Protein 2.3g

142. CURRIED CAULIFLOWER COCONUT SOUP

- Main Course/Appetizers - Prep time: 10 mins, Cook time: 20 mins, Total time: 30 mins, Servings: 8, Grill temp: 300°F

Ingredients

- 1 tbsp of grapeseed oil
- 1 medium yellow onion, finely chopped
- 1 large carrot, finely chopped
- 2 medium stalks of celery, finely chopped
- 1 clove of garlic, minced
- 1 tsp of kosher salt
- 1 medium head cauliflower, cut into florets
- 4 cups of vegetable stock
- 1- 15 oz. can of full-Fat coconut milk
- 1 tsp of curry powder
- ½ tsp of sambal oelek- chili garlic paste
- Juice of ½ lime
- Fresh cilantro leaves

Directions

1. In a medium soup pot over medium-high heat, heat grapeseed oil. Add yellow onion, carrot, celery, garlic, and kosher salt, and cook gently for about 5 mins or until the onion is softened.
2. Add cauliflower and vegetable stock. Reduce heat to medium-low, cover, and cook for about 10 mins or until cauliflower is tender.
3. Stir in coconut milk, curry powder, and sambal oelek, and cook for 2 more mins.
4. Remove from heat, and stir in lime juice.
5. Using an immersion blender, purée soup until smooth, or transfer it in batches to a blender to purée.
6. Serve immediately, garnished with a few whole cilantro leaves.

Nutritional Values

Calories 113, Fat 1.8g, Chol 0mg, Sodium 71.4mg, Potassium 67.7mg, Carbs 22g, Protein 2.3g

143. GIAMBOTTA- ITALIAN SUMMER VEGETABLE STEW

- Main Course/Appetizers - Prep time: 20 mins, Cook time: 60 mins, Total time: 1 hour 20 mins, Servings: 5, Grill temp: 300°F

Ingredients

- 1 medium eggplant, quartered and cut into ½ in.1.25cm slices
- 2 tsps of kosher salt
- ½ lb. of flat Italian green beans, trimmed
- 3 large white potatoes, unpeeled
- Twelve medium plum tomatoes
- ¼ cup of extra-virgin olive oil
- 2 large yellow onions, halved and thinly sliced
- 2 cloves of garlic smashed and roughly chopped
- 2 red bell peppers, ribs, and seeds were removed and thinly sliced
- 2 large zucchinis, halved and thinly sliced
- ½ tsp of freshly ground black pepper
- ¼ cup of fresh basil leaves

Directions

1. In a colander, toss eggplant with 1 tsp of kosher salt, and set aside to drain over a bowl. After 30 mins, discard the liquid, rinse the eggplant, and gently squeeze excess water. Set aside.
2. Bring a medium pot of salted water to a boil over high heat. Add Italian green beans, and cook for 5 mins. Using a slotted spoon, transfer beans to a bowl of ice water, immediately drain, and set aside.
3. In the same pot, cook white potatoes with boiling water to cover for about 15 mins or until tender. Remove to a cutting board to cool slightly.
4. Meanwhile, core plum tomatoes and score a small X at the bottom of each.
5. When potatoes are done, using the same pot of boiling water and adding a little more if necessary, work in batches to quickly blanch tomatoes, about 1 minute at a time, transferring them to an ice bath immediately after. Peel tomatoes and seeds, and cut them into slices, reserving tomatoes and juice in a bowl.
6. Heat extra-virgin olive oil in a 4-quart- 4L stockpot over medium-high heat. Add yellow onions, and cook for 5 mins.
7. Add garlic, and cook for 1 minute.
8. Stir in eggplant, and cook for another 5 mins, frequently stirring to avoid vegetables sticking while cooking.

9. Stir in tomatoes, red bell peppers, zucchini, green beans, and the remaining 1 tsp of kosher salt, reduce heat to medium-low, and simmer for 20 mins.
10. Meanwhile, peel potatoes and cut them into quarters. When vegetables are tender, stir in potatoes and black pepper, and cook for 5 mins. Remove from heat, stir in basil, and serve hot, warm, or cold.

Nutritional Values

Calories 193, Fat 1.8g, Chol 0mg, Sodium 61.4mg, Potassium 48.7mg, Carbs 22g, Protein 2.3g

144. GINGER KALE SOUP

- Appetizers/Main Course - Prep time: 10 mins, Cook time: 25 mins, Total time: 35 mins, Servings: 4, Grill temp: 300°F

Ingredients

- 1 tbsp of sesame oil
- 1- 2-in. piece fresh ginger, peeled and finely chopped
- 3 cloves of garlic, peeled and finely chopped
- 4 scallions, thinly sliced, white and green parts separated
- 1 large carrot, peeled and thinly sliced
- 2 large stalks of celery, thinly sliced
- 8 cups of vegetable stock
- 1 tsp of tamari
- 4 dried shiitake mushrooms rinsed well
- 6 oz. of fresh shiitake mushroom stems removed and thinly sliced
- 8 leaves of lacinato kale stemmed and sliced into thin ribbons
- Juice of 1 lemon
- 1 tsp of Sriracha, or to taste- optional
- 2 cups of cooked basmati or jasmine rice

Directions

1. In a medium saucepan over medium-high heat, heat sesame oil. Add ginger, garlic, and white parts of scallions, and stir for 1 minute.
2. Add carrot and celery, and stir for 1 minute.
3. Add vegetable stock, tamari, and dried shiitake mushrooms, and simmer the soup for 15 mins.

4. Add fresh shiitake mushrooms and kale, and simmer, covered, for 5 mins.
5. Remove dried shiitake mushrooms- compost them, or save them in the freezer for stock, and remove the pan from heat. Add lemon juice and a little Sriracha- if using.
6. Divide basmati rice among 4 bowls, and ladle soup over the top. Garnish each bowl with reserved green scallion slices, and serve.

Nutritional Values

Calories 113, Fat 1.8g, Chol 0mg, Sodium 71.4mg, Potassium 67.7mg, Carbs 22g, Protein 2.3g

145. GRANDMA'S CHICKEN NOODLE SOUP

- Main Course/Appetizers - Prep time: 10 mins, Cook time: 20 mins, Total time: 30 mins, Servings: 10, Grill temp: 300°F

Ingredients

- 2 oz. of spaghetti or fettuccine broken into small pieces
- 1 tbsp of extra-virgin olive oil
- 1 medium yellow onion, finely chopped
- 1 large carrot, cut into ¼ in. - 5cm dice
- 1 or 2 medium stalks of celery, cut in ¼ in.-.5cm dice
- 1 small parsnip, cut into ¼ in. .- 5cm dice
- 1 clove of garlic, minced
- 1 tsp of kosher salt
- 4 cups of Golden Chicken-y Stock or vegetable stock
- 1 tsp of nutritional yeast
- ½ tsp of reduced-Sodium tamari
- ¼ tsp of freshly ground black pepper
- 1 tbsp of finely chopped fresh Italian flat-leaf parsley
- 1 tbsp of finely chopped fresh dill

Directions

1. Bring a medium pot of salted water to a boil over high heat, add spaghetti, and cook according to the package directions until pasta is al dente- cooked but firm to the bite. Drain, rinse with cold water, and set aside.
2. In a large saucepan over medium-high heat, heat extra-virgin olive oil. Add onion,

reduce heat to medium, and cook, frequently stirring, for 5 to 10 mins, or until the onion is golden and softened.

3. Add carrot, celery, parsnip, garlic, and kosher salt, and cook for 3 mins.
4. Stir in Golden Chicken-y Stock, nutritional yeast, tamari, and black pepper. Increase heat to high, bring to a boil, reduce heat to medium, and simmer for 10 mins.
5. Stir in spaghetti, and cook for 1 more minute. 6 Stir in Italian flat-leaf parsley and dill, and serve immediately.

Nutritional Values

Calories 223, Fat 4.8g, Chol 1mg, Sodium 91.4mg, Potassium 44mg, Carbs 32g, Protein 6.3g

146. GREEN CURRY VEGETABLE STEW

- Appetizers/Main Course - Prep time: 10 mins, Cook time: 20 mins, Total time: 30 mins, Servings: 3 to 4, Grill temp: 300°F

Ingredients

- 2 tbsp of virgin coconut oil
- 2 cloves of garlic, finely chopped
- 1- 1-or 2-in. piece ginger, peeled and grated
- 2 tbsp of Thai green curry paste
- 1 hot chile pepper, such as Serrano, seeded and thinly sliced
- 1 medium yellow onion halved and thinly sliced
- 1- 8 oz. pkg. of shiitake mushrooms, stemmed and thinly sliced
- 1 tsp of kosher salt, plus more to taste
- 1- 14 oz. can full-Fat, best-quality Thai coconut milk
- 1 cup of vegetable stock or water
- 2 Kaffir lime leaves or 1 tbsp of grated lime zest
- 1 cup of carrot, thinly sliced
- 1 large zucchini, halved and thinly sliced
- 1- 10 oz. pkg. of baby spinach
- ½ cup of thinly sliced scallion, white and light green parts
- ¼ cup of finely chopped fresh cilantro

Directions

1. In a large saucepan over medium-high heat, heat virgin coconut oil. Add garlic,

ginger, Thai green curry paste, and hot chile pepper, and stir for 1 minute.
2. Add yellow onion, shiitake mushrooms, and kosher salt, and stir for 2 mins more.
3. Stir in coconut milk, vegetable stock, Kaffir lime leaves, and carrot. Bring to a boil, reduce heat to a simmer, and cook for 5 mins.
4. Stir in zucchini, and simmer for 5 mins.
5. Stir in baby spinach, scallion, and cilantro, and cook for 1 more minute. Remove from heat, and serve.

Nutritional Values

Calories 113, Fat 1.8g, Chol 0mg, Sodium 71.4mg, Potassium 67.7mg, Carbs 22g, Protein 2.3g

147. GUACAMOLE SOUP

- Appetizers - Prep time: 10 mins, Cook time: 10 mins, Total time: 20 mins, Servings: 4, Grill temp: 300°F

Ingredients

- 4 cups of veggie stock
- 3 smashed, ripe avocados
- 1 chopped onion
- 3 minced garlic cloves
- 1 tbsp of ground cumin
- 1 bay leaf
- 1 tsp of oregano
- ⅛ seeded and chopped small habanero
- 2 tsps of agave syrup
- Salt and pepper to taste

Directions

1. Heat 1 deep-bottomed saucepan/pot.
2. When hot, cook the onions and garlic for about 5 mins or until fragrant and the onions are clear.
3. Add the rest of the ingredients- minus the agave to the pot.
4. Cook on high heat for 10 mins.
5. Turn off the heat and let it stand for 5 mins.
6. Open the lid and pick out the bay leaf.
7. Blend the soup till smooth before adding the agave syrup and a squirt of lime juice.
8. Season more to taste, if necessary, before serving.

Nutritional Values

Calories 239, Fat 17g, Chol 0mg, Sodium 71.4mg, Potassium 67.7mg, Carbs 18g, Protein 3g

148. GUMBO FILÉ

- Appetizers/Main Course - Prep time: 25 mins, Cook time: 90 mins, Total time: 2 hours, Servings: 4 to 5, Grill temp: 300°F

Ingredients

- ½ cup of grapeseed oil
- ½ cup of all-purpose flour
- 1 large yellow onion, finely chopped
- 4 medium stalks of celery, finely chopped
- 1 medium green bell pepper, ribs, and seeds were removed and finely chopped
- 1 medium red bell pepper, ribs, and seeds were removed and finely chopped
- 6 cloves of garlic, chopped
- 6 cups of vegetable stock
- ¼ cup of extra-virgin olive oil
- 2 links veggie Andouille sausage, thinly sliced
- 1 lb. of oyster mushrooms, roughly chopped
- 1 tsp of sweet paprika
- 1 tsp of kosher salt
- ½ tsp of Creole seasoning
- ½ tsp of dried oregano
- ½ tsp of dried thyme
- ½ tsp of freshly ground black pepper
- ¼ tsp of ground allspice
- Pinch cayenne
- Twelve fl. oz. of amber beer
- 1- 14 oz. can dice fire-roasted tomatoes with juice
- 1 tbsp of balsamic vinegar
- 1 tbsp of vegan Worcestershire sauce
- 1 tsp of Louisiana hot sauce
- 2 tsps of filé powder
- ½ cup of thinly sliced scallions, white and green parts
- ¼ cup of finely chopped fresh Italian flat-leaf parsley
- 2 tbsp of dark rum- optional

Directions

1. In a large soup pot over medium heat, heat grapeseed oil. Whisk in all-purpose flour until well combined. Using a wooden spoon, stir roux over medium heat until the mixture is golden and caramel brown.
2. Stir in yellow onion, celery, green bell pepper, and red bell pepper, and cook, frequently stirring, for 10 more mins. Reduce heat to medium-low if necessary to prevent burning.
3. Add ½ of the garlic, stir for 1 minute, and bring to a simmer.
4. Stir in vegetable stock, bring to a boil, and reduce heat to a gentle simmer.
5. Meanwhile, heat extra-virgin olive oil over medium heat in a wide sauté pan. Add sliced veggie Andouille sausage, and stir for 1 minute. Using a slotted spoon, transfer the sausage to a bowl.
6. Add oyster mushrooms and remaining garlic to the sauté pan, and stir until mushrooms are golden.
7. Add sweet paprika, kosher salt, Creole seasoning, oregano, thyme, black pepper, allspice, and cayenne, and stir for 1 minute.
8. Add amber beer, increase heat to high, and stir vigorously to deglaze the pan, releasing any browned bits stuck to the pan.
9. Stir the mushroom mixture into the soup pot along with fire-roasted tomatoes with juice, balsamic vinegar, vegan Worcestershire sauce, and hot sauce. Bring to a boil, reduce heat to low or medium-low, and simmer for 1 hour, occasionally stirring and adjusting heat as necessary.
10. Stir in reserved Andouille sausage and filé powder, and simmer for 5 mins.
11. If using, stir in scallions, Italian flat-leaf parsley, and dark rum.
12. Ladle into bowls over hot, cooked rice, or serve with plenty of crusty French bread, passing additional filé powder and hot sauce at the table.

Nutritional Values

Calories 223, Fat 4.8g, Chol 1mg, Sodium 91.4mg, Potassium 44mg, Carbs 32g, Protein 6.3g

149. LIME-MINT SOUP

- Main Course/Appetizer - Prep time: 10 mins, Cook time: 20 mins, Total time: 30 mins, Servings: 4, Grill temp: 300°F

Ingredients

- 4 cups of vegetable broth
- ¼ cup of fresh mint leaves
- ¼ cup of scallions
- 3 garlic cloves, minced
- 3 tbsp of freshly squeezed lime juice

Directions

1. In a large stockpot, combine the broth, mint, scallions, garlic, and lime juice.
2. Bring to a boil over medium-high heat.
3. Cover, set heat to low, simmer for 15 mins, and serve.

Nutritional Values

Calories 214, Fat 2g, Chol 4mg, Sodium 71.4mg, Potassium 67.7mg, Carbs 7g, Protein 5g

150. MEATY MUSHROOM STEW

- Main Course/Appetizers - Prep time: 15 mins, Cook time: 30 mins, Total time: 45 mins, Servings: 6, Grill temp: 300°F

Ingredients

- 4 tbsp of extra-virgin olive oil
- 2 medium yellow onions, finely chopped
- 1 small shallot halved and finely chopped
- 2 medium stalks of celery, finely chopped
- 1 large carrot, finely chopped
- 1- 10 oz. pkg. of tiny white button mushrooms halved
- 8 oz. of hen of the woods mushrooms, sliced
- 8 oz. of fresh chanterelle mushrooms, sliced
- 3 cloves of garlic, finely chopped
- 1 tsp of kosher salt, plus more to taste
- ½ tsp of freshly ground black pepper, plus more to taste
- 1 tbsp of sweet Hungarian paprika
- 1 tsp of dried thyme
- 1 tsp of dried dill
- 2 tbsp of all-purpose flour
- 4 cups of Mushroom Stock
- 1 cup of dry red wine
- 1 large russet potato, peeled and diced
- ¼ cup of finely chopped fresh Italian flat-leaf parsley
- 1 tbsp of balsamic vinegar

Directions

1. In a 4-quart- 4L stockpot over medium-high heat, heat 2 tbsp extra-virgin olive oil. Add yellow onions and shallot, and cook, frequently stirring, for 5 mins.
2. Add celery, carrot, white button mushrooms, hen of the woods mushrooms, chanterelle mushrooms, and garlic, and cook, frequently stirring, for about 10 mins, or until mushrooms begin to turn golden. Add the remaining 2 tbsp of olive oil as mushrooms begin to stick to the pan.
3. Stir in kosher salt, black pepper, sweet Hungarian paprika, thyme, and dill.
4. Add all-purpose flour to the mushroom mixture, and stir for 2 mins.
5. Add 3 cups of Mushroom Stock, red wine, and russet potato, and bring to a boil. Reduce heat to medium, and cook, often stirring, for 10 mins, or until stew is thickened and vegetables are tender. Add additional stock if the stew is too thick for your liking.
6. Remove from heat, and stir in Italian flat-leaf parsley and balsamic vinegar. Taste, add more kosher salt and black pepper if needed, and serve.

Nutritional Values

Calories 223, Fat 4.8g, Chol 1mg, Sodium 91.4mg, Potassium 44mg, Carbs 32g, Protein 6.3g

151. VEGAN-MISO SOUP

- Appetizers - Prep time: 5 mins, Cook time: 10 mins, Total time: 15 mins, Servings: 4, Grill temp: 300°F

Ingredients

- 4 cups of water
- 1 cup of cubed silken tofu
- 2 chopped carrots
- 2 chopped celery stalks
- 1 sliced onion
- 2 tbsp of miso paste
- Dash of vegan-friendly soy sauce

Directions

1. Put the carrots, onion, celery, tofu, wakame, and water in a deep-bottomed saucepan with a lid.

2. Close and seal.
3. Cook on high pressure for 6 mins.
4. Turn off the heat and let it stand for 5 mins.
5. Open the lid and ladle out 1 cup of broth.
6. Add the miso paste to this broth and whisk until completely dissolved.
7. Pour back into pot and stir.
8. Season with soy sauce and serve!

152. MISO UDON BOWL

- Main Course/Appetizers - Prep time: 5 mins, Cook time: 20 mins, Total time: 25 mins, Servings: 4, Grill temp: 300°F

Ingredients

- 1- 8 oz. pkg. of udon noodles
- 4 cups of kombu stock or vegetable stock
- 1 tsp of grapeseed oil
- 1- 4 oz. pkg. of shiitake mushrooms, stemmed and thinly sliced
- 1- 1-in. piece fresh ginger, finely grated
- 1 clove of garlic, minced
- 1 cup of wakame- seaweed
- ½ pkg. of firm silken tofu, cut into ½ -in.- 1.25cm cubes
- 2 tbsp of white- Shiro miso paste
- 1- 5 oz. pkg. of baby spinach

Directions

1. Cook udon noodles in boiling water according to the package directions. Drain in a colander, rinse with cold water, and set aside.
2. In a small saucepan over medium-high heat, heat kombu stock until simmering. 3 In a medium saucepan over medium-high heat, heat grapeseed oil. Add shiitake mushrooms, and sauté for 1 minute.
3. Add ginger and garlic, and sauté for 30 seconds. Add heated stock, bring to a boil, and reduce heat to a simmer. Stir in wakame and tofu, and cook for 5 mins.
4. Ladle a ½ cup of soup into a small bowl, and whisk in white- Shiro miso paste.
5. Stir baby spinach and noodles into the soup, and cook for 1 minute or until

spinach is wilted. Remove from heat and stir in the miso mixture.
6. Serve immediately.

153. MUSHROOM AND CABBAGE BORSCHT

- Main Course/Appetizer - Prep time: 10 mins, Cook time: 70 mins, Total time: 1 hour 20 mins, Servings: 6, Grill temp: 400°F

Ingredients

- 4 small beets
- 1 tbsp plus 1 tsp of grapeseed oil
- 2 medium yellow onions, halved and thinly sliced
- 2 medium carrots, thinly sliced
- 3 large stalks of celery, thinly sliced
- 1- 10 oz. pkg. of white button mushrooms, thinly sliced
- 1 tbsp of sugar
- 2 tsps of kosher salt
- ¼ tsp of freshly ground black pepper
- 2 tbsp of tomato paste
- 8 cups of mushroom stock
- 1 small head of savoy cabbage, shredded
- 2 tbsp of freshly squeezed lemon juice, or apple cider vinegar
- ¼ cup of finely chopped fresh dill

Directions

1. Preheat the oven to 400°F - 200°C.
2. Scrub beets, but do not peel. Roast beets on a baking sheet lined with parchment paper for about 30 mins or until tender. Cool slightly, peel, and cut into 1 /4 -inch- .5cm dice.- Beets can be roasted 1 day in advance.
3. In a large soup pot over medium-high heat, heat the remaining 1 tbsp of grapeseed oil. Add yellow onions, carrots, celery, button mushrooms, sugar, and kosher salt. Cook, frequently stirring, for 5 to 10 mins, or until onions are softened and vegetables begin to color.
4. Stir in black pepper and tomato paste. Add mushroom stock and reserved beets.

5. Increase heat to high, boil, and stir in savoy cabbage. Reduce heat to medium-low, and cook, partially covered, occasionally stirring, for about 30 mins or until cabbage is tender.
6. Remove from heat, stir in lemon juice and fresh dill, and serve.

Nutritional Values

Calories 113, Fat 1.8g, Chol 0mg, Sodium 71.4mg, Potassium 67.7mg, Carbs 22g, Protein 2.3g

154. MUSHROOM BARLEY SOUP

- Main Course/Appetizers - Prep time: 20 mins, Cook time: 70 mins, Total time: 1 hour 20 mins, Servings: 4 to 5, Grill temp: 300°F

Ingredients

- 9 cups of vegetable stock
- 1 oz. of dried Borowik, porcini, or forest mix mushrooms
- 2 tbsp of grapeseed oil
- 2 large yellow onions, finely chopped
- 4 small stalks of celery, finely chopped
- 2 small carrots, finely chopped
- 3 cloves of garlic, finely chopped
- Twelve oz. of button mushrooms, thinly sliced
- ¾ cup of pearl barley
- 4 medium yellow potatoes- such as Yukon Gold, peeled and cut in ½ -in.- 1.25cm dice
- 1 bay leaf
- 4 tbsp of finely chopped fresh Italian flat-leaf parsley
- 1 tsp of kosher salt, plus more to taste
- ½ tsp of freshly ground black pepper
- Juice of ½ medium lemon

Directions

1. In a small saucepan over medium heat, bring 1 cup of vegetable stock to a simmer.
2. Rinse dried mushrooms, place in a small bowl, and pour the hot stock over the top. Set aside to soften for 10 mins.
3. When mushrooms are softened, lift them out of stock, gently agitating to loosen any remaining soil, and lightly squeeze dry and finely chop. Reserve mushroom-soaking liquid.

4. In a large, heavy soup pot over medium heat, heat grapeseed oil. Add yellow onions, celery, and carrots, and cook, frequently stirring, for 10 mins.
5. Add chopped dried mushrooms, garlic, and button mushrooms, and cook for 5 mins.
6. Line a fine-mesh strainer with cheesecloth, and pour reserved mushroom soaking liquid through the strainer into the soup pot. Add the remaining 8 cups of vegetable stock, increase heat to high, and bring to a boil.
7. Stir in the pearl barley, yellow potatoes, bay leaf, 2 tbsp of Italian flat-leaf parsley, kosher salt, and black pepper. Reduce heat to medium-low, and cook for about 45 minutes or until barley and vegetables are tender.
8. Remove soup from heat, and remove bay leaf. Stir in lemon juice and the remaining 2 tbsp of Italian flat-leaf parsley, taste to see if the soup needs more salt, and serve hot.

Nutritional Values

Calories 196, Fat 0g, Chol 0mg, Sodium 71.4mg, Potassium 67.7mg, Carbs 30g, Protein 10g

155. ROASTED TOMATO SOUP

- Main Course/Appetizers - Prep time: 20 mins, Cook time: 50 mins, Total time: 1 hour 10 mins, Servings: 6, Grill temp: 300°F

Ingredients

- 3 pounds of tomatoes in a halved manner
- 6 garlic-smashed
- 4 tsps of cooking oil or virgin oil
- Salt to taste
- ¼ cup of vegan heavy cream- optional
- Sliced fresh basil leaves for garnish

Directions

1. Oven medium heat of about 427°F; preheat the oven.
2. In your mixing bowl, mix the halved tomatoes, garlic, olive oil, salt, and pepper
3. Spread the tomato mixture on the already prepared baking sheet
4. For a process of 20-28 mins, roast and stir.

5. Then remove it from the oven, and the roasted vegetables should now be transferred to a soup pot.
6. Stir in the basil leaves.
7. Blend in small portions in a blender.
8. Serve immediately.

Nutritional Values

Calories 126, Fat 6g, Chol 0mg, Sodium 71.4mg, Potassium 67.7mg, Carbs 8g, Protein 3g

156. SMOKY WHITE BEAN AND TOMATO SOUP

- Appetizers - Prep time: 10 mins, Cook time: 60 mins, Total time: 1 hour 10 mins, Servings: 6, Grill temp: 300°F

Ingredients

- 2 cups of dry great northern beans or other small white beans soaked 6 hours or overnight
- 8 cups of vegetable stock or filtered water
- 4 cloves of garlic, thinly sliced
- 1 tbsp of finely chopped fresh rosemary
- 1 tsp of finely chopped fresh thyme or ½ tsp of dried
- ¼ cup of tomato paste
- 1 tsp of smoked sea salt
- 1 tsp of kosher salt
- 1 large yellow onion, chopped
- 4 small stalks of celery, cut in ¼ in.- .5cm dice
- 1- 28 oz. can of diced tomatoes with juice
- ¼ cup plus 2 tbsp of extra-virgin olive oil
- ¼ tsp of crushed red pepper flakes
- ¼ tsp of freshly ground black pepper
- 1 tbsp of apple cider vinegar

Directions

1. Drain soaked great northern beans, rinse well, and place in a large soup pot. Cover with vegetable stock, add garlic, rosemary, and thyme, and bring to a boil over high heat. Reduce heat to a simmer, and cook, partially covered, for 30 mins.
2. Taste beans for tenderness; they should be almost completely cooked but slightly al dente at this point. If not, cook for 10 to 15 more mins.

3. Place tomato paste in a small bowl, and ladle in a little of the hot stock.
4. Stir well, and add tomato paste mixture, smoked sea salt, kosher salt, yellow onion, celery, tomatoes with juice, ¼ cup of extra-virgin olive oil, crushed red pepper flakes, and black pepper. Increase heat to high, and return to a boil.
5. Reduce heat to medium-low, and simmer for 30 mins or until beans are completely tender.
6. Remove from heat, and stir in apple cider vinegar and the remaining 2 tbsp of olive oil. If desired, remove the ½ cup of soup to a blender, purée, return to the pot, and stir- or use an immersion blender to purée slightly. Serve hot.

Nutritional Values

Calories 383, Fat 7.8g, Chol 0mg, Sodium 71.4mg, Potassium 67.7mg, Carbs 42g, Protein 2.3g

157. TOM YUM SOUP

- Main Course/Appetizers - Prep time: 15 mins, Cook time: 10 mins, Total time: 25 mins, Servings: 4, Grill temp: 300°F

Ingredients

- 2 large stalks of fresh lemongrass
- 1 tsp of coconut oil or grapeseed oil
- 2 tbsp of finely chopped galangal or ginger
- 3 Kaffir lime leaves, fresh or frozen, or the zest of 1 medium lime
- 1 small fresh hot red chile pepper, such as Thai bird chile or Serrano, thinly sliced
- 2 tsps of sambal oelek-chili garlic sauce
- 5 cups of Golden Chicken-y Stock or vegetable stock
- 6 oz. of white button mushrooms, sliced
- ¼ lb. of firm silken tofu, cut into ½ in.- 1.25cm cubes
- 2 tbsp of reduced-Sodium tamari
- Juice of 1 ½ medium limes
- ¼ cup of finely chopped fresh cilantro

Directions

1. Peel the tough outer layer from lemongrass stalks and smash the stalks with the flat side of your knife to tenderize. Chop finely.

2. In a medium saucepan over medium-high heat, heat coconut oil.
3. Add lemongrass, galangal, Kaffir lime leaves, hot red chile pepper, and sambal oelek, and stir for 1 minute.
4. Add Golden Chicken-y Stock, button mushrooms, tofu, and tamari, and bring to a boil.
5. Reduce heat to medium, and cook for 10 mins or until mushrooms are tender.
6. Remove from heat, remove and discard lime leaves, stir in lime juice and cilantro, and serve.

Nutritional Values

Calories 196, Fat 0g, Chol 0mg, Sodium 78mg, Potassium 49.7mg, Carbs 30g, Protein 10g

158. ROSEMARY GARLIC POPCORN

- Snacks - Prep time: 6 mins, Cook time: 0 mins, Total time: 6 mins, Servings: 6, Grill temp: 0

Ingredients

- 1/8 tsp of salt
- ½ cup of popcorn kernels
- 1 tsp of rosemary
- 2 tbsp of olive oil
- Pinch of pepper
- 2 chopped garlic cloves

Directions

1. In a pan at medium flame, heat the olive oil and stir-fry the garlic.
2. Turn off the flame and mix rosemary with garlic.
3. Strain oil in a bowl and put popcorn in it.
4. Combine everything well, drizzle pepper and salt and serve.

Nutritional Values

Calories 122, Fat 5.4g, Chol 0mg, Sodium 71.4mg, Potassium 67.7mg, Carbs 17g, Protein 2.7g

159. CLASSIC HUMMUS

- Snack/Side - Prep time: 5 mins, Cook time: 18 mins, Total time: 23 mins, Servings: 8, Grill temp: 300°F

Ingredients

- 6 cups of water
- 1 cup of soaked chickpeas
- 3 to 4 crushed garlic cloves
- 1 bay leaf
- ¼ cup of chopped parsley
- 2 tbsp of tahini
- 1 juiced lemon
- ½ tsp of salt
- ¼ tsp of cumin
- Dash of paprika

Directions

1. Soak your chickpeas overnight in water.
2. When you're ready to make the hummus, rinse them and put them in the pressure cooker.
3. Pour in 6 cups of water.
4. Toss in the bay leaf and garlic cloves.
5. Close and seal the lid.
6. Cook for 18 mins on high pressure.
7. When the cooker is safe to open, drain the chickpeas, but save all the cooking liquid.
8. Remove the bay leaf before pureeing the chickpeas.
9. Add tahini, lemon juice, cumin, and ½ cup of cooking liquid to start.
10. Keep pureeing, and if the mixture isn't creamy enough, keep adding ½ cup of liquid at a time.
11. When it's the right level of creaminess, salt, and puree once more.
12. Serve with a sprinkle of paprika and fresh chopped parsley!

Nutritional Values

Calories 109, Fat 3.8g, Chol 0mg, Sodium 71.4mg, Potassium 67.7mg, Carbs 3.5g, Protein 4.1g

160. HERBED ZUCCHINI

- Sides/Snacks - Prep time: 10 mins, Cook time: 20 mins, Total time: 30 mins, Servings: 4, Grill temp: 400°F

Ingredients

- 2 large- about 8-inches zucchini
- ¼ cup of plant-based mayonnaise
- 2 cups of panko breadcrumbs
- ½ cup of finely chopped fresh mixed herbs such as parsley, chives, chervil, and/or tarragon
- ½ cup of extra-virgin olive oil
- 2 tsps of kosher salt

- 1 tsp of freshly ground black pepper
- 2 tsps of lemon zest

1. Preheat the oven to 400°F - 200°C.
2. Line a baking sheet with parchment paper.
3. Trim each zucchini, and cut into 1 /4 -inch- .5cm slices. Blot dry with paper towels, and brush both sides of each zucchini slice with mayonnaise.
4. In a small, shallow bowl, combine panko, herbs, extra-virgin olive oil, kosher salt, black pepper, and lemon zest.
5. Dredge each zucchini slice in panko mixture, coating both sides, and lay slices on the prepared baking sheet.
6. Bake for 20 mins, carefully turning with a spatula halfway through cooking, and serve immediately.

Nutritional Values

Calories 113, Fat 1.8g, Chol 0mg, Sodium 71.4mg, Potassium 67.7mg, Carbs 22g, Protein 2.3g

161. HOMEMADE MARINATED MUSHROOMS

- Sides/Snacks - Prep time: 5 mins, Cook time: 5 mins, Total time: 10 mins, Servings: 4, Grill temp: 400°F

Ingredients

- 8 twelve-ounce of white button mushrooms
- 5 tbsp of virgin olive oil
- 3 tbsp of white vinegar
- 3 chopped garlic cloves
- ½ chopped red bell pepper
- ½ tsps of dried basil
- ¼ tsp of dried thyme
- ¼ tsp of dried oregano
- ½ tsps of sugar
- 1/8 tsp of salt
- ½ tsps of red pepper flakes
- ½ tsps of Garlic Herb

Directions

1. Slightly cook the mushrooms by heating them in a microwave for 5 mins.

2. Whip up Marinade and emulsify with a whisk.
3. Pour hot mushrooms over them and seal them in a bag or covered bowl.
4. In the fridge, let the rest of your mushrooms for 24 hours to marinate.
5. Whatever floats the boat, enjoy cool or at room temperature.
6. Serve with toothpicks since food on a stick is even more enjoyable.

Nutritional Values

Calories 230, Fat 4g, Chol 0mg, Sodium 71.4mg, Potassium 67.7mg, Carbs 18g, Protein 2g

162. MUSHROOM BUN SLIDERS

- Snacks - Prep time: 10 mins, Cook time: 15 mins, Total time: 25 mins, Servings: 4, Grill temp: 300°F

Ingredients

- Twelve Portobello mushroom caps
- 2 tbsp of vegan butter
- 1 tbsp of olive oil
- 1 tbsp of vegan butter
- 1 tsp of Italian seasoning
- Pepper and salt according to taste
- Twelve slider buns

Directions

1. Cut the stems first from mushrooms and dust off the soil.
2. Heat the butter with some oil in a medium-sized saucepan over medium heat.
3. When the oil and butter are hot and bubbly, use a spatula to scatter oil uniformly in the skillet and add the mushrooms.
4. Sprinkle with the Italian seasoning, pepper, and salt on the mushrooms and roast for around 5 to 7 mins. Then Cook for another 7 mins or till the mushrooms are tender.
5. If you include vegan cheese, place a slice over each mushroom, then cook until it melts. You may place a cover on the pan to speed up the operation.
6. Place a mushroom on a bun and finish it off with your favorite topping.

Nutritional Values

Calories 137, Fat 5g, Chol 0mg, Sodium 71.4mg, Potassium 67.7mg, Carbs 19g, Protein 4g

163. BANH-MI-SANDWICH

- Snacks - Prep time: ready in about: 45 mins, Servings: 4, Grill temp: Medium-high

Ingredients

- olive oil, extra-virgin
- 1 firm tofu
- 4 pieces of baguette
- cilantro
- vegan mayo
- Sriracha
- 2 carrots, small
- 1 daikon
- ½ cucumber
- ¼ cup of white-wine-vinegar
- ½ jalapeño, sliced
- ¼ cup of rice vinegar
- salt
- sugar
- 1 tbsp olive oil
- ½ lime juice + zest
- 2 tbsp tamari
- 1 clove of garlic
- black pepper
- ½ tsp minced ginger

Directions

1. Prepare ahead of time: Combine the daikon, cucumbers, carrots, and jalapenos with rice vinegar, white wine vinegar, sugar, & salt in a small container. If liquids aren't enough to cover the vegetables, add 2 tbsp water and additional vinegar as needed.
2. Refrigerate for up to a week or chill for at least 1 hour. Drain & slice tofu into pieces of ½ -inch. To remove extra water, lay it on a towel & gently wipe it dry.
3. Mix together the tamari, olive oil, ginger, lime zest and, juice, garlic, pepper in a small bowl. In a small pan, place tofu & pour marinade over it. To properly cover the tofu, flip it and apply additional tamari if required. Give at least fifteen mins for the tofu to soak.

4. Preheat a nonstick pan o moderate heat. Proceeding in batches, if required, add a little oil to the pan and arrange tofu slices with plenty of space between them so that they don't become too crowded. Allow the tofu pieces to cook for some time on each side without tossing them around too much until they're caramelized around the edges.
5. Take off the flame and season as per taste. Assemble sandwiches with baguette, mayonnaise, tofu pieces, pickled vegetables, & cilantro, and enjoy with sriracha on the side.

Nutritional Values

Calories 272kcal, Carbs 30g, Protein 8g, Fat 15g, Sodium 786mg, Potassium 734mg, Chol 0mg

164. CHICKPEA-SALAD SANDWICH

- Snacks - Prep time: ready in about: 20 mins, Servings: 2, Grill temp: Medium

Ingredients

- 1 tbsp Maille Mustard
- 4 slices of bread/bagels
- 2 lettuce leaves
- 1 carrot, sliced
- 1 sliced cucumber
- 4 radishes sliced
- sprouts
- 1 avocado
- 1 can of chickpeas
- ¼ cup of chopped dill
- ¼ cup of chopped parsley
- 2 tbsp grain mustard
- salt & pepper
- 1–2 tbsp of Vegan Mayo

Directions

1. To make chickpea salad, add all ingredients to a large mixing bowl, mix well, then crush using a fork until well incorporated. Taste and season with salt & pepper.
2. Prepare the sandwiches by putting them together. On bread, a little amount of whole grain mustard. Add lettuce and a liberal helping of chickpea salad on top. Add cucumber slices, radishes, carrots, & avocado to a plate. Add a pile of sprouts & bread on top.

3. Cut it in ½ and eat it.

Calories 265kcal, Carbs 14g, Protein 14g, Fat 10g, Sodium 527mg, Potassium 834mg, Chol 0mg

165. CARROT-SMORREBROD-CRISPS

- Snacks - Prep time: ready in about: 30 mins, Servings: 4, Grill temp: Medium-low

Ingredients

- Sea salt
- 4 carrots
- 3 tbsp olive oil
- ½ tsp smoked paprika
- 1 tbsp rice vinegar
- lemon juice
- Wasa-Rye-Crispbreads
- black pepper
- Vegan-cream-cheese
- Radishes, sliced
- Persian cucumbers, sliced
- Capers
- Chopped dill
- Chives, chopped

Directions

1. Preheat the oven to 475°F and line parchment paper in a baking dish. C
2. over the bottom of the dish with a ¼-inch thick salt layer, then add the carrots and a generous quantity of salt. Don't worry; you won't have to consume all of this salt in the end. Roast carrots until they are tender but not mushy when probed using a fork.
3. Start checking them at 40 mins; my very big carrots needed 60-90 mins to cook. This step may be completed ahead of time. To make the marinade, follow these steps: Combine the lemon juice, rice vinegar, olive oil, paprika, and several pinches of black pepper in a small bowl. Allow the carrots to cool after removing them from the oven.
4. Remove any extra salt with your hands. Cut a thin strip of the carrot's skin horizontally with a knife, then peel the carrot in the shape of ribbons using a peeler.
5. Toss strips in the marinade to coat them. Build the sandwiches with crispbread, a smear of cream cheese, & cucumber &

radish slices. Add carrot ribbons, capers, and a dash of chives & dill to finish.

Nutritional Values

Calories 155kcal, Carbs 14g, Protein 7.4g, Fat 10g, Sodium 627mg, Potassium 834mg, Chol 0mg

166. BLT SANDWICH

- Snacks - Prep time: ready in about: 10 mins, Servings: 1, Grill temp: Medium

Ingredients

- 5-6 slices of Eggplant Bacon
- 2 slices of Vegan-Sandwich-Bread
- 2 Tbsp of Mayo/Hummus
- ½ ripe tomato, sliced
- ¼ onion
- 2 leaves of green lettuce

Directions

1. Toast the bread- optional. Meanwhile, preheat the pan over moderate heat. When the pan is heated, add the eggplant bacon and cook for 2 mins. Then turn and cook for 2 more mins.
2. Remove the pan from the heat and put it aside. Pour vegan mayo on toasted bread pieces to make the sandwich. Then add Eggplant, tomato, onion, and lettuce to 1 of the pieces.
3. Top with remaining bread, slice, and serve.

Nutritional Values

Calories 253kcal, Carbs 33g, Protein 10g, Fat 9g, Sodium 680mg, Potassium 834mg, Chol 0mg

167. JACKFRUIT-BBQ-SANDWICHES

- Snacks - Prep time: ready in about: 45 mins, Servings: 10, Grill temp: Medium

Ingredients

- 1 tbsp of olive oil, extra-virgin
- BBQ Sauce
- 1 yellow onion
- 1 20-ounce can of jackfruit
- ¼ tsp of sea salt
- ½ cup of water
- 8 slider buns, 6 hamburger buns
- 2 cups of shredded cabbage
- ½ tbsp of lime juice

- ¼ cup of cilantro, chopped
- Sea salt and black pepper
- ½ tsp of olive oil

Directions

1. Prepare jackfruit by shredding using your hands and eliminating any core chunks that are too firm. Heat 1 tbsp oil over medium heat in a large skillet.
2. Cook, sometimes stirring, for 10 mins, until sliced onion is tender, lowering the heat as needed. Cook for 5 mins, stirring intermittently, after adding the jackfruit.
3. Add a little bit of water if required to prevent it from clinging to the pan. ½ cup of water plus ½ of the BBQ sauce are combined in a mixing bowl.
4. Reduce to a low flame, cover, and cook for 20 mins.
5. Remove the lid and whisk in ½ of the leftover BBQ sauce, saving the other ½ for serving. To make the slaw, combine all of the ingredients in a large mixing bowl.
6. Combine cabbage, lime juice, cilantro, and olive oil with pinches of pepper and salt in a moderate mixing bowl.
7. Serve sliders with jackfruit, leftover BBQ sauce, slaw, and any additional toppings.

Nutritional Values

Calories 472kcal, Carbs 30g, Protein 8g, Fat 15.5g, Sodium 886mg, Potassium 734mg, Chol 0mg

168. NO-TUNA-SALAD-SANDWICH

- Snacks - Prep time: ready in about: 10 mins, Servings: 4, Grill temp: Medium

Ingredients

- 3 tbsp of tahini
- 1 can of drained and rinsed chickpeas
- 1 tsp of spicy brown or Dijon mustard
- ¼ cup of red onion, diced
- 1 tbsp of agave nectar or maple syrup
- ¼ cup of diced celery
- 1 tsp of capers
- ¼ cup of diced pickle
- Sea salt & black pepper
- 8 slices of bread, whole-wheat
- 1 tbsp of sunflower seeds
- Dijon mustard or spicy brown
- Tomato, sliced

- Romaine lettuce
- Sliced red onion

Directions

1. Mash the chickpeas with a fork in a mixing dish, leaving just a few beans intact.
2. In a bowl, combine the tahini, maple syrup, mustard, red onion, pickle, celery, capers, salt & pepper, & sunflower seeds- if using. To integrate, mix everything together. Season to taste & adjust spices as necessary. If desired, toast the bread & prepare any extra sandwich additions- such as tomato, lettuce, and onion.
3. Scoop approximately ½ cup of chickpea mixture onto 1 piece of bread, sprinkle with chosen toppings, then top with a second layer of bread.
4. Repeat with the remaining sandwiches.

Nutritional Values

Calories 125kcal, Carbs 14g, Protein 78.g, Fat 10g, Sodium 427mg, Potassium 425mg, Chol 0mg

169. GREENS & THINGS SANDWICHES

- Snacks - Prep time: ready in about: 20 mins, Servings: 4, Grill temp: Medium

Ingredients

- 2 tbsp of chopped shallot
- 2 thinly sliced carrots
- 1 minced clove of garlic
- 3 tbsp of lemon juice
- 1 15 oz. can of chickpeas, no-salt-added
- 1 tbsp of fresh dill, chopped
- 8 slices of toasted multigrain bread, country-style
- Black pepper
- 4 tsp of sunflower kernels, toasted
- ¼ cup of pickled and drained pepperoncini peppers sliced
- 1 cup of cucumber, thinly sliced
- 2 cups of kale & baby spinach

Directions

1. To make vegetarian hummus, mix carrots, garlic, shallot, and ¼ cup of water in a large pan. Bring to a low simmer.
2. Cook for 10 mins, on moderate, or till carrots is soft. Fill a blender halfway with the carrot mixture.

3. Combine chickpeas & lemon juice in a mixing bowl.
4. Cover and process until creamy, adding 1 tbsp of water at a time until the preferred consistency is reached. Place the ingredients in a mixing basin.
5. Add the dill & black pepper and mix well. Spread hummus on ½ of the bread pieces. Sunflower kernels, cucumber, pepperoncini, & kale on top.
6. Add the remaining bread pieces on top.

Nutritional Values
Calories 265kcal, Carbs 11g, Protein 10g, Fat 20g, Sodium 637mg, Potassium 345mg, Chol 0mg

170. JACKFRUIT-BARBECUE-SANDWICHES AND BROCCOLI-SLAW

- Snack - Prep time: ready in about: 3o mins, Servings: 6, Grill temp: Medium

Ingredients

- 2 tsp of lime juice
- ½ of an avocado, peeled and seeded
- 3 cups of shredded broccoli
- 1⅓ cups of tomato sauce; no added-salt
- ¼ cup of sliced scallions
- 3 whole dates pitted
- 2 cloves of garlic
- 1½ tsp of chili powder
- ½ tsp of smoked paprika
- 1 14 oz. can of chopped, drained, and rinsed green jackfruit
- 6 whole-wheat toasted hamburger buns
- ¼ tsp of black pepper, freshly ground
- 1 cup of cooked farro

Directions

1. To make the slaw, mash the avocado with the lime juice in a large mixing bowl.
2. Stir in the broccoli slaw mix & scallions to blend.
3. Cover and set aside while you make the filling. Inside a blender, mix the following 6 ingredients for the filling- through pepper.
4. Blend till smooth and covered. Fill a large saucepan halfway with water.
5. Combine the jackfruit & farro in a mixing bowl.

6. Cover and cook over medium heat until well heated, stirring periodically. Fill buns with jackfruit mixture.
7. Serve with slaw on the side.

Nutritional Values
Calories 165kcal, Carbs 14g, Protein 7g, Fat 10g, Sodium 627mg, Potassium 445mg, Chol 0mg

171. STACKED-VEGETABLE-SANDWICHES & CILANTRO-CHUTNEY

- Snack - Prep time: ready in about: 50 mins, Servings: 10, Grill temp: Medium

Ingredients

- 4 cups of tender stems and cilantro leaves
- 2 cups of green peas, frozen
- 2 tbsp of tahini
- ¼ cup of lime juice
- 1 seeded and stemmed jalapeño pepper
- 1 tsp of cumin seeds
- 1 small-sized coarsely chopped garlic clove
- ½ tbsp of date paste
- Sea salt
- 2 beets
- 2 russet potatoes
- Sea salt and black pepper
- 2 cucumbers
- 1 red onion
- 2 tomatoes
- 20 slices of bread, whole wheat

Directions

1. In a tiny saucepan, bring 1½ cups of water to a boil.
2. Cook, occasionally stirring, until peas are mushy, about 10 mins, over high heat. Rinse using cold water after draining.
3. In a blender, combine the peas, 1 cup of water, and the rest of the Chutney ingredients. Blend until smooth, then chill for 1 hour in a sealed container.
4. Put the potatoes with beets in a large saucepan with a steamer basket above 1 to 2 inches of water to create sandwiches. Bring the water to a simmer, cover the saucepan, and steam for 25 mins. Allow to cool fully before serving.
5. Thinly slice the potatoes, cucumbers, beets, tomatoes, & onion- preferably 18- to 14-

inch thick rounds. On 1 side of 10 bread pieces, spread chutney.

6. Beginning with potatoes, layer the veggies on top, followed by the beets, onion, cucumbers, and tomatoes. Season to taste with pepper and salt.
7. Top the sandwiches with Chutney on 1 side of the rest of the bread pieces.
8. Before serving, slice each sandwich in quarters.

Nutritional Values

Calories 365kcal, Carbs 10g, Protein 23g, Fat 10g, Sodium 427mg, Potassium 445mg, Chol 0mg

172. BUFFALO-CAULIFLOWER-PITA-POCKETS

- Snack - Prep time: ready in about: 30 mins, Servings: 8, Grill temp: Medium

Ingredients

- 2 tbsp of vinegar, white wine
- 2 15 oz. cans of no- added-salt chickpeas
- 1 tbsp of Dijon mustard
- 1 tbsp of no-added-salt tomato paste
- 1-2 tbsp of hot sauce
- 1 12-16 oz. package of frozen cauliflower
- ½ cup of chopped carrot
- ½ cup of chopped onion
- 3 minced cloves of garlic
- 8 leaves of lettuce
- Black pepper
- 4 pita bread, whole wheat rounds
- Lemon wedges
- ½ cup of celery, finely chopped

Directions

1. Drain and save the liquid from the garbanzo beans aquafaba.
2. Rinse the beans well. ½ cup of beans should be mashed in a small bowl, and the remaining beans should be kept aside. ¼ cup aquafaba- save remaining aquafaba for later use; vinegar, hot sauce, mustard, & tomato paste are whisked together in a separate bowl.
3. Combine with the mashed beans.
4. Cook cauliflower, carrot, onion, and garlic in a pan over medium heat for approximately 3 mins, turning frequently & adding water, 2–3 tbsp at a time, as required to avoid sticking. Combine the

entire beans and the mashed bean mixture in a mixing bowl.

5. Cook for 5 mins or until the liquid has almost evaporated and the cauliflower is soft. Season with salt and pepper.
6. Fill each pita ½ with 1 lettuce leaf, then fill with cauliflower filling and celery.
7. Garnish with lemon wedges & more hot sauce, if preferred.

Nutritional Values

Calories 265kcal, Carbs 12g, Protein 9.10g, Fat 10g, Sodium 647mg, Potassium 345mg, Chol 0mg

173. SUPER-SLOPPY-JOES

- Snack - Prep time: ready in about: 30 mins, Servings: 6, Grill temp: Medium-low

Ingredients

- ½ cup of yellow onion, finely chopped
- ⅓ cup of pitted dates
- ½ cup of celery, finely chopped
- ½ cup of green bell pepper, finely chopped
- 2 minced cloves of garlic
- 1 can of tomato purée
- 2 cups of wheat berries, cooked
- ¼ cup of ketchup
- Sea salt and black pepper
- 1 tbsp of vegan Worcestershire
- 6 hamburger buns, whole-grain

Directions

1. In a tiny saucepan, mix the dates and 1/3 cup of water, and cook over moderate heat for around 10 mins.
2. Drain and set aside the cooking liquid.
3. In a blender, puree dates until creamy; add cooking water as required. In a large pan, mix the celery, onion, and bell pepper and sauté for around 8 mins, over a moderate flame, turning regularly and adding water, 2 tbsp, as required to avoid sticking.
4. Cook, frequently stirring, for another minute after adding the garlic.
5. Combine the wheat berries, date paste, tomato purée, ketchup, & Worcestershire sauce in a large mixing bowl.
6. Cook, stirring periodically, for 10 mins.
7. Add Salt & pepper to taste. Serve inside buns.

Calories 465kcal, Carbs 14g, Protein 19g, Fat 10g, Sodium 4327mg, Potassium 445mg, Chol 0mg

174. SAUTÉED BRUSSELS-SPROUTS

- Snack - Prep time: ready in about: 25 mins, Servings: 4, Grill temp: Medium

Ingredients

- 1 tbsp of olive oil, extra-virgin
- 1 pound of Brussels sprouts
- ¼ tsp of sea salt
- Lemon wedge
- Vegan Parmesan or Grated Parmesan
- Black pepper
- Sea salt

Directions

1. In a big skillet, heat oil over moderate flame.
2. Place ½ of the Brussels sprouts in the pan cut-side on the bottom. Sear sprouts for 4 mins, without disturbing them, until they are thoroughly golden brown.
3. Toss, season with ½ salt & a few grinds of pepper, and simmer, occasionally turning, for 6 mins. Remove the sprouts from the pan, apply some more oil, and continue with the rest. When the second batch is done, return the first batch to the pan and cook until well heated.
4. Take off the heat, squeeze in the lemon, & season with extra sea salt to taste.
5. Serve immediately with a sprinkling of Parmesan.

Nutritional Values

Calories 272kcal, Carbs 30g, Protein 8.4g, Fat 15g, Sodium 886mg, Potassium 634mg, Chol 0mg

175. BABA GANOUSH

- Snack - Prep time: ready in about: 1 hr & 15 mins, Servings: 4, Grill temp: Medium

Ingredients

- ¼ cup of tahini
- 2 eggplant
- 3 tbsp lemon juice
- 2 cloves of garlic
- 2 tbsp olive oil

- Pita & Veggies
- ½ tsp sea salt
- smoked paprika
- parsley, chopped
- red-pepper-flakes- optional

Directions

1. Preheat the oven to 400°F and cover the eggplant with foil. Roast the eggplant for 60 mins.
2. Remove the baking sheet from the oven and put it aside. Take the skin off the eggplant after it has cooled, eliminating any large clusters of seeds.
3. To reduce the moisture content, drain the flesh in a sieve over a dish for 20 mins.
4. In a blender, blend the eggplant flesh, lemon juice, tahini, garlic, olive oil, and salt till smooth. Sprinkle with smoked paprika, chopped parsley, and red pepper flakes.
5. Serve with vegetables and pita bread.

Nutritional Values

Calories 272kcal, Carbs 30g, Protein 8g, Fat 15.8g, Sodium 886mg, Potassium 734mg, Chol 0mg

176. TOMATO BRUSCHETTA

- Snack - Prep time: ready in about: 10 mins, Servings: 4-6, Grill temp: Medium

Ingredients

- 2 cloves of garlic cloves
- 4 tomatoes, chopped
- ½ tsp red-wine-vinegar
- black pepper
- 2 tbsp capers
- ¼ tsp sea salt
- olive oil
- Fresh basil
- 6-8 slices of bread
- 6 olives, chopped

Directions

1. Combine the tomatoes, grated garlic, tomatoes, vinegar, salt, and a few grinds of pepper in a small mixing bowl. If using, add olives & capers.
2. Drizzle bread pieces using olive oil and toast.
3. Rub garlic on toast using the cut side of garlic halves.

4. Add tomato mixture & fresh basil over the top.

Calories 222kcal, Carbs 30g, Protein 8g, Fat 15g, Sodium 886mg, Potassium 734mg, Chol 0mg

177. GRILLED-RATATOUILLE-TARTINES

- Snack - Prep time: ready in about: 30 mins, Servings: 4, Grill temp: Medium

Ingredients

- 1 eggplant
- 1 sliced zucchini
- 1 red-bell-pepper
- - extra-virgin olive oil
- 3 scallions
- sea salt
- 1 clove of garlic
- 1 cup of cherry tomatoes
- 1 tsp sherry vinegar
- ¼ cup of chopped basil
- hummus
- 1 tsp herbs- de-Provence
- 8 slices of toasted bread

Directions

1. Preheat a grill over medium-high heat.
2. Drizzle olive oil and a bit of salt over the zucchini, red pepper, eggplant, &scallions.
3. Grill for 3 mins, on each side, until charred.
4. Remove veggies from the grill and set them aside to cool slightly before chopping them into 1-inch slices.
5. Toss them with cherry tomatoes, sherry vinegar, garlic, herbs de Provence, & basil in a mixing bowl. Season as per taste then enjoys with a dollop of goat cheese on toasted bread.

Nutritional Values

Calories 202kcal, Carbs 30g, Protein 8g, Fat 11g, Sodium 886mg, Potassium 734mg, Chol 0mg

178. SOCCA RECIPE

- Snack - Prep time: ready in about: 30 mins, Servings: 4, Grill temp: Medium

Ingredients

- 1 cup of water
- ½ tsp sea salt
- 1 cup of chickpea flour
- 1¾ tbsp olive oil

Directions

1. Preheat your oven to 475°F and place a 10-inch cast-iron pan inside.
2. Mix together the water, 1 tbsp olive oil, chickpea flour, and salt in a medium mixing bowl. Cover and put aside for 30 mins.
3. Take the hot skillet out of the oven with a potholder & brush the rest of ¾ tbsp olive oil all over the bottom & edges of the pan.
4. Bake for 20 mins. Don't undercook the potatoes; the crispier they are, the better.
5. Take out of the oven & cool slightly before loosening and transferring the socca from the pan to a serving platter with a spatula.

Nutritional Values

Calories 222kcal, Carbs 30g, Protein 8g, Fat 15g, Sodium 886mg, Potassium 634mg, Chol 0mg

179. LOADED-POTATO-SKINS

- Snack - Prep time: ready in about: 38 mins, Servings: 10, Grill temp: Medium

Ingredients

- olive oil
- 5 russet potatoes
- Sea salt & ground-black-pepper
- 1½ tbsp tamari
- 1½ cups of coconut flakes
- 1 tbsp maple syrup
- 1¼ cups of raw seeds of sunflower
- ½ tsp smoked paprika
- 1 cup of water
- 2 tbsp white-wine-vinegar
- 1 clove of garlic
- 1 tbsp lemon juice
- 1 can of black beans
- ½ tsp sea salt
- ¾ cup of corn kernels
- 1 clove of minced garlic
- ¼ cup of red onion
- 1 tbsp lime juice
- ½ cup of chopped cilantro
- ½ tsp chili powder
- ½ tsp sea salt
- Sliced, Cilantro
- Sliced, chives

- diced, Jalapeño pepper

1. Preheat the oven to 350°F and prepare a baking sheet using parchment.
2. On a baking sheet, mix the tamari, coconut flakes, maple syrup, & paprika together lightly to coat. Arrange in a thin layer & bake for 10 mins, or until rich golden brown and somewhat crunchy.
3. Preheat the oven to 400°F and line parchment paper on a baking sheet.
4. Scrub potatoes & poke holes in them with a fork before placing them on a baking pan.
5. Preheat the oven to 350°F and bake for 1 hour. Remove the baking sheet from the oven and raise the temperature to 450°F.
6. Slice every potato in ½ & scoop out the meat when cold enough to handle, leaving a ¼-inch line of potato in the shell. Brush the potato skins using olive oil, salt, & pepper before placing them cut side on the base of the baking sheet.
7. Roast for around 10 mins, then flip, brush with extra olive oil & a liberal pinch of salt, and continue to roast for another 10 mins. Save the potato flesh you scooped out for another recipe.
8. To make Sun Cheese, put sunflower seeds, garlic, water, vinegar, lemon juice, & salt in a blender & process until smooth, approximately 1 minute. Refrigerate until set to use.
9. To make the Black Bean and Corn Filling, combine black beans, red onion, corn, garlic, chili powder, lime juice, cilantro, &salt in a medium mixing bowl.
10. Fill potato skins with Black Bean and Corn mixture and season using salt & lime juice. Sun Cheese & Coconut Bacon go on top.
11. Garnish with jalapeno, chives, and cilantro, if desired.
12. Serve fresh lime wedges on the side.

Calories 282kcal, Carbs 30g, Protein 16g, Fat 15g, Sodium 886mg, Potassium 734mg, Chol 0mg

180. VEGAN PORTOBELLO-PIZZAS

- Snack - Prep time: ready in about: 30 mins, Servings: 3, Grill temp: Medium

- 3 Portobello mushrooms
- Olive oil
- ¼ tsp of garlic powder
- ¼ tsp of dried basil
- ¼ tsp of dried oregano
- 1 cup of pizza sauce
- ½ cup of mixed veggies
- Vegan-Parmesan-Cheese

1. Preheat the oven to 400°F.
2. Place the mushrooms on a baking sheet & sprinkle both sides with olive oil. Basil, Garlic powder, & oregano are sprinkled over the top.
3. After that, bake for around 5 mins.
4. Pull mushrooms from the oven after they've been par-baked & top with the required amount of pizza sauce, vegetables, & vegan parmesan.
5. Bake for 20 mins.

Calories 165kcal, Carbs 14g, Protein 7g, Fat 10g, Sodium 627mg, Potassium 834mg, Chol 0mg

181. VEGAN-LEMON-MUFFINS

- Snack - Prep time: ready in about: 40 mins, Servings: 9-10, Grill temp: Medium

- 1 tsp of Apple-Cider-Vinegar
- 1 cup of almond milk
- 1¾ cup of all-Purpose-Flour
- 2½ tsp Baking Powder
- ½ cup of almond flour
- ¼ tsp of Baking Soda
- ½ cup of Coconut Sugar
- ½ tsp sea Salt
- ⅓ cup of Olive Oil
- 3 tbsp lemon juice
- 2 tbsp lemon zest
- 1 tsp Vanilla Extract
- ½ cup of Cream Cheese, vegan
- 1 tbsp Chia Seeds
- 2 tbsp Maple Syrup

1. Preheat your oven to 375°F and gently grease a 12-cup muffin tray.
2. Combine the apple vinegar and almond milk in a small bowl. Place aside. Whisk flours, baking soda, baking powder, and salt in a large mixing bowl.
3. Whisk together olive oil, sugar, lemon juice, lemon zest, and vanilla in another mixing bowl. Add almond milk mixture and stir to combine.
4. Combine wet & dry ingredients and stir until just incorporated. Fold chia seeds in the mixture, then scoop batter into muffin pans using a 1/3 cup measuring cup. Cook for 16–17 mins.
5. Allow cooling in the pan for around 10 mins before transferring to a wire rack to cool completely.
6. Make the glaze by combining all of the ingredients in a food processor and pulse until smooth.
7. Place the chia seeds & lemon zest on top of the cooled muffins.

Nutritional Values
Calories 195kcal, Carbs 14g, Protein 18g, Fat 10g, Sodium 827mg, Potassium 834mg, Chol 0mg

182. HEALTHY BANANA-MUFFINS

- Snack - Prep time: ready in about: 30 mins, Servings: 10, Grill temp: Medium-low

Ingredients
- 1¾ cup of pastry flour
- 4 tbsp flaxseed + 4 tbsp warm water
- 1 tsp cinnamon
- 1 tsp baking powder
- ¼ tsp nutmeg
- ½ tsp baking soda
- ⅔ cup of almond milk
- ½ tsp sea salt
- 1 tbsp apple-cider-vinegar
- ⅓ cup of olive oil
- ⅓ cup of maple syrup
- 1 tsp vanilla
- ½ cup of chocolate chips
- 1 cup of mashed banana

Directions
1. Preheat your oven to 350°F and butter a 12-cup muffin tray gently.

2. Combine flaxseed with hot water in a small dish and put aside to thicken for about 5 mins.
3. Combine the cinnamon, flour, nutmeg, baking soda, baking powder, and salt in a large mixing bowl.
4. Blend the apple vinegar, almond milk, oil, maple syrup, and vanilla in a medium mixing bowl and toss to combine.
5. Stir flaxseed in the mixture.
6. Combine the wet & dry ingredients and whisk just until blended.
7. Do not over-mix the ingredients. If using, fold mashed banana & chocolate chips into the mixture.
8. To divide the batter into the muffin tray, use a 1/3 cup measuring scoop.
9. Bake for 20 mins. Allow cooling for 15 mins before transferring to a wire rack to finish cooling.

Nutritional Values
Calories 265kcal, Carbs 14g, Protein 7g, Fat 11g, Sodium 627mg, Potassium 834mg, Chol 0mg

183. MANGO-COCONUT-MUFFINS

- Snack - Prep time: ready in about: 30 mins, Servings: 12, Grill temp: Medium

Ingredients
- 3 tbsp water
- 1 tbsp flaxseed
- 2 tsp lime juice
- 2 cups of spelled flour
- ¾ cup of almond milk
- 2 tsp baking powder
- ½ tsp cinnamon
- ½ tsp salt
- ½ cup of cane sugar
- ½ - ¾ cup of coconut flakes
- 1 tsp vanilla
- ¼ cup of coconut oil
- 1 cup of diced mango

Directions
1. Preheat the oven to 350°F and line a muffin tray- 12-cup with paper liners.
2. Mix ground flaxseed & water in a bowl and place aside to thicken.
3. Add almond milk to lime juice in another bowl and place aside.

4. Mix the flour, salt, baking powder, cinnamon, and ½ cup of sugar in a big mixing bowl.
5. Mix together /the lime juice/almond milk combination, flaxseed mixture, coconut oil, & vanilla in a wide mixing bowl.
6. Pour wet ingredients into dry ingredients and whisk until everything is well incorporated.
7. Do not over-mix the ingredients. Toss in the sliced mango and mix well.
8. Divide batter evenly between muffin cups, packing them approximately 3-quarters full.
9. Scatter coconut flakes on top and bake for 20 mins, and finish with a little dusting of the remaining sugar.
10. Allow cooling for 10 mins before transferring to a wire rack to complete cooling.

Nutritional Values

Calories 265kcal, Carbs 11g, Protein 7g, Fat 10g, Sodium 621mg, Potassium 834mg, Chol 0mg

184. PORTOBELLO-MUSHROOM-BURGER

- Snack - Prep time: ready in about: 18 mins, Servings: 4, Grill temp: Medium

Ingredients

- olive oil
- 4 Portobello mushrooms
- Balsamic vinegar
- Sea salt & black pepper
- Tamari
- 4 hamburger buns, toasted
- Sliced tomato
- Lettuce
- red onion, sliced
- Ketchup, mustard, or mayo
- Pickles
- Pesto- optional

Directions

1. Remove the stems from the mushrooms and wipe the caps clean with a moist cloth.
2. Drizzle tamari, balsamic vinegar, olive oil, salt, & pepper over the mushrooms on a rimmed dish.

3. Use your hands to cover all sides of the mushrooms. Over moderate flame, preheat a grill pan.
4. Place mushrooms on the grill pan, gill side up. Cook for 7 mins, on each side, or until the mushrooms are soft.
5. Place mushrooms on buns and top with your favorite toppings.

Nutritional Values

Calories 325kcal, Carbs 14g, Protein 7g, Fat 10g, Sodium 627mg, Potassium 384mg, Chol 0mg

185. MAKI-SUSHI-RECIPE

- Snack - Prep time: ready in about: 80 mins, Servings: 3, Grill temp: Medium

Ingredients

- 1 tbsp olive oil
- 6 oz. of shiitake mushrooms
- 1 tbsp tamari
- ⅓ - ½ cup of water
- ½ cup of roasted carrots
- ¼ cup of olive oil
- 2 tsps of minced ginger
- 2 tbsp of rice vinegar
- ¼ tsp of sea salt
- 2 cups of water
- 1 cup brown rice
- 1 tsp olive oil
- 1 tbsp cane sugar
- 2 tbsp rice vinegar
- 1 tsp sea salt
- 1 cup red cabbage
- 3 nori-sheets
- 3 strips of cucumber
- Pickled ginger
- Sesame seeds
- ½ avocado,
- Tamari- for serving

Directions

1. To make roasted shiitake, follow these steps:
2. Preheat your oven to 400°F and prepare 2 baking sheets using parchment paper, 1 big and 1 little.
3. Combine the olive oil, shiitake mushrooms, and tamari in a mixing bowl and stir to coat. On a big baking sheet, distribute in an equal layer. Roast for 30 mins

4. Roast carrots for dipping sauce on the second sheet.
5. To make the ginger dipping sauce, follow these steps: Blend the water, roasted carrots, olive oil, ginger, rice vinegar, and salt until smooth in a blender. Set aside shiitakes.
6. To make sushi rice, follow these steps: Combine the water, rice, and olive oil in a saucepan & boil. Cover, lower the heat to low, and cook for 45 mins.
7. Take the rice off the heat and set aside for another 10 mins, covered.
8. Fold in the sugar, rice vinegar, and salt. Cover and set aside until ready to use. Put together the sushi rolls.
9. Place 1 nori sheet on a bamboo mat, shiny side down, and push a handful of rice into the bottom 2-thirds of the sheet.
10. Place the toppings at the base of the rice. Overfilling will make rolling more difficult.
11. To tuck & roll nori, use a bamboo mat. Use a bamboo mat to press & shape the roll after it's been rolled. Place the cut side of the roll to the side.
12. Repeat with the remaining rolls, cutting the sushi using a sharp chef's knife. Between cuts, wipe the knife clean using a moist cloth.
13. Sesame seeds may be sprinkled on top. If preferred, serve with tamari, dipping sauce, & pickled ginger.

Nutritional Values

Calories 265kcal, Carbs 11g, Protein 7g, Fat 16g, Sodium 627mg, Potassium 534mg, Chol 0mg

186. VEGAN-7-LAYER-DIP

- Snack - Prep time: ready in about: 40 mins, Servings: 6-8, Grill temp: Medium

Ingredients

- 1 Kale Guacamole pulsed
- 1 can of refried beans
- 1 cup of cherry tomatoes
- ½ cup of cilantro
- ½ bunch of scallions
- 1 jalapeño, sliced
- Tortilla Chips
- 1 cup of raw cashews
- 2 tbsp olive oil
- ½ cup of water
- 2 tbsp lemon juice
- ½ tsp sea salt
- 1½ cups of cooked-red-quinoa
- 1 tsp chili powder
- 1 clove of garlic
- 1 tsp smoked paprika
- ½ tbsp lime juice
- ½ tsp cumin
- 1 tsp olive oil
- ¼ tsp maple syrup
- ½ tsp sea salt

Directions

1. To make Cashew Cream, put the cashews, olive oil, water, lemon juice, & sea salt inside a blender and puree until smooth. Refrigerate until set to use.
2. To prepare the quinoa, combine the quinoa, chili powder, garlic, smoked paprika, lime juice, cumin, olive oil, sea salt, & maple syrup in a wide mixing bowl. Refrigerate until set to use.
3. Layer refried beans, cashew cream, kale guacamole, and spicy quinoa on an 8x12- or comparable serving dish.
4. Add the tomatoes, cilantro, scallions, extra cream, and, if desired, jalapenos to the top. Serve with chips.

Nutritional Values

Calories 272kcal, Carbs 30g, Protein 8.4g, Fat 15g, Sodium 886mg, Potassium 734mg, Chol 0mg

187. 2-MINS, STEAMED ASPARAGUS

- Sides - Prep time: 5 mins, Cook time: 5 mins, Total time: 10 mins, Servings: 4, Grill temp: 300°F

Ingredients

- 1 lb. trimmed asparagus
- 1 cup of water
- 2 tbsp of olive oil
- 1 tbsp of minced onion
- Sea salt and pepper to taste
- A squeeze of fresh lemon

Directions

1. Pour water into your pressure cooker and lower it to the steamer basket.
2. Put the asparagus in the basket.
3. Drizzle on a little olive oil and onion.
4. Close and seal the lid.
5. Select "steam" and adjust the time to 2 mins.
6. When time is up, hit "cancel" and quick-release the pressure.
7. Serve with salt, pepper, and a squeeze of lemon juice.

Nutritional Values

Calories 84, Fat 0g, Chol 0mg, Sodium 51.4mg, Potassium 47.7mg, Carbs 5g, Protein 3g

188. SUN-DRIED-TOMATO & CHICKPEA SLIDERS

- Sides - Prep time: ready in about: 35 mins, Servings: 8, Grill temp: Medium

Ingredients

- ½ cup of fresh mushrooms, coarsely chopped
- ½ cup of chopped onion
- ½ cup of zucchini, coarsely chopped
- ¾ cup of chickpeas, no-added-salt
- 1 minced clove of garlic,
- ¼ cup of tomatoes, chopped and sun-dried
- ½ tsp of lemon zest
- 1 tsp of crushed Italian seasoning
- Sea salt and black pepper
- 8 slices of Roma tomato
- 1 zucchini
- ¼ cup of cornmeal
- 2 tbsp of balsamic vinegar

Directions

1. Cook the initial 4 ingredients- through garlic in a large pan over medium heat for 3 to 4 mins, turning periodically and adding water as required to avoid sticking.
2. Combine the chickpeas, tomatoes, Italian spice, & lemon zest in a food processor. Seal and process until the mixture is lumpy but not completely pureed. If the filling seems dry or isn't adhering together, add 2 tbsp of aquafaba.
3. It's important that the mixture be damp but not wet. Salt & pepper to taste.

4. Form the bean filling into 8 patties using damp hands. Allow at least 20 mins for chilling.
5. To coat the patties, lightly dredge them in cornmeal.
6. Preheat the grill pan to medium-high heat. Cook sliders for 8 to 10 mins, flipping once until browned and cooked thoroughly.
7. Brush some balsamic vinegar on the zucchini planks.
8. Cook 6 mins on a pan, rotating once until crisp-tender & grill marks emerge. For the "buns, " cut the planks into 6teen pieces.
9. Sliders & tomato slices should be sandwiched between plank slices. Pour any leftover vinegar on top.

Nutritional Values

Calories 158kcal, Carbs 12g, Protein 44g, Fat 10g, Sodium 427mg, Potassium 245mg, Chol 0mg

189. MEXICAN CAULIFLOWER RICE

- Sides - Prep time: 10 mins, Cook time: 10 mins, Total time: 20 mins, Servings: 3, Grill temp: 300°F

Ingredients

- 1 large cauliflower florets
- 2 garlic cloves, minced
- 1 tbsp of olive oil
- ¼ cup of vegetable broth
- 3 tbsp of tomato paste
- ½ tsps of cumin
- 1 tsp of salt

Directions

1. Stir in cauliflower in a food processor until it looks like rice.
2. Cook oil in a pan over medium heat.
3. Cook onion and garlic for 3 mins.
4. Add cauliflower rice, cumin, and salt and stir well.
5. Add broth and tomato paste and stir until well combined.
6. Serve and enjoy.

Nutritional Values

Calories 90, Fat 5g, Chol 0mg, Sodium 71.4mg, Potassium 67.7mg, Carbs 11g, Protein 3g

190. MINTED PEAS AND BABY POTATOES

- Sides - Prep time: 10 mins, Cook time: 10 mins, Total time: 20 mins, Servings: 3, Grill temp: 300°F

Ingredients

- 1 lb. of very small new potatoes
- 2 tbsp of extra-virgin olive oil
- 1 shallot, thinly sliced
- 1 tsp of kosher salt
- 4 cups of shelled fresh peas, or 1- 10 oz. pkg. frozen peas, thawed
- 2 tbsp of water
- 2 tbsp of finely chopped fresh mint
- Juice of ½ lemon
- ½ tsp of freshly ground black pepper

Directions

1. In a large pot with a tight-fitting lid, bring 1 inch- 2.5cm water to a boil over medium heat. Place new potatoes in a steamer basket, set in the pot, and steam for about 10 mins, or until potatoes are tender and easily pierced with a fork. Drain and cool slightly. If potatoes are larger than 1 inch- 2.5cm in diameter, cut them in ½.
2. Meanwhile, in a large saucepan over medium-high heat, heat extra-virgin olive oil. Add shallots and kosher salt, and cook for about 5 mins or until softened.
3. Stir in peas and water, and cook for 2 mins.
4. Add reserved potatoes, increase heat to high, and stir for 1 minute.
5. Remove from heat. Add mint, lemon juice, and black pepper, and serve.

Peas
1. For Herbed Peas and Potatoes, replace mint with chervil, parsley, chives, French tarragon, or any combination of these herbs.

Nutritional Values

Calories 223, Fat 3.8g, Chol 0mg, Sodium 71.4mg, Potassium 67.7mg, Carbs 32g, Protein 2.3g

191. MUSHROOM RISOTTO

- Sides - Prep time: 10 mins, Cook time: 20 mins, Total time: 30 mins, Servings: 4 to 6, Grill temp: 300°F

Ingredients

- 4 cups of veggie stock
- 1 ½ pounds of mixed, chopped mushrooms
- 1 ounce of dried porcini mushrooms
- 2 cups of Arborio rice
- 1 cup of chopped yellow onion
- ¾ cups of dry white wine
- 4 tbsp of olive oil
- 4 tbsp of vegan butter
- 1 tbsp of miso paste
- 2 tsps of soy sauce
- 2 tsps of minced garlic
- ½ cup of chopped herbs

Directions

1. Microwave the dried mushrooms in broth for 5 mins.
2. Chop the porcini and set it aside for now. Keep the broth separate.
3. Heat olive oil in a deep-bottomed saucepan/pot with a lid.
4. Add the fresh mixed mushrooms and cook for about 8 mins, until brown.
5. Season with salt and pepper.
6. Add the onion, garlic, porcini, and butter.
7. Stir until the onions are soft.
8. Add the rice and stir to coat in oil.
9. When toasty after 3-4 mins, add the soy sauce and miso paste.
10.   Pour in the wine and cook for 2 mins.
11.   Pour the broth through a strainer into the pot and deglaze.
12.   Close and seal the pot.
13.   Cook on high flame for 5 mins.
14.   Open the lid and stir.
15.   Add herbs and season with salt and pepper before serving.

Nutritional Values

Calories 431, Fat 17g, Chol 0mg, Sodium 71.4mg, Potassium 67.7mg, Carbs 58g, Protein 10g

192. RED CABBAGE WITH APPLES AND PECANS

- Sides - Prep time: 20 mins, Cook time: 15 mins, Total time: 35 mins, Servings: 8, Grill temp: 350°F

Ingredients

- 2 tbsp of extra-virgin olive oil
- 1 large red onion halved and thinly sliced
- 1 tsp of kosher salt

- ¼ cup of apple cider vinegar
- 1 tsp of whole-grain Dijon mustard
- 1 large, crisp apple, such as Fuji, skin on, cored, and thinly sliced
- 1 small red cabbage, cored, quartered, and thinly sliced
- 1 or 2 tbsp of water
- ½ tsp of freshly ground black pepper
- ½ cup of toasted, chopped pecans

Directions

1. In a large nonstick sauté pan or wide, large saucepan over medium-high heat, heat extra-virgin olive oil. Add red onion and kosher salt, and cook, frequently stirring, for 4 or 5 mins, or until the onion is limp.
2. Reduce heat to medium, and remove the pan from the burner for about 30 seconds.
3. Stir in apple cider vinegar and whole-grain Dijon mustard, and stir to coat onions.
4. Return the pan to the burner, and cook for 30 seconds to 1 minute to reduce slightly if needed.
5. Stir in apple and red cabbage. If the mixture looks dry, add 1 tbsp of water. Cover, reduce heat to medium, and cook for 5 mins, stirring once or twice and adding more water as needed.
6. Uncover, stir, and continue to cook until cabbage is crisp-tender.
7. Season with black pepper, and sprinkle with pecans. Serve hot, warm, or cold.
8. To make Toasted Nuts, preheat the oven to 350°F - 180°C. Spread pecans or your favorite nuts on a baking sheet lined with parchment paper and bake, stirring once or twice, for 6 or 7 mins, or until nuts are fragrant and toasty.

Nutritional Values

Calories 113, Fat 1.8g, Chol 0mg, Sodium 71.4mg, Potassium 67.7mg, Carbs 22g, Protein 2.3g

193. FRAGRANT CAULIFLOWER RICE

- Sides - Prep time: 10 mins, Cook time: 1 hour 40 mins, Total time: 1 hour 50 mins, Servings: 4, Grill temp: 350°F

Ingredients

- ¼ cup of chopped onion

- 1 tbsp of vegetable oil
- 1 cup of long-grain rice
- 1 tbsp of minced garlic
- Fourteen ½ ounces of beef broth
- 1 fifteen-ounces can of black beans
- 2 lb. of ground turkey
- 1 cup of whole-kernel corn
- ½ cup of Picante sauce
- ½ cup of crushed tortilla chips
- 1 tsp of taco seasoning
- Cilantro to taste- optional
- Shredded Mexican cheese- optional
- 1 chopped tomato- optional
- Jalapeño pepper as required- optional

Directions

1. Fry the onion in hot oil over medium heat in a large skillet for 5 mins or till tender.
2. Mix in the garlic and rice. For 5 mins, cook and mix until the rice is brown. Include broth of beef. Get it to a boil, and lower the flame.
3. Simmer, covered, until the rice is soft, or for 10 to 15 mins. Mix in the beans, and put down for around 20 mins to cool slightly.
4. Heat the oven to 350° F. Use parchment paper to line a 15x10x1-inch baking pan, and set aside.
5. Combine the turkey, Picante sauce, corn, and taco seasoning crushed chips in a large mixing bowl. Stir in a mixture of rice. Lightly pat the turkey mixture into the 10x5-inch loaf in a prepared baking tray.
6. Put in the oven for 1-¼ to 1-½ hours or till the thermometer registers 165°F when inserted in the loaf center.
7. Let the meatloaf rest for 10 mins. Sprinkle with tomato, cheese, coriander, and sliced jalapeño if needed, and serve with lemon.

Nutritional Values

Calories 343, Fat 11g, Chol 0mg, Sodium 71.4mg, Potassium 67.7mg, Carbs 33g, Protein 28g

194. GARLIC SAUTÉED SPINACH

- Sides - Prep time: 6 mins, Cook time: 10 mins, Total time: 16 mins, Servings: 6, Grill temp: 300°F

Ingredients

- 1 tsp of olive oil
- 6 cups of spinach
- 5 cloves garlic
- 1/8 cup of feta cheese
- 4 tbsp of chopped walnuts

Directions

1. Sauté walnuts garlic in olive oil for around 5 mins, or till garlic is fragrant and tender.
2. Include around ½ of the spinach and mix till spinach is wilted on low heat.
3. Again add the remaining spinach and the cheese, and keep stirring until all is wilted, for about 2 to 3 mins or more. Then It's ready to serve.

Nutritional Values

Calories 109, Fat 13g, Chol 0mg, Sodium 71.4mg, Potassium 67.7mg, Carbs 13g, Protein 3g

195. ROASTED TOMATOES

- Sides - Prep time: 20 mins, Cook time: 60 mins, Total time: 1 hour 20 mins, Servings: 4, Grill temp: 300°F

Ingredients

- 2 lb. of cherry tomatoes halved
- 3 cloves of garlic, sliced very thin
- 2 tbsp of olive oil
- 1 tsp of kosher salt
- ½ tsp of freshly ground black pepper

Directions

1. Preheat the oven to 300°F - 150°C. Arrange 2 racks in the lower third of the oven.
2. Divide cherry tomatoes, cut side up, between 2 rimmed baking sheets. Insert 1 garlic slice into each ½, drizzle with olive oil, and season lightly with kosher salt and black pepper.
3. Bake for about 1 hour, stirring once or twice, or until tomatoes are reduced and very soft. Serve warm or at room temperature. Leftovers will keep in the refrigerator for up to 3 days.

Nutritional Values

Calories 223, Fat 3.8g, Chol 0mg, Sodium 71.4mg, Potassium 67.7mg, Carbs 32g, Protein 2.3g

196. SAUTÉED BROCCOLI RABE

- Sides - Prep time: 5 mins, Cook time: 10 mins, Total time: 15 mins, Servings: 4, Grill temp: 300°F

Ingredients

- 1 large bunch of broccoli rabe, about 1 lb.
- 1 tsp of kosher salt
- 2 tbsp of extra-virgin olive oil
- 3 cloves of garlic, thinly sliced
- ½ tsp of crushed red pepper flakes

Directions

1. Wash broccoli rabe, and trim off the tough bottom end of each stem- about ½ inch, 1.25cm.
2. In a medium saucepan over high heat, bring enough water to cover the broccoli rabe by 1 inch- 2.5cm to a boil. Add ½ tsp kosher salt and broccoli rabe, blanch for 1 minute, transfer to an ice bath to cool quickly, drain, and set aside.
3. In a medium sauté pan over medium heat, heat extra-virgin olive oil, and garlic. When garlic begins to sizzle and turns a golden color- but before it browns, add broccoli rabe, toss to combine, and cook, frequently stirring, for 5 mins, or until broccoli rabe is tender.
4. Season with the remaining 1 tsp of kosher salt and crushed red pepper flakes, and serve immediately.

Nutritional Values

Calories 113, Fat 1.8g, Chol 0mg, Sodium 71.4mg, Potassium 67.7mg, Carbs 22g, Protein 2.3g

197. SAUTÉED ZUCCHINI AND CHERRY TOMATOES

- Sides - Prep time: 15 mins, Cook time: 15 mins, Total time: 30 mins, Servings: 4, Grill temp: 300°F

Ingredients

- 2 tbsp of olive oil
- 1 tsp of salt
- 1 chopped red onion
- 1 tbsp of chopped basil
- 1-pint cherry tomatoes
- 1 lb. of zucchini

- 2 chopped garlic cloves
- ¼ tsp of powdered black pepper

Directions

1. Heat the olive oil in a saucepan. Add red onions and cook until soft and pale purple, frequently stirring, for 8 mins. Don't transform brown.
2. Add the tomatoes, zucchini, garlic, pepper, and salt and cook for 4 mins, frequently stirring, until the tomatoes have started to create a little bit of sauce.
3. Stir in the basil, then, if necessary, taste and adjust the seasoning.
4. Transfer to a serving dish and garnish with more fresh basil.- if needed.

Nutritional Values

Calories 104, Fat 7g, Chol 0mg, Sodium 71.4mg, Potassium 67.7mg, Carbs 9g, Protein 2g

198. SESAME ASPARAGUS

- Sides - Prep time: 5 mins, Cook time: 40 mins, Total time: 45 mins, Servings: 4, Grill temp: 400°F

Ingredients

- 1 lb. of slender asparagus spears
- 1 tbsp of dark sesame oil
- 1 tsp of kosher salt
- ½ tsp of freshly ground black pepper
- 1 tbsp of toasted sesame seeds or gomasio

Directions

1. Preheat the oven to 400°F -200°C, or preheat a grill for direct, high heat. Line a baking sheet with parchment paper.
2. Grasp an asparagus spear and gently bend to snap off the tough bottom of the spear. Trim the remaining spears to this length, and peel lower 2/3 of the asparagus stem. Place on the baking sheet, and toss with sesame oil, kosher salt, and black pepper.
3. Roast for 8 mins, or grill over direct heat, turning once or twice, for about 5 mins or until asparagus is tender.- When you pick up a single spear with a pair of tongs, and it droops slightly, it's done. Serve hot, warm, or cold, sprinkled with toasted sesame seeds.

Nutritional Values

Calories 223, Fat 3.8g, Chol 0mg, Sodium 76.4mg, Potassium 54mg, Carbs 32g, Protein 2.3g

199. SESAME GINGER BROCCOLI

- Sides - Prep time: 10 mins, Cook time: 10 mins, Total time: 20 mins, Servings: 5, Grill temp: 300°F

Ingredients

- 1 large head of fresh broccoli
- 1 tsp of kosher salt
- 2 tbsp of light sesame oil
- 2 cloves of garlic, thinly sliced
- 1 tsp of freshly grated ginger
- 1 tsp of gomasio

Directions

1. Wash broccoli and separate florets into small pieces. Peel broccoli stem and slice into 1 /4 -inch- .5cm rounds.
2. Prepare an ice-water bath for broccoli.
3. Bring a medium pot of water to a boil over high heat, and add kosher salt. Blanch broccoli and stems for 2 mins, or just until crisp-tender. Using tongs, immediately remove from boiling water and plunge into an ice bath. Drain and set aside.
4. In a large sauté pan over medium-high heat, heat sesame oil. Add garlic and ginger, and stir for 1 minute.
5. Add broccoli, and cook for 2 mins. 6 Sprinkle with gomasio and serve immediately.

Nutritional Values

Calories 214, Fat 3.8g, Chol 0mg, Sodium 71.4mg, Potassium 67.7mg, Carbs 22g, Protein 2.3g

200. SMOKY LIMA BEANS

- Sides - Prep time: 25 mins, Cook time: 40 mins, Total time: 1 hour 5 mins, Servings: 12, Grill temp: 300°F

Ingredients

- Twelve cups of water
- 2 pounds of dry large lima beans
- ⅛ cup of Colgin liquid smoke
- 1 tsp of onion powder

- 1 tsp of garlic powder
- Salt and pepper to taste

1. Rinse beans before putting them into the pot with water.
2. Add onion and garlic powder, and close the lid.
3. Cook for about 25 mins.
4. Add salt and liquid smoke.
5. Taste and add more seasonings if necessary.
6. Bring to boil for 10 mins.
7. Simmer for 20-30 mins until thickened.

Nutritional Values

Calories 213, Fat 0g, Chol 0mg, Sodium 71.4mg, Potassium 67.7mg, Carbs 40g, Protein 16g

201. SOUTHERN SWEET POTATOES WITH PECAN STREUSEL

- Sides/Main course - Prep time: 10 mins, Cook time: 50 mins, Total time: 60 mins, Servings: 8, Grill temp: 350°F

Ingredients

- 2 lb. of sweet potatoes, peeled and cut into 2-in.- 5cm chunks
- 2 tbsp plus ¼ cup of plant-based butter
- 2 tbsp of plus ¼ cup of brown sugar, lightly packed
- ½ tsp of ground cinnamon
- ½ tsp of kosher salt
- ¼ tsp of freshly ground black pepper
- ¼ cup of all-purpose flour
- ¼ cup of chopped walnuts
- Pinch cayenne

Directions

1. Preheat the oven to 350°F - 180°C. Line a baking sheet with parchment paper. Lightly coat an 8×8-inch- 20×20cm baking pan with cooking spray.
2. In a large pot fitted with a steamer basket over medium-high heat, bring 1 inch- 2.5cm water to a boil. Place sweet potatoes in the basket, cover, and cook for 10 mins, or until potatoes are tender. Cool slightly.
3. Place sweet potatoes in a medium bowl, and using a potato masher, mash until smooth.

4. Stir in 2 tbsp of butter, 2 tbsp of brown sugar, cinnamon, kosher salt, and black pepper. Spread the sweet potato mixture evenly on the bottom of the baking pan.
5. To make the streusel, in a medium bowl, combine all-purpose flour, the remaining quarter cup of brown sugar, walnuts, and cayenne.
6. Cut the remaining quarter cup of butter into small chunks, sprinkle over the flour mixture, and use your hands to rub the mixture until it begins to stick together.
7. Sprinkle streusel over sweet potatoes, and bake for about 20 mins or until golden.
8. Serve immediately.

Nutritional Values

Calories 223, Fat 3.8g, Chol 0mg, Sodium 61.4mg, Potassium 57.7mg, Carbs 32g, Protein 2.3g

202. SOUTHERN-STYLE BRAISED GREENS

- Sides - Prep time: 15 mins, Cook time: 35 mins, Total time: 50 mins, Servings: 4 to 6, Grill temp: 300°F

Ingredients

- 4 cups of vegetable stock
- ¼ cup of extra-virgin olive oil
- 1 tsp of smoked sea salt
- ½ tsp of freshly ground black pepper
- 2 cloves of garlic, crushed and finely chopped
- 1 large bunch of collard greens, tough stems removed, cut into small pieces
- 1 large bunch of mustard greens, tough stems removed, cut into small pieces
- 1 large bunch of curly kale, tough stems removed, cut into small pieces
- 1 tbsp of apple cider vinegar or juice of a ½ lemon

Directions

1. In a large saucepan or soup pot over high heat, combine vegetable stock, extra-virgin olive oil, smoked sea salt, black pepper, and garlic. Bring to a boil.
2. Stir in collard greens, mustard greens, and curly kale. Reduce heat to medium, and cook, uncovered and occasionally stirring, for about 35 mins or until greens are

tender. Adjust heat to maintain a gentle simmer.

3. Season greens with apple cider vinegar, and serve with a little of the liquid that remains in the pot-pot liquor.

Calories 113, Fat 1.8g, Chol 0mg, Sodium 71.4mg, Potassium 67.7mg, Carbs 22g, Protein 2.3g

203. STEAMED ARTICHOKES

- Sides - Prep time: 10 mins, Cook time: 20 mins, Total time: 30 mins, Servings: 6, Grill temp: 300°F

Ingredients

- 6 long, narrow artichokes
- 3 smashed garlic cloves
- 2 cups of water
- 2 cups of olive oil
- Juice of 1 lemon
- 1 sliced lemon
- 1 tbsp of whole peppercorns

Directions

1. Pour 2 cups of water, lemon juice, lemon slices, and peppercorns into a pressure cooker.
2. Prepare artichokes by tearing off the tough leaves on the outside, peeling the stem, cutting off the end of the stem, and cutting the top ½ off of the leaves horizontally, so you end up with what looks like a hat. Pry open the leaves and take out the hairy, hard part to access the heart, leaving the dotty part where the hairy part was attached.
3. Open the leaves up a bit more and dip them in the pressure cooker, head down, and swirl around before putting them in the steamer basket.
4. Put a basket with artichokes in the pressure cooker.
5. Close and seal the lid.
6. Cook on high pressure for 5 mins.
7. When time is up, quick-release the pressure after turning off the cooker.
8. Shake the artichokes and put them in a strainer for 15 mins to dry out.

9. In a pan, heat up about 2 centimeters of oil and just fry the artichokes head down until their edges start to turn golden.
10. Plate and dab with a paper towel to remove excess oil before serving.

Nutritional Values

Calories 40, Fat 2g, Chol 0mg, Sodium 71.4mg, Potassium 67.7mg, Carbs 3g, Protein 1g

204. SWEET THAI COCONUT RICE

- Sides - Prep time: 10 mins, Cook time: 25 mins, Total time: 35 mins, Servings: 4, Grill temp: 300°F

Ingredients

- 1 ½ cups of water
- 1 cup of Thai sweet rice
- ½ can of full-Fat coconut milk
- 2 tbsp of sugar
- Dash of salt

Directions

1. Mix rice and water in your pressure cooker.
2. Cook for just 3 mins on high pressure.
3. When time is up, turn it off and wait 10 mins for a natural release.
4. In the meanwhile, heat coconut milk, sugar, and salt in a saucepan.
5. When the sugar has melted, remove it from the heat.
6. When the cooker has released its pressure, mix the coconut milk mixture into your rice and stir.
7. Put the lid back on and let it rest for 5-10 mins without returning it to pressure.
8. Serve and enjoy!

Nutritional Values

Calories 269, Fat 8g, Chol 0mg, Sodium 71.4mg, Potassium 67.7mg, Carbs 47g, Protein 4g

205. VEGAN-WELSH-RAREBIT & MUSHROOMS

- Snack - Prep time: ready in about: 30 mins, Servings: 8, Grill temp: Medium

Ingredients

- 1 thinly sliced onion
- 1 8 oz. packages of cremini mushrooms

- ¼ tsp of crushed dried thyme
- 2 tbsp of English mustard or Dijon-style
- 1 15 oz. can of beans
- 2 tbsp of nutritional yeast
- Sea salt and black pepper
- 2 tbsp of almond butter or cashew butter
- 4 sprouted toasted and split English muffins
- Chopped parsley
- Paprika

Directions

1. Combine onion, mushrooms, thyme, & 1 cup of water in a large pan.
2. Bring to a low simmer, covered, over medium heat.
3. Cook for 10 mins, or until the mushrooms & onion pieces are soft. Uncover and heat for another 1 to 2 mins or until the liquid has almost evaporated.
4. Meanwhile, put the following 4 ingredients- through the nut butter and ½ cup of boiling water in a blender.
5. Cover and puree until smooth. In a mixing bowl, combine the mushrooms and the sauce.
6. Cook for 1 to 2 mins or until the sauce has thickened. Salt & pepper to taste.
7. Preheat the oven to broil. Set toasted muffins on a baking sheet to assemble. Add the mushroom mixture on top.
8. Broil for 5 - 6 mins, or until gently browned on the surface, at 4 to 5 inches from the flame.
9. Paprika & parsley are sprinkled over the top.

Nutritional Values

Calories 245kcal, Carbs 18g, Protein 16g, Fat 10g, Sodium 427mg, Potassium 442mg, Chol 0mg

206. AIR-FRYER ONION-RINGS

- Snack - Prep time: ready in about: 35 mins, Servings: 4, Grill temp: Medium

Ingredients

- ½ tsp of garlic powder
- 1¼ cup of bread crumbs
- ½ tsp of onion powder
- 2 eggs
- ½ tsp of sea salt

- ½ cup of flour, all-purpose
- Olive oil, Extra-virgin
- 1 yellow onion
- Tartar Sauce

Directions

1. Combine the panko, onion powder, garlic powder, and salt on the rimmed tray.
2. Gently beat eggs in a shallow bowl. In a separate small bowl, put the flour.
3. Preheat the air fryer to a temperature of 370°F.
4. Every onion ring should be dipped in flour and then tapped to remove extra flour.
5. Place it on a big plate after dipping it in egg and coating it with panko mixture.
6. Spray onion rings using olive oil and place them in a thin layer in an air fryer basket with some space between them.
7. Make sure the basket isn't too full. If necessary, work in bunches.
8. Cook for around 11 min.
9. Repeat with the rest of the onion rings. If preferred, serve with tartar sauce.

Nutritional Values

Calories 272kcal, Carbs 30.2g, Protein 8g, Fat 15g, Sodium 886mg, Potassium 714mg, Chol 0mg

207. WASABI-GINGER-BEET & AVOCADO WITH TARTINES

- Snack - Prep time: ready in about: 15 mins, Servings: 4, Grill temp: Medium-low

Ingredients

- 1 tsp of fresh ginger, grated
- 2½ tsp of unseasoned apple cider or rice vinegar
- 1 shredded beet
- 2 seeded and halved avocados
- Sea salt and black pepper
- 1-2 tsp of wasabi paste
- ¾ cup of alfalfa sprouts or broccoli sprouts
- 4 slices of toasted rye

Directions

1. Combine 1½ tsp Vinegar as well as ginger in a mixing dish.
2. Toss in the beets to coat. Salt & pepper to taste.

3. Remove the avocado flesh and place it in a separate dish. Avocado, wasabi paste, as well as the remaining 1 tsp vinegar, are mashed together.
4. Salt & pepper to taste.
5. To finish, spoon the avocado mixture onto the bread pieces. Beets & sprouts go on top.

Nutritional Values

Calories 212kcal, Carbs 14g, Protein 14.2g, Fat 10g, Sodium 637mg, Potassium 425mg, Chol 0mg

208. ROASTED-KABOCHA SQUASH

- Snack - Prep time: ready in about: 50 mins, Servings: 4-6, Grill temp: Medium

Ingredients

- 2 tbsp of olive oil, extra-virgin
- 1 kabocha squash
- Sea salt and black pepper
- Microgreens
- ¼ cup of chopped scallions
- Ginger Sesame Dressing
- Sesame seeds

Directions

1. Preheat your oven to 425°F and cook the squash for around 10 mins in the oven to make slicing easier.
2. Line 2 baking pans using parchment paper.
3. Dice squash lengthwise in ½, remove the ribbing and seeds, then slice into 112-inch slices.
4. The olive oil over the slices, season with salt & pepper, & roast for around 30 mins, turning halfway through. On a shallow dish, position the squash.
5. Drizzle using dressing and top with sesame seeds, scallions, and microgreens, if desired.
6. Serve with additional salt & pepper to taste.

Nutritional Values

Calories 282kcal, Carbs 30g, Protein 8.9g, Fat 15g, Sodium 888mg, Potassium 734mg, Chol 0mg

209. ROASTED PUMPKIN-SEEDS

- Snack - Prep time: ready in about: 65 mins, Servings: 4, Grill temp: Medium-high

Ingredients

- ½ tsp of olive oil, extra-virgin
- Chili Powder
- 1 cup of pumpkin seeds
- ¼ tsp of sea salt

Directions

1. To detach the seeds from the flesh, scoop the seeds from the pumpkin and immerse them in a bucket of water.
2. Rinse seeds in a sieve to remove any extra flesh.
3. To dry the seeds, place them in 1 layer on a kitchen towel.
4. Preheat your oven to 300°F and line parchment paper on a baking sheet.
5. Drizzle olive oil & salt over the seeds in a dish and stir to coat.
6. Roast for 45 mins, mixing halfway through.
7. Serve with a pinch of chili powder on top.

Nutritional Values

Calories 262kcal, Carbs 20g, Protein 8g, Fat 15g, Sodium 886mg, Potassium 934mg, Chol 0mg

210. AVOCADO FRIES

- Snack - Prep time: ready in about: 30 mins, Servings: 4, Grill temp: Medium

Ingredients

- 1 tsp of coriander
- ¾ cup of bread crumbs
- 1 tsp of cumin
- ½ cup of flour, all-purpose
- 1 tsp of sea salt
- 2 beaten eggs
- Olive oil, Extra-virgin
- 2 avocados
- Chipotle Ranch

Directions

1. Preheat your oven to 425°F and place parchment paper on a baking pan.
2. Combine the panko, cumin, coriander, and salt in a shallow dish.
3. Put the flour in 1 bowl and the egg in another small 1.
4. Peel avocados & cut them into 8 pieces lengthwise.

5. After coating each piece in flour and brushing off any excess, dip it in egg, then into the panko mixture.
6. Sprinkle with olive oil & place on a baking sheet.
7. Bake for around 14 mins.

Calories 212kcal, Carbs 30g, Protein 9g, Fat 10g, Sodium 886mg, Potassium 734mg, Chol 0mg

211. BAKED POTATO-WEDGES

- Snack - Prep time: ready in about: 55 mins, Servings: 4, Grill temp: Medium

Ingredients

- 2 tbsp of olive oil, extra-virgin
- 4 russet potatoes
- 1½ tsp of garlic powder
- ¾ tsp of onion powder
- 1 tsp of sea salt
- ¾ tsp of smoked paprika
- Chopped parsley
- Ketchup, Tartar Sauce, and/or mustard
- Black pepper
- Parmesan cheese, grated

Directions

1. Preheat your oven to 425°F and line 2 baking sheets using parchment paper.
2. Toss potatoes with olive oil, salt, garlic powder, smoked paprika, onion powder, and a few grinds of pepper in a big mixing bowl, then lay them out equally on baking sheets.
3. Roast for 45 mins, tossing and rotating pans in the oven at the 20-minute mark.
4. Sprinkle fresh parsley & Parmesan cheese, if desired. Season with a pinch of salt.
5. Serves with the dipping sauces of your choice.

Nutritional Values

Calories 272kcal, Carbs 30g, Protein 8g, Fat 15g, Sodium 886mg, Potassium 734mg, Chol 0mg

212. INSTANT-POT MASHED-POTATOES

- Snack - Prep time: ready in about: 25 mins, Servings: 8, Grill temp: Medium-low

Ingredients

- 6 cups of water
- 4 pounds of Yukon gold potatoes
- 4 tsp of sea salt
- ⅓ cup of olive oil, extra-virgin
- 3 grated cloves of garlic
- ¼ cup of unsalted butter
- Chives
- Black pepper

Directions

1. In the Instant Pot bowl, combine the water, potatoes, and 2 tbsp of salt.
2. Place the cover on Instant Pot and set the pressure to high.
3. Cook for around 12 mins.
4. Quickly release pressure & drain, reserving ¾ cup of boiling water.
5. Add the olive oil, garlic, butter, as well as the leftover 2 tbsp sea salt to the saucepan.
6. Mash the potatoes well using a potato masher. Using a rubber spatula, whisk & mash potatoes till creamy, adding the leftover cooking water ¼ cup at a time. As required, stir in the remaining cooking water to get the appropriate consistency.
7. Garnish using chives & fresh black pepper.

Nutritional Values

Calories 372kcal, Carbs 20g, Protein 8g, Fat 15g, Sodium 886mg, Potassium 634mg, Chol 0mg

213. HOMEMADE GRANOLA

- Snack - Prep time: ready in about: 40 mins, Servings: 4-6, Grill temp: Medium

Ingredients

- ½ cup of chopped walnuts
- 2 cups of oats, whole rolled
- ½ cup of coconut flakes
- ½ tsp of sea salt
- 2 tsp of cinnamon
- 2 tbsp of coconut oil, melted
- 2 tbsp of almond butter, creamy
- ¼ cup of maple syrup
- 1/3 cup of dried cranberries

Directions

1. Preheat the oven to 300°F and line parchment paper on a baking sheet.

2. Combine the walnuts, oats, coconut flakes, cinnamon, & salt in a medium mixing bowl.
3. Add almond butter once the coconut oil & maple syrup has been drizzled in. Stir until everything is well blended.
4. Scoop granola onto a baking sheet and shape it into an oval of 1-inch thickness with your hands. This will facilitate the formation of clumps.
5. Bake for around 15 mins, flip the pan at ½ time through baking, and carefully break up the granola with a fork.
6. Bake for a further 15 mins. If desired, top with cranberries. Allow 15 mins to cool before serving.

Nutritional Values
Calories 282kcal, Carbs 30g, Protein 8g, Fat 10g, Sodium 886mg, Potassium 734mg, Chol 0mg

214. HOMEMADE TAQUITOS

- Snack - Prep time: ready in about: 55 mins, Servings: 6-8, Grill temp: Medium

Ingredients
- 1 tsp of olive oil, extra-virgin
- 1 can of Jackfruit
- 2 grated garlic cloves
- 1 tsp of coriander
- 1 tsp of cumin
- Pinch of cayenne pepper
- Black pepper
- ½ tsp of sea salt
- 1 can of green chilies
- ¾ cup of refried beans
- 12-14 flour tortillas
- ½ cup of jack cheese
- Olive oil
- ¼ cup of chopped scallions
- Guacamole, cilantro, Pico de Gallo, serranos

Directions
1. Preheat the oven to 400°F and line parchment paper on a baking sheet.
2. Toss jackfruit with olive oil, cumin, garlic, coriander, salt, cayenne, and a few grinds of pepper on the baking sheet. Stir in the green chilies. On a baking sheet, distribute in a thin layer.
3. Bake for 18 mins. Remove pan from heat.

4. Heat the tortillas on a baking sheet lined with parchment paper for 5 mins. Place a refried bean strip at the tortilla's left edge.
5. Sprinkle part of the jackfruit mixture, cheese, & scallions.
6. Tuck & roll the tortillas into taquitos, then gently place them on the baking sheet. If required, toothpicks may be used to keep them in place.
7. Cook for 20 mins, sprayed liberally with cooking spray.

Nutritional Values
Calories 282kcal, Carbs 30g, Protein 8g, Fat 19g, Sodium 886mg, Potassium 734mg, Chol 0mg

215. SHEET-PAN-NACHOS

- Snack - Prep time: ready in about: 30 mins, Servings: 2, Grill temp: Medium

Ingredients
- Cheese, vegan
- Tortilla-Chips
- Taco-Meat
- 2 tbsp chopped scallions
- Pico-de-Gallo, chopped
- 1 jalapeno, sliced
- Pickled Onions
- Lime wedges- for serving
- Sliced avocado/Guacamole
- 1 tbsp cilantro, chopped

Directions
1. On a dish, arrange tortilla chips.
2. Drizzle cheese sauce and top with taco "meat, " scallions, tomato, serrano, radishes, avocado, and pickled onions.
3. Serve using lime wedges for juicing and a garnish of cilantro.

Nutritional Values
Calories 332kcal, Carbs 30g, Protein 8g, Fat 15g, Sodium 686mg, Potassium 834mg, Chol 0mg

216. CRISPY-ROASTED-CHICKPEAS

- Snack - Prep time: ready in about: 35 mins, Servings: 2 cups, Grill temp: Medium

Ingredients
- olive oil

- Paprika or curry powder-optional
- 1 ½ cups of cooked chickpeas
- Sea salt

Directions

1. Preheat the oven to 425°F and line parchment paper on a baking sheet.
2. To dry chickpeas, lay them out on a kitchen towel.
3. Discard any skins that have come loose.
4. Toss dry chickpeas with a splash of olive oil and a few pinches of salt on the baking sheet.
5. Roast for 30 mins or. Take out of the oven and stir with your preferred spices.
6. Roasted chickpeas should be kept at room temperature in a container.

Nutritional Values

Calories 222kcal, Carbs 30g, Protein 8g, Fat 15g, Sodium 886mg, Potassium 734mg, Chol 0mg

217. ROASTED CAULIFLOWER & LEMON ZEST

- Snack - Prep time: ready in about: 32 mins, Servings: 4, Grill temp: Medium

Ingredients

- olive oil, extra-virgin
- 1 cauliflower
- sea salt and black pepper
- ¼ cup of chopped parsley
- 1 lemon, zest

Directions

1. Preheat the oven to 425°F and line parchment paper on a baking sheet.
2. Cauliflower should be broken into florets of bite-size.
3. Spread equally on a baking sheet after tossing with salt, olive oil, and pepper.
4. Roast for 30 mins. Season using pepper and salt to taste, then mix with lemon zest & parsley.

Nutritional Values

Calories 272kcal, Carbs 30g, Protein 9.8g, Fat 15g, Sodium 886mg, Potassium 734mg, Chol 0mg

218. HOMEMADE SALSA

- Snack - Prep time: ready in about: 10 mins, Servings: 4, Grill temp: Medium

Ingredients

- 1 clove of garlic
- ¼ white onion, chopped
- 1 lb. tomatoes, chunks
- ¼ cup of cilantro
- 1 jalapeño
- Juice & zest of a lime
- ¼ tsp cumin
- ½ tsp sea salt
- Sugar, a pinch

Directions

1. Combine onion & garlic in a blender. Pulse until everything is finely chopped.
2. Combine tomatoes, jalapeño, cilantro, lime zest, lime juice, cumin, salt, and sugar in a large bowl.
3. Pulse until everything is well blended yet still chunky. The texture of this salsa is determined by the amount of water in the tomatoes.
4. Filter ½ of it to eliminate part of the liquid if it's overly watery.
5. Combine the leftover salsa with a chunky strained mixture. If you still want a chunkier texture, squeeze out additional liquid until you have the texture you want.

Nutritional Values

Calories 292kcal, Carbs 30g, Protein 8g, Fat 15g, Sodium 786mg, Potassium 734mg, Chol 0mg

219. MANGO SALSA

- Snack - Prep time: ready in about: 20 mins, Servings: 3-4, Grill temp: Medium

Ingredients

- ¼ cup red onion
- 2 ripe mangos
- ¼ cup chopped cilantro
- ¼ tsp sea salt
- 1 clove of garlic
- Juice + zest of a lime
- ½ minced jalapeño

Directions

1. Peel & dice the mangos.

2. Combine the onion, mango, cilantro, garlic, lime juice, jalapeno, & salt in a medium mixing basin. Refrigerate until set to use.

Calories 272kcal, Carbs 30g, Protein 7.9g, Fat 15g, Sodium 886mg, Potassium 734mg, Chol 0mg

220. FRENCH-ONION-DIP

- Snack - Prep time: ready in about: 30 mins, Servings: 4, Grill temp: Medium

Ingredients

- ½ cup of Onions, caramelized and cooled
- 1 Cashew-Sour-Cream
- ¼ tsp onion powder
- black pepper
- Potato chips
- ½ tsp sea salt
- 2 tbsp chives, chopped

Directions

1. Combine the sour cream, caramelized onions, salt, onion powder, and several pinches of pepper in a mixing bowl.
2. Refrigerate for 1 hour, covered.
3. Serve with chives and potato chips on top of the cooling dip.

Nutritional Values

Calories 375kcal, Carbs 15g, Protein 7g, Fat 17g, Sodium 527mg, Potassium 834mg, Chol 0mg

221. TOMATILLO-SALSA-VERDE

- Snack - Prep time: ready in about: 30 mins, Servings: 2, Grill temp: Medium

Ingredients

- ¼ onion chunks form
- 6 tomatillos
- 1 jalapeño pepper
- 1 ½ tbsp olive oil
- 2 cloves of garlic cloves
- 1 ½ tbsp lime juice
- ½-¾ tsp sea salt
- ¼ cup of chopped cilantro

Directions

1. Preheat your oven to 450°F and prepare a baking sheet using parchment paper.

2. Eliminate the tomatillos' husks and rinse them under cold water.
3. Toss the onion, tomatillos, and pepper with olive oil on the baking sheet and add salt.
4. Place garlic cloves covered in foil on the pan.
5. Tomatillos should be tender after 15 mins of roasting.
6. Remove garlic cloves from the foil and set them in a food processor.
7. Add roasted veggies, lime juice, & cilantro & pulse. If your salsa is overly thick, thin it up with 2 tbsp water until it reaches the required consistency. Season as per taste. Serve with tortilla chips or your favorite Mexican dish.

Nutritional Values

Calories 155kcal, Carbs 14g, Protein 16g, Fat 10g, Sodium 627mg, Potassium 544mg, Chol 0mg

222. COWBOY CAVIAR

- Snack - Prep time: ready in about: 25 mins, Servings: 8, Grill temp: Medium

Ingredients

- 1 ½ cups of black-eyed peas, cooked
- 1 ½ cups of black beans, cooked
- 2 cups of cherry tomatoes
- 1 bell pepper
- 1 cup of corn kernels
- ½ cup of diced onion
- juice of lime
- 1 jalapeño pepper, chopped
- 2 avocados, diced
- tortilla chips
- ¼ cup of cilantro
- 2 tbsp red-wine-vinegar
- 1 tsp cumin
- 2 tbsp of olive oil
- ½ tsp cayenne
- ½ tsp black pepper
- 1 clove of garlic
- ½ tsp honey
- 1 ½ tsp of sea salt

Directions

1. Combine the peas, black beans, tomatoes, bell pepper, corn, onion, jalapeño, & lime juice in a mixing bowl.

2. Mix together the oil, vinegar, cumin, honey, cayenne, garlic, salt, & pepper in a separate bowl. Overbean mixture, pour dressing. Season as per taste after adding the avocado & cilantro. Chill for 1 hour.
3. Serve with tortilla chips before serving.

223. AIR FRYER-FRENCH-FRIES

- Snack - Prep time: ready in about: 30 mins, Servings: 4, Grill temp: Medium

Ingredients

- olive oil
- 2 potatoes
- sea salt

Directions

1. Preheat your air fryer to 380°F. Drizzle olive oil over the potatoes, season with salt, & toss to coat.
2. Place potatoes in a thin layer in the air fryer basket, making sure they are not touching. You'll need to work in groups.
3. Air fried for 15 mins, turning halfway through. If your fries aren't crisp enough, air-fry them for a few mins longer.
4. Serve with dips & spices.

224. BAKED-SWEET-POTATO-FRIES

- Snack - Prep time: ready in about: 80 mins, Servings: 4-5, Grill temp: Medium

Ingredients

- olive oil
- 2 lb. sweet potatoes
- Sea salt
- fresh herbs
- Chipotle-Sauce- for dipping
- Red-pepper-flakes

Directions

1. Preheat the oven to 450°F and line 2 rimmed baking sheets with parchment paper. Soak sweet potatoes for 30 mins in a big dish of cold water. Afterward, drain and pat dry.
2. Drizzle a little amount of olive oil over the top and stir to coat.
3. Place the potatoes on sheets in an equal layer, leaving space between each fry. Cook for around 38 mins. Flip the potatoes midway through.
4. Remove the pan from the oven & season with sea salt.
5. Mix with herbs & red pepper flakes, then season to taste with mustard/ketchup.

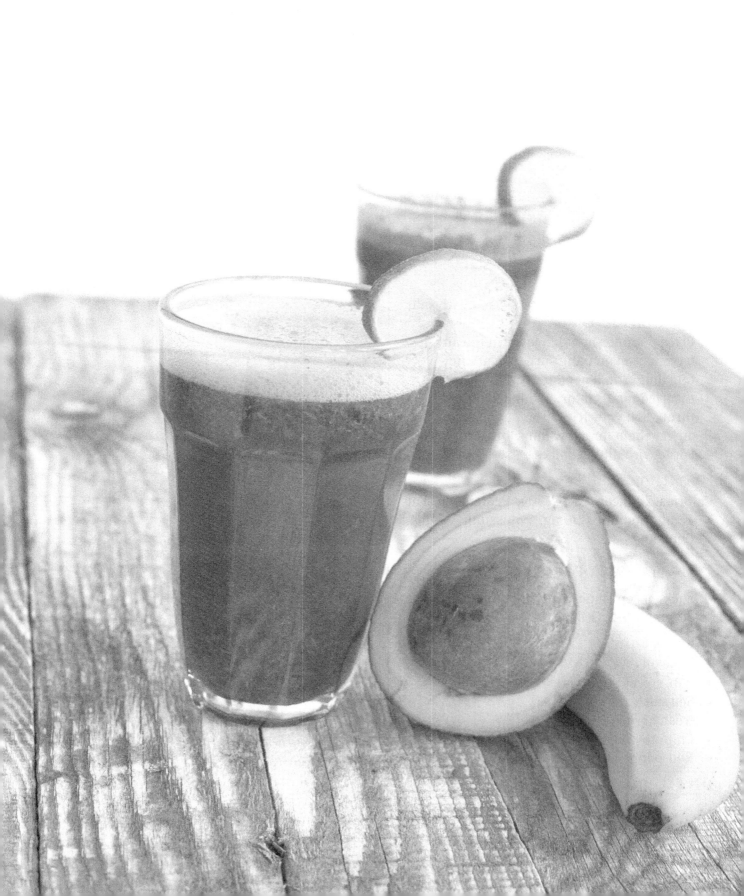

Chapter 8.

Supper & Savory Bowls

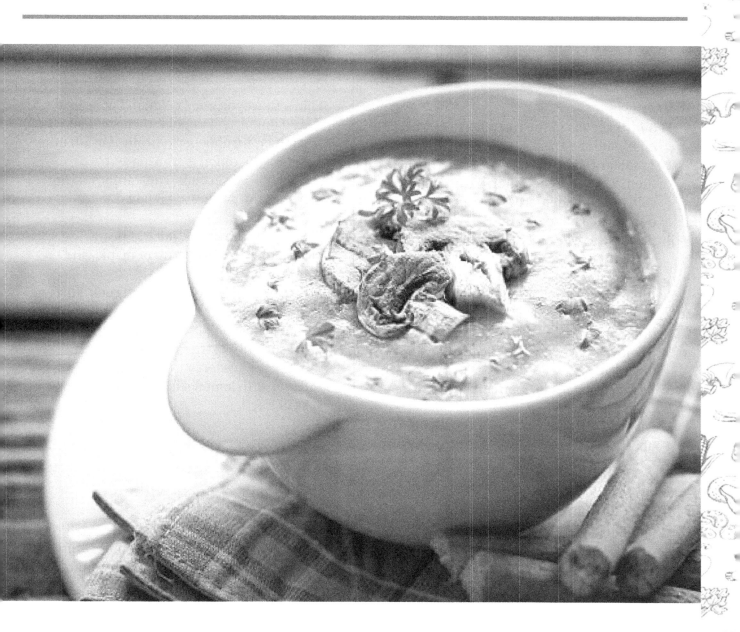

225. INSTANT-POT-BLACK-BEANS

- Lunch - Prep time: ready in about: 45 mins, Servings: 8, Grill temp: Medium

Ingredients

- 6 cups of water
- 2 cups of black beans
- ½ cup of onion- diced
- 2 tsp of salt
- 2 cloves of garlic
- juice of lime, optional
- 1 tsp of chili powder
- 1 tsp of oregano
- 1 tsp of cumin
- black pepper

Directions

1. Sift the beans in the colander to extract and eliminate the trash.
2. Transfer the beans to a Pot after rinsing them. Combine the water, garlic, onion, salt, chili powder, oregano, salt, and black pepper in a bowl.
3. Place the cover on Pot and set the pressure to high. Cook for about 25 mins on high flame.
4. Allow the Pot to automatically release pressure. It will take between 20 to 30 mins.
5. Remove the cover after the float lever has dropped.
6. Use these beans in your current favorite bean recipe.
7. Season with extra salt, peppers, and lime if necessary.

Nutritional Values

Calories 325kcal, Carbs 14g, Protein 7g, Fat 10g, Sodium 627mg, Potassium 384mg, Chol 0mg

226. BLACK-BEAN-CHILI

- Lunch - Prep time: ready in about: 40 mins, Servings: 8, Grill temp: Medium

Ingredients

- 1 onion, chopped
- 1 tbsp of olive oil- extra-virgin
- 1 diced bell pepper
- 3 cloves of garlic
- 1 ½ tsp of salt
- 3 tbsp of chili powder
- 1 can of roasted tomatoes
- 3 cups of black beans
- 1 can of green chilies
- black pepper
- 1 tsp of maple syrup
- 1 tbsp of lime juice
- Greek yogurt
- ¼ tsp of cayenne- optional
- Tortilla chips
- Avocado
- Cilantro
- Sliced jalapeños
- Pickled onions

Directions

1. In a saucepan over medium flame, heat oil. Add onion, and pepper, then salt and simmer, turning periodically, for 5-8 mins before the onion is transparent.
2. Cook for 30 seconds, constantly stirring, before the garlic & chili powder are aromatic.
3. Combine the beans, juice of beans, tomatoes, chilies, syrup of maple, and pepper in a bowl.
4. Reduce the flame to low and cook, stirring periodically, for twenty mins or when the chili is thickened.
5. Season with extra salt, chili powder, & pepper, if preferred.
6. Serve with lemon slices and other toppings as desired.

Nutritional Values

Calories 265kcal, Carbs 11g, Protein 7g, Fat 10g, Sodium 621mg, Potassium 834mg, Chol 0mg

227. ROASTED-GOLDEN-BEETS

- Lunch - Prep time: ready in about: 1 hr & 15 mins, Servings: 4, Grill temp: Medium

Ingredients

- Lemon Vinaigrette
- 4-5 beets
- ¾ tsp of coriander
- ¼ tsp of cumin
- ½ tsp of honey
- 2 cups of arugula
- 2 tbsp of toasted pistachios
- ¼ cup of crumbled feta

- Sea salt
- Microgreens- optional
- black pepper

Directions

1. Preheat your oven to 400°F.
2. Put every beet on the aluminum foil, spray with olive oil, and season with salt and ground pepper.
3. Cover your beets in foil and bake for 40- 90 mins. The amount of time it takes to boil the beets depends on their size and quality.
4. Remove your beets from the oven, discard the foil, & then let it cool.
5. Peels off beets when they are cold enough to handle.
6. Place the beets in your fridge, sliced into 2 equal parts or bite-sized chunks.
7. On a dish, place the beets, feta, pistachios, and arugula.
8. Sprinkle with salt.
9. Serve with the microgreens on top, if preferred.

Nutritional Values

Calories 165kcal, Carbs 14g, Protein 16g, Fat 10g, Sodium 627mg, Potassium 434mg, Chol 0mg

228. BUTTERNUT-SQUASH-RISOTTO

- Lunch - Prep time: ready in about: 55 mins, Servings: 4, Grill temp: Medium

Ingredients

- 1 chopped onion
- 1 tbsp of olive oil- extra virgin
- ½ tsp of salt
- 2 cups of butternut squash
- black pepper
- 2 cloves of garlic
- 1 cup of Arborio rice
- 1 tsp of rosemary
- ½ cup of wine
- Chopped parsley for garnish
- 4 cups of vegetable broth
- ½ cup of Parmesan cheese for serving

Directions

1. Heat oil on medium flame in a skillet.
2. Simmer for 2 - 3 mins with onion, pepper, and salt.

3. Simmer for another 6- 8 mins with butternut squash.
4. Garlic cloves, rosemary, & rice should all be added at this point. Stir in the wine and simmer for 1 min.
5. Heat for 1–3 mins, and stir occasionally.
6. Pour the broth into a third of a cup and constantly stir to ensure that every round of liquid is soaked before pouring the next.
7. Season with salt to taste.
8. Serve with the cheese if preferred and topped with parsley.

Nutritional Values

Calories 265kcal, Carbs 14g, Protein 7g, Fat 11g, Sodium 627mg, Potassium 834mg, Chol 0mg

229. ARUGULA-SALAD WITH LEMON-VINAIGRETTE

- Lunch - Prep time: ready in about: 20 mins, Servings: 4, Grill temp: Medium

Ingredients

- 1 cup of red grapes- seedless
- ½ cup of almonds
- ¼ cup olive oil- Extra-virgin
- ½ tbsp of tamari
- salt and black pepper
- 6 cups of arugula
- ¼ cup of Lemon vinaigrette
- Parmesan

Directions

1. Preheat your oven to 400°F and line 2 baking pans with parchment paper.
2. In the first pan, arrange the almonds, and in the second pan, arrange the grapes.
3. Sprinkle olive oil over the nuts and grapes, then season with some salt and pepper.
4. Roast your almonds with tamari for 7-10 mins.
5. Bake the grapes for about 7-15 mins. The time will be determined by the size of the grapes.
6. Toss the arugula with the vinaigrette in a bowl.
7. Add your almonds, Parmesan, and grapes to the top.
8. Season with salt and pepper to taste, and then serve.

Nutritional Values

Calories 155kcal, Carbs 14g, Protein 7.4g, Fat 10g, Sodium 627mg, Potassium 834mg, Chol 0mg

230. BROWN RICE

- Lunch - Prep time: ready in about: 60 mins, Servings: 4, Grill temp: Medium

Ingredients

- 2 cups of water
- 1 cup of brown rice, rinsed
- 1 tsp of olive oil- extra-virgin

Directions

1. In a saucepan, bring the washed rice, water, plus olive oil to a boil.
2. Cover, turn to low flame, and cook for about 45 mins.
3. Turn off the heat, then set aside for another 10 mins, undisturbed.
4. Using a fork, fluff the mixture.

Nutritional Values

Calories 155kcal, Carbs 14g, Protein 8g, Fat 10g, Sodium 627mg, Potassium 834mg, Chol 0mg

231. KIMCHI-BROWN-RICE-BLISS-BOWLS

- Lunch - Prep time: ready in about: 40 mins, Servings: 2-3, Grill temp: Medium

Ingredients

- ¼ cup of kimchi
- 1 cup of brown rice
- 1 cucumber
- ½ avocado
- ½ cup of red cabbage
- 8 oz. of Tempeh
- ½ tsp of sesame seeds
- ½ recipe of Peanut Sauce
- 2 Thai chilies
- Microgreens, optional
- Lime wedges for serving

Directions

1. Toss the cucumber, kimchi, rice, cabbage, tempeh, and avocado into the bowls.
2. Top with a considerable quantity of peanut sauce, sesame seeds, as well as chilies.

3. Serve with leftover peanut sauce and lime wedges on the table. If preferred, garnish using microgreens.

Nutritional Values

Calories 265kcal, Carbs 14g, Protein 14g, Fat 10g, Sodium 527mg, Potassium 834mg, Chol 0mg

232. BOX-BUDDHA-BOWLS

- Lunch - Prep time: ready in about: 35 mins, Servings: 4-6, Grill temp: Medium

Ingredients

- Massaged kale
- Brown rice
- Chickpeas, or edamame
- Radishes, cabbage, carrot
- sweet potatoes
- Sauerkraut and pickled ginger
- Sesame seeds
- Lemon sauce

Directions

1. Make your bowls with grain, kale, legumes, cooked vegetable, uncooked vegetable, and fermented vegetables.
2. Drizzle the tahini sauce and sesame seeds on top.
3. Serve with extra tahini sauce.

Nutritional Values

Calories 253kcal, Carbs 33g, Protein 10g, Fat 9g, Sodium 680mg, Potassium 834mg, Chol 0mg

233. CURRIED-LENTIL-SALAD

- Lunch - Prep time: ready in about: 40 mins, Servings: 4, Grill temp: Medium

Ingredients

- 2 tbsp of lemon juice
- 2 ½ cups of green lentils
- 2 garlic cloves
- 1 tsp of cumin
- ½ tbsp of fresh ginger
- 1 tsp of cardamom
- Dressing of Cilantro Lime
- ½ tsp of sea salt
- 1-2 serrano chilies
- Florets from 1 cauliflower
- 4 baked Tofu

- olive oil- Extra-virgin
- 4 cups of spinach
- ¼ tsp of turmeric
- black pepper

Directions

1. Preheat your oven to 425°F and line 2 baking pans using parchment paper.
2. Mix the lime juice, ginger, cumin, garlic, salt, and pepper in the mixing bowl.
3. Toss in the lentils, then whisk to combine. While cooking the original dish, add the chilies of serrano to the processor and prepare the Lime cilantro dressing. Some of the sauce should be mixed into lentils.
4. Place the cauliflower in the second baking pan and the paneer in the first pan.
5. Drizzle each with olive oil, a bit of salt, and pepper.
6. Paneer should be roasted for 15 mins, while cauliflower should be roasted for 20-25 mins.
7. Mix the cauliflower with turmeric as it gets out of the oven.
8. Mix the lentils with the spinach.
9. Add the cauliflower, then bake tofu on top.
10. Sprinkle some more sauce on the top and serve the rest on the table.

Nutritional Values

Calories 558 kcal, Carbs 76.3g, Protein 16.2g, Fat 23.5g, Sodium 607mg, Potassium 834mg, Chol 0mg

234. CINNAMON-ROASTED-SWEET-POTATO-SALAD WITH WILD-RICE

- Lunch - Prep time: ready in about: 40 mins, Servings: 4, Grill temp: Medium

Ingredients

- 1 onion
- 12 ounces of sweet potatoes
- 4 tbsp of olive oil
- ½ tsp of black pepper
- 1 tsp of salt
- ¼ tsp of cinnamon
- 1 tbsp of curry powder
- 2 tbsp of rice vinegar
- 2 tbsp of honey
- ¼ tbsp of black pepper
- ½ tbsp of salt
- ¼ cup of cilantro

- 2 cups of rice
- ¼ cup of raisins
- 4 ounces of chicken
- 2 peeled carrots

Directions

1. Preheat the oven to 400°F. Cover a pan using cooking spray.
2. Toss potato, onions, oil, salt, pepper, and cinnamon in a bowl to mix.
3. Place the mixture on the tray that has been prepared.
4. Roast for approximately 20 mins. Meanwhile, whisk together the remaining oil, vinegar, powder of curry, honey, salt, and pepper in a dish.
5. Fill jars halfway with rice.
6. Baked potatoes, poultry, raisins, and carrots go on top.
7. The dressing should be drizzled over the salad, and cilantro should be sprinkled on top.
8. Refrigerate for up to 3 days if covered.

Nutritional Values

Calories 403 kcal, Carbs 32.3g, Protein 14g, Fat 16g, Sodium 395mg, Potassium 834mg, Chol 0mg

235. SHIITAKE BACON

- Lunch - Prep time: ready in about: 45 mins, Servings: 4, Grill temp: Medium

Ingredients

- 2 tbsp of olive oil- extra-virgin
- 8 oz. of shiitake mushrooms
- 1 tbsp of tamari

Directions

1. Preheat your oven to 300°F and prepare a pan with the parchment paper to prepare your shiitake bacon.
2. Clean the mushrooms thoroughly with a moist towel.
3. Remove the stems and slice your mushrooms, then mix using olive oil & tamari.
4. Spread the mushrooms in a uniform layer on the baking pan and heat for 30- 40 mins.

Nutritional Values

Calories 165kcal, Carbs 14g, Protein 7g, Fat 10g, Sodium 627mg, Potassium 834mg, Chol 0mg

236. COCONUT BACON

- Lunch - Prep time: ready in about: 40 mins, Servings: 4, Grill temp: Medium

Ingredients

- ¾ tbsp of tamari
- ¾ cup of coconut flakes
- ¼ tsp of paprika- smoked
- ½ tbsp of maple syrup

Directions

1. Preheat your oven to 350°F and prepare a pan using parchment paper to make the coconut bacon.
2. Mix gently to cover the flakes of coconut, tamari, syrup of maple, and paprika in the pan.
3. Pour in a fine layer on the pan and bake for 6-10 mins.
4. Keep an eye on the flakes as the temperature of the oven might fluctuate, and they can burn rapidly.

Nutritional Values

Calories 282kcal, Carbs 30g, Protein 16g, Fat 15g, Sodium 886mg, Potassium 734mg, Chol 0mg

237. AVOCADO-SWEET-POTATO-TACOS

- Lunch - Prep time: ready in about: 30 mins, Servings: 2-3, Grill temp: Medium

Ingredients

- olive oil- Extra-virgin
- 1 cubed sweet potato
- ½ tsp of chili powder
- 1 cup of black beans, rinsed
- 4-6 tortillas
- Lime wedges for serving
- Sauce of Avocado yogurt
- Salt and black pepper
- ½ cup of Greek yogurt
- ½ clove of garlic
- 1 avocado
- 1 lime juice
- 2 scallions
- Pickled onions
- Crumbled feta

- fresh cilantro

Directions

1. Preheat your oven to 400°F and prepare a baking pan with parchment paper.
2. Spread the potatoes on the pan after tossing them with olive oil, chili flakes, salt, & pepper.
3. Bake for twenty mins. To prepare the avocado cream sauce, Add the yogurt, avocados, lemon juice, garlic, and sprinkles of salt & pepper in a processor, then Pulse.
4. Season with salt and pepper to taste.
5. Put it in the fridge.
6. Make the tacos by layering the sauce, roasted potatoes, beans, and chosen toppings on the top.
7. Serve your meal.

Nutritional Values

Calories 222kcal, Carbs 30g, Protein 8g, Fat 15.5g, Sodium 886mg, Potassium 734mg, Chol 0mg

238. MACRO-VEGGIE-BOWL

- Lunch - Prep time: ready in about: 40 mins, Servings: 4, Grill temp: Medium

Ingredients

- Lemon squash
- 1 watermelon
- 1 cup of mung beans
- 1 head of broccoli florets
- 6 carrots
- 8 leaves of kale
- ¾ cup of sauerkraut
- 2 cups of brown rice
- 2 tbsp of sesame seeds
- Salt and black pepper
- micro greens, optional
- Turmeric Tahini
- 1 tbsp of lemon juice
- 1 tbsp of olive oil- extra-virgin
- ½ tbsp of tahini
- ½ clove of garlic
- ½ tbsp of water
- ¼ tsp of turmeric

Directions

1. Prepare the sauce.
2. Combine olive oil, lime juice, water, garlic, tahini, turmeric, salt, and pepper in a bowl.

3. Toss the radish slices with a squeeze of lime after thinly slicing.
4. Sauté the beans in the salted water and Drain.
5. Boil your carrots, covered, inside a steamer over a saucepan of boiling water for 7-10 mins.
6. Remove the item and place it away. After that, heat the broccoli for 4-5 mins.
7. Finally, heat the kale for 30 seconds and -1 minute. Assemble the rice, beans, carrots, kale, sauerkraut, broccoli, sesame seeds, and microgreens in a separate bowl.
8. Serve with Tahini Sauce, which has been seasoned with salt & pepper.

Nutritional Values

Calories 322kcal, Carbs 30g, Protein 8g, Fat 15g, Sodium 586mg, Potassium 734mg, Chol 0mg

239. FALAFEL FLATBREAD

- Lunch - Prep time: ready in about: 60 mins, Servings: 2, Grill temp: Medium

Ingredients

- 1 tsp of sea salt
- 2 cups of chickpea flour
- 4 garlic cloves, minced
- 2 tbsp of cilantro
- 2 tbsp of parsley
- 1 tsp of cumin
- ¼ tsp of chili powder
- ½ tsp of coriander
- 2 tsp of lemon juice
- Yogurt
- 8 tbsp of olive oil 9 extra-virgin
- cucumbers
- Diced onion
- Sliced tomatoes
- Fresh herbs
- Muhammara red pepper
- Lemon slices
- Salt and black pepper

Directions

1. Mix the flour of chickpea, salt, garlic, cilantro, parsley, coriander, cumin, chili flakes, lime juice, 2 cups of water, and 6 tbsp of olive oil together in a basin.
2. To hydrate your flour, soak this mixture for about 30- 60 mins.

3. Preheat your broiler with a middle rack in place.
4. Preheat the oven to 350°F and place a pan in the oven for 5 mins. Take out the pan with care.
5. Put in ½ of the mixture after swirling in 1 tbsp of oil to grease the bottom.
6. Rotate the pan to ensure that the batter is properly distributed.
7. Transfer the pan to your oven and bake for over 5-15 mins.
8. Take the flatbread out from the oven and place it on a platter carefully. To create other flatbreads, repeat the process with the leftover batter.
9. Spread yogurt on the flatbreads and garnish with the muhammara, if desired.
10. Spray with the olive oil and sprinkle some salt & pepper to taste.

Nutritional Values

Calories 222kcal, Carbs 30g, Protein 8g, Fat 15g, Sodium 886mg, Potassium 634mg, Chol 0mg

240. VEGAN-EGG-SALAD

- Lunch - Prep time: ready in about: 15 mins, Servings: 3, Grill temp: Medium

Ingredients

- 1 tsp of olive oil- extra-virgin
- ¼ cup of mayonnaise
- 2 tsp of Dijon mustard
- 1 tsp of lemon juice
- 1 tsp of capers
- 1 clove of garlic
- ¼ tsp of salt
- ¼ tsp of turmeric
- black pepper
- celery seed
- 7.5 oz. of tofu
- 2 tbsp fresh dill
- 6 pieces of sandwich bread
- 2 tbsp of fresh chives
- Watercress, optional
- slices of radish, optional
- Pickled onion

Directions

1. Mix together mayonnaise, olive oil, capers, mustard, lime juice, cloves of garlic,

turmeric, a pinch of salt, and pepper in a bowl.

2. Stir in tofu, then crush it softly using your hands, leaving some cubes behind.
3. Make an egg salad consistency rather than scrambled eggs.
4. Combine celery seeds, dill, then chives in a bowl.
5. Put it in the fridge.
6. Top the sandwiches using watercress, and a dollop of egg salad, if preferred.

Nutritional Values

Calories 212kcal, Carbs 30g, Protein 8g, Fat 15g, Sodium 786mg, Potassium 734mg, Chol 0mg

241. ADZUKI-BEAN-BOWLS

- Dinner - Prep time: ready in about: 50 mins, Servings: 4, Grill temp: Medium-high

Ingredients

- 3 carrots
- ½ cabbage head
- 1 cup of snap peas
- 1 cup of brown rice- cooked
- 2 tbsp of sesame seeds
- 2 tbsp of cilantro leaves
- 2 avocados
- 1 ½ cups of adzuki beans
- 1 red chili
- ¼ cup of white miso
- Dressing of sesame Miso
- 1/3 cup of rice vinegar
- 3 tbsp of tamari
- ¼ cup of olive oil
- 1 tbsp of sesame oil

Directions

1. Prepare your salad dressing.
2. Mix together miso, vinegar, olive oil, and sesame oil in a bowl.
3. Combine your vegetables in a bowl.
4. Fold some cilantro into the cabbage before serving.
5. Using 4 dishes, divide the rice, salad of cabbage, beans, then avocados.
6. Sprinkle with additional dressing, if needed, and then top with chili, cilantro, plus sesame seeds, as wanted.

Nutritional Values

Calories 272kcal, Carbs 30g, Protein 8g, Fat 15g, Sodium 186mg, Potassium 734mg, Chol 0mg

242. ROASTED-VEGGIE-GRAIN-BOWL

- Dinner - Prep time: ready in about: 45 mins, Servings: 4, Grill temp: Medium-high

Ingredients

- 1¾ cup of water
- 1 cup of quinoa
- ½ cup of pepitas
- 1 cup of chopped kale
- 2 garlic cloves
- 1 cup of cilantro
- ½ tsp of salt
- ¼ cup of lemon juice
- black pepper
- ½ cup of water
- ½ cup of olive oil
- ½ tsp of maple syrup
- ½ cauliflower florets
- 2 parsnips
- ½ bunch of broccolini
- 1 can of chickpeas
- pepitas
- 1½ cups of Brussels
- sauerkraut scoop

Directions

1. Preheat your oven to 425°F and, using parchment paper, prepare 2 baking trays.
2. Make quinoa first. In a saucepan, combine the washed quinoa and some water.
3. Bring to the boil, then low your flame and let it cook for about 15 mins.
4. Remove the heat and set aside for another 10 mins, undisturbed. Using a fork, smooth the mixture.
5. Make your sauce.
6. Inside a blender, puree together pepitas, cilantro, kale, lime juice, salt, olive oil, some water, and syrup of maple. The veggies should next be roasted.
7. On a tray, combine Brussels sprouts, parsnips, and then cauliflower.
8. On the other tray, arrange the broccolini.
9. Toss the veggies with olive oil and some salt & pepper, and lay them out equally on pans.

10. Bake this for 20-25 mins. Broccolini should be roasted for 10-12 mins. When the stems of broccolini are cold enough to handle, cut them up. Fill dishes with quinoa, roasted veggies, chickpeas, and a tsp of sauerkraut, then sprinkle with pepitas.
11. Pour the sauce on top. If preferred, season with more salt & pepper before serving.
12. Refrigerate the leftover.

Nutritional Values

Calories 202kcal, Carbs 30g, Protein 8g, Fat 11g, Sodium 886mg, Potassium 734mg, Chol 0mg

243. SWEET-POTATO-QUINOA-BOWL

- Dinner - Prep time: ready in about: 25 mins, Servings: 2-3, Grill temp: Medium-high

Ingredients

- olive oil- Extra-virgin
- 1 sweet potato
- ½ cup of chickpeas
- 2 scallions
- 1 cup of quinoa
- ¼ cup of red cabbage
- ¼ cup of almonds
- ⅓ cup of feta cheese
- 2 cups of salad greens
- Salt and black pepper
- ½ lemon juice

Directions

1. Preheat the oven to 400°F and prepare a tray using parchment paper.
2. Combine the potatoes with salt and black pepper and a spritz of olive oil.
3. Roast for 25-35 mins.
4. Mix the chickpeas, quinoa, feta, scallions, cabbage, nuts, and salad leaves with the roasted potatoes.
5. Sprinkle the olive oil, lime juice, and salt as well as pepper to taste. Season with extra lemon juice.
6. Toss everything together and pour into bowls.

Nutritional Values

Calories 222kcal, Carbs 30g, Protein 8g, Fat 15g, Sodium 886mg, Potassium 734mg, Chol 0mg

244. MANGO-GINGER-RICE-BOWL

- Dinner - Prep time: ready in about: 25 mins, Servings: 2, Grill temp: Medium-high

Ingredients

- 1-2 cups of white rice
- 2 snap peas
- 2 cups of green cabbage
- ½ cucumber
- 1 carrot
- 1 ripe mango
- 2 tbsp of pickled ginger
- ½ cup of black beans
- ¼ cup of basil
- sesame seeds
- ¼ cup of peanuts
- ¼ - ½ avocado
- 2 tbsp of rice vinegar
- 2 tbsp of tamari
- 2 tbsp of lime juice
- 2 tsp of cane sugar
- 2 cloves of garlic, minced
- ½ tsp of sriracha

Directions

1. To make your dressing, Mix tamari, vinegar, lemon juice, garlic, sugar cane, and then sriracha in a bowl.
2. Bring a saucepan of water to a boil, and have an ice bucket near.
3. Place the peas in hot water, then take them out and place them in freezing water to halt the cooking.
4. Strain, dry thoroughly, and cut once cool.
5. Put rice, cabbage, carrots, cucumber, mango, beans, ginger, and basil in the bowls. If desired, top with peanut, seeds, & avocado.
6. ½ of the dressing should be drizzled into the bowls, and the remainder should be served on the table if preferred.

Nutritional Values

Calories 272kcal, Carbs 30g, Protein 8g, Fat 15g, Sodium 686mg, Potassium 734mg, Chol 0mg

245. SESAME-SOBA-NOODLES

- Dinner - Prep time: ready in about: 20 mins, Servings: 4, Grill temp: Medium-high

Ingredients

- ¼ cup of rice vinegar
- Sesame Dressing
- 2 tbsp of tamari
- 1 tsp of ginger
- ½ tsp of sesame oil
- 1 clove of garlic
- Soba Noodles
- ½ tsp of maple syrup
- 2 avocados
- Sesame oil
- Lemon squashes
- ¼ cup of edamame
- 2 cups of snap peas
- 1 watermelon
- Sesame seeds
- ¼ cup of mint leaves

Directions

1. To make a dressing, combine all ingredients in a bowl.
2. Mix the vinegar, tamari, oil, garlic, and honey in a bowl.
3. Bring a saucepan of water to boil, and then cook the noodles according to the Directions.
4. Drain and thoroughly rinse with cold water. This aids in the removal of clump-causing starches.
5. Mix your noodles in the dressing, then split them into 2 to 4 bowls.
6. Drizzle lemon juice over the diced avocado and toss with the peas, radish, mint, and seeds in the bowls. If preferred, drizzle with extra tamari and sesame oil.

Nutritional Values

Calories 222kcal, Carbs 30g, Protein 8.9g, Fat 15g, Sodium 886mg, Potassium 734mg, Chol 0mg

246. VEGAN-BURRITO-BOWL

- Dinner - Prep time: ready in about: 50 mins, Servings: 2, Grill temp: Medium-high

Ingredients

- 1-2 chopped peppers
- 1 cup of pinto beans, rinsed
- ½ tsp of olive oil- extra-virgin

- 2 cups of arugula
- 1 cup of lime rice
- ½ cup of guacamole
- ¼ cup of cilantro
- ½ cup of pineapple salsa
- Salt and black pepper
- olive oil- Extra-virgin
- 2 caps of the mushroom
- Adobo sauce
- 1 jalapeno pepper, optional
- 1 bell pepper
- Salt and black pepper
- 1 green pepper

Directions

1. Put the beans, peppers, olive oil, lemon juice, salt, and pepper in a bowl.
2. Prepare the vegetables as follows:
3. Preheat a pan inside the grill to medium flame.
4. The mushrooms will be grilled simply on the grill, while the chopped peppers will be grilled on a pan.
5. Using olive oil and adobo sauce, coat the entire mushroom caps. Use sauce to thoroughly cover the mushrooms from both sides.
6. Season to taste with salt & pepper.
7. Heat the Portobello for 4-5 mins on each side. Just before arranging the bowls, cut.
8. Combine the pepper with olive oil, then salt & pepper to taste.
9. Grill for 8-10 mins, flipping regularly.
10. Mix the rice, beans, arugula, mushrooms, guacamole, salsa, and cilantro into the bowls.
11. On the table, serve with additional salsa and lime slices.

Nutritional Values

Calories 272kcal, Carbs 33g, Protein 8g, Fat 15g, Sodium 686mg, Potassium 734mg, Chol 0mg

247. CAULIFLOWER-RICE-KIMCHI-BOWLS

- Dinner - Prep time: ready in about: 40 mins, Servings: 4, Grill temp: Medium-high

Ingredients

- 2 tbsp of miso paste
- ⅓ cup of coconut milk
- 1 tbsp of vinegar

- sea salt
- 1 tsp of ginger
- 1 cauliflower head
- ½ clove of garlic
- ½ cup of scallions
- 7 oz. of shiitake mushrooms
- ½ tsp of tamari
- ½ tsp of vinegar
- 6 leaves of kale
- 1 avocado
- 14 oz. of baked tofu
- ½ cup of kimchi
- sesame seeds
- ¼ cup of microgreens
- olive oil- Extra-virgin
- Lime wedges for serving

Directions

1. To prepare coconut sauce, combine coconut milk, miso sauce, lemon juice, ginger, and salt in a dish.
2. Warm olive oil in a pan over low flame.
3. Simmer for 3 mins to remove the raw taste of cauliflower, adding the cauliflower rice, scallions, garlic, and salt.
4. Remove the pan from heat and mix in coconut sauce.
5. Divide the rice into 4 dishes.
6. Remove any residual cauliflower parts from the pan with a paper towel. With a few drops of olive oil, return the dish to medium flame.
7. Simmer, about 5 mins. Take the pan off the heat, then add vinegar and tamari.
8. Fill the cauliflower dishes with mushrooms. Wipe out your pan, add a splash of water and kale, and simmer, undisturbed, for 1 minute.
9. Drizzle coconut sauce over every chunk of cauliflower to finish arranging the bowls.
10. In the bowls, combine kale, tofu, avocados, as well as microgreens and seeds, if desired.
11. Serve with lime slices and leftover sauce on the table.

Nutritional Values

Calories 242kcal, Carbs 30g, Protein 8.16g, Fat 15g, Sodium 886mg, Potassium 734mg, Chol 0mg

248. SPAGHETTI SQUASH

- Dinner - Prep time: ready in about: 40 mins, Servings: 4, Grill temp: Medium

Ingredients

- olive oil- Extra-virgin
- 1 squash of spaghetti
- salt and black pepper

Directions

1. Scoop off the seeds & ribbing from spaghetti squash by cutting it in ½.
2. Season the interior of the squash with pepper and salt after drizzling it with olive oil.
3. Poke holes in the spaghetti cut side down above a pan with a fork.
4. Bake for 30-40 mins. Based on the size of the squash, the time varies.
5. Remove the squash from your oven and place it chopped side up.
6. When the squash is cold enough to handle, peel and puff the threads off the sides with a fork.

Nutritional Values

Calories 272kcal, Carbs 30g, Protein 8g, Fat 15g, Sodium 888mg, Potassium 734mg, Chol 0mg

249. STUFFED-ACORN SQUASH

- Dinner - Prep time: ready in about: 40 mins, Servings: 4, Grill temp: Medium

Ingredients

- 1 package of tempeh
- 2 squash of Acron
- 1 tbsp of olive oil- extra-virgin
- 8 oz. of cremini mushrooms
- ½ onion
- ⅓ cup of walnuts
- 3 cloves of garlic
- 1 tbsp of tamari
- ½ tbsp of rosemary
- 1 tbsp of vinegar
- ¼ cup of sage
- Parsley and pomegranate arils
- ⅓ cup of cranberries
- Salt and black pepper

Directions

1. Preheat your oven to 425°Fand place parchment paper on a pan.
2. Scoop out all seeds from the squash and toss them away.
3. Spray the squash pieces using olive oil, then sprinkle salt on the tray.
4. Cook for 40 mins.
5. Slice the tempeh into pieces, put it inside a steamer, and arrange it over a saucepan filled with water.
6. Raise water to a boil, then cover and cook for 10 mins.
7. Take the tempeh out first from the pot, remove the excess water, then crumble it with your hands in a pan; heat olive oil on moderate flame.
8. Cook for 5 mins with the onion, salt, and black pepper.
9. Cook for approximately 8 mins.
10. Cook for another 2 - 3 mins, stirring in the crushed tempeh, cloves, nuts, tamari, vinegar, rosemary, or sage as needed.
11. Season with salt and pepper to taste after adding the cranberries.
12. Fill the cooked acorn squash slices and decorate with parsley & pomegranates.

Nutritional Values

Calories 272kcal, Carbs 30g, Protein 10g, Fat 15g, Sodium 886mg, Potassium 734mg, Chol 0mg

250. STUFFED-POBLANO-PEPPERS

- Dinner - Prep time: ready in about: 40 mins, Servings: 4, Grill temp: Medium

Ingredients

- olive oil- Extra-virgin
- 4 peppers of poblano
- 1/3 cup of onion
- ½ cup of bell pepper
- 1 cup of cauliflower florets
- ½ tsp of cumin
- ½ tsp of oregano
- ½ tsp of coriander
- 1 clove of garlic
- 1 cup of brown rice
- 1 cup of black beans, rinsed
- 3 cups of spinach
- ¼ cup of tomatillo salsa
- 2 tbsp of lime juice

- Salt and black pepper
- avocado slices
- green cashew cream
- tomatillo salsa

Directions

1. Preheat your oven to 400°F and prepare a tray using parchment paper.
2. Remove your seeds and cut peppers by slicing them in ½.
3. Place on a tray, sprinkle using olive oil, and season with salt.
4. Roast for about 15 mins, sliced side up. 1 tbsp of oil, heated in a pan over medium flame.
5. Combine the onion, cabbage, pepper, coriander, cumin, garlic, salt, and pepper in a bowl.
6. Cook for 5-8 mins.
7. Mix in the beans, spinach, lemon juice, rice, and salsa after removing the pan from the heat.
8. Season with salt and pepper to taste.
9. Fill the peppers with the filling and roast for about 15 mins.
10. On the table, serve the avocado slices, cilantro, salsa, cashew cream, & lime wedges.

Nutritional Values

Calories 272kcal, Carbs 30g, Protein 8.4g, Fat 15g, Sodium 886mg, Potassium 734mg, Chol 0mg

251. AVOCADO-CUCUMBER-SUSHI-ROLL

- Dinner - Prep time: ready in about: 75 mins, Servings: 4, Grill temp: Medium

Ingredients

- 2 cups of water
- 1 cup of brown rice
- 2 tbsp of rice vinegar
- 1 tsp of sea salt
- 1 tbsp of sugar
- 1 cucumber
- 1 avocado
- 1 ripe mango
- ⅓ cup of microgreen
- 4 sheets of nori
- sauce of Coconut peanut
- 2 tbsp of sesame seeds
- tamari sauce

1. To prepare your sushi rice, put the water, rice, and olive oil in a pot and boil it.
2. Cover, lower the heat to low, and cook for 45mins. Take the rice out from the heat and set it aside for another 10 mins, wrapped.
3. Fold in the sugar, rice vinegar, and salt after fluffing with a fork.
4. Cover and set aside until set to use.
5. Prepare the rolls of sushi as follows: Because your hands will become sticky, have a small water pot and a towel near the work area.
6. Place 1 nori sheet on a bamboo mat, shiny side down, and compress a scoop of rice into the bottom 2/3 of your sheet.
7. Place the toppings at the base of the rice. Overfilling will make rolling more difficult. To wrap and fold the nori, utilize the wooden mat and press gently and mold the roll after it's been rolled. Put the cut side of the rolls to the side.
8. Continue with the other rolls. To cut your sushi, utilize a fine chef's knife.
9. Between cuts, clean the knife with a moist cloth.
10. Serve right away with ponzu or tamari sauce.

Nutritional Values

Calories 412kcal, Carbs 30g, Protein 8g, Fat 19g, Sodium 886mg, Potassium 734mg, Chol 0mg

252. SPICY-MANGO & AVOCADO-RICE-BOWL

- Dinner - Prep time: ready in about: 60 mins, Servings: 4, Grill temp: Medium

Ingredients

- 1 14 ounces of tofu
- 2 cups of rice
- olive oil
- 1 mango
- tamari
- 1 scallion
- radishes
- 1 cup of cabbage
- ½ cup of cucumber
- lime slices
- 1 avocado
- chopped cilantro
- ⅓ cup of coconut milk
- 2 tsp of soy sauce
- 2 tbsp of peanut butter
- 2 tsp of lime juice
- minced garlic
- 1 tsp of sriracha

Directions

1. Prepare black rice in the same manner as brown rice. 1 cup of rice and 2 cups of water is the ratio.
2. Preheat the oven to 400°F, and line a baking paper.
3. Toss tofu with a sprinkle of tamari and olive oil after patting it dry.
4. Bake it until it becomes golden brown from the edges on a baking tray. It takes around 20-25 mins.
5. Take the tofu out from the oven and sprinkle it with sriracha to cover the exterior.
6. Combine the sauce items while the tofu is baking.
7. Season with salt and pepper to taste. Mango, shredded red cabbage, scallions, radishes, cucumber, avocado, tofu, and cilantro, go into bowls.
8. Serve with more sriracha and lime pieces on the side.

Nutritional Values

Calories 272kcal, Carbs 30g, Protein 7.9g, Fat 15g, Sodium 886mg, Potassium 734mg, Chol 0mg

253. QUINOA-PILAF-RECIPE

- Dinner - Prep time: ready in about: 40 mins, Servings: 4, Grill temp: Medium

Ingredients:

- 1/2 Tbsp of olive oil
- 1 cup of quinoa
- 1/2 onion
- 3 cups of vegetable broth
- 1 carrot
- 2 Tbsp of pine nuts
- 1/2 cup of parsley
- 1/4 cup of raisins
- Salt and pepper

1. Wash the quinoa. Drain the water completely. In a saucepan, add the oil on moderate heat.
2. Simmer the onion & carrot until cooked, then add quinoa, then cook for 3 mins, or until gently toasted and smelling nutty.
3. Bring the stock to a low simmer. Lower the heat, then cover and cook for approximately 20 mins.
4. Mix the quinoa in a mixing dish using a fork.
5. Combine the raisins, pine nuts, and parsley.

Nutritional Values

Calories 230kcal, Carbs 30g, Protein 7.9g, Fat 7g, Sodium 320mg, Potassium 734mg, Chol 0mg

254. RADISH-SALAD W/RADISH-TOP-PESTO

- Dinner - Prep time: ready in about: 25 mins, Servings: 6, Grill temp: Medium

Ingredients

- ¼ cup of Lemon Vinaigrette
- 1 ½ cups of beans
- 9 radishes
- ¼ cup of pine nuts
- 2-3 red radishes
- 1 tbsp of capers
- ¼ cup of mint leaves
- ¼ cup of Pesto
- 2 tbsp of pecorino
- Salt and black pepper
- lemon juice

Directions

1. Toss your beans with 2 tbsp of Lemon Vinaigrette in a medium basin.
2. Arrange the beans, sliced raw radishes, roasted radishes, pine nuts, dollops of pesto, and capers, on a tray.
3. Drizzle it with the additional dressing and, if desired, fresh mint as well as pecorino.
4. Add salt and pepper, as well as some lemon squeezes, if preferred.

Nutritional Values

Calories 292kcal, Carbs 30g, Protein 8g, Fat 15g, Sodium 786mg, Potassium 734mg, Chol 0mg

255. KALE-SALAD W/CARROT-GINGER-DRESSING

- Dinner - Prep time: ready in about: 40 mins, Servings: 4, Grill temp: Medium

Ingredients

- 1/3- ½ cup of water
- ½ cup of carrots- roasted
- ¼ cup of olive oil- extra-virgin
- 2 tsp of ginger
- 2 tbsp of vinegar
- ¼ tsp of salt
- 1 bunch of kale
- 1 batch of Chickpeas
- 1 tsp of lemon juice
- 1 carrot
- ½ tsp of olive oil- extra-virgin
- 1 red beet
- 1 avocado
- ½ watermelon radish
- 2 tbsp of cranberries
- 1 tsp of sesame seeds
- ¼ cup of pepitas
- Salt and black pepper

Directions

1. Preheat your oven to 400°F, and by using parchment paper, line your baking sheet.
2. Mix your chickpeas with olive oil and a sprinkling of salt and black pepper before serving. To roast with the chickpeas, put the carrot slices for the salad in their corner on the oven sheet.
3. Grill for 25 to 30 mins or when the carrots are tender and the chickpeas are colored browned and crunchy. Set aside the roasted chickpeas.
4. Toss the carrots with water, rice vinegar, olive oil, salt, and ginger, in a blender.
5. Mix the dressing till it's smooth, then refrigerate until prepared to use.
6. In a mixing bowl, combine the lemon juice, kale leaves, 12 tsp of olive oil, and a couple pinches of salt.
7. Massage the leaves with your hands until they are limp and wilted. The amount of liquid in the dish has been reduced by roughly ½.
8. Mix in the carrots, beets, ½ cubed avocado, watermelon radish, pipits, cranberries, and some pinches of pepper and salt.

9. Drizzle the ginger carrot dressing over the top.
10. Top with the leftover avocado, roasted chickpeas, more dressing, and some sesame seeds.
11. Season with salt and pepper to taste, then serve.

Nutritional Values

Calories 272kcal, Carbs 30g, Protein 8g, Fat 15.8g, Sodium 886mg, Potassium 734mg, Chol 0mg

256. ROASTED-CAULIFLOWER-SALAD

- Lunch - Prep time: ready in about: 40 mins, Servings: 2, Grill temp: Medium

Ingredients

- olive oil- Extra-virgin
- 1 cauliflower head
- 2 cups of arugula
- Lemon wedges
- ½ cup of Lemon-Herb
- ½ cup of Tahini Sauce
- ¼ cup of pine nuts
- ¼ cup of Pickled Onions
- 4 apricots, diced
- Microgreens
- ¼ cup of olives
- Salt and black pepper

Directions

1. Cauliflower should be roasted.
2. Preheat your oven to 425°F, and with parchment paper, line a baking sheet.
3. Roast cauliflower florets for 20-25 mins, or till brown color around the sides, with a sprinkle of olive oil and a sprinkling of pepper and salt.
4. Mix the roasted cauliflower and arugula with a drizzle of a lemon squeeze, olive oil, and salt in a medium mixing bowl.
5. Drizzle a third of your tahini sauce over the top and serve.
6. Combine the lentils, pine nuts, pickled onions, olives, and apricots in a mixing bowl.
7. Sprinkle with the leftover tahini dressing.
8. Add salt and pepper to taste, then serve.

Nutritional Values

Calories 272kcal, Carbs 30g, Protein 9.8g, Fat 15g, Sodium 886mg, Potassium 734mg, Chol 0mg

257. TACO SALAD

- Lunch - Prep time: ready in about: 25 mins, Servings: 2-3, Grill temp: Medium-low

Ingredients

- olive oil- Extra-virgin
- 2 corn of tortillas
- 1 head of romaine lettuce
- ½ cup of black beans
- 1 cup of red cabbage
- 2 radishes
- 1 avocado
- ½ cup of cherry tomatoes
- Jalapeno slices
- Sea salt
- Dressing of Cilantro Lime
- Lime wedges
- 1 tbsp of olive oil
- Shiitake meat
- 8 oz. of shiitake mushrooms
- 1 tbsp of tamari
- 1 cup of walnuts
- 1 tsp of chili powder
- Salt and black pepper
- ½ tsp of balsamic vinegar

Directions

1. Preheat your oven to 400°F and line the baking sheet using parchment paper.
2. Combine the tortilla pieces with a sprinkle of salt and a drizzle of olive oil.
3. Cook for 10-14 mins, or till crispy, on the baking sheet. Heat some olive oil in a pan over medium-high heat.
4. Cook, stirring just periodically, for 3-4 mins, or till the mushroom begin to color brown and soften. 1-2 mins; after adding the walnuts, gently toast them.
5. Combine the tamari & chili powder in a mixing bowl. Stir in some balsamic vinegar.
6. Remove the pan from heat and add pepper and salt.
7. Arrange the cabbage, romaine lettuce, taco meat, black beans, tomatoes, radishes, jalapenos, avocado, if using, and cilantro lime and avocado dressing on top of the salad.

8. Spray with some olive oil and season with salt and pepper.
9. Serve it with lime slices and a side of additional dressing.

Nutritional Values

Calories 272kcal, Carbs 30g, Protein 8g, Fat 15g, Sodium 786mg, Potassium 734mg, Chol 0mg

258. COCONUT CURRY

- Lunch - Prep time: ready in about: 50 mins, Servings: 4, Grill temp: Medium

Ingredients

- 1 cup of onion
- 1 tbsp of coconut oil
- 2 cloves of garlic
- ½ tsp of cumin
- ½ tsp of ginger
- ¼ tsp of coriander
- ¼ tsp of cardamom
- ¼ tsp of turmeric
- 1 tsp of sea salt
- 3 Thai chilies
- 2 cups of butternut squash
- 2 cups of cauliflower
- 1 tbsp of lemon juice
- 1 can of coconut milk
- 1 tbsp of lime juice
- ½ cup of peas
- 4 cups of spinach
- black pepper
- basil
- 2 cups of basmati rice
- Naan bread

Directions

1. In your Dutch oven, heat oil over moderate flame.
2. Cook for approximately 10 mins till the onion is tender and browned, decreasing the temperature to low midway through.
3. Combine the ginger, garlic, coriander, cumin, cardamom, turmeric, and salt in a bowl. Take the equation.
4. Cook it for 5mins after adding the chilies and butternut squash to the pan.
5. After that, add coconut milk, cauliflower, and spice mixture.
6. Cook for 20mins, or till the veggies are cooked and covered.

7. Stir the lime juices and lemon, peas, and spinach.
8. Season to taste spices, if needed, with more lime juice, pepper, and salt.
9. Serve your curry with lime slices and rice on the side, as well as naan bread and fresh basil, if preferred.

Nutritional Values

Calories 282kcal, Carbs 30g, Protein 8g, Fat 19g, Sodium 886mg, Potassium 734mg, Chol 0mg

259. BIBIM-BAP

- Dinner - Prep time: ready in about: 50 mins, Servings: 2, Grill temp: Medium

Ingredients

- ½ cucumber
- Bowls
- ½ tsp of rice vinegar
- 1 cup of mung bean
- 1¼ tsp of sesame oil
- 1 cup of shredded carrots
- ½ tsp of tamari
- 4 cups of baby spinach
- 2 cups of white rice, cooked
- 4 oz. of shiitake mushrooms
- 2 eggs- fried
- 1 Gochujang sauce
- Sea salt
- Chopped scallions
- Sesame seeds
- Kimchi, optional

Directions

1. Mix the slices of cucumber slices with rice vinegar, sesame oil, and salt in a dish.
2. Set it aside. A small saucepan of water should be brought to a boil.
3. Boil for 1 min after adding bean sprouts. Drain the water and put it aside in a pan; heat sesame oil on moderate flame. With salt, toss in some carrots.
4. Sauté for 1- 2 mins, occasionally stirring, until slightly softened, then remove it from the pan, then put aside. In the same pan, heat sesame oil, then add some spinach & tamari. Heat for thirty seconds, occasionally stirring.
5. Take the spinach out from the pan and drain off any extra liquid.

6. Arrange the cucumber slices, rice, carrots, bean sprouts, and spinach in the bowls.
7. Serve it with baked tofu or fried egg as a topping. Garnish with preferred toppings.

Nutritional Values

Calories 465kcal, Carbs 14g, Protein 19g, Fat 10g, Sodium 4327mg, Potassium 445mg, Chol 0mg

260. TAMAGO-KAKE-GOHAN

- Dinner - Prep time: ready in about: 50 mins, Servings: 2, Grill temp: Medium

Ingredients

- 2-3 cups of brown rice, cooked
- olive oil- Extra-virgin
- 2 eggs
- 1 scallion, chopped
- tamari splashes
- sesame seeds
- sliced nori
- egg yolks, extra
- Japanese pickles
- rice vinegar splashes
- roasted broccoli
- microgreens
- avocado slices

Directions

1. Distribute the prepared brown rice evenly between 2 dishes. While the rice is still hot, crack 1 egg into each dish, then add tamari, stirring quickly to cook the egg, giving a creamy texture to the rice.
2. Add sesame seeds, onions, and any other preferred toppings to every dish.
3. Toss with a side of tamari for seasoning.

Nutritional Values

Calories 265kcal, Carbs 11.2g, Protein 7.4g, Fat 10g, Sodium 437mg, Potassium 245mg, Chol 0mg

261. VEGAN-POKE-BOWL

- Dinner - Prep time: ready in about: 60 mins, Servings: 2-4, Grill temp: Medium

Ingredients

- 2 cloves of garlic
- 1 tbsp of tamari
- 2 tsp of lime juice

- 1 tbsp of cane sugar
- 2 tsp of rice vinegar
- ½ tsp of sesame oil
- ¼ cup of scallions
- 5 cups of watermelon
- 1 sliced cucumber
- 2 tbsp of pickled ginger
- ¼ cup of macadamia nuts
- 1 jalapeno
- Furikake
- ½ avocado- ripped
- microgreens
- 1 nori sheet
- 2 tbsp of sesame seeds
- ¼ tsp of sugar
- ¼ tsp of sea salt

Directions

1. Flapping the nori sheet on your gas burner till it's browned and crunchy is a good way to cook it.
2. Cut the chicken into tiny pieces.
3. Combine the sesame seeds, toasted nori, salt, & sugar in a blender.
4. Blend until all of the ingredients are finely minced.
5. Mix the garlic, tamari, rice vinegar, lime juice, sesame oil, and sugar in a small bowl.
6. Mix watermelon with a little flavoring and some scallions.
7. Prepare the cucumber, watermelon, pickled ginger, macadamia nuts, avocado, jalapeno, and micro greens, in bowls.
8. Mix in some additional dressing and toss lightly. Furikake should be drizzled.

Nutritional Values

Calories 212kcal, Carbs 14g, Protein 14.2g, Fat 10g, Sodium 637mg, Potassium 425mg, Chol 0mg

262. AVOCADO-CRISPBREADS W/EVERYTHING-BAGEL-SEASONING

- Dinner - Prep time: ready in about: 50 mins, Servings: 2, Grill temp: Medium

Ingredients

- 1 ripe avocado
- 4 Rye Crispbreads
- 2 tsp of bagel seasoning
- 2 radishes
- 1 lemon slice

- Fresh dill

Directions:

1. Remove the pit from the avocado, then cut it in ½. Slice thinly and arrange it on every crisp bread.
2. Add the entire bagels seasoning, lemon juice, and fresh dill and radish slices to each crispbread.

Nutritional Values

Calories 265kcal, Carbs 11g, Protein 10g, Fat 20g, Sodium 637mg, Potassium 345mg, Chol 0mg

263. MIXED-GREENS-SALAD W/PUMPKIN-VINAIGRETTE

- Dinner - Prep time: ready in about: 50 mins, Servings: 6, Grill temp: Medium

Ingredients

- 3 tbsp of canned pumpkin
- ¼ cup of cider vinegar
- 2 tbsp of maple syrup
- 1 tsp of Dijon mustard
- 2 tbsp of olive oil
- ¼ tsp of salt
- 9 cups of mixed greens
- ¼ tsp of black pepper
- 2 pears- sliced
- 12 Medjool dates
- ½ cup of red onion
- ½ cup of walnut pieces

Directions:

1. To make the vinaigrette, whisk together the pumpkin, vinegar, maple syrup, mustard, oil, salt, & pepper into a twist container.
2. Cover then shake. Place veggies in a large mixing dish.
3. Mix with a 1-third cup of the vinaigrette and toss to coat. Arrange the greens on the serving platters.
4. Pears, dates, onions, and walnuts go on top.
5. Pass the leftover vinaigrette.

Nutritional Values

Calories 312 kcal, Carbs 11g, Protein 4g, Fat 11g, Sodium 131mg, Potassium 345mg, Chol 0mg

264. VEGGIE-RICE-BOWL RECIPE

- Dinner - Prep time: ready in about: 50 mins, Servings: 1, Grill temp: Medium

Ingredients

- 1 vegetable pouch- steam-in
- 1 package of instant rice
- 1 egg
- Butter
- 1 tsp of soy sauce
- Sriracha

Directions:

1. Follow the package directions for cooking the rice.
2. Cook the veggies after that. In a pan, melt a tiny quantity of butter.
3. Prepare the egg until it is done to your taste.
4. Fry the egg just on 1 side till the white is not runny. In a mixing bowl, combine the rice, veggies, and soy sauce.
5. On top of it, place your egg. If desired, season with Sriracha.

Nutritional Values

Calories 195kcal, Carbs 14g, Protein 16g, Fat 12g, Sodium 547mg, Potassium 440mg, Chol 0mg

265. GRILLED-VEGETABLE-WRAP W/BALSAMIC-MAYO

- Dinner - Prep time: ready in about: 50 mins, Servings: 4, Grill temp: Medium

Ingredients

- 2 mushroom caps
- 12 spears of asparagus
- 1 bell pepper
- Salt and pepper
- 1 tbsp of olive oil
- 2 tbsp of mayonnaise
- 1 clove of garlic
- 1 tbsp of balsamic vinegar
- 4 spinach
- 3/4 cup of crumbled goat
- 2 cups of arugula

Directions

1. Prepare a grill by preheating it. With pepper and salt, mix the mushrooms, asparagus, and also bell pepper with some olive oil.

2. Cook, frequently turning, till lightly browned and cooked on the highest section of the grill. Using a sharp knife, cut the mushroom tops into small slices.
3. Slice the pepper.
4. Stir together the vinegar, mayonnaise, and garlic until fully combined.
5. Heat your tortillas for thirty seconds on the grill or in the oven.
6. Top each tortilla with the balsamic mayo, then greens & cheese.
7. To make the wraps, divide the cooked veggies among tortillas, fold them up securely, and cut them in ½.

Nutritional Values

Calories 240 kcal, Carbs 14g, Protein 16g, Fat 13g, Sodium 450mg, Potassium 440mg, Chol 0mg

266. MUSHROOM-CHEESESTEAK RECIPE

- Dinner - Prep time: ready in about: 50 mins, Servings: 4, Grill temp: Medium

Ingredients

- Portobello mushrooms
- tbsp of canola oil
- 1 onion
- 1 tbsp of soy sauce
- 1 bell pepper
- 1 tbsp of Worcestershire sauce
- slices provolone
- Salt and pepper
- hoagie rolls

Directions

1. In a sauté pan, warm ½ tbsp Oil on moderate flame.
2. Cook, stirring periodically, for approximately 5mins, till the slices of Portobello are well browned. Place on a platter to cool.
3. In this pan, heat the leftover ½ tbsp Oil. Cook for 5mins, until the onion and pepper are mellow and starting to brown.
4. Stir in some soy sauce & Worcestershire sauce after returning your mushrooms to the pan.

5. Heat for 2 mins.
6. Add salt and black pepper after removing it from the fire. In your pan, split the veggies into 4 heaps and cover with a piece of cheese for each.
7. Tuck the veggie heaps inside the rolls after the cheese starts to melt.

Nutritional Values

Calories 340 kcal, Carbs 20g, Protein 16g, Fat 14g, Sodium 740mg, Potassium 440mg, Chol 0mg

267. NUTRIENT PACKED-SIMMERED-LENTILS RECIPE

- Dinner - Prep time: ready in about: 50 mins, Servings: 6, Grill temp: Medium

Ingredients

- 1 tbsp of olive oil
- 1 1/2 cups of lentils
- 1/2 chopped onion
- 2 cloves of garlic
- 2 diced carrots
- 1 1/2 cups of vegetable broth
- 1/2 tbsp of wine vinegar
- 2 leaves of bay
- Salt and pepper

Directions

1. Wash lentils. In a medium-sized saucepan, heat some olive oil.
2. Heat the carrots, onion, and garlic for 5-7 mins or until tender.
3. Combine the broth, lentils, and bay leaves.
4. Cook for 15 - 20 mins, or till the lentils become soft.
5. Add the salt, vinegar, and pepper to taste.
6. Remove the bay leaves.

Nutritional Values

Calories 160 kcal, Carbs 14g, Protein 16g, Fat 4.5g, Sodium 540mg, Potassium 440mg, Chol 0mg

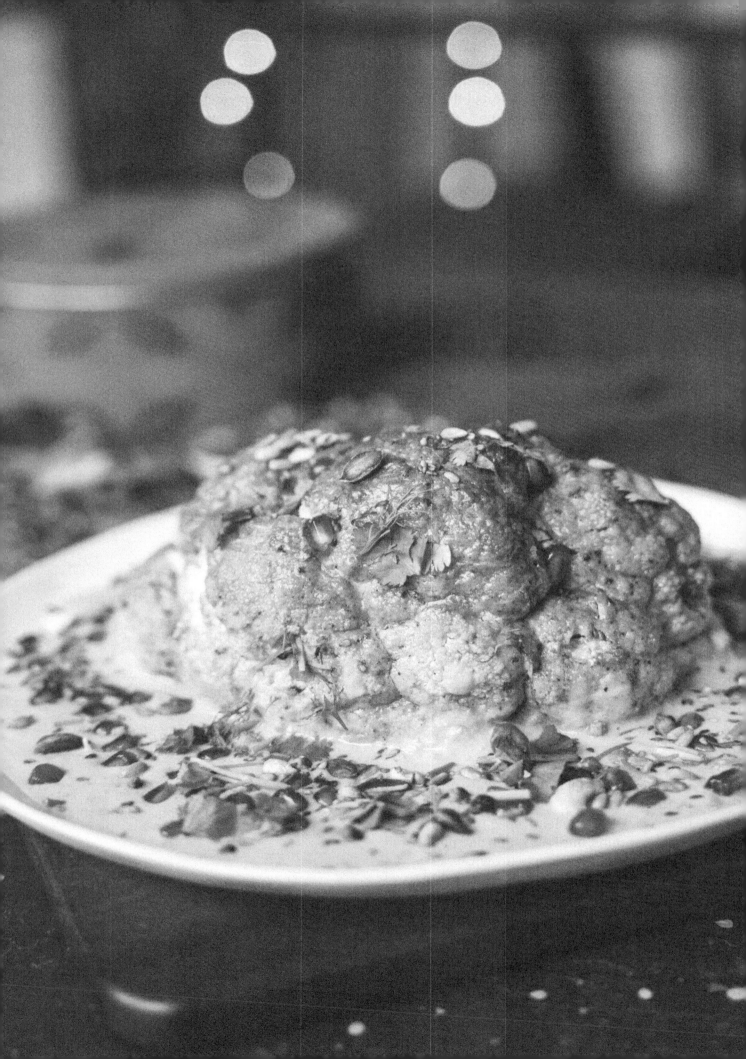

Chapter 9.

Soups & Stews Recipes

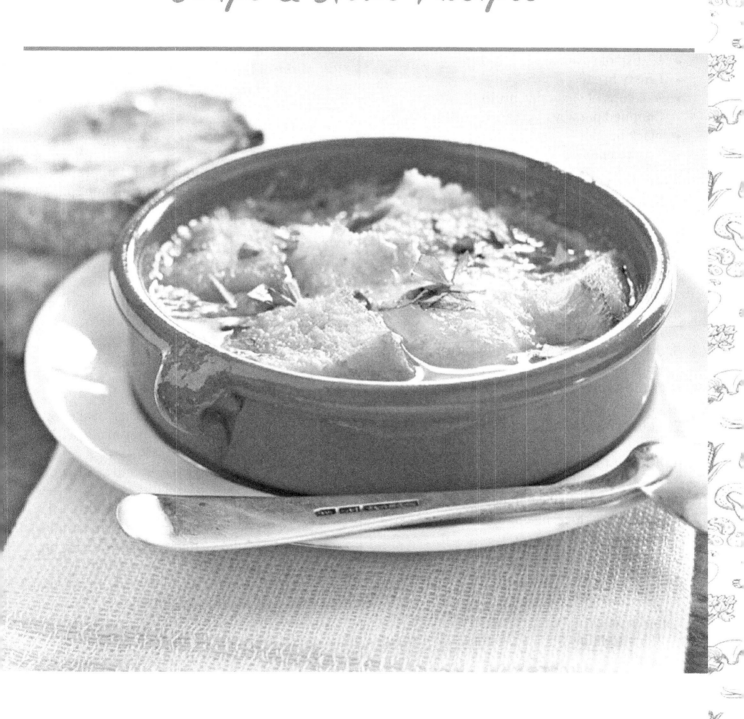

268. BUTTERNUT-SQUASH-SOUP

- Lunch - Prep time: ready in about: 45 mins, Servings: 6, Grill temp: Medium

- 1 onion
- 2 tbsp of olive oil- extra-virgin
- ½ tsp of sea salt
- 3 cloves of garlic
- 1 squash of butternut
- 1 tbsp of sage
- 1 tsp of ginger
- ½ tbsp of rosemary
- Crusty bread
- 3- 4 cups of vegetable broth
- Chopped parsley
- black pepper
- Toasted pepitas

Directions

1. In a saucepan over medium-high heat, warm up the oil.
2. Add the salt, onion, and pepper and cook for 5-8 mins or until tender.
3. Cook, turning regularly, for 8-10 mins, till the squash starts to soften.
4. Combine the sage, garlic, ginger, and rosemary, in a mixing bowl.
5. Stir and heat for 30 seconds to 1 minute, or until scented, adding 3 cups broth.
6. Bring it to a boil, then cover & keep to low heat.
7. Cook for 20-30 mins or till the squash is soft.
8. Allow it to cool somewhat before transferring it to a blender and blending until smooth, using batches if required. If the soup is thick, mix in up to 1 cup of extra broth.
9. Season it to taste with parsley, crusty bread, and pepitas.

Nutritional Values

Calories 222kcal, Carbs 30g, Protein 8g, Fat 15g, Sodium 886mg, Potassium 734mg, Chol 0mg

269. VEGAN-BROCCOLI-SOUP

- Lunch - Prep time: ready in about: 50 mins, Servings: 4, Grill temp: Medium

Ingredients

- 1 onion
- 2 tbsp of olive oil- extra-virgin
- ½ cup of celery
- 1 pound of broccoli
- ⅓ cup of carrots
- 1 potato
- black pepper
- 4 cups of vegetable broth
- 4 cloves of garlic
- 3 cups of bread
- 1½ tsp of vinegar
- ½ cup of raw cashews
- ½ tsp of Dijon mustard
- 1 tbsp of lemon juice
- ¼ cup of fresh dill
- ¾ tsp of sea salt

Directions

1. Preheat your oven to 350°F and prepare 2 small baking pans using parchment paper.
2. In a saucepan, heat oil over medium-high heat.
3. Sauté the celery, onion, broccoli stems, carrots, pepper, and salt for approximately 10 mins, or till softened.
4. Mix in some potatoes & garlic, then cover and cook for 20 mins, or till potatoes are tender.
5. Allow cooling slightly before serving. 1 cup of broccoli florets should be set aside to grill as a stew topping.
6. Put the leftover florets inside a basket of steamer over 1 inch of water inside a saucepan.
7. Allow water to boil, cover, and steam your broccoli for 5 mins, till it is tender.
8. Place the saved bread cubes and broccoli floret on the baking pans in the meantime.
9. Roast for 10-15 mins, tossing with a drop of olive oil as well as a bit of salt till the bread is crunchy and the broccoli is soft and brown all around the sides.
10. In a blender, combine the cashews, soup, mustard, and apple cider vinegar and mix until smooth. If needed, work in groups.
11. Pulse in the cooked broccoli florets, lemon juice, and dill until the broccoli is evenly distributed but still lumpy. If the

soup is thick, dilute it with ½ cup of water to get the required consistency.

12. Mix roasted broccoli & croutons, and then serve it in bowls.

Calories 332kcal, Carbs 30g, Protein 8g, Fat 15g, Sodium 686mg, Potassium 834mg, Chol 0mg

270. TOMATO-BASIL SOUP

- Lunch - Prep time: ready in about: 90 mins, Servings: 8, Grill temp: Medium

Ingredients

- ¼ cup of olive oil- extra-virgin
- 2½ lb. of tomatoes
- 1 onion
- 4 cloves of garlic
- ⅓ cup of carrots
- 3 cups of vegetable broth
- Salt and black pepper
- 1 tsp of thyme leaves
- 1 tbsp of vinegar
- 1 basil leaves

Directions

1. Preheat your oven to 350°F, and using parchment paper, line a baking sheet.
2. Put tomatoes on your baking sheet split side up, sprinkle with 2 tbsp Olive oil, & season with pepper and salt.
3. Roast it for 1 hour or till the sides begin to shrivel, but the inside remains moist. In a saucepan, heat the leftover 2 tbsp of olive oil on moderate heat.
4. Cook, occasionally stirring, until the carrots, onions, garlic, & 1/2 tsp salt are tender,4 approximately 8 mins.
5. Boil for twenty mins after adding the tomatoes, vinegar, vegetable broth, and some thyme leaves.
6. Allow it to cool somewhat before blending the soup in portions if required.
7. Blend till completely smooth. Blend in basil until it's completely mixed.
8. Serve with basil leaves and crusty bread on top.

Nutritional Values

Calories 472kcal, Carbs 30g, Protein 8g, Fat 15.5g, Sodium 886mg, Potassium 734mg, Chol 0mg

271. CREAMY-MUSHROOM-SOUP

- Lunch - Prep time: ready in about: 40 mins, Servings: 4-6, Grill temp: Medium

Ingredients

- 2 leeks
- 2 tbsp of olive oil- extra-virgin
- 2 stalks of celery
- 2 tbsp of tamari
- 16 oz. of cremini mushrooms
- ¼ cup of white wine
- 2 tbsp of thyme leaves
- 2 cloves of garlic
- 4 cups of vegetable broth
- 1 tsp of Dijon mustard
- 1 lb. of cauliflower
- 1 tbsp of balsamic vinegar
- Salt and black pepper
- coconut milk
- Additional mushrooms
- Microgreens
- Crusty bread
- pine nuts

Directions

1. In a saucepan on moderate heat, warm up the oil.
2. Cook for 5 mins with the celery, leeks, and a quarter tsp salt.
3. Cook for another 8-10mins, or till the mushrooms are tender.
4. Cook it for 15 to 30 sec, just until the liquid has evaporated, after adding the wine, tamari, thyme, and garlic.
5. Add some cauliflower as well as a broth to the pot.
6. Cook for 20mins, open, or till cauliflower is very tender.
7. Add the vinegar and mustard to a blender and mix till smooth.
8. Season with salt and pepper to taste, and serve with chosen toppings.

Nutritional Values

Calories 282kcal, Carbs 30g, Protein 8g, Fat 10g, Sodium 886mg, Potassium 734mg, Chol 0mg

272. WILD RICE

- Lunch - Prep time: ready in about: 45 mins, Servings: 4, Grill temp: Medium

Ingredients

- ⅓ cup of cashews
- 1 cup of almond milk
- ¼ cup of cannellini beans
- 2 tsp of Dijon mustard
- 2 tbsp of miso paste
- 2 tbsp of olive oil extra-virgin
- 1 stalk of celery
- 1 bunch of scallions
- 1 carrot
- 1 tsp of sea salt
- 8 oz. of cremini mushrooms
- 4 cloves of garlic
- 1 thyme bunch
- 2 tbsp of rosemary
- 1¼ cup of cannellini beans
- 4 cups of water
- ½ tsp of black pepper
- pepper flakes
- 1 cup of wild rice- cooked
- 4 cups of chopped kale
- 1-2 tbsp of lemon juice
- Chopped parsley

Directions

1. Inside a blender, combine the cashews, almond milk, miso paste, white beans, Dijon mustard, and miso paste, and mix till smooth.
2. Set it aside. In a medium-sized Dutch oven, heat some olive oil over a moderate flame.
3. Stir in the celery, mushrooms, scallions, carrots, and salt until all ingredients are well combined.
4. Cook, stirring, for 8 -10 mins.
5. Stir with rosemary, garlic, rosemary, and thyme, as well as the pepper, cannellini beans, the water.
6. Cook for 20mins with the lid on.
7. Remove your thyme bundle, then combine the rice, cashew mixture, lemon juice, & kale in a mixing bowl.
8. Cook, stir to combine, till the kale is softened, approximately 5 mins.
9. Salt to taste and top with additional parsley, lemon juice, and red pepper if preferred.

Nutritional Values

Calories 372kcal, Carbs 20g, Protein 8g, Fat 15g, Sodium 886mg, Potassium 634mg, Chol 0mg

273. POTATO-LEEK-SOUP

- Lunch - Prep time: ready in about: 60 mins, Servings: 8, Grill temp: Medium

Ingredients

- 4 cups of leeks
- 3 tbsp of olive oil- extra-virgin
- ¾ tsp of sea salt
- 1 tbsp of wine vinegar
- 4 cloves of garlic
- 4 cups of vegetable broth
- 1½ cups of white beans
- pepper flakes
- 1 lb. of potatoes
- ½ tbsp of lemon juice
- black pepper
- ½ tbsp of Dijon mustard
- Nuts of pine and parsley

Directions

1. In a Dutch oven, heat 2 tsp oil over a moderate flame.
2. Combine the salt, leeks, and pepper in a mixing bowl. Sauté for 6-8 mins.
3. Stir in garlic and simmer for another 2 mins.
4. Heat for thirty seconds while tossing in the wine vinegar, then add potatoes, broth, and white beans.
5. Bring it to a boil, then lower it to low heat and let to boil for thirty mins, open.
6. Allow cooling before blending with the other 1 tbsp oil, mustard, and lemon juice in a blender.
7. Mix until completely smooth.
8. Season with pepper and salt to taste, then top with pine nuts, chopped parsley, olive oil, and red pepper, if preferred.

Nutritional Values

Calories 272kcal, Carbs 30g, Protein 8.4g, Fat 15g, Sodium 886mg, Potassium 634mg, Chol 0mg

274. PUMPKIN-TORTILLA-SOUP

- Lunch - Prep time: ready in about: 40 mins, Servings: 4, Grill temp: Medium

Ingredients

- 1 onion, sliced
- 4 tomatoes
- 3 whole cloves of garlic
- 5 corn of tortillas
- 1 pasilla
- ½ tsp of sea salt
- 2 tbsp of olive oil- extra-virgin
- 2½ cups of vegetable broth
- 1 tsp of cumin
- 2 cups of pumpkin- sliced
- ½ tsp of oregano
- 1½ cups of black beans
- ground pepper
- Lime slices
- Sliced avocado
- 2 jalapenos, sliced
- 3 radishes, sliced
- ½ cup of cilantro

Directions

1. Preheat your oven to 450°F and prepare 2 baking pans with baking parchment.
2. Put the onions, tomatoes, and garlic on just a baking tray and roast for 20-25 mins, or till the covers of both tomatoes and the sides of onions are browned.
3. Next, soak your dried chili in boiling water for 10 mins or until tender.
4. Toss the onion, tomatoes, peeled garlic, 1 split tortilla, softened dry chili, 1 cup of vegetable broth, and salt in a blender.
5. Blend till the mixture is smooth and not completely pureed. Inside a large saucepan on moderate heat, warm up the olive oil.
6. Mix in the oregano and cumin for thirty seconds.
7. Combine the mixed tomato mix, cubed pumpkin, 1 ½ cups more broth, and some black beans in a bowl.
8. Cook for approximately 25 mins. Decrease the oven temperature to 300°F in the meantime.
9. Spread the other 4 tortillas on the other baking sheet in thin slices. With a splash of oil on olives and a sprinkling of pepper and salt, toss the vegetables.
10. Bake for 8-14 mins.
11. Add pepper and salt to taste. If your soup is overly thick, thin it up with a little additional broth. If that's too thin, cook it for a few mins or more till it thickens.
12. Add several squeezes of lime to make the soup extra tangy.
13. Serve with avocado, crunchy tortilla strips, jalapenos, cilantro, radishes, and lime slices on top of the soup. Throw a twist of lime as well as salt on avocado slices if preferred.

Nutritional Values

Calories 272kcal, Carbs 30g, Protein 8g, Fat 15g, Sodium 886mg, Potassium 734mg, Chol 0mg

275. TOMATO-BASIL-SOUP

- Lunch - Prep time: ready in about: 90 mins, Servings: 6-8, Grill temp: Medium

Ingredients

- ¼ cup of olive oil- extra-virgin
- 2½ lb. of Roma tomatoes
- 1 yellow onion
- 4 cloves of garlic
- ⅓ cup of carrots
- 3 cups of vegetable broth
- 1 tsp of thyme leaves
- Salt and black pepper
- 1 tbsp of balsamic vinegar
- 1 cup of basil leaves

Directions

1. Preheat your oven to 350°F, and using parchment paper, line a baking sheet.
2. Put your tomatoes onto the baking sheet, trim up, spray with 2 tbsp Oil, and season with pepper and salt.
3. Cook for 60 mins.
4. In a saucepan, heat the leftover 2 tbsp of olive oil on moderate flame.
5. Cook, occasionally stirring, until the carrots, onions, garlic, and ½ tsp salt are tender, approximately 8 mins.
6. Cook for 20mins after adding the tomatoes, vinegar, vegetable broth, & thyme leaves.
7. Allow it to cool somewhat before blending the broth in batches if required.
8. Blend until completely smooth.
9. Blend in some basil until it's completely mixed.

10. Serve your soup with crispy bread & basil leaves on top.

Nutritional Values

Calories 212kcal, Carbs 30g, Protein 9g, Fat 10g, Sodium 886mg, Potassium 734mg, Chol 0mg

276. CARROT-SOUP-RECIPE W/GINGER

- Lunch - Prep time: ready in about: 55 mins, Servings: 3-4, Grill temp: Medium

Ingredients

- 1 cup of onions
- 1 tbsp of olive oil- extra-virgin
- 3 cloves of garlic
- 1½ tsp of ginger
- 2 cups of carrots
- 1 tbsp of vinegar- Apple cider
- Salt and black pepper
- 3-4 cups of vegetable broth
- 1 tsp of maple syrup
- pesto dollops
- coconut milk optional

Directions

1. In a saucepan on medium heat, heat some olive oil.
2. Cook, stirring periodically, for approximately 8mins, till the onions have softened as well as pepper and salt has been added.
3. Cook for another 8mins, stirring regularly, after adding the crushed garlic cloves.
4. Add ginger, apple cider vinegar, and 3-4 cups of broth, based on the thickness you want. Lower to low heat and cook for 30 mins or till the carrots are tender.
5. Allow cooling somewhat before blending.
6. Blend until completely smooth.
7. Season with salt and pepper to taste. If desired, drizzle with maple syrup.

Nutritional Values

Calories 262kcal, Carbs 20g, Protein 8g, Fat 15g, Sodium 886mg, Potassium 934mg, Chol 0mg

277. ROASTED-RED-PEPPER-SOUP

- Lunch - Prep time: ready in about: 45 mins, Servings: 4, Grill temp: Medium

Ingredients

- 1 chopped onion
- ¼ cup of olive oil- extra-virgin
- 2 cloves of garlic
- 3 carrots
- 1 fennel bulb
- 1 tbsp of thyme leaves
- 3 jarred bell peppers
- 2 tbsp of balsamic vinegar
- ¼ cup of cannellini beans, cooked
- 4 cups of vegetable broth
- 2 tbsp of tomato paste
- ½ - 1 tsp of sea salt
- ½ tsp of pepper flakes
- ½ tsp of black pepper
- 1 red pepper
- Warm baguette
- flakes of pepper
- parsley chopped
- Microgreens

Directions

1. In a saucepan, heat 2 tbsp Oil on moderate heat.
2. Cook, occasionally stirring, until the onion is translucent, approximately 5 mins.
3. Combine the fennel, garlic, thyme leaves, and carrots in a large bowl.
4. Cook, occasionally stirring, until the carrots are tender, approximately 10 mins.
5. ½ tsp salt, red peppers, balsamic vinegar, tomato paste, beans, and broth Cook for 15-20 mins or till carrots are soft.
6. Puree the simmering soup with leftover 2 tbsp Of olive oil in a high-powered blender until smooth.
7. Add pepper and salt.
8. Add ½ tsp of red pepper seasoning if you want it to be a bit spicier.
9. Serve the baguette immediately with drizzles of some olive oil and chosen toppings.

Nutritional Values

Calories 282kcal, Carbs 30g, Protein 8.9g, Fat 15g, Sodium 888mg, Potassium 734mg, Chol 0mg

278. CAULIFLOWER SOUP

- Lunch - Prep time: ready in about: 55 mins, Servings: 6, Grill temp: Medium

Ingredients

- 2 shallots, sliced
- 1 head of cauliflower
- 4 garlic cloves
- 5 Leaves of thyme
- 4 cups of vegetable broth
- ½ tbsp of miso paste
- 3 tbsp of olive oil- extra-virgin
- ½ tsp of Dijon mustard
- 1 tbsp of lemon juice
- Microgreens, optional
- Salt and black pepper

Directions

1. Preheat your oven to 400°F, and using parchment paper, line a baking sheet. Cauliflower, along with the core portions, should be chopped.
2. Mix the cauliflower with olive oil, then a bit of pepper and salt on the baking sheet.
3. Cover the garlic cloves and shallot in aluminum foil and lay them on a baking sheet along with the veggies and olive oil, as well as a bit of salt.
4. Cook for 30-35 mins. Bring the veggie broth to a moderate boil in a large saucepan.
5. Cook, covered, for 15mins with roasted cauliflower, peeled garlic, shallots, and thyme. Allow cooling just before blending.
6. Combine the mustard, miso paste, olive oil, & lemon juice in a mixing bowl.
7. Blend until completely smooth.
8. Add another quarter to ½ a tsp of salt and additional lime juice to taste.
9. If preferred, garnish with some microgreens before serving.

Nutritional Values

Calories 272kcal, Carbs 30.2g, Protein 8g, Fat 15g, Sodium 886mg, Potassium 714mg, Chol 0mg

279. RED-CURRY-LEMONGRASS-SOUP

- Lunch - Prep time: ready in about: 50 mins, Servings: 4-6, Grill temp: Medium

Ingredients

- 5 cups of vegetable broth
- 1 stalk of lemongrass
- 1 2-inch ginger
- 2 tbsp of cane sugar
- 2 tbsp of tamari
- Juice of 2 limes
- 1 onion
- 1 tbsp of coconut oil
- 4 cups of shiitake mushrooms
- 1 tomato
- ½ - 1 tbsp of curry paste
- 5-6 cups of bok choy
- jasmine rice, cooked
- Sea salt

Directions

1. Bash lemongrass with the back of the chef's knife to help set free the flavor.
2. Chop this into 1" pieces after slicing in ½. Simmer for 15mins with the broth, ginger, tamari, lemongrass, lime juice, sugar, and lime zest in a saucepan.
3. Set it aside. Return the saucepan to the stovetop over moderate heat and melt the coconut oil.
4. Cook, occasionally stirring, till the onion is pink and tender.
5. Add some mushrooms as well as a bit of salt to taste.
6. Cook, occasionally stirring, for approximately 15 mins or till mushrooms are tender.
7. Stir in your paste of curry till well combined, then add the tomatoes.
8. Cook for 5mins with the saved broth before adding bok choy.
9. Cook for 5-7 mins, or until the bok choy is soft but it's still bright green.
10. Add additional tamari and lime juice.
11. Add additional red curry if you want it spicier.
12. Serve immediately with baked tofu.

Nutritional Values

Calories 274kcal, Carbs 30g, Protein 12g, Fat 15g, Sodium 786mg, Potassium 634mg, Chol 0mg

280. CARROT-COCONUT-SOUP

- Lunch - Prep time: ready in about: 15 mins, Servings: 4, Grill temp: Medium

Ingredients

- 16 oz. of carrots
- 1 stalk of lemongrass

- 1 can of coconut milk
- 2 tbsp of olive oil- extra-virgin
- 1 clove of garlic
- 2 tbsp of sherry vinegar
- ½ tsp of sea salt
- 1 tsp of curry paste
- ½ cup of water
- Optional, hemp seeds
- sea salt and black pepper

Directions

1. Cut the root end and the rough top stem of lemongrass to clean it.
2. Combine the carrots, lemongrass, garlic, coconut milk, sherry vinegar, olive oil, red curry paste, water, sherry vinegar, salt, & pepper in a high-powered blender.
3. Blend until completely smooth.
4. Refrigerate it for 4 hours.
5. If your soup hardens in the refrigerator, add a bit of extra cold water to thin it down.
6. Alternatively, you may reheat the soup inside a pot and serve it warm.
7. Salt and black pepper to taste.
8. Garnish with chosen toppings and a sprinkle of olive oil.

Nutritional Values

Calories 272kcal, Carbs 30g, Protein 8g, Fat 15g, Sodium 886mg, Potassium 734mg, Chol 0mg

281. FRENCH-ONION-SOUP

- Dinner - Prep time: ready in about: 100 mins, Servings: 4-6, Grill temp: Medium

Ingredients

- 3 lb. of onions
- 6 tbsp of olive oil
- ¾ tsp of sea salt
- 1½ tbsp of tamari
- 1½ tbsp of balsamic vinegar
- 1½ tbsp of thyme leaves
- 3 tbsp of white flour
- 3 cloves of garlic
- 1 cup of wine
- black pepper
- 6 cups of vegetable broth
- Baguette slices
- Fresh thyme
- Gruyère cheese and aged cheddar

- pepper flakes

Directions

1. In a Dutch oven, heat oil on a moderate flame.
2. Toss in the salt, onions, and pepper to mix. Lower the heat and cook, occasionally stirring, for approximately 40mins, or till the onions seem to be very soft.
3. Raise the temperature to be medium and continue to cook, often turning, for another 15-20 mins or till golden brown.
4. Stir in the tamari, thyme, vinegar, thyme, and garlic.
5. Cook it for 2mins after adding the flour to the onions.
6. Cook for 2 mins.
7. Add remaining broth and cook for thirty mins on moderate flame.
8. Preheat your oven to 450°F and prepare a baking tray.
9. Place the slices of baguette onto the baking sheet, covered with cheese, then bake for 8-10 mins, or till the pieces are browned and the cheese has melted.
10. Serve the stew in bowls with baked baguette slices, red pepper flakes, and fresh thyme on top, if preferred.

Nutritional Values

Calories 115kcal, Carbs 14g, Protein 7g, Fat 10g, Sodium 627mg, Potassium 445mg, Chol 0mg

282. OYSTER-MUSHROOM-SOUP

- Dinner - Prep time: Dinner, ready in about: 70 mins, Servings: 6-8, Grill temp: Medium

Ingredients

- 3 cups of leeks
- 3 tbsp of olive oil- extra-virgin
- 1 cup of celery
- 2 tbsp of ginger
- ¼ cup of garlic
- 1½ tbsp of miso paste
- 1 tbsp of onion powder
- 1 tbsp of garlic powder
- 5 cups of vegetable broth
- 3 cups of oyster mushrooms
- 5 cups of filtered water
- 2 cups of carrot
- 1 stalk of lemongrass

- 5 leaves of bay
- 2 tbsp of tamari
- 1 tbsp of rice vinegar
- 1½ tbsp of lemon juice
- 1-inch of kombu
- 8 oz. of tofu
- black pepper

Directions

1. Heat olive oil in a saucepan on moderate heat.
2. Sauté the leeks & celery for approximately 10mins, or until transparent. Ginger and garlic should be added now.
3. Cook for 5 mins. Cook for yet another 5mins after adding the garlic powder, miso, & onion powder.
4. Add the water, vegetable broth, carrots, oyster mushrooms, lemongrass, bay leaves, tamari, vinegar, lemon juice, and kombu, as well as the lemongrass vinegar, bay leaves, lemon juice, tamari, and kombu.
5. Mix thoroughly.
6. Boil, then lower the heat and simmer for 5mins. Lower the heat and continue cooking for an additional thirty mins.
7. Add tofu, if preferred, and season with salt & black pepper.
8. Remove the kombu and bay leaves before serving. If desired, garnish with sesame seeds, scallions, and flakes of red pepper.

Nutritional Values

Calories 265kcal, Carbs 14g, Protein 18g, Fat 10g, Sodium 627mg, Potassium 245mg, Chol 0mg

283. Tortellini Soup

- Dinner - Prep time: ready in about: 50 mins, Servings: 4, Grill temp: Medium

Ingredients

- 1 onion
- 2 tbsp of olive oil- extra-virgin
- 2 carrots
- ½ tsp of sea salt
- 1 fennel bulb
- black pepper
- 2 cloves of garlic
- 2 tsp of balsamic vinegar
- 1 can of tomatoes
- 1 tbsp of thyme leaves

- 3½ cups of vegetable broth
- ½ cup of parsley
- ¼ - ½ tsp of pepper flakes
- 5 cups of torn kale
- 9- 12 oz. of cheese tortellini
- Kale Pesto

Directions

1. In a big saucepan on moderate heat, warm up the oil.
2. Cook, occasionally stirring, until the carrots, onion, salt, fennel, and black pepper soften for approximately 8 mins.
3. Combine the garlic, balsamic vinegar, tomatoes, thyme, broth, and flakes of red pepper in a large mixing bowl.
4. Cook for thirty mins. Meanwhile, prepare tortellini till al dente as per package guidelines in a saucepan of boiling water with salt.
5. Cook for 2mins longer after adding the tortellini & greens to the broth.
6. Season with salt and pepper to taste.
7. Serve in dishes with kale pesto & fresh parsley on top.

Nutritional Values

Calories 265kcal, Carbs 14g, Protein 7.5g, Fat 10g, Sodium 527mg, Potassium 445mg, Chol 0mg

284. Vegetarian Pho

- Dinner - Prep time: ready in about: 50 mins, Servings: 2, Grill temp: Medium

Ingredients

- 1 stick of cinnamon
- 2 anise
- 1 tbsp of whole peppercorns
- 5 cups of water
- ¼ tsp of whole cloves
- ½ onion
- 1 2-inch of ginger
- 2 cloves of garlic
- 4 oz. of shiitake mushrooms
- 1 tbsp of rice vinegar
- ¼ cup of tamari
- 2 scallions
- ½ cup of frozen edamame
- 2 bok choy
- 4 oz. of rice noodles- cooked
- Lime slices

- Fresh herbs, mint,
- Mung bean
- Sriracha

Directions

1. Mix the peppercorns, cinnamon stick, star anise, and cloves in a saucepan on less heat, then stir until aromatic, approximately 30 seconds.
2. Add the onion, water, ginger, garlic, and stems of the shiitake mushroom to the pot.
3. Cook for twenty mins, then drain the fluid and return it to the saucepan.
4. Add the caps of shiitake mushroom, rice vinegar, tamari, and scallions to the saucepan and mix well.
5. Cook for 15 mins. Heat until the edamame, and bok choy are soft about 5 to 8 mins.
6. Add more tamari to have flavor and more vinegar for tang.
7. Over the boiled rice noodles, pour the soup into 2 bowls. Garnish with sprouts, Chile peppers, lime slices, sriracha, herbs, and extra tamari.

Nutritional Values

Calories 212kcal, Carbs 14g, Protein 18.25g, Fat 10g, Sodium 627mg, Potassium 435mg, Chol 0mg

285. SPIRALIZED-ZUCCHINI-VEGETABLE-NOODLE SOUP

- Dinner - Prep time: ready in about: 50 mins, Servings: 6, Grill temp: Medium

Ingredients

- 1 onion
- 2 tbsp of olive oil- extra-virgin
- 2 chopped carrots
- 1 can of diced tomatoes
- ½ tsp of sea salt
- 3 cloves of garlic
- 15-20 sprigs of thyme
- 3 sprigs of rosemary
- 6 cups of vegetable broth
- 1½ cups of chickpeas, rinsed
- 3 cups of cannellini beans, cooked
- 1 potato- sweet
- black pepper
- 2 spiralized zucchini
- parmesan cheese, optional

Directions

1. In a saucepan over moderate heat, warm up the oil.
2. Combine the carrots, onion, and ½ tsp salt & pepper in a mixing bowl.
3. Cook, occasionally stirring, for approximately 8 mins or till the onions are tender.
4. Combine the rosemary, garlic, tomatoes, rosemary, and thyme in a mixing bowl.
5. Stir in the broth, sweet potato, chickpeas, zucchini noodles, and salt and pepper to taste.
6. Cook, occasionally stirring, for 20-30 mins.
7. Season with salt and pepper to taste, then top with parmesan cheese, finely grated, or pesto, if preferred.

Nutritional Values

Calories 265kcal, Carbs 14g, Protein 17g, Fat 10g, Sodium 627mg, Potassium 445mg, Chol 0mg

286. GINGER-MISO-SOUP

- Dinner - Prep time: ready in about: 50 mins, Servings: 2, Grill temp: Medium

Ingredients

- 4 cups of water
- dried kombu piece
- 4 cups of dashi
- 1 tsp of ginger
- 3-4 tbsp of miso paste
- ¼ cup of scallions- chopped
- 4 turnips
- ½ cup of shiitake mushrooms
- few tsps of soy sauce
- ½ carrots
- 4 oz. of soba noodles
- ½ cup of tofu cubes
- 1 cup of turnip greens

Directions

1. Wash the kombu slice gently.
2. Put in a medium saucepan containing 4 cups of water and cook for 10mins on low heat. If you allow it to boil, the kombu taste will become bitter.
3. Take the kombu out when it has softened and boil the water. Lower the heat, then add another cup of water. Whisk the miso

paste and part of the dashi water together in the basin, then stir it in soup stock.

4. Simmer over low heat till the turnips become soft & fork-tender, then add the scallions, ginger, and turnips, shiitake mushrooms, and carrots.
5. Toss in the soba noodles and tofu.
6. Now taste, and adjust spices, if desired, by adding a few tbsp of soy sauce.

Nutritional Values

Calories 158kcal, Carbs 12g, Protein 44g, Fat 10g, Sodium 427mg, Potassium 245mg, Chol 0mg

287. CABBAGE SOUP

- Dinner - Prep time: ready in about: 50 mins, Servings: 6, Grill temp: Medium

Ingredients

- 2 carrots
- 2 tbsp of olive oil extra-virgin
- 1 onion
- 2 tbsp of wine vinegar
- 1 rib of celery
- 2 cans of tomatoes
- 1 can of white beans, rinsed
- 4 cups of vegetable broth
- 4 cloves of garlic
- 1 green cabbage
- 2 diced potatoes
- 1 tsp of thyme-dried
- black pepper
- ¾ tsp of sea salt
- Fresh parsley

Directions

1. In a saucepan on moderate heat, add the oil.
2. Heat for 8mins, stirring regularly, with the celery, onion, carrots, salt, and pepper.
3. Add the broth, cabbage, tomatoes, beans, potatoes, garlic, and thyme, stirring to combine.
4. Cook for 20-30 mins, covered.
5. Add salt and pepper to taste, then serve some fresh parsley as a garnish.

Nutritional Values

Calories 365kcal, Carbs 14g, Protein 34g, Fat 10g, Sodium 627mg, Potassium 545mg, Chol 0mg

288. RIBOLLITA TUSCAN BEAN SOUP

- Dinner - Prep time: ready in about: 60 mins, Servings: 2-3, Grill temp: Medium

Ingredients

- 1 chopped onion
- 2 tbsp of olive oil- extra-virgin
- 3 chopped carrots
- 2 cloves of garlic
- 1 tbsp of rosemary- chopped
- 3 Roma, diced
- 2 tbsp of white wine
- ½ tsp of pepper flakes- red
- 1½ cups of cannellini beans, rinsed
- 3 kale leaves
- 4 cups of vegetable broth
- 4 slices of ciabatta bread
- ¼ cup of Parmesan cheese
- balsamic vinegar
- salt and black pepper

Directions

1. In a saucepan on moderate heat, heat olive oil.
2. Cook, turning periodically, until the onions are tender, approximately 4mins, with pepper and salt.
3. Combine the rosemary, carrots, and garlic in a mixing bowl.
4. Cook for another 4mins, lowering the temperature if required to protect the garlic from burning.
5. Add the red pepper flakes, tomatoes, salt & pepper to taste.
6. Cook for approximately 15 mins, stirring often.
7. Cook for 1 minute after adding the wine. After that, add beans and vegetable broth.
8. Cook, stirring periodically, for 30-35 mins.
9. Stir in cubed bread, kale, and balsamic vinegar after the carrots are soft.
10. Cook until the kale has wilted. Serve in big bowls. If desired, grate some Parmesan cheese.

Nutritional Values

Calories 365kcal, Carbs 10g, Protein 23g, Fat 10g, Sodium 427mg, Potassium 445mg, Chol 0mg

289. VEGGIE SOUP

- Dinner - Prep time: ready in about: 40 mins, Servings: 6, Grill temp: Medium

Ingredients

- 1 diced onion
- 2 tbsp of olive oil- extra-virgin
- Salt and black pepper
- 1 potato
- 1 diced carrot
- ¼ cup of white wine
- 4 cloves of garlic
- 1 14.5 oz. can of tomatoes
- 2 tsp of oregano
- 4 cups of vegetable broth
- ¼ tsp of pepper flakes
- 2 leaves of bay
- 1 cup of green beans
- 1 cup of cherry tomatoes
- 1 diced zucchini
- 2 tbsp of wine vinegar
- 1 15 oz. can of chickpeas
- 1½ cups of chopped kale

Directions

1. In a saucepan on moderate heat, heat oil.
2. Heat, stirring regularly, for 8mins with some onion, ½ tsp salt & pepper.
3. Cook for another 2mins after adding the sweet potato and carrot.
4. Heat for thirty seconds to decrease the wine by 50% before adding the tinned tomatoes, oregano, garlic, and flakes of red pepper.
5. Combine the broth & bay leaves in a mixing bowl.
6. Boil it, then lower to low heat for twenty mins, covered.
7. Cover and simmer for 10-15 mins longer, stirring in the zucchini, green beans, cherry tomatoes, and chickpeas.
8. Add the kale, vinegar, salt & pepper to taste.

Nutritional Values

Calories 265kcal, Carbs 12g, Protein 14g, Fat 6g, Sodium 627mg, Potassium 845mg, Chol 0mg

290. VEGETABLE STOCK

- Lunch - Prep time: ready in about: 60 mins, Servings: 8, Grill temp: Medium

Ingredients

- 4 carrots, chopped
- 2 onions, halved
- 1-2 celery stalks
- 1 garlic, halved
- Leek tops, chopped
- fresh parsley
- 3 leaves of bay
- fresh thyme
- tsp of sea salt
- 10-12 cups of water
- 1 tsp of peppercorns

Directions

1. In a saucepan, bring the onions, celery, carrot, leek tips, cloves, thyme, bay leaf, parsley, salt, pepper, & water to boiling over high temperature. If the pot doesn't accommodate Twelve cups of water, use 10 cups.
2. Reduce heat to low and cook for about 1 hour, undisturbed. Vegetables should be strained and discarded.
3. Season with salt and pepper to taste, then use with your best soup recipes.

Nutritional Values

Calories 375kcal, Carbs 15g, Protein 7g, Fat 17g, Sodium 527mg, Potassium 834mg, Chol 0mg

291. CREAMY-POTATO-SOUP

- Lunch - Prep time: ready in about: 40 mins, Servings: 4-6, Grill temp: Medium

Ingredients

- 1 white onion
- 3 tbsp of olive oil- extra-virgin
- ½ tsp of sea salt
- 1 tbsp of wine vinegar- white
- 4 cloves of garlic
- 4 cups of vegetable broth- homemade
- 1½ cups of white beans, rinsed
- 1½ lb. potatoes- chopped
- ½ tsp of Dijon mustard
- ¼ tsp of paprika
- 1 tbsp of lemon juice
- Black pepper- grounded
- Chives - optional, Greek yogurt
- Coconut bacon
- Cheddar cheese

Directions

1. In a saucepan, melt 2 tsp of oil over moderate flame. Combine the onions, pepper, and salt in a bowl. Cook for 6-8 mins before the vegetables are softened. Whisk in the garlic and simmer for another 2 mins.
2. Cook for thirty seconds while tossing with the white vinegar, and pour the broth, white beans, and potatoes. Bring to the boil, then lower the heat and continue to cook for 30 mins.
3. Allow cooling before blending ½ portion of the soup with the other 1 tsp of olive oil, mustard, lime juice, & paprika in a mixer.
4. Put the blended soup in a pot after blending before smoothing.
5. Carefully crush the potato slices and beans with the potato masher.
6. Sprinkle some salt & pepper, and then serve with the chosen toppings.

Nutritional Values

Calories 265kcal, Carbs 11g, Protein 7g, Fat 16g, Sodium 627mg, Potassium 534mg, Chol 0mg

292. SWEET-POTATO-SOUP

- Lunch - Prep time: ready in about: 30 mins, Servings: 4, Grill temp: Medium

Ingredients

- 1 yellow onion, sliced
- 2 tbsp of olive oil- extra virgin
- 1 tsp of salt
- 3 cubed potatoes
- Black pepper
- 1 chopped apple
- 1 tsp of ginger
- 3 cloves of garlic
- 1 tsp of coriander
- 1 tsp of vinegar
- ½ tsp of paprika- smoked
- 3-4 cups of vegetable broth
- Pepitas
- 1 can of coconut milk
- Fresh cilantro
- Crispy bread
- pepper for garnishing

Directions

1. In a saucepan over medium flame, heat oil.
2. Add the salt and fresh pepper and cook for 5-8 mins. Simmer, occasionally stir, before the potatoes & apple start to soften, approximately 8-10 mins.
3. Stir in the garlic, coriander, paprika, and ginger. Then, add vinegar, broth, and coconut milk.
4. Bring to the boil, then cover and low flame.
5. Cook for 20-30 mins before the potatoes are cooked.
6. Allow it to cool before transferring to a mixer and working in portions if required. If the soup is thick, mix in 1 cup of extra stock. If preferred, garnish with coconut milk, cilantro, and pepper.
7. With the crusty bread, serve.

Nutritional Values

Calories 155kcal, Carbs 14g, Protein 16g, Fat 10g, Sodium 627mg, Potassium 544mg, Chol 0mg

293. INSTANT-POT-LENTIL-SOUP

- Lunch - Prep time: ready in about: 60 mins, Servings: 8, Grill temp: Medium

Ingredients

- 1 chopped onion
- 2 tbsp of olive oil- extra virgin
- 2 stalks of celery
- 6 leaves of kale
- 2 cups of carrots
- 4 cloves of garlic
- ¾ cup of green lentils
- 1 can of roasted tomatoes
- 2 tbsp of vinegar- white
- 1½ tsp of sea salt
- 12 sprigs of thyme
- ½ tsp of cumin
- 6 cups of vegetable broth
- black pepper
- Red pepper
- Grated Parmesan, optional
- ½ cup of parsley
- Crispy bread for the serving

Directions

1. In your Pot, choose the Sauté setting.
2. Set the timer to 8 mins and level to moderate. Spray the oil in the Pot and add

onion, carrots, and celery when the pot has been warmed.
3. Cook for another 8 mins.
4. Stir in the kale, garlic, tomato, wine, thyme, salt, cumin, and then pepper.
5. Fill the Pot ½ with veggie liquid and cover it. Cook for 15 mins, in a cooker on high.
6. Allow the Pot to automatically release pressure. It will take around 20-30 mins.
7. Remove the cover and mix in the leaves of kale when the floating nozzle lowers.
8. Sprinkle with salt and red pepper.
9. Discard the bundle of thyme and, if preferred, top with parsley and Parmesan.
10. With the crusty bread, serve.

Nutritional Values

Calories 195kcal, Carbs 14g, Protein 18g, Fat 10g, Sodium 827mg, Potassium 834mg, Chol 0mg

294. BARLEY WITH WINTER VEGETABLE SOUP

- Main Course - Prep time: 5 mins, Cook time: 10 mins, Total time: 15 mins, Servings: 6 to 8, Grill temp: 300°F

Ingredients

- 6 cups of veggie broth
- 3 cups of water
- 2 cups of chopped winter vegetables
- 1 ½ cups of chopped carrots
- 1 cup of sliced onions
- 1 cup of peeled, chopped parsnip
- 1 cup of pearled barley
- 1 chopped potato
- ½ cup of chopped celery
- 2 tbsp of tamari
- 1 tbsp of olive oil
- 1 tbsp of miso- dissolved in 3 tbsp of water
- Salt and pepper to taste

Directions

1. Pour oil into a deep-bottomed saucepan with a lid and heat it.
2. When hot, cook celery, carrots, and onions until the onions are browning.
3. Pour in the broth, and add potato, tamari, parsnip, and barley.
4. Close and seal the lid.
5. Cook on high heat for 8 mins.

6. Turn off the heat and let it stand for some time.
7. Check the barley, and if it isn't cooked through, bring the pot back to pressure for 3-5 mins.
8. When ready, add the miso- dissolved in water.
9. Season and serve!

Nutritional Values

Calories 233, Fat 2g, Chol 0mg, Sodium 71.4mg, Potassium 67.7mg, Carbs 29g, Protein 4g

295. BLACK BEAN SOUP

- Main Course - Prep time: 5 mins, Cook time: 20 mins, Total time: 25 mins, Servings: 6, Grill temp: 300°F

Ingredients

- 4 tbsp of sour cream
- 1 chopped onion
- 1 tbsp of. chili powder
- Fifteen ounces of black beans
- 1 tbsp of canola oil
- 1 tsp of cumin
- ½ cup of prepared salsa
- ¼ tsp of salt
- 1 tbsp of lime juice
- 3 cups of water
- 2 tbsp of chopped cilantro

Directions

1. In a saucepan, heat oil and add onion.
2. Cook the onions for 3 mins,
3. Add cumin and chili powder while stirring.
4. Then, add salt, water, salsa, and beans and boil at low heat for 10 mins.
5. Turn off the heat and add lime juice.
6. Later, blend the mixture in a blender and make a puree.
7. Afterward, slightly cook the puree in a pan for 5 mins.
8. Serve it with cilantro or sour cream.

Nutritional Values

Calories 191, Fat 4g, Chol 0mg, Sodium 71.4mg, Potassium 67.7mg, Carbs 31g, Protein 9g

296. VEGAN CHILI SOUP

- Main course - Prep time: 30 mins, Cook time: 10 mins, Total time: 40 mins, Servings: 8, Grill temp: 300°F

Ingredients

- 6 cups of tomato juice
- 7 cups of canned kidney beans
- 2 cups of textured soy protein
- 2 cans of diced tomatoes
- 1 cup of water
- 5 minced garlic cloves
- 1 diced onion
- 2 tbsp of vegetable oil
- 1 tbsp plus 1 tsp of chili powder
- 1 tsp of garlic powder
- 1 tsp of sea salt
- ½ tsp of cumin
- Salt to taste

Directions

1. In a deep-bottomed saucepan/pot, heat the veggie oil.
2. When hot, cook onions until they're soft and about to become clear.
3. Add the garlic and cook for a minute or so. Scoop out the onions and garlic.
4. Add the tomato juice and seasonings.
5. Puree the onion/garlic mixture before returning it to the pot.
6. Add the rest of the ingredients.
7. Close and seal the lid.
8. Let it cook for around 7 mins.
9. Turn off the flame and let it stand for 5 mins.
10. Taste and season before serving!

Nutritional Values

Calories 331, Fat 5g, Chol 0mg, Sodium 71.4mg, Potassium 67.7mg, Carbs 51g, Protein 25g

297. CREAMY BROCCOLI SOUP WITH "CHICKEN" AND RICE

- Main Course - Prep time: 30 mins, Cook time: 10 mins, Total time: 40 mins, Servings: 8 to 10, Grill temp: 300°F

Ingredients

- 2 boxes of mushroom broth
- 2 bunches' worth of broccoli florets
- 1 head's worth of cauliflower florets
- 1 medium-sized, diced Yukon Gold potato
- 2 cups of cooked brown rice
- 1 package of vegan chicken strips
- 1 vegan, chicken-flavored bouillon cube
- 1 cup of water
- 1 cup of unsweetened almond milk
- 3 minced garlic cloves
- 1 diced white onion
- 2 tbsp of tamari
- 1 tbsp of vegetable oil
- Dash of salt
- Dash of black pepper

Directions

1. Heat the oil in a deep bottomed saucepan with a lid.
2. Toss in the onion and cook until soft.
3. Add garlic and cook for another minute or so.
4. Add the broccoli, cauliflower, and potato.
5. Season with the tamari, salt, pepper, and bouillon cube.
6. Pour in the liquids- water, milk, and broth and stir.
7. Close and seal the lid.
8. Cook on high pressure for 6 mins.
9. Turn off the flame and let it stand for 5 mins.
10. Puree when the soup has cooled a little.
11. Before serving, add the vegan chicken strips and cooked rice.

Nutritional Values

Calories 193, Fat 5g, Chol 0mg, Sodium 71.4mg, Potassium 67.7mg, Carbs 28g, Protein 8g

298. LENTIL AND VEGETABLE DAL

- Main Course - Prep time: 10 mins, Cook time: 30 mins, Total time: 40 mins, Servings: 4, Grill temp: 300°F

Ingredients

- 2 tbsp of coconut oil
- 1 large yellow onion, finely chopped
- 1 tbsp of finely chopped fresh ginger
- 2 cloves of garlic, minced
- 6 cups of vegetable stock
- 1 cup of red lentils picked over and rinsed
- 1 /3 small head cauliflower, separated into florets and finely chopped

- 1 tbsp of ground turmeric
- 1 tsp of ground coriander
- ½ tsp of ground cumin
- ¼ tsp of ground cinnamon
- ¼ tsp of cayenne
- 2 tbsp of tomato paste
- 1 bunch of spinach washed well, stemmed, and thinly sliced
- 1 tsp of kosher salt
- Juice of 1 medium lime
- 2 tbsp of finely chopped fresh cilantro
- ½ cup of plant-based plain yogurt

Directions

1. In a large soup pot over medium-high heat, heat coconut oil. Add yellow onion, ginger, and garlic, and cook, frequently stirring, for 5 mins. Reduce heat if necessary to prevent burning.
2. Stir in vegetable stock, red lentils, cauliflower, turmeric, coriander, cumin, cinnamon, and cayenne. Bring to a boil, reduce heat, and simmer for 20 mins.
3. When lentils and cauliflower are tender, place tomato paste in a small bowl. Ladle a little bit of broth into the bowl, stir until smooth, and stir the mixture back into the soup pot.
4. Add spinach, kosher salt, lime juice, and 1 tbsp of cilantro, and simmer for 5 mins.
5. Whisk the remaining 1 tbsp of cilantro into yogurt, and serve dal warm with a dollop of cilantro yogurt.
6. Make Naan served with dal.
7. Before making dal, in a large bowl, whisk together 2 ½ cups of all-purpose flour with 1 package of fast-acting instant yeast, 2 tsps of kosher salt, and 1 tsp of baking powder.
8. In a medium bowl, whisk together ¾ cup of warm water, 3 tbsp of plain plant-based yogurt, and 2 tbsp melted coconut oil. Stir wet ingredients into dry, and knead with your hands for 1 or 2 mins, to form a sticky dough. Let dough rise at room temperature for 45 mins or until doubled.
9. Heat a large cast-iron frying pan over medium heat for 10 mins before serving.
10. Divide dough into 6 balls and stretch into teardrop shapes about 5 inches-

12.5cm long. Dampen dough with a little water, add to the hot pan a few at a time, and cook for about 1 minute per side.
11. Brush the pan with ½ tsp grapeseed oil to keep naan from sticking if necessary.

Nutritional Values

Calories 323, Fat 4.8g, Chol 1mg, Sodium 91.4mg, Potassium 44mg, Carbs 56g, Protein 6.3g

299. LENTIL SOUP WITH CUMIN AND CORIANDER

- Breakfast - Prep time: 10 mins, Cook time: 20 mins, Total time: 30 mins, Servings: 8, Grill temp: 300°F

Ingredients

- 8 cups of veggie broth
- 2 cups of uncooked brown lentils
- 2 sliced carrots
- 2 cubed big Yukon gold potatoes
- 2 bay leaves
- 2 minced garlic cloves
- 1 chopped onion
- 1 chopped celery rib
- 1 tsp of ground coriander
- ½ tsp of ground cumin
- Black pepper to taste

Directions

1. First, pick through the lentils and throw out any stones, and then rinse.
2. Pour the broth into a pressure cooker and heat it up.
3. Prepare the vegetables. Add to the pressure cooker, along with everything else.
4. Close and seal the pressure cooker.
5. Cook on high pressure for 10 mins. After, wait for 5 mins before quick-releasing.
6. Check the tenderness of the lentils and potatoes.
7. If not done, turn the pot back and finish cooking with the lid on but not sealed or at pressure.
8. Pick out the bay leaves and salt to taste.
9. Serve with a squirt of lemon juice.

Nutritional Values

Calories 228, Fat 0g, Chol 0mg, Sodium 71.4mg, Potassium 67.7mg, Carbs 41g, Protein 14.4g

300. MEATY SEITAN STEW

- Main Course - Prep time: 10 mins, Cook time: 10 mins, Total time: 20 mins, Servings: 6 to 8, Grill temp: 300°F

Ingredients

- 4 cups of veggie broth
- 2 cups of cubed seitan
- 6 quartered baby potatoes
- 3 chopped carrots
- 1 15-ounce can of corn
- 1 15-ounce can of green beans
- 1 chopped sweet onion
- 2 bay leaves
- 2 tbsp of vegan-friendly Worcestershire sauce
- 2 tbsp of arrowroot powder
- 1 tbsp of tomato paste
- 1 tbsp of cumin
- 1 tsp of garlic powder
- 1 tsp of onion powder
- 1 tsp of paprika

Directions

1. Dissolve the arrowroot powder in a little bit of water.
2. Pour- along with everything else in the pressure cooker and stir.
3. Close and seal the lid.
4. Cook on high pressure for 10 mins.
5. Pick out the bay leaves before serving.
6. Add some black pepper if desired.

Nutritional Values

Calories 213, Fat 2g, Chol 0mg, Sodium 71.4mg, Potassium 67.7mg, Carbs 29g, Protein 19g

301. MEXICAN BAKED POTATO SOUP

- Main Course - Prep time: 5 mins, Cook time: 15 mins, Total time: 20 mins, Servings: 4, Grill temp: 300°F

Ingredients

- 4 cups of veggie broth
- 4 cups of diced potatoes
- 4 diced garlic cloves

- 1 diced onion
- ½ cup of salsa
- ½ cup of nutritional yeast
- ⅛ cup of seeded jalapeno peppers
- 1 tsp of cumin
- ¼ tsp of oregano
- Black pepper to taste

Directions

1. Heat up a deep-bottomed saucepan with a lid.
2. When hot, add the onion, jalapeno, and garlic. Stir until browning.
3. Add potatoes, salsa, cumin, and oregano, and pour the broth over everything. Stir.
4. Close and seal the lid.
5. Cook for 10 mins on high heat.
6. Turn off the heat and let it stand for 10 mins.
7. To make the soup creamy, run through a blender.
8. Add nutritional yeast and pepper.
9. Serve!

Nutritional Values

Calories 196, Fat 0g, Chol 0mg, Sodium 71.4mg, Potassium 67.7mg, Carbs 30g, Protein 10g

302. MINESTRONE

- Main Course - Prep time: 15 mins, Cook time: 60 mins, Total time: 1 hour 15 mins, Servings: 4 to 5, Grill temp: 300°F

Ingredients

- 4 tbsp of extra-virgin olive oil
- 1 large red onion, cut into small dice
- 3 medium carrots, cut into small dice
- 4 large stalks of celery, cut into small dice
- 5 cloves of garlic, minced
- 3 tbsp of tomato paste
- 6 cups of vegetable stock
- 1 large russet potato, peeled and cut into small dice
- 1 bay leaf
- 1 tsp of kosher salt, plus more to taste
- ½ small head of savoy cabbage, thinly sliced
- 1- 14 oz.. can of cannellini beans, rinsed and drained

- 1- 14 oz.. can of cranberry beans, rinsed and drained
- 1- 28 oz. can of diced tomatoes, with juice
- 4 tbsp of finely chopped fresh Italian flat-leaf parsley
- 1 tbsp of red wine vinegar
- ½ tsp of freshly ground black pepper

Directions

1. In a large soup pot over medium-high heat, heat 2 tbsp of extra-virgin olive oil. Add red onion, carrots, and celery, and cook, often stirring, for 5 mins.
2. Add 2 cloves of garlic, and stir for 1 minute more.
3. Stir in tomato paste, mix well, and add vegetable stock. Bring to a boil.
4. Add russet potato, bay leaf, and kosher salt. Reduce heat to a simmer, and cook for 15 mins.
5. Meanwhile, in a wide sauté pan over medium-high heat, heat the remaining 2 tbsp of extra-virgin olive oil. Add remaining 3 cloves of garlic, and stir for 30 seconds.
6. Add savoy cabbage, and cook, frequently stirring, for about 10 mins, or until cabbage is softened.
7. Add cabbage to the soup pot along with cannellini beans, cranberry beans, tomatoes with juice, and 2 tbsp of Italian flat-leaf parsley, and simmer for 30 mins.
8. Stir in red wine vinegar and black pepper. Allow soup to rest for 10 mins, remove bay leaf, stir in the remaining 2 tbsp of Italian flat-leaf parsley, and serve.

Nutritional Values

Calories 411, Fat 8.8g, Chol 5mg, Sodium 61.4mg, Potassium 89.7mg, Carbs 55g, Protein 5.3g

303. MUSHROOM & JALAPEÑO STEW

- Main Course - Prep time: 20 mins, Cook time: 50 mins, Total time: 1 hour 10 mins, Servings: 4, Grill temp: 300°F

Ingredients

- 2 tsps of olive oil
- 1 cup of leeks, chopped
- 1 garlic clove, minced
- ½ cup of celery stalks, chopped
- ½ cup of carrots, chopped
- 1 green bell pepper, chopped
- 1 jalapeño pepper, chopped
- 2 ½ cups of mushrooms, sliced
- 1 ½ cups of vegetable stock
- 2 tomatoes, chopped
- 2 thyme sprigs, chopped
- 1 rosemary sprig, chopped
- 2 bay leaves
- ½ tsps of salt
- ¼ tsp of ground black pepper
- 2 tbsp of vinegar

Directions

1. Set a pot over medium heat and warm oil.
2. Add in garlic and leeks and sauté until soft and translucent.
3. Add in the black pepper, celery, mushrooms, and carrots.
4. Cook as you stir for 12 mins, stirring in a splash of vegetable stock to ensure there is no sticking.
5. Stir in the rest of the ingredients.
6. Set heat to medium, allow to simmer for 25 to 35 mins, or until cooked through.
7. Divide into individual bowls and serve warm.

Nutritional Values

Calories 65, Fat 2.7g, Chol 0mg, Sodium 71.4mg, Potassium 67.7mg, Carbs 1g, Protein 2.8g

304. RED CURRY-COCONUT MILK SOUP

- Main Course - Prep time: 5 mins, Cook time: 6 mins, Total time: 11 min, Servings: 4, Grill temp: 300°F

Ingredients

- 2 cups of veggie broth
- 1 ½ cups of red lentils
- 1 15-ounce can of coconut milk
- 1 14-ounce can of diced tomatoes- with liquid
- 1 diced onion
- 3 minced garlic cloves
- 2 tbsp of red curry paste
- ⅛ tsp of ground ginger
- Dash of red pepper

- Handful of spinach

Directions

1. Heat a deep-bottomed saucepan/pot.
2. When hot, cook onion and garlic until they're beginning to brown.
3. Add the curry paste, ground ginger, and red pepper.
4. Stir to coat the onion and garlic in spices.
5. Pour in the diced tomatoes with their liquid, coconut milk, veggie broth, and lentils.
6. Stir before closing and sealing the lid.
7. Cook for 6 mins, on high.
8. Turn off the heat and let it stand for 10 mins.
9. When the pressure is all gone, throw in the spinach and serve when the leaves have wilted.

Nutritional Values

Calories 553, Fat 24g, Chol 0mg, Sodium 71.4mg, Potassium 67.7mg, Carbs 60g, Protein 23g

305. ROOT VEGGIE SOUP

- Main Course - Prep time: 10 mins, Cook time: 30 mins, Total time: 40 mins, Servings: 8, Grill temp: 300°F

Ingredients

- 7 cups of veggie broth
- 6 cups of peeled and chopped russet potatoes
- 3 cups of peeled and chopped carrots
- 1 cup of Italian-style tomatoes- canned
- 1 cup of chopped yellow onion
- ½ cup of coconut oil
- 2 tbsp of garlic powder
- 1 tbsp of mild chili powder
- 1 tbsp of salt

Directions

1. Pour everything into a deep pot with a lid.
2. Stir before closing the lid.
3. Let it boil and cook for around 30 mins.
4. Turn off the heat and let it stand for around 10 mins.
5. To make the soup creamy, blend until smooth.
6. Taste and season more if necessary.

Nutritional Values

Calories 256, Fat 14g, Chol 0mg, Sodium 71.4mg, Potassium 67.7mg, Carbs 31g, Protein 24g

306. SPICY CHILI WITH RED LENTILS

- Main Course - Prep time: 15 mins, Cook time: 20 mins, Total time: 35 mins, Servings: 5, Grill temp: 300°F

Ingredients

- 7 cups of water
- 2 cups of red lentils
- 2 diced red peppers
- 1 diced onion
- 14-ounce can of diced tomatoes
- 5 minced garlic cloves
- ¼ cup of brown sugar
- 6-ounce can of tomato paste
- 2 tbsp of apple cider vinegar
- 1 tbsp of paprika
- 1 tbsp of chili powder
- 1 tsp of cayenne

Directions

1. Prepare your ingredients.
2. Throw everything in the dee pot and seal the lid.
3. Cook for 17 mins on high pressure.
4. Turn down the flame and wait for 15 mins before opening up the lid.
5. Stir and serve over rice!

Nutritional Values

Calories 420, Fat 2g, Chol 0mg, Sodium 77mg, Potassium 62mg, Carbs 76g, Protein 24g

307. SPLIT-PEA SOUP

- Main Course - Prep time: 10 mins, Cook time: 45 mins, Total time: 55 mins, Servings: 6, Grill temp: 300°F

Ingredients

- 6 cups of veggie broth
- 1 pound of split peas
- 3 diced carrots
- 3 diced celery ribs
- 1 diced yellow onion
- 2 minced garlic cloves
- 2 tbsp of coconut oil
- 1 bay leaf

- ½ tbsp of smoked paprika
- ¼ tsp of dried thyme
- Black pepper

Directions

1. Prepare your vegetables.
2. Put everything in a deep pot and seal the lid.
3. Cook on high pressure for 15 mins.
4. Turn down the flame and let it stand for around 10 mins.
5. Open and stir the soup.
6. Season to taste.

Nutritional Values

Calories 180, Fat 1g, Chol 0mg, Sodium 71.4mg, Potassium 67.7mg, Carbs 32g, Protein 12g

308. TOFU STIR FRY WITH ASPARAGUS STEW

- Main Course - Prep time: 15 mins, Cook time: 30 mins, Total time: 45 mins, Servings: 4, Grill temp: 300°F

Ingredients

- 1 pound of asparagus cut-off stems
- 2 tbsp of olive oil
- 2 blocks of tofu pressed and cubed
- 2 garlic cloves, minced
- 1 tsp of Cajun spice mix
- 1 tsp of mustard
- 1 bell pepper, chopped
- ¼ cup of vegetable broth
- Salt and black pepper to taste

Directions

1. Using a huge saucepan with lightly salted water, place in asparagus and cook until tender for 10 mins, drain.
2. Set a wok over high heat and warm olive oil, stir in tofu cubes, and cook for 6 mins.
3. Place in garlic and cook for 30 seconds until soft.
4. Stir in the remaining ingredients, including reserved asparagus, and cook for an additional 4 mins.
5. Divide among plates and serve.

Nutritional Values

Calories 138, Fat 9g, Chol 0mg, Sodium 71.4mg, Potassium 67.7mg, Carbs 12g, Protein 7g

309. TOMATO RICE SOUP

- Main Course - Prep time: 10 mins, Cook time: 20 mins, Total time: 30 mins, Servings: 8, Grill temp: 300°F

Ingredients

- 3 tbsp of extra-virgin olive oil
- 2 medium leeks, thinly sliced
- 1 large carrot, finely chopped
- 4 medium stalks of celery, finely chopped
- 2 cloves of garlic, finely chopped
- 1 tsp of kosher salt
- 1 tsp of sweet Hungarian paprika
- ½ tsp of freshly ground black pepper
- ¼ tsp of smoked paprika
- ¼ tsp of ground allspice
- ¼ tsp of ground cloves
- 1 bay leaf
- 1- 28 oz. can of plum tomatoes, with juice, crushed by hand
- 4 cups of vegetable stock or filtered water
- ½ cup of white basmati rice
- ¼ cup of dry white wine
- ½ tsp of hot sauce- optional

Directions

1. In a medium soup pot over medium-high heat, heat extra-virgin olive oil. Add leeks, carrot, and celery, and cook for about 5 mins, or until leeks are reduced and softened.
2. Add garlic, kosher salt, sweet Hungarian paprika, black pepper, smoked paprika, allspice, cloves, and bay leaf, and stir for 1 minute.
3. Add crushed tomatoes with juice and vegetable stock, bring to a boil, and stir in white basmati rice. Reduce heat to medium, cover, and cook, occasionally stirring, for 15 mins or until rice is tender.
4. Remove bay leaf, and stir in white wine and hot sauce- if using. Serve immediately, or freeze in an airtight container for up to 3 months.

Nutritional Values

Calories 216, Fat 2.7g, Chol 0mg, Sodium 78mg, Potassium 49.7mg, Carbs 30g, Protein 10g

310. TURKISH SOUP

- Main Course - Prep time: 5 mins, Cook time: 10 mins, Total time: 15 mins, Servings: 10, Grill temp: 300°F

Ingredients

- 1 cup of red lentils
- 1 chopped carrot
- 1 chopped potato
- 1 chopped onion
- ½ cup of celery
- 3 minced garlic cloves
- ½ tbsp of rice
- 3 tsps of olive oil
- ½ tsp of paprika
- ½ tsp of coriander
- Salt to taste

Directions

1. Heat a deep-bottomed pot with a lid, and add oil.
2. While that heats up, prepare your veggies.
3. When the oil is hot, cook the garlic for a few mins until fragrant.
4. Rinse off the rice and lentils, and put them in the pot.
5. Add 2 ½ cups of water, paprika, salt, and veggies.
6. Close and seal the lid.
7. Cook on high pressure for 10 mins.
8. Turn down the flame and let it rest for 10 mins.
9. Let the mixture cool for a little while before pureeing in a blender.
10. Serve!

Nutritional Values

Calories 531, Fat 9g, Chol 0mg, Sodium 71.4mg, Potassium 67.7mg, Carbs 73g, Protein 29g

311. VEGGIE-QUINOA SOUP

- Main Course - Prep time: 5 mins, Cook time: 5 mins, Total time: 10 mins, Servings: 6, Grill temp: 300°F

Ingredients

- 3 cups of boiling water
- 2 bags of frozen mixed veggies- 12 ounces each
- 1 15-ounce can of white beans
- 1 15-ounce can of fire-roasted diced tomatoes
- 1 15-ounce can of pinto beans
- ¼ cup of rinsed quinoa
- 1 tbsp of dried basil
- 1 tbsp of minced garlic
- 1 tbsp of hot sauce
- ½ tbsp of dried oregano
- Dash of salt
- Dash of black pepper

Directions

1. Put everything in the pot and stir.
2. Close and seal the lid.
3. Cook for 2 mins on high pressure.
4. Turn down the heat and let it stand for some time.
5. When all the pressure is gone, open the pot and season to taste.
6. Serve!

Nutritional Values

Calories 201, Fat 1.1g, Chol 0mg, Sodium 71.4mg, Potassium 67.7mg, Carbs 37g, Protein 11g

312. WEEKNIGHT 3-BEAN CHILI

- Breakfast - Prep time: 10 mins, Cook time: 6 mins, Total time: 16 mins, Servings: 6 to 8, Grill temp: 300°F

Ingredients

- 3 ½ cups of vegetable broth
- 1 can of black beans
- 1 can of red beans
- 1 can of pinto beans
- 1 14.5-ounce can of diced tomatoes
- 1 14.5-ounce can of tomato sauce
- 2 cups of chopped onion
- ¾ cup of chopped carrots
- ¼ cup of chopped celery
- 1 chopped red bell pepper
- 2 tbsp of mild chili powder
- 1 tbsp of minced garlic
- 1 ½ tsps of ground cumin
- 1 ½ tsps of dried oregano
- 1 tsp of smoked paprika

Directions

1. Rinse and drain the canned beans.

2. Heat a pressure cooker before throwing in the onion and garlic to sauté for 5 mins or so.
3. Add the rest of the ingredients except the tomatoes and tomato sauce. Stir.
4. Close and seal the lid.
5. Cook on high pressure for 6 mins.
6. Let the pressure come down naturally. When the pressure is gone, stir in the tomato sauce and diced tomatoes.
7. If you want a thicker chili, spoon out 2 cups of the chili and blend before returning to the pot.
8. Serve with fresh parsley if desired.

Nutritional Values

Calories 167, Fat 1g, Chol 0mg, Sodium 71.4mg, Potassium 67.7mg, Carbs 32g, Protein 11g

313. VEGETABLE DETOX SOUP

- Prep time: 20 mins, Cook time: 20 mins, Total time: 40 mins, Servings: 6

Ingredients

- 2 cloves garlic minced
- 1 cup purple cabbage chopped
- 1 tbsp fresh ginger peeled and minced
- 2 cups kale de-stemmed and torn into pieces
- 2 cups chopped celery
- fresh cracked black pepper to taste
- 1 cup chopped carrots
- pink Himalayan salt or sea salt to taste
- 3 cups broccoli florets
- 1 tsp Italian seasoning
- 1 cup cauliflower florets
- 4 cups water
- olive oil
- 1 can 14.5 oz. can of no-salt diced tomatoes- preferably organic
- a handful of chopped parsley for serving
- juice from ½ of a small lemon
- ½ of a red onion diced
- ½ tsp turmeric optional or to taste

Directions

1. Add the oil to a big saucepan and set the heat to medium-high. Combine the onion, garlic, and ginger in a mixing bowl. Cook, occasionally stirring, for 2 mins. Combine the celery, carrots, broccoli, and cauliflower in a large mixing bowl. Cook, occasionally stirring, for 2-3 mins, or until slightly softened. Combine the turmeric & diced tomatoes in a mixing bowl.
2. Bring the water to a boil. Reduce the heat to low and cook for 15-20 mins or until the veggies are soft. Near the end of the simmering time, add the Italian spice, salt & pepper to taste the kale, cabbage, and lemon juice.
3. Serve with chopped parsley on the side.

Nutritional Values

Calories 39kcal, Carbohydrates-8g, Protein 3g, Fat 1g, Sodium 41mg

314. MEAN GREEN DETOX VEGETABLE SOUP

- Prep time: 15 mins, Cook time: 45 mins, Total time: 60 mins, Servings: 6

Ingredients

- 4 carrots chopped
- 4 cloves of garlic minced or grated
- 2 cups broccoli florets
- 1-inch piece of ginger grated
- 4 cups roughly torn kale
- kosher salt + pepper
- 1 cup green lentils
- ½ tsp cayenne pepper
- 1 tbsp apple cider vinegar
- 2 tbsp olive oil
- ¼ cup of low-sodium soy sauce
- zest + juice of 1 lemon
- ¼ cup fresh parsley plus cilantro
- 1 leek halved + sliced
- ¼ head of purple cabbage shredded
- 2 quarts low sodium vegetable broth

Directions

1. In a large saucepan over medium heat, heat the olive oil. Add the leeks & carrots when the oil begins to shimmer. Cook for 5 mins, occasionally stirring. Cook for another 30 - 60 seconds after adding the garlic and ginger. Add salt & pepper to taste. Combine the cayenne pepper, broth, soy sauce, & vinegar in a mixing bowl. Bring the pot to a boil over high temperature with 2 cups of water. Reduce heat to medium-low and cook the lentils for 20 mins. Add the

broccoli, kale, and cabbage and simmer for another 10-15 mins, or until the lentils and broccoli are soft.

2. Mix in the lemon juice, parsley, and cilantro just before serving. If necessary, season with additional salt.

3. Serve the soup in dishes with vegan Parmesan on top.

Nutritional Values

Calories 70kcal, Carbohydrates-14g, Protein 3g, Fat 0.5g, Sodium 200mg

315. CLEANSING DETOX SOUP

- Prep time: 15 mins, Cook time: 15 mins, Total time: 30 mins, Servings: 4

Ingredients

- 1 cup purple cabbage, chopped
- 2 cloves garlic, minced
- 2 cups kale, de-stemmed and torn into pieces
- 3 celery stalks, diced
- 6 cups water- or 4 cups vegetable broth + 2 cups water
- 3 medium carrots, diced
- fine-grain sea salt and black pepper, to taste
- 1 small head of broccoli, florets
- 1/8 tsp cayenne pepper, or to taste-optional
- 1 cup chopped tomatoes
- ½ of red onion, diced
- ¼ cup water- or vegetable broth
- 1 tbsp fresh ginger, peeled and minced
- 1 tsp turmeric
- ¼ tsp cinnamon
- juice from ½ of a small lemon

Directions

1. Add the water to a big saucepan and set the heat to high. Add the garlic and onion once it's heated. Cook, stirring periodically, for 2 mins. Combine the carrots, celery, tomatoes, broccoli, and fresh ginger in a large mixing bowl. Cook for 3 mins, occasionally stirring and adding more water or broth as required- another ¼ cup. Combine the cinnamon, turmeric, and cayenne pepper, as well as salt and pepper to taste, in a mixing bowl.

2. Bring to a boil with water or veggie broth. Reduce the heat to low and cook for another 10-15 mins or until the veggies are tender. Near the end of the simmering time, add the kale, cabbage, and lemon juice.

3. Enjoy!

Nutritional Values

Calories 114kcal, Carbohydrates-27.4g, Protein 3.3g, Fat 0.8g, Sodium 955mg

316. VEGAN TURMERIC CAULIFLOWER CHICKPEA STEW

- Prep time: 7 mins, Cook time: 23 mins, Total time: 30 mins, Servings: 6

Ingredients

- 2 shallots, diced
- 2 tbsp coconut oil
- 1 can of chickpeas
- 2 stalk celery, chopped
- 4 cups cauliflower florets- about 1 head of cauliflower
- 1 whole lemon, juiced
- 1 can of full-Fat coconut milk
- 2 tsp turmeric powder
- 4 cups of reduced-Sodium vegetable broth
- 2 tsp ginger powder
- ¼ cup fresh Italian parsley, chopped
- ½ tsp salt
- ½ tsp fresh ground black pepper

Directions

1. In a soup pot over low heat, combine the coconut oil, shallots, and celery. 3 mins of sautéing

2. Season with salt and pepper, then add the lemon juice, vegetable broth, coconut milk, and cauliflower. Bring to a boil, then reduce to low heat for 20 mins.

3. Use a blender to mix the soup partly so it is creamy but still has some cauliflower chunks.

4. To finish heating, add the chickpeas & parsley & simmer for 8-10 mins.

5. Enjoy!

Nutritional Values

Calories 276kcal, Carbohydrates-28g, Protein 8.9g, Fat 15.5g, Sodium 243mg

317. CHICKEN DETOX SOUP

- Prep time: 20 mins, Cook time: 35 mins, Total time: 55 mins, Servings: 12

Ingredients

- 2 quarts of chicken broth
- 2 ½ cups sliced carrots
- 3 tbsp fresh ginger, shredded or grated
- 1 large onion, peeled and chopped
- ¼ tsp ground turmeric
- ¼ - ½ tsp crushed red pepper
- 3 cups broccoli florets
- 1 tbsp apple cider vinegar
- 2 cups chopped celery
- 2 tbsp olive oil
- 1 ½ cup frozen peas
- 4 garlic cloves minced
- 1 ½ pounds boneless skinless chicken breast
- ¼ cup chopped parsley
- salt and pepper

Directions

1. Place a large sauce saucepan on the stove over medium heat. Combine the chopped onions, olive oil, ginger, celery, and garlic in a large mixing bowl. To soften, cook for 5-6 mins. The raw chicken breasts, carrots, broth, crushed red pepper, apple cider vinegar, turmeric, and 1 tsp sea salt are added.
2. Bring to a boil, then reduce to low heat and cook for 20+ mins or until the boneless breasts are fully cooked. The chicken should then be removed with tongs and placed on a chopping board to cool.
3. Toss in the broccoli, peas, & parsley. Continue to cook until the broccoli is tender. Meanwhile, using 2 forks, shred the chicken pieces and return them to the soup. Taste the broccoli after it's soft, and season with salt and pepper as required. Warm the dish before serving.

Nutritional Values

Calories 91kcal, Carbohydrates-6g, Protein 9g, Fat 2g, Sodium 456mg

318. SLIMMING DETOX SOUP

- Prep time: 10 mins, Cook time: 20 mins, Total time: 30 mins, Servings: 4

Ingredients

- 1 large shallot peeled and thinly sliced
- a handful of pea pods of any type, halved if large
- a handful of small grape tomatoes cut in ½
- 2 cloves garlic minced
- 1 hot chili pepper
- 2 tbsp olive oil
- a handful of baby kale and or spinach leaves
- 1 thumb-sized piece of fresh ginger peeled and grated
- salt and black pepper to taste
- A 32-ounce carton of Swanson® Unsalted Chicken Broth
- 1 bell pepper any color, cut into strips
- 1 large carrot peeled and thinly sliced
- a handful of shredded red cabbage
- a handful of small broccoli florets
- several mushrooms sliced
- 1 medium golden beet or several baby beets, peeled and sliced
- a handful of small cauliflower florets
- a sprinkling of grated Parmesan or other hard Italian cheese

Directions

1. In a big heavy-bottomed pan, heat the olive oil. Soften the garlic, shallot, and ginger in a skillet for a few mins.
2. Bring the broth to a low simmer in the pan. Simmer for a few mins after adding the carrots and beets.
3. Simmer for a few mins, more after adding the broccoli & cauliflower florets, as well as the hot pepper, if using. The vegetables should be just soft enough to eat. If not, cook for a few mins longer.
4. The red cabbage, mushrooms, pea pods, and bell pepper will be added next. Bring to a boil again, then reduce the heat to low; these vegetables don't need much cooking. Season with salt and pepper to taste.
5. When ready to serve, toss in the leafy greens & tomatoes and whisk everything together. Add a sprinkle of cheese to each bowl.

Nutritional Values

Calories 300kcal, Carbohydrates-56g, Protein 2g, Fat 3g, Sodium 550mg

319. CLEANSING CARROT AUTUMN SQUASH SOUP

- Prep time: 15 mins, Cook time: 25 mins, Total time: 40 mins, Servings: 4

Ingredients

- ½ white onion, chopped
- ½ cup vegetable broth- low-sodium or water- for sautéing
- fresh juice from ½ lemon
- 1 to 2 cloves minced garlic
- ½ cup unsweetened almond milk- or light coconut milk
- 2 medium-sized chopped carrots
- 4 cups of low-Sodium vegetable broth
- 1 apple, chopped
- black pepper, to taste
- 1 ½ tbsp fresh ginger, minced
- ¼ tsp cinnamon
- 1 small butternut squash, peeled and chopped
- 2 tbsp pure maple syrup
- 1 tsp sea salt
- ½ tsp turmeric
- ½ tsp dried thyme

Directions

1. Heat the vegetable broth- or water in a soup pot over medium-high heat. For 2-3 mins, sauté the garlic and onion.
2. Combine the carrots, apple, and ginger in a mixing bowl. Cook for approximately 5 mins.
3. Add the butternut squash, turmeric, thyme, cinnamon, and pepper to the pan. Cook for another 5 mins after thoroughly mixing.
4. Combine the vegetable broth & almond milk in a mixing bowl. Bring to a boil, then lower to low heat and cover to keep warm. Cook for 20 mins or until all of the veggies are tender.
5. Remove from heat and mix in the maple syrup and fresh lemon juice.
6. Puree the soup with a hand blender until smooth and creamy. A standard blender may also be used, but be cautious! To avoid a soup explosion, be sure to let out hot air from the top.
7. Taste the dish and adjust the seasonings as required.
8. Serve right away. Fresh apples, pumpkin seeds, hemp seeds, raisins, or nuts make great garnishes!
9. Freeze for up to 3 days before serving. It freezes quite nicely.
10. Enjoy!

Nutritional Values

Calories 323kcal, Carbohydrates-52g, Protein 8g, Fat 11g, Sodium 325mg

320. TOMATO BASIL SOUP

- Prep time: 10 mins, Cook time: 1 hr, Total time: 1 hr 10 mins, Servings: 4

Ingredients

- 2 tbsp extra virgin olive oil divided
- 1 pound tomatoes heirloom
- ½ tsp kosher or sea salt
- 1 carrot diced
- 1 bay leaf
- 1 celery stalk diced
- dash of cayenne pepper
- 2 garlic cloves minced
- 2 cups vegetable broth low-sodium
- 2 medium shallots chopped
- ¼ cup chopped basil

Directions

1. Preheat the oven to 400°F.
2. Split the tomatoes and set them on a foil-lined baking sheet. 1 tbsp oil drizzled over tomatoes to catch any liquid; gently fold the foil's edges toward the tomatoes. 20 mins are required to roast tomatoes.
3. Meanwhile, sauté chopped carrot & celery in the leftover 1 tbsp of oil in a small pan over medium-low heat until soft, 10–15 mins. Turn heat to low & continue to sauté for another 4 mins, with the bay leaf, garlic, and shallots.
4. Remove the tomatoes from the oven and set them aside to cool for 15 mins or until they are safe to handle. The peeling should simply peel away from the tomatoes. Peelings should be discarded. To remove any seeds, press tomatoes through a sieve

if preferred.- Removing seeds is a personal choice, not a must.

5. Remove bay leaf, then puree all ingredients- except broth in a food processor or with an emulsion blender.
6. In a medium saucepan, combine the tomato purée and broth, bring to a boil, lower to a low simmer, and cook for 15–20 mins. Remove the bay leaf before serving.

321. LENTIL AND KALE SOUP

- Prep time: 10 mins, Cook time: 1 hr, Total time: 1 hr 10 mins, Servings: 8

Ingredients
- 3 cups vegetable broth
- 1 onion medium, coarsely chopped
- ½ tsp pepper
- 1 carrot medium, peeled and coarsely chopped
- ½ tsp salt
- 1 celery stalk coarsely chopped
- 2 cups lite coconut milk canned
- 1 cup chopped kale
- 1 cup of water to water it down
- ½ cup lentils
- 1 tbsp extra virgin olive oil
- 2 bay leaves torn in ½

Directions
1. Sauté the onions for 2 mins in a saucepan with olive oil over medium-low heat, then add the celery and carrots. 5 mins in the oven
2. Cook for a further 10 mins after adding the kale.
3. Toss the lentils into the pot and cook for 2 mins.
4. Combine the vegetable broth & bay leaves in a large mixing bowl. Bring to a boil, then reduce to low heat and cook for 20 mins.
5. Cook for a further 10 mins after adding the coconut milk.
6. Season with salt & pepper, then remove and discard the bay leaves.
7. Blend the soup with an immersion blender until it is smooth and creamy.

8. Cook for a further 5 mins. With the water, adjust the soup's consistency.
9. Pour them into individual cups and finish with a sprinkle of olive oil.

322. ROASTED CAULIFLOWER SOUP

- Prep time: 5 mins, Cook time: 1 hr, Total time: 1 hr 5 mins, Servings: 4

Ingredients
- 1 onion medium, roughly chopped
- 14 ounces cauliflower head small, florets separated
- ½ tsp rosemary fresh, finely chopped
- pepper to taste
- 4 cups vegetable broth
- 1 tbsp extra virgin olive oil
- ½ cup water to water it down
- ½ tsp salt
- 1 celery stalk roughly chopped

Directions
1. Preheat the oven to 390°F.
2. Scatter the cauliflower on a baking tray lined with parchment paper. Drizzle with olive oil after seasoning with salt and pepper. Preheat the oven to 350°F and bake for 30 mins.
3. After 30 mins, sautè the onions & celery in olive oil in a saucepan over medium heat.
4. Toss in the roasted cauliflower and cook for 5 mins.
5. Cook for a further 15 mins after adding the veggie broth and rosemary.
6. In a saucepan, mix the soup with an immersion blender until smooth and creamy. Cook for another 5 mins, after seasoning with salt and pepper.
7. Drizzle olive oil over the top before serving in cups.

323. CREAMY BUTTERNUT SQUASH SOUP

- Prep time: 5 mins, Cook time: 55 mins, Total time: 60 mins, Servings: 4

Ingredients

- 2/3 cup of coconut milk canned, whole, not light, is preferred
- 1 pound diced squash
- 1 tsp nutmeg grated
- 4 cups vegetable broth
- ground pepper
- 1 white onion medium, coarsely chopped
- extra virgin olive oil
- Salt
- thyme fresh

Directions

1. Sauté the onion in olive oil in a large saucepan over medium heat.
2. Add the squash after the onion has cooked through, approximately 3 mins. Cook for 10 mins, constantly stirring.
3. Cover and cook for approximately 20 mins on low heat with the veggie broth.
4. Add the nutmeg after seasoning with salt and pepper.
5. Puree the soup in the pot with an immersion blender while it's still hot.
6. Cook for another 10 mins after adding the coconut milk.
7. Before switching off the heat, add the thyme.
8. Serve immediately.

Nutritional Values

Calories 308kcal, Carbs 33g, Protein 8g, Fat 17g, Sodium 250mg

324. RAW RED PEPPER SOUP

- Prep time: 10 mins, Cook time: 0 mins, Total time: 10 mins, Servings: 3

Ingredients

- 3 cups red bell pepper chopped, ½ cup reserved
- 2/3 cup raw cashews
- 1 ½ cups water
- basil, parsley, or cilantro chopped for garnish

Directions

1. Blend all of the ingredients until smooth, excluding ½ cup reserved red pepper.

2. Add the rest of ½ cup of red bell pepper to a mixing bowl. Serve with basil, parsley, or cilantro as a garnish.

Nutritional Values

Calories 213kcal, Carbohydrates-17g, Protein 6g, Fat 15g, Sodium 209mg

325. BROCCOLI BASIL CREAM SOUP

- Prep time: 15 mins, Cook time: 8 mins, Total time: 23 mins, Servings: 4

Ingredients

- 2 tbsp extra virgin olive oil or virgin coconut oil
- ½ cup broccoli sprouts are optional but are potent detoxifiers
- 1 cup zucchini squash organic, diced- leave the skin on
- 6 to 8 basil leaves fresh
- sea salt unrefined, to taste
- 1/3 cup walnuts raw, soak for 3 hours in filtered water, rinsed well, and drained
- 4 cups broccoli florets organic, steamed
- 1 tbsp lemon juice fresh
- 4 cups vegetable broth organic or vegetable stock
- 2 garlic cloves grated
- ½ cup white onion diced
- black pepper fresh ground, to taste

Directions

1. In a medium-size saucepan with a cover, heat the olive oil/coconut oil until hot.
2. Add the chopped onions and zucchini cubes, and season with salt and pepper to taste. Cook for 7-8 mins, or until zucchini and onions are soft.
3. In a high-powered blender, combine steamed broccoli, cooked veggies, ½ cup vegetable broth, black pepper to taste, grated garlic, and drained walnuts. Blend on high speed until the mixture is smooth and creamy.
4. Pour the vegetable-walnut combination back into the saucepan where the zucchini was cooked, along with the remaining vegetable stock and salt to taste. Cover the saucepan with a lid and stir to combine everything.

5. Broccoli Basil Cream Soup should be heated but not boiled when served. Put into a serving dish after tasting and adjust seasoning if necessary. If using, garnish the hot soup with lemon juice, fresh basil leaves, and broccoli sprouts.
6. Place any remaining soup in a heatproof container with a cover and set it aside to cool slightly before putting it in the fridge. For supper, reheat the leftover soup over low heat.

Nutritional Values

Calories 329kcal, Carbohydrates-37g, Protein 11g, Fat 17g, Sodium 532mg

326. CREMINI MUSHROOM SOUP

- Prep time: 0 mins, Cook time: 20 mins, Total time: 20 mins, Servings: 6

Ingredients

- 1 garlic clove minced
- ½ cup diced onion
- salt to taste
- 1 tbsp olive oil
- ½ tsp black pepper
- 4 cups of chicken broth with low sodium
- 1 ½ pounds cremini mushrooms diced
- ¼ cup flat-leaf parsley fresh, chopped
- parmesan grated for garnish

Directions

1. Sauté the onion & garlic in olive oil in a medium soup pot until translucent, approximately 6 mins. Add the chicken broth, parsley, mushrooms, salt & pepper to taste. Cook, occasionally stirring, until the mushrooms get wilted, about 10 mins. Season with salt to taste.
2. You may also purée the soup if you like a smoother texture. To puree the soup, put an immersion/hand blender in the pot or fill the blender halfway with water each time, cover with a towel, & puree until smooth, beginning on low and progressing to high. For a creamier consistency, add a splash of milk to the pureed soup.
3. Serve with a sprinkling of Parmesan cheese & fresh parsley as a garnish.

Nutritional Values

Calories 71kcal, Carbohydrates-8g, Protein 4g, Fat 3g, Sodium 86mg

327. PROTEIN PACKED BLACK BEAN AND LENTIL SOUP

- Prep time: 10 mins, Cook time: 35 mins, Total time: 45 mins, Servings: 8

Ingredients

- 2 garlic cloves minced
- 1 tbsp olive oil
- ½ tsp crushed red pepper
- 1 yellow onion diced small
- ½ tsp kosher salt
- 2 carrots peeled and diced small
- ½ tsp black pepper
- 15 ounces diced tomatoes can
- ½ tsp cumin
- 1 cup dried lentils
- 4 cups vegetable broth
- 15 ounces of black beans can- drained
- 1 tsp chili powder

Directions

1. Add olive oil to a big saucepan and sauté garlic for 1 minute. Continue to sauté the diced onions & carrots until the onion is soft, about 5 mins. Cover and mix in the remaining ingredients.
2. Bring to a boil over medium heat, then lower to low heat and cook for 25 to 30 mins, or until lentils & carrots are cooked.

Nutritional Values

Calories 171kcal, Carbohydrates-29g, Protein 10g, Fat 2g, Sodium 3640mg

328. THAI ROASTED SWEET POTATO SOUP

- Prep time: 5 mins, Cook time: 55 mins, Total time: 60 mins, Servings: 6

Ingredients

- ½ tsp sea salt
- 1 pound of sweet potatoes peeled and cubed
- 2 cups vegetable broth
- ½ tsp yellow curry powder
- 1 cup of coconut milk canned
- ¼ tsp cumin
- 1 tsp lemon juice

- ½ inch ginger root peeled and finely chopped
- ½ cup water to water it down
- 1 onion medium, roughly chopped
- 1 tbsp extra virgin olive oil
- ½ tsp black pepper

Directions

1. Preheat the oven to 395°F.
2. Place the potatoes on a baking sheet, drizzle with olive oil, and add salt and pepper. Preheat oven to 350°F and cook for 30 mins.
3. Sauté the onions in olive oil in a medium skillet over medium heat before adding the sweet potatoes. Cook for approximately 5 mins.
4. Toss in the curry, cumin, and ginger, and cook for 1 minute.
5. Allow boiling after adding the veggie broth and lemon juice. Cook for 5 mins at a low temperature.
6. Cook for a further 5 mins after adding the coconut milk. Salt & pepper to taste.
7. Blend the soup with an immersion blender until it is smooth. With the water, adjust the consistency to your liking. Cook for a further 5 mins.
8. Before serving, drizzle with olive oil.

Nutritional Values

Calories 230kcal, Carbohydrates-29g, Protein 4g, Fat 12g, Sodium 153mg

329. SLOW COOKER SAVORY SUPERFOOD SOUP

- Prep time: 5 mins, Cook time: 8 hrs, Total time: 8 hrs 5 mins, Servings: 8

Ingredients

- 1 garlic clove minced
- 2 cups sliced carrots
- 2 cups vegetable broth low-sodium, water as a substitute
- 1 cup green beans, fresh or frozen
- kosher or sea salt to taste
- ½ cup fresh cilantro chopped
- 1 tsp cumin
- 1 onion small, diced
- 2 cups tomato-based vegetable juice, no sugar added, similar to V8 juice

- 1 sweet potato large, cut into ½-inch cubes
- 1 tsp chili powder
- 30 ounces of black beans cans, drained and rinsed
- ½ tsp crushed red pepper flakes
- ½ tsp black pepper

Directions

1. In a slow cooker, combine all ingredients, cover, and simmer on low for 8 hours or until soft vegetables. If preferred, top with a spoonful of reduced-Fat cheddar cheese.
2. Add 2 cups roughly chopped kale in the final 5 mins of simmering, or until wilted, to make this a Superfood Soup.

Nutritional Values

Calories 157kcal, Carbohydrates-32g, Protein 7g, Fat 1g, Sodium 174mg

330. FLUSH THE FAT AWAY VEGETABLE SOUP

- Prep time: 0 mins, Cook time: 8 hrs, Total time: 8 hrs mins, Servings: 8

Ingredients

- 3 carrots large, peeled, and sliced
- 1 sweet potato medium, peeled and cut into 1-inch cubes
- 4 cups baby spinach loosely packed- optional 2 zucchini, sliced
- 14 ½ ounces diced tomatoes can- no salt added
- 1 celery stalk diced
- 4 cups vegetable broth low-sodium
- 1 yellow onion small, diced
- 1 tbsp plus 1 tsp extra-virgin olive oil optional, for serving- ½ tsp per serving
- 1 garlic clove minced
- 30 ounces navy beans cans, drained and rinsed- optional black beans
- pinch of kosher or sea salt, more or less to taste
- 1 tsp paprika
- ½ tsp black pepper
- 1 bay leaf
- 1/8 tsp allspice

Directions

1. In a slow cooker, combine all ingredients except the spinach and olive oil. Cook for 6

to 8 hours on low or until the veggies are soft.
2. Stir in the spinach and simmer for another 5 mins or until it has wilted.
3. Serve and have fun!

Nutritional Values
Calories 181kcal, Carbohydrates-31g, Protein 9g, Fat 3g, Sodium 603mg

331. SLOW COOKER BUTTERNUT SQUASH & KALE STEW

- Prep time: 10 mins, Cook time: 3 hrs, Total time: 3 hrs 10 mins, Servings: 6

Ingredients
- 2 cups vegetable broth low-sodium
- 1 sweet potato cut into ½-inch cubes
- 2 cups vegetable juice
- ½ cup cilantro fresh, chopped
- kosher or sea salt to taste
- 1 onion small, diced
- 1 tsp cumin
- 1 garlic clove minced
- 1 tsp chili powder
- 30 ounces of black beans cans, drained and rinsed
- ½ tsp black pepper
- 2 cups sliced carrots
- 8 ounces kale coarsely chopped
- 1 butternut squash small, cut into ½-inch cubes
- ½ tsp crushed red pepper flakes

Directions
1. In a slow cooker, combine all of the ingredients except the kale.
2. Cover and simmer for 6-8 hours on low, 3-4 hours on high, or until soft vegetables.
3. Cover for 5 mins or until kale has wilted.

Nutritional Values
Calories 229kcal, Carbohydrates-46g, Protein 13g, Fat 1g, Sodium 413mg

332. SLOW COOKER CHICKEN ENCHILADA STEW

- Prep time: 10 mins, Cook time: 3 hrs 10 mins, Total time: 3 hrs 20 mins, Servings: 6

Ingredients
- 10 ounces red enchilada sauce can, sugar-free
- 1 cup Greek yogurt Fat-free
- 15 ounces of kidney beans can, drained and rinsed
- 1 tsp cumin
- 15 ounces black beans can, drained and rinsed
- 1 tsp paprika
- 1 cup corn frozen or fresh
- 1 tsp salt
- 3 boneless and skinless chicken breasts
- ½ tsp pepper
- 2 cups chicken stock
- ½ tsp cayenne pepper
- 1 tbsp lime juice
- 2 tbsp chopped cilantro
- 14 ½ ounces petite diced tomatoes with green chiles can
- 2 tbsp chili powder

Directions
1. A large slow cooker combines undrained tomatoes, enchilada sauce, black beans, corn, kidney beans, and uncooked chicken breasts. Combine the chicken stock with all of the ingredients in a large mixing bowl. Mix thoroughly.
2. Cover and cook for 3-5 hours on high or 5-8 hours on low or until the chicken is readily shreddable. Remove the chicken and shred it with 2 forks in a separate dish. In the meanwhile, mix the Greek yogurt into the slow cooker until it is well incorporated. Return the shredded chicken to the slow cooker. Stir in the chicken until everything is well-mixed.
3. Serve with a garnish of chopped cilantro.

Nutritional Values
Calories 304kcal, Carbohydrates-42g, Protein 27g, Fat 4g, Sodium 1170mg

333. SLOW COOKER BLACK BEAN & VEGGIE SOUP

- Prep time: 10 mins, Cook time: 8 hrs, Total time: 8 hrs 10 mins, Servings: 6

Ingredients
- ½ cup cilantro fresh, chopped
- 2 garlic cloves minced

- 1 sweet onion small, diced
- 3 carrots sliced into ¼-inch pieces
- 1 sweet potato medium, cut into ½ -inch cubes
- 14 ½ ounces of fire-roasted tomatoes canned, regular diced is optional
- 4 ounces of green chili peppers canned, diced
- 30 ounces of black beans canned, drained
- 1 tsp chili powder
- 1 tsp cumin
- ½ tsp crushed red pepper flakes, more or less to taste
- ¼ tsp black pepper freshly ground
- kosher or sea salt to taste
- 2 ½ cups of vegetable broth low sodium

Directions

1. Stir together all of the ingredients in the slow cooker. Cook for 6-8 hours on low or until the carrots are soft.
2. Top with low-Fat cheddar cheese and a dollop of Fat-free sour cream, if preferred.

Nutritional Values

Calories 245kcal, Carbohydrates-46g, Protein 12.5g, Fat 2g, Sodium 349mg

334. PESTO WHITE BEAN SOUP

- Prep time: 10 mins, Cook time: 4 hrs, Total time: 4 hrs 10 mins, Servings: 6

Ingredients

- 2 cloves garlic minced
- 1 onion medium, diced
- ½ cup prepared pesto plus more for serving, Pesto recipe
- 1 tbsp Italian seasoning
- 1 cup brown rice cooked
- ¼ tsp red pepper flakes
- 1 lemon juiced
- 1 tsp sea salt
- 6 cups chicken stock or vegetable stock
- ½ tsp ground black pepper
- parmesan cheese grated for serving
- 28 ounces diced tomatoes cans
- 30 ounces of white beans cans, rinsed and drained

Directions

1. In a slow cooker, combine all ingredients except the pesto, cooked rice, and Parmesan. Cook for 8 hours on low or 4 hours on high in the slow cooker.
2. Stir the rice & pesto into the soup when you're ready to eat. If preferred, top with a dollop of pesto and a dusting of Parmesan cheese.

Nutritional Values

Calories 391kcal, Carbohydrates-74g, Protein 20g, Fat 2g, Sodium 332mg

335. SKINNY DETOX SOUP

- Prep time: 25 mins, Cook time: 1 hr 25 mins, Total time: 1 hr 50 mins, Servings: 2

Ingredients

- 3 cups of baby carrots, sliced
- 2 tsp extra virgin olive oil
- 1 tsp salt
- 4 celery stalks, diced
- ½ cup of fresh cilantro, chopped
- 3 small turnips, peeled + diced
- 1 zucchini, diced
- 1 cup yellow onion, diced
- 1 bunch of kale, finely chopped
- 3 cloves garlic, crushed
- 15 oz. can Pinto beans, rinsed + drained
- 7 cups of reduced-sodium vegetable broth
- 1 tsp black pepper
- 2 large tomatoes, diced
- 15 oz. can Cannellini beans, rinsed + drained

Directions

1. In a large saucepan over medium heat, warm the olive oil. Simmer for 5 mins over low heat with carrots, celery, turnips, and onion.
2. Simmer for 3 mins, longer after adding the garlic.
3. Simmer for 1 hour, or until veggies are soft, with the stock, white beans, tomatoes, and pinto beans.
4. Add the kale, zucchini, and cilantro for about 20 mins before serving and mix thoroughly.
5. Before serving, add salt and black pepper.

Nutritional Values

Calories 133kcal, Carbohydrates-27g, Protein 7g, Fat 1g, Sodium 495mg

336. WEIGHT LOSS SOUP

- Prep time: 20 mins, Cook time: 2 hrs, Total time: 2 hrs 20 mins, Servings: 2

Ingredients

- 2 cloves garlic, minced
- black pepper, to taste
- 1- 5-ounce package of shiitake mushrooms, sliced
- salt, to taste
- 3 whole carrots, peeled and sliced
- 1 tsp Italian seasoning
- 3 cups of low-Sodium tomato juice
- 3 cups purple cabbage, chopped
- 2 cups low-sodium chicken broth
- 1- 15-ounce can of kidney beans, drained and rinsed
- 2- 14.5-ounce cans of no-salt-added fire-roasted diced tomatoes
- 1- 8-ounce bag of frozen green beans
- 1 zucchini, sliced in rounds and quartered
- ½ tsp crushed red pepper flakes
- 1 small white onion, diced
- 1 yellow squash, sliced in rounds and quartered

Directions

1. Coat a large skillet with cooking spray and heat over medium-low heat. Cook the onion, mushrooms, garlic, and carrots for approximately 5 mins or until they begin to soften.
2. Combine the chicken broth, tomato juice, cooked veggies, tomatoes, and the remaining vegetables in a slow cooker. Season to taste with Italian seasoning, salt, and pepper.
3. Cook on low for 2 to 3 hours or until veggies are soft.

Nutritional Values

Calories 204kcal, Carbohydrates-42g, Protein 9g, Fat 1g, Sodium 217mg

337. SUPERFOODS DETOX SOUP

- Prep time: 20 mins, Cook time: 40 mins, Total time: 60 mins, Servings: 8

Ingredients

- 1 onion, diced
- 4 cups kale, coarsely chopped
- 1 large sweet potato, peeled and cubed
- 1- 15-ounce can cannellini beans, drained and rinsed
- 1 red bell pepper, diced
- 2 cups cabbage, shredded
- 4 cups water
- black pepper, to taste
- 2 cups low-sodium chicken broth
- ¼ tsp salt
- 1 cup lentils, dried
- ¼ tsp red pepper flakes
- 2 tsp extra virgin olive oil
- 2 tsp cumin

Directions

1. Heat the oil, sweet potato, onion, and red bell pepper in a large stockpot over medium heat. Cook for 10 mins, or until the potatoes are softened, and color has developed.
2. Bring the water, chicken stock, lentils, cumin, salt, and black pepper to a boil, lower to low heat, and cook for 20 to 25 mins, or until the potatoes & lentils are cooked.
3. Simmer for 4-6 mins after adding the cabbage and beans.
4. Season with salt and pepper, then add the kale and red pepper flakes and cook for 5 mins or until the kale has wilted.

Nutritional Values

Calories 201kcal, Carbohydrates-37g, Protein 11g, Fat 2g, Sodium 212mg

338. CREAMY NUTMEG BROCCOLI SOUP

- Prep time: 20 mins, Cook time: 10 mins, Total time: 30 mins, Servings: 4

Ingredients

- ½ cup scallions, chopped
- 1-quart low-sodium vegetable broth
- ¼ tsp cayenne pepper
- 1 tbsp coconut oil
- 1 tsp ground nutmeg
- 4 large broccoli stalks, chopped- use both the stems and florets

- 1 cup rice milk
- 1 or 2 garlic cloves, peeled and chopped

Directions

1. In a large saucepan over high heat, bring the broth to a boil. Reduce the heat and add the broccoli. Cover and cook for approximately 10 mins or until the vegetables are soft.
2. Meanwhile, in a small pan over medium heat, heat the oil. Cook, occasionally stirring, until the scallions & garlic are soft.
3. In a large mixing bowl, combine the scallions and garlic. Allow it cool for 15 mins after removing it from the heat.
4. In a blender, purée in batches until smooth. Put the purée back in the saucepan.
5. In a small bowl, mix the nutmeg and cayenne, then mix in the rice milk. Add this mixture into the purée gradually.
6. Return the soup to medium heat and simmer, occasionally stirring, until heated through. Serve immediately.

Nutritional Values

Calories 125kcal, Carbohydrates-18.6g, Protein 5.3g, Fat 4.5g, Sodium 206mg

339. BROCCOLI AND ARUGULA SOUP

- Prep time: 13 mins, Cook time: 12 mins, Total time: 25 mins, Servings: 2

Ingredients

- 2 ½ cups water
- 1 tbsp olive oil
- ¾ cup arugula- watercress would be good, too
- ½ yellow onion, roughly diced
- ¼ tsp black pepper, freshly ground
- 1 head broccoli, cut into small florets- about 2/3 pound
- ½ lemon
- 1 clove of garlic, thinly sliced
- ¼ tsp coarse salt

Directions

1. In a medium clean saucepan, heat the olive oil over medium heat. Sauté for about a minute or until the garlic & onion are aromatic.
2. Cook for 4 mins or until the broccoli is brilliant green.

3. Bring the water, salt, & pepper to a boil, then reduce the heat and cover. Cook until the broccoli is just cooked, for about 8 mins.
4. Pour the soup into a blender with the arugula and purée until smooth. Start carefully and work in batches if required while mixing hot liquids.
5. Serve with a squeeze of fresh lemon.

Nutritional Values

Calories 129kcal, Carbohydrates-14.1g, Protein 4.9g, Fat 7.7g, Sodium 301mg

340. DETOX DELICIOUSLY: GINGER-CARROT SOUP

- Prep time: 10 mins, Cook time: 25 mins, Total time: 35 mins, Servings: 8

Ingredients

- 1 cup chopped sweet onion
- 1 tsp honey
- 1 tbsp minced garlic
- 1 1/3 cups plain low-Fat Greek yogurt
- 2 tbsp minced peeled ginger
- ¼ cup pine nuts
- 2 pounds carrots, peeled and chopped
- Freshly ground pepper
- 2 tbsp extra-virgin olive oil
- 6 cups low-Sodium chicken or vegetable stock
- 1 tsp minced fresh thyme
- Kosher salt
- 1 medium russet potato, peeled and chopped

Directions

1. In a Dutch oven or heavy saucepan over medium-high heat, combine the olive oil & onion. Sprinkle with ½ tsp salt and heat, occasionally stirring, for 10 mins, or until the sugars are just beginning to caramelize.
2. Cook for another 2 mins, constantly stirring, taking care not to burn the mixture. Combine the potato, carrots, and chicken/vegetable stock in a mixing bowl. Bring to a low simmer, cover, and cook for 20 to 25 mins, or until the carrots & potato be very soft. Keep yourself warm.

3. Meanwhile, gently cook the pine nuts in a medium sauté pan over medium-high heat. Allow cooling before serving.
4. Combine the yogurt, thyme, honey, and ½ tsp pepper in a small bowl.
5. Using an immersion blender, purée the soup until it is completely smooth. Season with salt and pepper, then top with a dollop of the yogurt mixture and pine nuts to serve.

Nutritional Values
Calories 262kcal, Carbohydrates-31.4g, Protein 10.2g, Fat 10.2g, Sodium 349mg

341. SPRING DETOX SOUP

- Prep time: 25 mins, Cook time: 20 mins, Total time: 45 mins, Servings: 8

Ingredients

- 2 large yellow onions, chopped
- Big pinch of cayenne pepper
- 1 bunch of asparagus tips
- 4 cups vegetable broth, store-bought or homemade
- 1 tsp salt, divided
- 14 cups gently packed spinach- about 12 ounces, any tough stems trimmed
- 2 tbsp plus 3 cups water, divided
- 1 tbsp lemon juice, or more to taste
- ¼ cup quinoa
- 2 tbsp extra-virgin olive oil, plus more for garnish
- 1 bunch of green chard- about 1 pound

Directions

1. Take a large skillet and heat 2 tbsp oil over high heat. Add the onions and ¼ tsp salt and simmer, constantly turning, for approximately 5 mins, or until the onions start to brown. Reduce heat to low and cover with 2 tbsp water. Cook, stirring regularly, until the pan cools down, then periodically, always covering the pot again, for 25 to 30 mins, or until the onions are reduced and have a rich caramel color.
2. Bring a kettle of water to a boil while the onions are cooking. Blanch the asparagus tips for 1 minute before draining and transferring them to a dish of cold water.

3. In a soup pot, mix 3 cups water & ¾ tsp salt, and add quinoa. Bring the water to a boil. Reduce to a low heat setting, cover, & cook for 15 mins. Remove the chard's white ribs and discard. Cut the chard greens & spinach coarsely.
4. Mix in the chard greens after 15 mins of cooking the quinoa. Return to low heat, cover, and cook for an additional 10 mins. Stir a bit of the boiling liquid into the caramelized onions before adding them to the quinoa, along with the asparagus, spinach, cayenne, and broth. Return to a simmer, cover, and cook for another 5 mins, mixing once until the spinach is soft but still brilliant green.
5. Using an immersion blender, mix the soup in the pot until completely smooth or in stages in a conventional blender- return it to the pot.

Nutritional Values
Calories 97kcal, Carbohydrates-12.9g, Protein 4.2g, Fat 4g, Sodium 719mg

342. VEGAN BLACK BEAN SOUP

- Prep time: 5 mins, Cook time: 25, Total time: 30 mins, Servings: 6

Ingredients

- 1 medium onion diced
- 1 can- 14.5 ounces diced tomatoes
- 1 red bell pepper seeded and diced
- 3 cans- 15 ounces each of black beans rinsed and drained
- 1 tsp cumin
- ½ tsp salt or to taste
- ½ tsp dried oregano
- 3-4 cups of low-sodium vegetable broth
- 2 cloves minced garlic
- ½ tsp smoked paprika

Directions

1. Cook the garlic and onion in ¼ cup water in a soup saucepan over medium heat until tender and translucent, approximately 5 to 6 mins.
2. Sauté the red bell pepper for 2 to 3 mins or until it begins to soften.

3. Sauté for another minute or 2 until the smoked paprika, oregano, cumin, and salt are aromatic.
4. Combine the black beans, tomatoes, and vegetable broth in a large mixing bowl. Transfer to a boil over high heat, then lower the heat to medium-low and cook for 15 to 20 mins.
5. Purée as much of the soup as you want with an immersion blender. If you prefer a thinner soup, add the remaining cup of stock.
6. Serve hot with your preferred toppings.

343. TUSCAN PORTOBELLO STEW

- Prep time: 20 mins, Cook time: 20 mins, Total time: 40 mins, Servings: 4

Ingredients

- ½ cup white wine or vegetable broth
- 2 large Portobello mushrooms, coarsely chopped
- ¼ tsp pepper
- 3 garlic cloves, minced
- ¼ tsp salt
- 2 tbsp olive oil
- 2 cans- 15 ounces each of cannellini beans, rinsed and drained
- 1 medium onion, chopped
- ½ tsp dried rosemary, crushed
- 1 can- 28 ounces of diced tomatoes, undrained
- ½ tsp dried basil
- 2 cups chopped fresh kale
- 1 bay leaf
- 1 tsp dried thyme

Directions

1. Sauté the mushrooms, onion, and garlic in oil in a large pan until soft. Pour in the wine or broth, whatever you like. Bring to a boil, then cook until the liquid has been reduced by ½.
2. Combine the tomatoes, greens, and spices in a mixing bowl. Bring the water to a boil. Reduce the heat to low, cover, and cook for 8-10 mins.

3. Heat through the beans. Bay leaf should be discarded.

344. BRAISED PORK STEW

- Prep time: 30 mins, Cook time: 0 mins, Total time: 30 mins, Servings: 4

Ingredients

- ½ tsp salt
- 1 pound pork tenderloin, cut into 1-inch cubes
- 1 tsp dried thyme
- ½ tsp pepper
- 2 tsp stone-ground mustard
- 5 tbsp all-purpose flour, divided
- 2 garlic cloves, minced
- 1 tbsp olive oil
- 2 tbsp water
- 16 ounces of assorted frozen vegetables
- 1-½ cups reduced-Sodium chicken broth

Directions

1. Season pork with pepper and salt, then toss with 3 tbsp flour to coat. Heat the oil in a large skillet over medium heat. Pork should be browned. If required, drain. In a large mixing bowl, mix the veggies, broth, garlic, mustard, and thyme. Bring the water to a boil. Reduce heat to low, cover and cook for 10-15 mins, or cook until pork and veggies.
2. Combine the remaining flour & water in a small dish until smooth, and stir into the stew. Bring to a boil, frequently stirring, for 1-2 mins or until the sauce has thickened.

345. PORK AND GREEN CHILE STEW

- Prep time: 40 mins, Cook time: 7 hrs, Total time: 7 hrs 40 mins, Servings: 8

Ingredients

- 1 large onion, cut into ½ -in. pieces
- 2 pounds boneless pork shoulder butt roast, cut into 3 /4-in. cubes

- 1 cup minced fresh cilantro
- 2 tbsp canola oil
- ½ tsp ground cumin
- 1 tsp salt
- ½ tsp dried oregano
- 1 tsp coarsely ground pepper
- 2 garlic cloves, minced
- 4 large potatoes, peeled and cut into 3 /4-in. cubes
- 2 tbsp quick-cooking tapioca
- 3 cups water
- 2 cans- 4 ounces each chopped green chiles
- 1 can- 16 ounces hominy, rinsed and drained
- Optional: Sour cream and additional cilantro

Directions

1. Brown pork & onion in batches in oil in a big pan. Season to taste with salt & pepper. Fill a 5-quart slow cooker halfway with water.
2. Combine the water, potatoes, chiles, hominy, garlic, tapioca, cumin, and oregano in a large mixing bowl. Cover and simmer on low for 7-9 hours, or until meat is cooked, tossing in cilantro in the final 30 mins. Serve with sour cream and more cilantro, if preferred.

Nutritional Values

Calories 322kcal, Carbohydrates-25g, Protein 21g, Fat 15g, Sodium 723mg

346. MOROCCAN VEGETARIAN STEW

- Prep time: 20 mins, Cook time: 30 mins, Total time: 50 mins, Servings: 8

Ingredients

- 1 large onion, chopped
- 1 tbsp olive oil
- 2 small zucchini, cut into 1-inch cubes
- 2 tsp ground cumin
- 3 cups water
- 2 tsp ground cinnamon
- 3 plum tomatoes, chopped
- 1 tsp ground coriander
- 4 medium carrots, sliced
- ½ tsp ground allspice

- 2 medium potatoes, peeled and cut into 1-inch cubes- about 4 cups
- ½ tsp cayenne pepper
- 1 can- 15 ounces garbanzo beans or chickpeas, rinsed and drained
- ¼ tsp salt
- 1 small butternut squash, peeled and cut into 1-inch cubes- about 4 cups

Directions

1. Heat oil in a 6-quart stockpot over medium-high heat and sauté onion until tender. Season with salt and pepper, simmer and stir for 1 min.
2. Bring to a boil with the squash, potatoes, carrots, tomatoes, and water. Reduce heat to low and cook, uncovered, for 15-20 mins, or until squash & potatoes are nearly soft.
3. Bring the zucchini and beans to a boil. Reduce heat to low and cook, uncovered, for 5-8 mins, or until soft veggies.

Nutritional Values

Calories 180kcal, Carbohydrates-36g, Protein 5g, Fat 3g, Sodium 174mg

347. WINTERTIME BRAISED BEEF STEW

- Prep time: 40 mins, Cook time: 2 hrs, Total time: 2 hrs 40 mins, Servings: 8

Ingredients

- 2 tbsp all-purpose flour
- 2 pounds boneless beef sirloin steak or chuck roast, cut into 1-inch pieces
- 1 can- 15 ounces of cannellini beans, rinsed and drained
- 2 tsp Montreal steak seasoning
- 2 fresh oregano sprigs
- 2 tbsp olive oil, divided
- 2 bay leaves
- 1 large onion, chopped
- 2 tbsp red currant jelly
- 2 celery ribs, chopped
- 1 cup dry red wine or reduced-Sodium beef broth
- 2 medium parsnips, peeled and cut into 1-½ -inch pieces
- Minced fresh parsley, optional
- 2 medium carrots, peeled and cut into 1-½ -inch pieces

- 2 garlic cloves, minced
- 1 can- 14-½ ounces diced tomatoes, undrained

1. Preheat the oven to 350°F. Combine the meat, flour, and steak seasoning in a mixing bowl.
2. Heat the remaining oil in the same pan over medium heat. Cook and whisk in the onion, celery, parsnips, and carrots until the onion is soft. Cook for a further minute after adding the garlic. Bring the wine, tomatoes, bay leaves, jelly, meat, and oregano to a boil.
3. Preheat oven to 350°F and bake for 1 ½ hours, covered. Add the beans and bake for another 30-40 mins, covered, or until the meat and veggies are cooked. Remove the bay leaves & oregano sprigs from the pot. Sprinkle with parsley if desired.

Nutritional Values

Calories 310kcal, Carbohydrates-26g, Protein 25g, Fat 9g, Sodium 373mg

348. BEEFY CABBAGE BEAN STEW

- Prep time: 20 mins, Cook time: 6 hrs, Total time: 6 hrs 20 mins, Servings: 6

Ingredients

- 3 cups shredded cabbage or angel hair coleslaw mix
- ½ pound lean ground beef- 90% lean
- 1 tsp ground cumin
- 1 can- 16 ounces of red beans, rinsed and drained
- 3 garlic cloves, minced
- 1 can- 14-½ ounces diced tomatoes, undrained
- 1 small onion, chopped
- 1 can- 8 ounces tomato sauce
- ½ tsp pepper
- ¾ cup salsa or Picante sauce
- 1 medium green pepper, chopped

Directions

1. Cook beef in a large pan over low-medium heat until it is no longer pink, about 4-6 mins, breaking it up into crumbles, and drain.

2. Place the beef in a 4-quart slow cooker. Combine the beans, cabbage, tomato sauce, tomatoes, green pepper, Picante sauce, garlic, onion, pepper, and cumin in a large mixing bowl. Cook on low for 6-8 hours, covered, or until cabbage is soft. Top with chopped cheddar cheese and jalapeño peppers, if preferred.

Nutritional Values

Calories 177kcal, Carbohydrates-23g, Protein 13g, Fat 4g, Sodium 591mg

349. CHICKEN MUSHROOM STEW

- Prep time: 20 mins, Cook time: 4 hrs, Total time: 4 hrs 20 mins, Servings: 6

Ingredients

- 2 tbsp canola oil, divided
- 2 tsp each of dried thyme, oregano, marjoram, and basil
- 8 ounces fresh mushrooms, sliced
- ¾ cup water
- 1 medium onion, diced
- 1 can- 6 ounces tomato paste
- 3 cups diced zucchini
- 3 medium tomatoes, chopped
- 1 cup chopped green pepper
- 6 boneless skinless chicken breast halves- 4 ounces each
- 4 garlic cloves, minced
- Chopped fresh thyme, optional

Directions

1. Cut the chicken into 1-inch pieces and brown them in a large pan with 1 tbsp of oil. Fill a 3-quart slow cooker halfway with water. In the same skillet, sauté the mushrooms, onion, zucchini, and green pepper until crisp-tender; add the garlic and cook for another minute.
2. Put everything in the slow cooker. Combine the tomatoes, water, tomato paste, and spices in a large mixing bowl. Cook for 4-5 hours on low or until the beef is no longer pink & the veggies are soft. Top with finely chopped thyme, if preferred.

Nutritional Values

Calories 237kcal, Carbohydrates-15g, Protein 27g, Fat 8g, Sodium 82mg

350. 1-POT BEEF & PEPPER STEW

- Prep time: 10 mins, Cook time: 30 mins, Total time: 40 mins, Servings: 8

Ingredients

- 3 cans- 14-½ ounces each of diced tomatoes, undrained
- 2 cups uncooked instant rice
- 4 large green peppers, coarsely chopped
- ¼ tsp salt
- 1 large onion, chopped
- 1 tsp pepper
- 2 cans- 4 ounces each chopped green chiles
- Hot pepper sauce, optional
- 1 pound lean ground beef- 90% lean
- 3 tsp garlic powder

Directions

1. Cook beef in a 6-quart stockpot over medium heat, about 6-8 mins; crumble steak, and drain. Bring to a boil with the green peppers, tomatoes, chiles, onion, and spices. Reduce to low heat and cook, covered, for 20-25 mins, or until veggies are soft.
2. Cook the rice according to the package directions.
3. Serve with stew & pepper sauce, if preferred.

Nutritional Values

Calories 244kcal, Carbohydrates-35g, Protein 15g, Fat 5g, Sodium 467mg

351. MANCHESTER STEW

- Prep time: 25 mins, Cook time: 8 hrs, Total time: 8 hrs 25 mins, Servings: 6

Ingredients

- 2 medium onions, chopped
- 2 garlic cloves, minced
- ½ tsp salt
- 1 tsp dried oregano
- 1 tsp dried thyme
- 1 cup dry red wine
- 1 can- 14-½ ounces diced tomatoes, no-salt-added
- 1 pound of small red potatoes, quartered
- 2-½ cups water
- 1 can- 16 ounces of kidney beans, rinsed and drained
- 1 cup fresh baby carrots
- ½ pound sliced fresh mushrooms
- Fresh basil leaves
- 2 tbsp olive oil
- ¼ tsp pepper
- 2 medium leeks- white portions only, sliced

Directions

1. Heat the oil in a large skillet over medium-high heat. Cook & stir until onions are soft, about 2-3 mins. Cook and stir for another minute after adding the garlic and oregano. Pour in the wine. Bring to a boil, and simmer for 3-4 mins, or until liquid is decreased by ½.
2. Fill a 5- or 6-quart slow cooker halfway with water. Potatoes, beans, mushrooms, onions, and carrots are all good additions. In a large mixing bowl, combine the water, tomatoes, thyme, salt, and pepper. Cook for 8-10 hours on low, covered until potatoes are soft. Garnish with basil.

Nutritional Values

Calories 221kcal, Carbohydrates-38g, Protein 8g, Fat 5g, Sodium 354mg

352. TERIYAKI BEEF STEW

- Prep time: 20 mins, Cook time: 6 hrs 30 mins, Total time: 6 hrs 50 mins, Servings: 6

Ingredients

- 2 tbsp cornstarch
- 2 pounds of beef stew meat
- Hot cooked rice, optional
- ¼ cup teriyaki sauce
- 2 cups frozen peas, thawed
- 2 garlic cloves, minced
- 2 tbsp sesame seeds
- 1 bottle- 12 ounces of ginger beer or ginger ale
- 2 tbsp cold water

Directions

1. Brown the meat in batches in a large nonstick pan. Fill a 3-quart slow cooker halfway with water.
2. In a small dish, combine the garlic, teriyaki sauce, ginger beer, and sesame seeds and pour over the meat. Cook on medium for 6-8 hours or until meat is cooked covered.

3. To make the cornstarch, whisk the cold water and cornstarch until smooth, and gradually mix into the stew. Add the peas and mix well. Cook for 30 mins, on high, or until the sauce has thickened. If preferred, serve with rice.

Nutritional Values

Calories 310kcal, Carbohydrates-17g, Protein 33g, Fat 12g, Sodium 528mg

353. WEST AFRICAN CHICKEN STEW

- Prep time: 20 mins, Cook time: 30 mins, Total time: 50 mins, Servings: 8

Ingredients

- ½ tsp salt
- 1-½ tsp minced fresh thyme or ½ tsp dried thyme, divided
- ¼ tsp pepper
- ¼ cup creamy peanut butter
- 3 tsp canola oil divided
- 1 cup of reduced-sodium chicken broth
- 1 medium onion, thinly sliced
- 1 large sweet potato, peeled and cut into 1-inch cubes
- 6 garlic cloves, minced
- 1 can- 28 ounces of crushed tomatoes
- 2 tbsp minced fresh ginger root
- ¼ tsp cayenne pepper
- 1 pound boneless skinless chicken breasts, cut into 1-inch cubes
- 2 cans- 15-½ ounces each of black-eyed peas, rinsed and drained
- Hot cooked brown rice, optional

Directions

1. Season the chicken with pepper and salt before serving. Cook chicken in 2 tbsp oil in a Dutch oven over medium heat for 4-6 mins or until no longer pink.
2. In the same pan, sauté the onion until soft in the remaining oil. Cook for a further minute after adding the garlic and ginger.
3. In a large mixing bowl, combine the tomatoes, peas, broth, sweet potato, 1-¼ tsp thyme, peanut butter, and cayenne pepper. Bring the water to a boil. Reduce the heat to low, cover, and cook for 15-20 mins, or until the potatoes are cooked. Heat through the chicken.

4. If preferred, serve with rice. Finish with the remaining thyme.

Nutritional Values

Calories 275kcal, Carbohydrates-32g, Protein 22g, Fat 7g, Sodium 636mg

354. SLOW-COOKED LENTIL STEW

- Prep time: 45 mins, Cook time: 6 hrs, Total time: 6 hrs 45 mins, Servings: 8

Ingredients

- 2 tbsp canola oil
- 1 tsp cumin seeds
- 2 tbsp minced fresh ginger root
- 2 tbsp butter
- 3 garlic cloves, minced
- ¾ cup heavy whipping cream
- 8 plum tomatoes, chopped
- 1 can- 4 ounces chopped green chiles
- 2 tsp ground coriander
- 2 cups dried lentils, rinsed
- 1-½ tsp ground cumin
- 2 cups water
- ¼ tsp cayenne pepper
- 6 cups hot cooked basmati or jasmine rice
- 2 large onions, thinly sliced, divided
- 3 cups vegetable broth

Directions

1. ½ of the onions should be sauteed in oil in a large pan until soft. Sauté for 1 minute with the ginger and garlic. Cook and mix in the tomatoes, coriander, cumin, and cayenne for another 5 mins.
2. Combine the water, tomato mixture, vegetable broth, green chiles, lentils, and remaining onion in a 4-5 quart slow cooker. Cover and simmer on low for 6-8 hours or until lentils are cooked.
3. Stir cream into the slow cooker just before serving. Melt butter in a small pan over medium heat. Cook, constantly stirring, until the cumin seeds are golden brown, about 1-2 mins. Toss in the lentils.
4. Spoon over rice to serve. Top with green onions or cilantro, if preferred.

Nutritional Values

Calories 499kcal, Carbohydrates-72g, Protein 17g, Fat 16g, Sodium 448mg

355. ROOT STEW

- Prep time: 30 mins, Cook time: 2 hrs, Total time: 2 hrs 30 mins, Servings: 8

Ingredients

- 2 tbsp canola oil, divided
- 2 tbsp cornstarch
- 1-½ pounds of beef stew meat
- ¼ cup cold water
- ½ tsp pepper
- 2 medium parsnips
- 1 medium onion, chopped
- 2 medium turnips
- 6 garlic cloves, minced
- 3 medium carrots
- 2 bay leaves
- 1 small rutabaga
- 1 tsp dried thyme
- 1-½ tsp salt
- 3 cups of reduced-Sodium beef broth

Directions

1. Preheat the oven to 325°F. 1 tbsp oil. Brown the meat in small batches. Remove the pan from the heat and season with salt & pepper.
2. Heat the remaining oil in the same pan over medium heat. Cook, occasionally stirring, until the onion is soft, about 4-6 mins. Cook for 1 minute, constantly stirring. Bring to a boil with the bay leaves, thyme, meat, and broth. 1 hour in the oven, covered.
3. Add the remaining veggies to the Dutch oven, peel, and cut into 1-inch pieces. 1 to 1-¼ hour in the oven, covered, until meat and veggies are cooked.
4. Combine cornstarch and water in a small dish until smooth, and add into stew. Bring to a boil, then simmer and stir for 1-2 mins or until the sauce has thickened. Bay leaves should be discarded.

Nutritional Values

Calories 227kcal, Carbohydrates-16g, Protein 18g, Fat 1g, Sodium 676mg

356. CURRIED BEEF STEW

- Prep time: 15 mins, Cook time: 2 hrs, Total time: 2 hrs 15 mins, Servings: 4

Ingredients

- ¼ tsp salt
- 1/8 tsp pepper
- 2 large carrots, thinly sliced
- 2 tbsp all-purpose flour
- 1-½ pounds potatoes- about 3 medium, cut into 1-inch cubes
- 1 tbsp canola oil
- 3 cups beef stock
- 1 large onion, cut into 3/4-inch pieces
- 2 bay leaves
- 2 tbsp curry powder
- Hot cooked brown rice, optional
- ¾ pound beef stew meat- 1- to 1-½ -inch pieces
- 1 tbsp white vinegar
- 2 tsp reduced-Sodium soy sauce

Directions

1. Season the beef with pepper and salt, then coat it with flour. Heat oil in a Dutch oven over medium heat; sauté meat and onion, turning periodically until lightly browned. Bring to a boil with curry powder, soy sauce, bay leaves, and stock. Reduce heat to low and cook for 45 mins, covered.
2. Return to a boil after adding the potatoes and carrots. Reduce heat to low and cook, covered, for 1 to 1-¼ hours, or until meat & vegetables are cooked, occasionally stirring. Remove the bay leaves and add the vinegar.
3. Serve with rice if preferred.

Nutritional Values

Calories 362kcal, Carbohydrates-44g, Protein 24g, Fat 10g, Sodium 691mg

357. SWEET POTATO LENTIL STEW

- Prep time: 15 mins, Cook time: 5 hrs, Total time: 5 hrs 15 mins, Servings: 6

Ingredients

- 1-½ cups dried lentils, rinsed
- 1-¼ pounds sweet potatoes- about 2 medium, peeled and cut into 1-inch pieces
- 1 carton- 32 ounces of vegetable broth
- 3 medium carrots, cut into 1-inch pieces
- ¼ tsp cayenne pepper
- 1 medium onion, chopped

- ¼ tsp ground ginger
- 4 garlic cloves, minced
- ½ tsp ground cumin
- ¼ cup minced fresh cilantro

Directions

1. Combine the first 9 ingredients in a 3-quart slow cooker.
2. Cook for 5-6 hours on low, covered until veggies and lentils are soft.
3. Add the cilantro and mix well.

Nutritional Values

Calories 290kcal, Carbohydrates-58g, Protein 15g, Fat 1g, Sodium 662mg

358. SPICY CHICKEN STEW

- Prep time: 10 mins, Cook time: 20 mins, Total time: 30 mins, Servings: 6

Ingredients

- 2 tsp minced garlic
- 2 pounds boneless skinless chicken thighs, cut into ½ -inch pieces
- 1 cup lime-garlic salsa
- 2 tbsp olive oil
- 1/3 cup minced fresh cilantro
- 1 can- 15 ounces garbanzo beans or chickpeas, rinsed and drained
- Sour cream, optional
- 1 can- 14-½ ounces diced tomatoes with onions, undrained
- 1 tsp ground cumin

Directions

1. Cook chicken & garlic in oil for 5 mins in a Dutch oven. Combine the beans, tomatoes, salsa, and cumin in a mixing bowl.
2. Cover and cook for 15 mins, or until the chicken is no longer pink.
3. Add the cilantro and mix well. If preferred, serve with sour cream on top.

Nutritional Values

Calories 359kcal, Carbohydrates-18g, Protein 31g, Fat 17g, Sodium 622mg

359. SPICY BEEF VEGETABLE STEW

- Prep time: 10 mins, Cook time: 8 hrs, Total time: 8 hrs 10 mins, Servings: 8

Ingredients

- 1 pound lean ground beef- 90% lean
- 1 cup sliced celery
- 1 cup chopped onion
- 1 package- 16 ounces of frozen mixed vegetables
- 1 tsp beef bouillon granules
- 1 can- 10 ounces diced tomatoes and green chiles
- 1 jar- 24 ounces of meatless pasta sauce
- 1 tsp pepper
- 3-½ cups water

Directions

1. Cook beef and onion in a large pan over medium heat until no longer pink, for 5-10 mins, breaking meat into pieces, then drain.
2. Fill a 5-quart slow cooker halfway with water. Combine the remaining ingredients in a mixing bowl.
3. Cook for 8 hours on low or until the veggies are soft.

Nutritional Values

Calories 177kcal, Carbohydrates-19g, Protein 15g, Fat 5g, Sodium 675mg

360. SWEET POTATO STEW

- Prep time: 20 mins, Cook time: 20 mins, Total time: 40 mins, Servings: 4

Ingredients

- 2 cans- 14-½ ounces each reduced-Sodium beef broth
- ½ tsp dried thyme
- 2 medium sweet potatoes, peeled and cut into ½ -inch cubes
- 1 garlic clove, minced
- 1 small onion, finely chopped
- Dash cayenne pepper
- ½ cup V8 juice
- ¾ pound lean ground beef- 90% lean
- 1 tbsp golden raisins

Directions

1. Bring broth to a boil in a large saucepan. In a large mixing bowl, crumble the meat and add it to the liquid. Cook for 3 mins, covered, stirring periodically. Return to a boil with the remaining ingredients.

2. Reduce heat to low and cook uncovered for 15 mins, or until the meat is no longer pink & potatoes are soft.

Nutritional Values

Calories 265kcal, Carbohydrates-29g, Protein 20g, Fat 7g, Sodium 532mg

361. APPLE CHICKEN STEW

- Prep time: 35 mins, Cook time: 3 hrs, Total time: 3 hrs 35 mins, Servings: 8

Ingredients

- ¾ tsp dried thyme3 hrs
- Minced fresh parsley
- ½ tsp pepper
- 1 tbsp cider vinegar
- ¼ to ½ tsp caraway seeds
- 1 large tart apple, peeled and cut into 1-inch cubes
- 1-½ pounds potatoes- about 4 medium, cut into 3/4-inch pieces
- 1 bay leaf
- 4 medium carrots, cut into ¼-inch slices
- 2 tbsp olive oil
- 1 medium red onion, halved and sliced
- 1-¼ cups apple cider or juice
- 1 celery rib, thinly sliced
- 1-½ tsp salt
- 2 pounds boneless skinless chicken breasts, cut into 1-inch pieces

Directions

1. Combine the first 4 ingredients in a bowl. Layer the veggies in a 5-quart slow cooker and season with ½ of the salt mixture.
2. Toss the chicken with the remaining salt mixture and the oil. Cook chicken in batches in a large pan over medium-high heat. Toss everything into the slow cooker. Garnish with a bay leaf and an apple. Pour in the vinegar and cider.
3. 3 to 3-½ hours on high, covered, until it is no longer pink & veggies are cooked. Bay leaf should be discarded. Before serving, give it a good stir.
4. Serve with a parsley garnish.

Nutritional Values

Calories 284kcal, Carbohydrates-31g, Protein 26g, Fat 6g, Sodium 533mg

362. BEEFLESS STEW

- Prep time: 20 mins, Cook time: 20, Total time: 40 mins, Servings: 6

Ingredients

- 6 cloves minced garlic
- sea salt and pepper to taste- optional
- 3 large stalks of celery cut into 3/4″ chunks
- 2 cups low-Sodium vegetable broth
- 3 large carrots cut into 3/4″ chunks
- ½ tsp smoked paprika
- 16 ounces mushrooms, if large, cut into ¾ inch chunks or left whole
- 1 tbsp fresh rosemary chopped
- 2 lbs potatoes cut into 1″ chunks- peeling is an option
- 1 tbsp Italian herbs
- 2 cups frozen peas thawed
- ½ cup water or more as needed
- 1 large yellow onion cut in ½ and sliced
- ½ 6 oz. can tomato paste mixed with a little water to thin

Directions

1. In a big soup pot, cook onion, celery, and carrots for a few mins with ¼ cup of water. Sauté for several mins, longer with the garlic and mushroom.
2. Add the tomato paste, potatoes, herbs, salt, smoked paprika, and pepper to the vegetable broth.
3. Cook, covered, over medium heat for 15-20 mins, or until the potatoes & carrots are soft. If the stew becomes too thick, add up to a ½ cup of water or more as required.
4. Blend approximately 1 ½ cups of broth with some of the veggies until smooth in a blender.
5. Transfer the blended sauce to the saucepan and whisk until everything is well combined.
6. Heat for approximately 5 mins after adding the thawed peas.
7. For a full dinner, serve with crusty bread as well as a salad.

Nutritional Values

Calories 246kcal, Carbohydrates-53g, Protein 10g, Fat: 0.8, Sodium 154mg

Chapter 10.

Lunch & Dinner Recipes

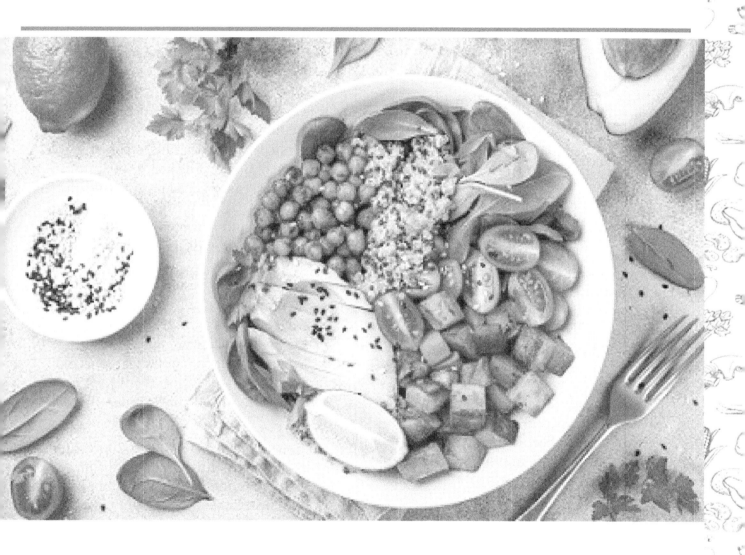

363. ARANCINI- RISOTTO BALLS

- Main Course - Prep time: 45 mins, Cook time: 10 mins, Total time: 55 mins, Servings: 6, Grill temp: 375°F

Ingredients

- 1 cup of all-purpose flour
- ½ cup of water
- 1 ½ cups of panko breadcrumbs
- ½ batch Risotto Milanese, or 5 cups of your favorite risotto, chilled overnight
- 10- ½ -in., 1.25cm cubes of plant-based mozzarella cheese
- ¼ cup of frozen peas
- Grapeseed oil
- Tomato Sauce

Directions

1. Line 2 baking sheets with parchment paper.
2. Place all-purpose flour, water, and panko breadcrumbs in separate small, shallow bowls.
3. Scoop out a ½ cup of portions of chilled Risotto Milanese. Using wet hands, form each portion into a ball, tucking 1 mozzarella cheese cube and a few peas into the center. Place balls on a baking sheet.
4. Working 1 at a time, quickly roll each ball in flour, dip in the water, and roll in panko breadcrumbs, being sure to thoroughly coat each ball. Roll once more in flour, shake off excess, and set aside on the second baking sheet. When all balls are breaded, chill for 30 mins or overnight.
5. Just before you're ready to serve, preheat the oven to 250°F - 120°C.
6. In a wide saucepan over medium-high heat, heat 3 or 4 inches- 7.5 to 10cm - grapeseed oil. Use a deep-frying thermometer to bring oil to 375°F - 190°C, and add balls, 3 or 4 at a time. Cook, frequently turning, for about 3 mins, or until golden brown all over. Transfer to a metal cooling rack set over a baking pan to keep balls crisp, and keep warm in the oven as you fry subsequent batches.
7. Serve hot with Tomato Sauce for dipping.

Nutritional Values

Calories 216, Fat 2.7g, Chol 0mg, Sodium 78mg, Potassium 49.7mg, Carbs 30g, Protein 10g

364. BISTEEYA- MOROCCAN PHYLLO PIE

- Main Course - Prep time: 55 mins, Cook time: 45 mins, Total time: 1 hour 40 mins, Servings: 6, Grill temp: 400°F

Ingredients

- 6 tbsp of extra-virgin olive oil
- 2 large red onions, finely chopped
- 2 cloves garlic, finely chopped
- 1 tbsp of grated fresh ginger
- 1 small hot green chile, seeded and finely chopped
- 1 tsp of ground cinnamon, plus more for dusting
- ½ tsp of saffron threads, crushed
- 1 cup of Golden Chicken-y Stock
- 2- 14 oz. cans of chickpeas, rinsed and drained
- 1 russet potato, peeled and finely chopped
- 1 preserved lemon, peel only, finely chopped
- 2 tbsp of finely chopped fresh cilantro
- ½ tsp of kosher salt
- ½ tsp of freshly ground black pepper
- 1 cup of blanched almonds
- 1 tbsp of confectioners' sugar, plus more for dusting
- 6- 9×14-in. sheets phyllo dough

Directions

1. Preheat the oven to 400°F - 200°C. Line a baking sheet with parchment paper.
2. In a wide sauté pan over medium-high heat, heat 2 tbsp extra-virgin olive oil. Add red onions, garlic, ginger, and hot green chile, and cook, frequently stirring, for 10 mins.
3. Add ½ a tsp of cinnamon, saffron threads, and Golden Chicken-y Stock, and bring to a boil. Stir in chickpeas, russet potato, and preserved lemon peel. Reduce heat to medium, and cook, often stirring, for about 10 mins, or until vegetables are very tender and most of the liquid has evaporated.

4. Stir in cilantro, kosher salt, and black pepper, and set aside to cool.
5. Spread almonds on the prepared baking sheet and toast in the oven for 6 mins. Remove from the oven and cool.
6. In a food processor fitted with a chopping blade, pulse together almonds, remaining ½ tsp of cinnamon, and confectioners' sugar until the mixture resembles fine crumbs.
7. Brush a 9-inch- 23cm round cake pan with a little extra-virgin olive oil. Lay 1 phyllo sheet in the pan and sprinkle with 1/5 almond mixture. Brush the second sheet of phyllo with extra-virgin olive oil, and lay it oiled side up on top of the second sheet in a criss-cross direction.
8. Sprinkle with ¼ remaining almond mixture, and continue to layer the remaining phyllo and almonds, placing phyllo, so the overhang is evenly spaced around the pan- first in a cross shape, then in an X shape, then a slightly offset X shape. Spoon vegetable-chickpea mixture into the pan and spread evenly. Gather overhanging phyllo to cover the top of the pie, and brush with a little more extra-virgin olive oil.
9. Place the pan on a rimmed baking sheet, and bake for about 35 mins, or until crisp and golden. Cool slightly, remove carefully from the pan, and dust with a little more confectioners' sugar and cinnamon.
10. Cut into wedges, and serve.

Nutritional Values

Calories 113, Fat 1.8g, Chol 0mg, Sodium 71.4mg, Potassium 67.7mg, Carbs 22g, Protein 2.3g

365. BUTTERNUT SQUASH TAGINE

- Main Course - Prep time: 20 mins, Cook time: 25 mins, Total time: 45 mins, Servings: 4, Grill temp: 300°F

Ingredients

- 2 tbsp of extra-virgin olive oil
- 1 medium butternut squash, peeled and cut into ½ -in.- 1.25cm cubes
- 1 large yellow onion halved and thinly sliced
- 2 cloves of garlic, finely chopped
- ½ preserved lemon, peel only, finely chopped
- 1 tbsp of tomato paste
- 1 tsp of ground cumin
- 1 tsp of ground coriander
- ½ tsp of ground cinnamon
- ½ tsp of freshly ground black pepper
- 1 tsp of kosher salt
- 2 cups of vegetable stock
- 1- 14 oz. can chickpeas, rinsed and drained
- ½ cup of dried apricots, chopped
- ½ cup of pitted green olives
- ¼ cup of finely chopped fresh cilantro

Directions

1. In a tagine or a large skillet with a lid over medium-high heat, heat extra-virgin olive oil. Add butternut squash and yellow onion, and cook, stirring, for 5 mins.
2. Add garlic, preserved lemon peel, tomato paste, cumin, coriander, cinnamon, and black pepper, and stir for 1 minute.
3. Stir in kosher salt, vegetable stock, chickpeas, and apricots. Cover, reduce heat to low or medium-low, and cook at a brisk simmer, occasionally stirring, for 15 to 20 mins, or until squash is tender but not mushy.
4. Add green olives, garnish with cilantro, and serve.

Nutritional Values

Calories 256, Fat 7g, Chol 0mg, Sodium 73.5mg, Potassium 58.9mg, Carbs 31g, Protein 9g

366. CASSOULET

- Main Course - Prep time: 15 mins, Cook time: 3 hours 45 mins, Total time: 4 hours, Servings: 4, Grill temp: 300°F

Ingredients

- 2 cups of dried white beans, such as flageolet or great northern
- 4 cups of vegetable stock, preferably homemade
- ½ cup of extra-virgin olive oil
- 2 medium leeks, white and light green parts, cut into 1 /8 -in.- 3mm pieces
- 3 medium stalks of celery, cut into 1 /8 -in.- 3mm pieces

- 1 medium carrot halved and cut into 1 /8 - in.- 3mm slices
- 2 medium shallots, minced
- 2 cloves of garlic, thinly sliced
- 1 tbsp of fresh thyme leaves
- 1 tsp of herbes de Provence
- 2 tbsp of tomato paste
- 1 ½ cups of dry red wine
- 1 tsp of kosher salt
- ½ tsp of freshly ground black pepper
- ½ cup of finely chopped fresh Italian flat-leaf parsley

Directions

1. Preheat the oven to 300°F - 150°C.
2. Rinse white beans, pick over, and drain.
3. In a heavy earthenware or cast-iron Dutch oven with a lid, combine beans and vegetable stock.- Alternatively, you can use a heavy stainless-steel Dutch oven with a lid. Set aside.
4. In a medium sauté pan over medium-high heat, heat extra-virgin olive oil. Add leeks, celery, carrot, and shallot, and stir for 5 mins.
5. Stir in garlic, thyme, and herbes de Provence, and cook for 1 minute.
6. Stir in tomato paste, followed by red wine, kosher salt, and black pepper. Combine thoroughly, and remove from heat.
7. Pour vegetable mixture over beans, stir gently, and bake, covered, stirring once or twice, for 3 ½ hours or until beans are tender. Remove the lid during the last hour of cooking.
8. Remove from the oven, stir in Italian flat-leaf parsley, and serve.

Nutritional Values

Calories 113, Fat 1.8g, Chol 0mg, Sodium 71.4mg, Potassium 67.7mg, Carbs 22g, Protein 2.3g

367. CLEAN VEGAN PAD THAI

- Main Course - Prep time: 5 mins, Cook time: 25 mins, Total time: 30 mins, Servings: 2, Grill temp: 300°F

Ingredients

- 2 tbsp of natural peanut butter
- 2 tbsp of rice vinegar

- 2 tsps of tomato paste
- 2 tsps of low-Sodium soy sauce or tamari sauce
- Chili flakes
- 2 medium-sized zucchini end trimmed
- 1 cup of mixed bell peppers and carrots
- 1 cup of snap peas
- 2 small scallions, sliced
- 1 cup of shelled edamame

Directions

1. In a small bowl, stir together tomato paste, rice vinegar, soy sauce, peanut butter, and chili flakes to taste until smooth.
2. Spiralizer the zucchini or peel the julienne peeler, potato peeler, or mandolin into ribbons. Placed the zucchini noodles in the sauce in a wide tub.- If you can boil the zucchini in peanut sauce for at least 20 mins, this recipe tastes much better. Substitute the remaining vegetables and toss to blend.
3. If wanted, serve topped with avocado, peanuts, coriander, and lime wedges.

Nutritional Values

Calories 305, Fat 12g, Chol 0mg, Sodium 71.4mg, Potassium 67.7mg, Carbs 34g, Protein 18g

368. CREAMY PASTA WITH SWISS CHARD AND TOMATOES

- Main Course - Prep time: 5 mins, Cook time: 10 mins, Total time: 15 mins, Servings: 4 to 5, Grill temp: 300°F

Ingredients

- 1 lb. of fettuccine
- ¼ cup of extra-virgin olive oil
- 3 cloves of garlic, thinly sliced
- 1 bunch of Swiss chard washed well and torn into small pieces
- ½ tsp of kosher salt
- 2 large tomatoes, cored, seeded, and cut into 1 /4 -in.- .5cm strips
- ½ cup of plant-based sour cream
- ½ tsp of crushed red pepper flakes

Directions

1. Cook fettuccine in well-salted water according to the package directions.

2. Meanwhile, in a large sauté pan over medium heat, heat extra-virgin olive oil. Add garlic, and cook, stirring, for 30 seconds.
3. Add Swiss chard and kosher salt, and cook, stirring once or twice or until tender. Remove from heat, and cover to keep warm while pasta finishes cooking.
4. When pasta is ready, reserve a ½ cup of the cooking water, and drain the pasta. Add pasta to Swiss chard along with tomatoes, sour cream, and crushed red pepper flakes. Toss well, add a little reserved pasta water if the dish seems dry, and serve immediately.

Nutritional Values
Calories 256, Fat 7g, Chol 0mg, Sodium 73.5mg, Potassium 58.9mg, Carbs 31g, Protein 9g

369. CRISPY QUINOA CAKES

- Main Course - Prep time: 25 mins, Cook time: 25 mins, Total time: 50 mins, Servings: 4 to 6, Grill temp: 400°F

Ingredients
- 2 tbsp of flax meal- ground flaxseeds
- 6 tbsp of warm water
- 3 tbsp of extra-virgin olive oil
- ¼ medium red onion, finely chopped
- 2 cloves of garlic, finely chopped
- 1 bunch of lacinato kale stemmed and finely chopped
- 2 cups of cooked quinoa
- 1 ½ cups of cooked brown or green lentils
- ¼ cup of roasted pumpkin seeds, roughly chopped
- ¼ cup of finely chopped fresh Italian flat-leaf parsley
- 2 tbsp of finely chopped fresh cilantro
- 2 tbsp of tahini
- Juice of 1 lemon
- 2 tbsp of all-purpose flour
- 1 tsp of kosher salt
- 1 tsp of ground cumin
- ½ tsp of freshly ground black pepper

Directions
1. Preheat the oven to 400°F - 200°C. Line a baking sheet with parchment paper.

2. In a small bowl, whisk together flax meal and warm water. Set aside.
3. In a medium sauté pan over medium-high heat, heat 2 tbsp of extra-virgin olive oil. When oil begins to shimmer, add red onion and cook, frequently stirring, for about 3 mins, or until the onion is translucent and just beginning to turn golden around the edges.
4. Add garlic, reduce heat to medium, and stir for 30 seconds. Add lacinato kale, and cook, occasionally stirring, for about 5 mins. Remove from heat, and set aside to cool slightly.
5. In a large bowl, combine quinoa, lentils, pumpkin seeds, Italian flat-leaf parsley, and cilantro.
6. Whisk tahini, lemon juice, and all-purpose flour into flax mixture until smooth, and add to quinoa mixture. Stir in kosher salt, cumin, black pepper, and kale mixture, and combine well.
7. Using wet hands, divide the mixture into 12 even-size balls, and flatten them into 1-inch- 2.5cm cakes, spacing them evenly on the baking sheet.- If desired, you can use a ring mold to form perfectly round cakes.
8. Brush each cake lightly with remaining extra-virgin olive oil, and bake for 20 mins, or until golden brown and crisp.
9. Serve immediately.

Nutritional Values
Calories 256, Fat 7g, Chol 0mg, Sodium 73.5mg, Potassium 58.9mg, Carbs 31g, Protein 9g

370. EGGPLANT AND ROASTED TOMATO POLENTA LASAGNA

- Main Course - Prep time: 45 mins, Cook time: 45 mins, Total time: 1 hour 30 mins, Servings: 6, Grill temp: 400°F

Ingredients
- 1 cup of coarse polenta- not instant
- 1 large Italian eggplant, cut into 1-in.- 2.5cm cubes
- 3 cloves of garlic, thinly sliced
- 1 ½ cups of Tomato Sauce
- 6 large basil leaves, cut into thin ribbons- chiffonade

- 5 cups of water
- 1 ½ tsps of kosher salt
- Twelve oz. of cherry tomatoes halved
- 4 tbsp of extra-virgin olive oil
- 1 cup of Summer Pesto
- ½ cup of pine nuts, toasted

Directions

1. Brush a 9-inch- 23-cm baking pan with olive oil after lining it with parchment paper.
2. Bring water to a boil in a large saucepan over high heat. Add the polenta in a thin stream, constantly stirring. Reduce heat to medium and continue to whisk until polenta is thoroughly cooked, about ½ tsp kosher salt.- When you taste it, it will be creamy and smooth, with no "bite."
3. Allow cooling somewhat before pouring the polenta into the prepared baking pan. Refrigerate for at least 2 hours or overnight, or until completely set.
4. Preheat the oven to 400°F - 200°C.
5. Sprinkle ½ tsp kosher salt over Italian eggplant chunks and drain for 30 mins in a colander. After rinsing, gently squeeze out any excess water.
6. Toss eggplant cubes and cherry tomatoes with sliced garlic and 3 tbsp extra-virgin olive oil on a large rimmed baking sheet. Spread evenly and roast for 30 mins, stirring once or twice. Reduce the temperature to 375°F - 190°C after removing the pan from the oven.
7. Carefully remove the polenta from the pan once it has been set. To make 9 polenta "lasagna noodles, " cut each third into thirds and slice each third horizontally into 3 equal pieces. Use a spatula to carefully handle them, but don't worry if they break—just reassemble them in the pan.
8. Brush the baking pan with the leftover sauce before assembling the lasagna. Extra-virgin olive oil, 1 tbsp. Cover the bottom of the skillet with ½ a cup of tomato sauce and 3 pieces of polenta. ½ of the tomato-eggplant mixture and ½ of the Summer Pesto are layered on top, then another layer of polenta is added.

9. Add the remaining ½ cup of Tomato Sauce, the eggplant-tomato mixture, and the remaining Summer Pesto.
10. Spread the leftover Tomato Sauce equally over the top of the final layer of polenta. Bake for about 40 mins, or until hot and bubbling, covered.
11. Sprinkle basil and toasted pine nuts on top of lasagna just before serving.
12. Serve immediately.

Nutritional Values

Calories 113, Fat 1.8g, Chol 0mg, Sodium 71.4mg, Potassium 67.7mg, Carbs 22g, Protein 2.3g

371. FARRO RISOTTO WITH ROASTED FENNEL AND MUSHROOMS

- Main Course - Prep time: 10 mins, Cook time: 35 mins, Total time: 45 mins, Servings: 4, Grill temp: 400°F

Ingredients

- 2 cups of farro
- 1 ½ tsps of kosher salt
- 1- 10 oz. pkg. of small cremini- Baby Bella mushrooms, quartered
- 2 medium bulbs fennel tops removed, cut into ½ -in.- 1.25cm chunks
- 2 cloves garlic, finely chopped
- 4 tbsp of extra-virgin olive oil
- 2 cups of vegetable stock
- 1 bunch of scallions, white and light green parts separated from dark green parts, thinly sliced
- ½ cup of dry white wine

Directions

1. Preheat the oven to 400°F - 200°C. Line a rimmed baking sheet with parchment paper.
2. In a medium saucepan over high heat, combine farro with 1 tsp kosher salt and enough water to cover by 1 inch- 2.5cm. Bring to a boil, reduce heat to medium, and cook, occasionally stirring, for 20 mins.- Adjust heat as necessary to maintain a brisk simmer. Drain and set aside.
3. On the baking sheet, toss cremini mushrooms, fennel, and garlic with 2 tbsp

of extra-virgin olive oil. Roast, stirring once or twice, for 20 mins. Set aside.

4. In a small saucepan over medium-high heat, bring vegetable stock to a simmer.

5. In a large sauté pan over medium-high heat, heat the remaining 2 tbsp of extra-virgin olive oil. Add white and light green parts of scallions, and stir for 1 minute.

6. Add drained farro and white wine, stir until wine is evaporated, and add 1 cup of vegetable stock. Cook, stirring until the stock is absorbed.

7. Add remaining 1 cup of vegetable stock along with roasted vegetables, and stir until the stock is absorbed.

8. Stir in reserved dark green parts of scallions, season to taste with remaining ½ tsp kosher salt, and serve.

Nutritional Values

Calories 243, Fat 8.8g, Chol 2mg, Sodium 64mg, Potassium 87mg, Carbs 22g, Protein 9.3g

372. GRILLED TOFU CAPRESE

- Main Course - Prep time: 30 mins, Cook time: 10 mins, Total time: 40 mins, Servings: 4, Grill temp: 300°F

Ingredients

- 1 small eggplant, skin on, trimmed, and cut into 8 even slices
- 1 tsp of kosher salt
- 5 tbsp of extra-virgin olive oil
- 2 cloves of garlic, finely chopped
- ½ tsp of dried oregano
- 3 tbsp of balsamic vinegar
- ½ lb. of a firm or extra-firm tofu, cut into 8 slices
- 2 large beefsteak tomatoes, each cored and cut into 4 slices
- 6teen large, fresh basil leaves
- ½ tsp of freshly ground black pepper

Directions

1. Sprinkle eggplant with ½ tsp kosher salt, and set aside on paper towels for 5 mins. Rinse and pat dry.

2. In a shallow bowl, whisk 2 tbsp extra-virgin olive oil, garlic, oregano, and 1 tbsp

of balsamic vinegar. Add eggplant, and marinate for 15 mins.

3. Heat a grill to high, or set a grill pan over high heat.

4. Brush tofu with 1 tbsp of extra-virgin olive oil, and sprinkle with a pinch of kosher salt. Add to the grill or grill pan, and cook for about 2 mins, per side or until nicely marked. Brush grill grates with 1 tbsp of olive oil, and grill eggplant for about 3 mins, per side or until tender.

5. Stack 1 slice eggplant, 1 slice beefsteak tomato, 1 slice tofu, and 1 basil leaf on each of 4 plates, and repeat. Drizzle with the remaining 1 tbsp of olive oil and remaining 2 tbsp balsamic vinegar, season with black pepper, and serve.

Nutritional Values

Calories 313, Fat 4.8g, Chol 6mg, Sodium 65.4mg, Potassium 87.7mg, Carbs 32g, Protein 2.3g

373. HEARTY SEITAN ROAST

- Main Course - Prep time: 15 mins, Cook time: 30 mins, Total time: 45 mins, Servings: 6, Grill temp: 375°F

Ingredients

- 2 tbsp of olive oil
- ½ batch of Basic Seitan
- 1 tsp of kosher salt
- ½ tsp of freshly ground black pepper
- 1 large yellow onion, cut in ½ -in.- 1.25cm wedges
- 2 medium carrots, peeled and cut into 1-in.- 2.5cm chunks
- 2 medium parsnips, peeled and cut into 1-in.- 2.5cm chunks
- 2 cloves of garlic, thinly sliced
- 1 tsp of herbes de Provence
- 1 cup of vegetable stock- preferably Basic Seitan cooking stock
- ½ cup of dry red wine
- 2 tbsp of ketchup
- 1 tbsp of reduced-Sodium tamari
- 1 tbsp of balsamic vinegar

Directions

1. Preheat the oven to 375°F - 190°C.

2. In a large, preferably cast-iron skillet over medium-high heat, heat 1 tbsp of olive oil.
3. Season Basic Seitan evenly with ½ a tsp of kosher salt and ¼ tsp of black pepper. Add seitan to the skillet, and brown on all sides, turning every 1 or 2 mins, or until evenly browned.
4. In a small roasting pan, toss yellow onion, carrots, parsnips, and garlic with the remaining 1 tbsp of olive oil, herbes de Provence, remaining ½ tsp of kosher salt, and ¼ tsp of black pepper. Place browned roast on top of vegetables.
5. In a small saucepan over high heat, whisk vegetable stock, red wine, ketchup, tamari, and balsamic vinegar. Cook, often stirring, for about 10 mins, or until the mixture is thickened slightly and reduced to 1 cup of liquid. Pour over roast and vegetables.
6. Cover the roasting pan with aluminum foil, and bake for 20 mins. Uncover, and bake for 10 more mins.
7. Using a sharp, serrated knife, cut the roast into paper-thin slices, place it on a serving dish, and spoon some vegetables and sauce over the slices.
8. Serve immediately.

Nutritional Values

Calories 243, Fat 8.8g, Chol 2mg, Sodium 64mg, Potassium 87mg, Carbs 22g, Protein 9.3g

374. MIXED VEGETABLE COTTAGE PIE

- Main Course - Prep time: 30 mins, Cook time: 60 mins, Total time: 1 hour 30 mins, Servings: 4, Grill temp: 375°F

Ingredients

- 1 tbsp of vegetable oil
- 1 medium yellow onion, finely chopped
- 4 oz. of white mushrooms, sliced
- 2 medium carrots, grated
- 2 small turnips, grated
- 2 oz. of shelled fresh or thawed frozen peas
- 2- 14 oz. cans of pinto beans, rinsed and drained
- 2 cups of vegetable stock
- 1 tbsp of soy sauce
- 1 tbsp of vegan Worcestershire sauce
- 1 tsp of herbes de Provence
- ½ tsp of kosher salt
- ¼ tsp of freshly ground black pepper, plus more to taste
- ¼ cup of all-purpose flour
- ¼ cup of water
- 1 small rutabaga, cut into small chunks
- 1 lb. of russet potatoes, peeled and cut into small chunks
- 2 tbsp of plant-based butter
- ¼ cup of rice milk
- Grated nutmeg
- 2 oz. of grated plant-based cheddar-style cheese- optional

Directions

1. In a large saucepan over medium-high heat, heat vegetable oil. Add yellow onion, and sauté, stirring, for 3 mins, or until lightly golden.
2. Add white mushrooms, carrots, turnips, peas, and pinto beans. Stir in vegetable stock, soy sauce, vegan Worcestershire sauce, herbes de Provence, kosher salt, and black pepper. Bring to a boil, reduce heat to medium, cover, and simmer gently for 10 mins, or until vegetables are tender.
3. In a small bowl, blend all-purpose flour with water. Stir mixture into the saucepan, and cook, constantly stirring, for 2 mins, to thicken.
4. Meanwhile, cook rutabaga and potatoes in a large saucepan of salted, boiling water over medium-high heat for 15 mins or until tender. Drain and return vegetables to the saucepan, reduce heat to low, and cook to dry out slightly.
5. Add plant-based butter, rice milk, a generous grating of nutmeg, and a generous grinding of black pepper and mash. Beat well with a wooden spoon until smooth.
6. Preheat the oven to 375°F - 190°C.
7. Spoon vegetable and bean mixture into a 2-quart- 2L ovenproof baking dish or 4 ramekins. Top with rutabaga mash and fluff with a fork. Sprinkle cheddar-style cheese- if using over the top, and bake for about 40 mins, or until golden.
8. Serve hot.

Nutritional Values

Calories 277, Fat 8.8g, Chol 2mg, Sodium 64mg, Potassium 87mg, Carbs 52g, Protein 10g

375. MOROCCAN COUSCOUS

- Main Course - Prep time: 10 mins, Cook time: 30 mins, Total time: 40 mins, Servings: 4, Grill temp: 300°F

Ingredients

- 2 tbsp of extra-virgin olive oil
- 1 medium yellow onion halved and thinly sliced
- ½ tsp of ground cumin
- ½ tsp of ground turmeric
- ½ tsp of kosher salt
- 1- 3-or 4-in. cinnamon stick
- ½ tsp of saffron threads, lightly crushed
- 2 ½ cups of Golden Chicken-y Stock or vegetable stock
- ¼ cup of chopped dried apricots
- ¼ cup of currants
- 1 cup of instant couscous
- ½ cup of toasted pine nuts
- 1 tbsp of finely chopped fresh cilantro

Directions

1. In a medium saucepan over medium heat, heat extra-virgin olive oil. Add yellow onion, and cook, occasionally stirring, for 10 mins.
2. Stir in cumin, turmeric, kosher salt, cinnamon stick, and saffron threads, and cook for 30 seconds.
3. Add Golden Chicken-y Stock, reduce heat to low, and simmer for 10 mins.
4. In a small bowl, place apricots and currants. Add ¼ cup of hot stock, cover, and set aside.
5. Measure remaining stock to be sure you have exactly 2 cups. Return stock to the saucepan, and bring to a boil over high heat. Remove from heat, stir in couscous, cover, and set aside for 10 mins.
6. Drain apricots and currants. Remove cinnamon stick from couscous, and fluff couscous with a fork. Stir fruit and pine nuts into couscous, garnish with cilantro, and serve immediately.

Nutritional Values

Calories 257, Fat 7.8g, Chol 2mg, Sodium 88mg, Potassium 57mg, Carbs 32g, Protein 6.9g

376. MUSHROOM LASAGNA

- Main Course - Prep time: 30 mins, Cook time: 50 mins, Total time: 1 hour 20 mins, Servings: 8, Grill temp: 375°F

Ingredients

- ½ oz. of dried porcini mushrooms
- ½ cup of boiling water
- ¼ cup of extra-virgin olive oil
- 3 cloves of garlic, minced
- 1- 8 oz. pkg. of cremini- Baby Bella mushrooms, thinly sliced
- 1- 4 oz. pkg. of shiitake mushrooms, stemmed and thinly sliced
- 1 tsp of chopped fresh rosemary or ½ tsp of dried
- 1 tsp of kosher salt, or to taste
- ½ tsp of dried oregano
- ½ tsp of freshly ground black pepper, or to taste
- ¼ cup of dry red wine
- 4 cups of Tomato Sauce
- 9 no-boil lasagna noodles
- 2 cups of Cashew Ricotta

Directions

1. Preheat the oven to 375°F - 190°C. Lightly coat a 9×13-inch- 23×33cm baking dish with cooking spray.
2. Place porcini mushrooms in a small bowl, pour boiling water over the top, and soak for about 5 mins, or until softened. Lift porcini from soaking water, agitating gently to release any soil. Reserve soaking liquid. Chop mushrooms, and set them aside.
3. In a large sauté pan over medium-high heat, heat extra-virgin olive oil. Add garlic, and cook, stirring continuously, for 1 minute.
4. Add porcini mushrooms, cremini mushrooms, shiitake mushrooms, rosemary, kosher salt, oregano, and black pepper, and cook, occasionally stirring, for 10 mins or until mushrooms begin to brown.

5. Strain mushroom soaking liquid, leaving the last few tsps behind to eliminate grit, and add to mushrooms along with red wine, stirring vigorously to deglaze the pan. Stir until liquid has evaporated, and set mushrooms aside.
6. Spread 1 cup of Tomato Sauce evenly over the bottom of the baking dish, and lay 3 lasagna noodles over the sauce.
7. Spoon ½ of the mushroom mixture and ½ of Cashew Ricotta evenly over the noodles. Pour ¾ cup Tomato Sauce over Cashew Ricotta, layer 3 more noodles, and add the remaining mushrooms and Cashew Ricotta, followed by another cup of Tomato Sauce. Finish with another 3 noodles and 1 cup of Tomato Sauce. Cover the pan with heavy-duty aluminum foil, folding back 1 corner slightly to vent. Reserve the remaining ½ cup of sauce for serving.
8. Bake for 50 mins, or until hot and bubbly. Remove from the oven and set aside to rest for 5 mins before cutting. Reheat the remaining sauce to pass at the table.

Nutritional Values

Calories 261, Fat 7g, Chol 2mg, Sodium 68mg, Potassium 75mg, Carbs 32g, Protein 9g

377. 1-PAN PASTA PRIMAVERA

- Main Course - Prep time: 10 mins, Cook time: 20 mins, Total time: 30 mins, Servings: 4 to 6, Grill temp: 300°F

Ingredients

- ¼ cup of extra-virgin olive oil
- 1 medium yellow onion halved and thinly sliced
- 2 cloves garlic, thinly sliced
- Twelve oz. of thin spaghetti
- 4 ½ cups of vegetable stock or water
- 1- 14 oz. can of diced tomatoes, with juice
- 2 cups of fresh or frozen broccoli florets
- 1 medium carrot, peeled, halved, and thinly sliced
- 1 tsp of kosher salt
- 1- 5 oz. pkg. of baby spinach
- ½ cup of fresh or frozen baby peas
- ½ tsp of freshly ground black pepper

Directions

1. In an extra-large sauté pan with a lid over medium-high heat, heat extra-virgin olive oil. Add yellow onion, and sauté for 2 mins.
2. Add garlic, spaghetti, vegetable stock, tomatoes with juice, broccoli, carrot, and kosher salt. Bring to a boil, reduce heat to medium-low, cover, and cook for 3 mins.
3. Uncover, stir, and continue cooking, constantly stirring and adjusting heat as necessary to maintain a brisk simmer for about 8 mins, or until stock is absorbed and pasta is tender.
4. Stir in baby spinach, peas, and black pepper, toss for 1 minute, and serve immediately.

Nutritional Values

Calories 257, Fat 7.8g, Chol 2mg, Sodium 88mg, Potassium 57mg, Carbs 32g, Protein 6.9g

378. QUINOA VEGETABLE SALAD

- Main Course - Prep time: 10 mins, Cook time: 25 mins, Total time: 35 mins, Servings: 4, Grill temp: 300°F

Ingredients

- 1 cup of quinoa
- 1 ½ cups of water
- 1 tsp of kosher salt
- 1 bunch of curly kale leaves only
- Juice of 1 lemon
- 3 tbsp of extra-virgin olive oil
- 1 clove of garlic, finely chopped
- 2 tbsp of apple cider vinegar
- 2 tbsp of tahini
- 1 small jicama, cut in 1 /4 -in.- .5cm dice
- 1 cup of frozen, fully cooked edamame, thawed
- ½ small red onion, very thinly sliced
- ½ cup of toasted sliced almonds
- ½ cup of dried cranberries

Directions

1. In a dry, medium saucepan with a tight-fitting lid over medium-high heat, toast quinoa, constantly stirring, for 1 minute.
2. Add water and ½ tsp of kosher salt. Bring to a boil, reduce heat to low, and cook, covered, for 15 mins. Let stand covered for 10 mins, and fluff with a fork.

3. In a large bowl, toss curly kale leaves with 1 tbsp of lemon juice, 1 tbsp of extra-virgin olive oil, and a pinch of kosher salt. Using clean hands, massage kale for 5 mins, or until softened and reduced. Stir in garlic, and set aside.
4. In a small bowl, whisk the remaining 1 tbsp of lemon juice, remaining 2 tbsp of extra-virgin olive oil, remaining ½ tsp of kosher salt, apple cider vinegar, and tahini. Set aside.
5. Add quinoa, jicama, edamame, red onion, almonds, cranberries, and reserved dressing to kale, and toss. Serve warm or cold.

Nutritional Values

Calories 113Kcal, Fat 1.8g, Chol 0mg, Sodium 71.4mg, Potassium 67.7mg, Carbs 22g, Protein 2.3g

379. RISOTTO MILANESE

- Main Course - Prep time: 5 mins, Cook time: 35 mins, Total time: 40 mins, Servings: 4 to 6, Grill temp: 300°F

Ingredients

- 3 tbsp of extra-virgin olive oil
- 4 small shallots, finely minced
- 1 tsp of kosher salt, plus more to taste
- 8 cups of Golden Chicken-y Stock or homemade vegetable stock
- ¼ tsp of saffron threads
- 2 cups of Arborio or carnaroli rice
- 1 cup of dry white wine
- 2 tbsp of nutritional yeast
- 1 tbsp of plant-based butter
- 1 tbsp of finely chopped fresh Italian flat-leaf parsley
- 1 tbsp of finely chopped fresh chives
- ½ tsp of freshly ground black pepper

Directions

1. In a large, wide saucepan over medium heat, heat extra-virgin olive oil. Add shallots and kosher salt, and cook, frequently stirring, for about 10 mins, or until shallots are softened and just beginning to turn a light golden color-without browning.

2. In a large saucepan over medium-high heat, heat Golden Chicken-y Stock. Reduce heat to a simmer.
3. In a small bowl, place saffron threads. Ladle about 1 tbsp of stock over saffron, and set aside to steep.
4. Increase heat under shallots to high, add Arborio rice all at once, and cook, constantly stirring, for 2 mins, or until rice smells nutty.
5. Add white wine and saffron, reduce heat to medium, and stir until most of the wine has been absorbed.
6. Add 2 cups of simmering stock to the pan, and reduce heat to low or medium-low.- Adjust heat as needed to keep risotto at a gentle simmer as you cook it. Cook, constantly stirring, until the stock is almost completely absorbed, and add another cup of stock. Continue in this manner until rice is tender but al dente- still a bit firm to the bite and risotto is creamy.
7. Remove from heat and stir in nutritional yeast, butter, Italian flat-leaf parsley, chives, and black pepper.
8. Taste and add more kosher salt if desired, and serve immediately.

Nutritional Values

Calories 267, Fat 8g, Chol 2mg, Sodium 85mg, Potassium 67mg, Carbs 32g, Protein 9g

380. SAVORY STUFFED CABBAGE

- Main Course - Prep time: 15 mins, Cook time: 40 mins, Total time: 1 hour 55 mins, Servings: 4, Grill temp: 400°F

Ingredients

- Twelve large napa cabbage leaves, bottom 3 in.- 7.5cm of stem removed, frozen for at least 1 hour
- 2 tbsp of extra-virgin olive oil
- 1 small yellow onion, finely chopped
- 1 tsp of kosher salt
- ¼ tsp of freshly ground black pepper
- 1- 8 oz. pkg. of cremini- Baby Bella mushrooms, finely chopped
- 1 tbsp of finely chopped fresh dill
- 1 tbsp of finely chopped fresh Italian flat-leaf parsley
- ½ tsp of dried thyme leaves

- 1 cup of cooked brown rice
- 2 cups of vegetable stock
- 4 tbsp of tomato paste
- 2 tbsp of sugar
- ½ tsp of ground allspice
- ¼ cup of dry white wine

Directions

1. Preheat the oven to 400°F - 200°C.
2. Lightly coat a 9×13-inch- 23×33cm glass baking pan with cooking spray.
3. Thaw napa cabbage leaves at room temperature and squeezes excess moisture from each leaf. Set aside on a paper towel-lined surface.
4. In a large sauté pan over medium-high heat, heat extra-virgin olive oil. Add yellow onion, kosher salt, and black pepper, and stir for 2 mins.
5. Add cremini mushrooms, and cook, often stirring, until they begin to color. Remove from heat, and stir in dill, Italian flat-leaf parsley, thyme, and brown rice.
6. In a small saucepan over medium-high heat, combine vegetable stock, tomato paste, sugar, allspice, and white wine. Bring to a boil, reduce heat to medium, and cook, stirring to dissolve tomato paste and white wine for about 10 mins, or until sauce is reduced and slightly thickened. Keep warm while you fill cabbage rolls.
7. Working with 1 cabbage leaf at a time, spoon a few tbsp filling in the center and roll up like a burrito, tucking up short ends first, then rolling each into a long cylinder. Place each finished cabbage roll in the prepared baking dish, and repeat with the remaining ingredients.
8. Pour sauce over cabbage rolls, cover the pan with heavy-duty aluminum foil, and bake for 30 mins.
9. Serve hot.

Nutritional Values

Calories 257, Fat 7.8g, Chol 2mg, Sodium 88mg, Potassium 57mg, Carbs 32g, Protein 6.9g

381. SEITAN AND DUMPLINGS

- Main Course - Prep time: 25 mins, Cook time: 40 mins, Total time: 1 hour 5 mins, Servings: 4 to 6, Grill temp: 300°F

Ingredients

- 2 tbsp of grapeseed oil
- 1 loaf of Basic Seitan pulled into small chunks before simmering, or 1- 1-lb. pkg. of seitan pieces
- 1 large yellow onion halved and thinly sliced
- 2 large carrots, peeled and cut into ½ -in.- 1.25cm rounds
- 1- 8 oz. pkg. of button mushrooms, quartered
- 2 large stalks of celery, cut in ½ -in.- 1.25cm slices
- 2 tsps of kosher salt
- 1 tsp of freshly ground black pepper
- 1 ½ cups of soy or hemp milk
- 1 tsp of apple cider vinegar
- 3 tbsp plus 1 ½ cups of all-purpose flour
- ½ cup of coarse yellow cornmeal
- 2 tbsp of baking powder
- 2 tbsp of finely chopped fresh Italian flat-leaf parsley
- ½ tsp of dried thyme
- ½ tsp of Bell's seasoning or poultry seasoning
- 5 cups of vegetable stock 1 cup of fresh or frozen tiny green peas

Directions

1. In a Dutch oven over medium-high heat, heat 1 tbsp of grapeseed oil. Add Basic Seitan chunks in batches, and sauté, stirring gently, for 5 mins or until browned. Set aside on a plate, and cover to keep warm while you cook the remaining seitan.
2. Add remaining 1 tbsp of grapeseed oil to the pan, along with yellow onion, carrots, button mushrooms, celery, 1 tsp of kosher salt, and ½ tsp black pepper. Cook, stirring frequently and adjusting heat as needed to prevent burning, for 5 mins.
3. In a medium bowl, whisk soy milk with apple cider vinegar. Set aside to curdle slightly.
4. In a large bowl, whisk together 1 ½ cups of all-purpose flour, yellow cornmeal, baking

powder, Italian flat-leaf parsley, thyme, Bell's seasoning, remaining 1 tsp kosher salt, and remaining ½ tsp black pepper. Pour in soy milk mixture, and stir just until combined—do not knead. Set aside for 10 mins.

5. Add remaining 3 tbsp of all-purpose flour to vegetables, and stir for 1 minute. Add vegetable stock, and stir vigorously to release any browned bits from the bottom of the pan.

6. Stir in seitan and tiny green peas, and bring to a boil. Drop-in dumpling batter by the heaping spoonfuls, spacing evenly- you'll have about 10 dumplings, which will cover the surface of the stew.

7. Cover, reduce heat to low, and cook—without opening the lid—for 15 mins. Uncover, remove from heat, and serve.

Nutritional Values

Calories 269, Fat 8.9g, Chol 2mg, Sodium 89mg, Potassium 76.7mg, Carbs 32g, Protein 11g

382. SEITAN SATAY

- Main Course - Prep time: 2 hours 30 mins, Cook time: 15 mins, Total time: 1 hour 45 mins, Servings: 4, Grill temp: 300°F

Ingredients

- 1 loaf of Basic Seitan, cut into 1-in.- 2.5cm chunks
- ¼ cup of plus 2 tbsp of reduced-Sodium tamari
- ¼ cup of water
- 1 tbsp of toasted sesame oil
- 1 tbsp of melted coconut oil
- 3 tbsp of grated fresh ginger
- 2 cloves of garlic, finely chopped
- 2 tbsp of tamarind paste
- 2 tbsp of hot- not boiling water
- ½ cup of chunky peanut butter
- ½ cup of full-Fat coconut milk, well shaken
- 1 tsp of crushed red pepper flakes

Directions

1. Place Basic Seitan chunks in a baking dish large enough to hold it in a single layer.
2. In a small bowl, whisk together ¼ cup of tamari, water, sesame oil, coconut oil, 1

tbsp of ginger, and garlic. Pour over seitan, and stir well. Cover and refrigerate for 2 hours or overnight.

3. Soak 8 bamboo skewers in warm water for at least 30 mins. Drain.

4. Preheat a broiler, a grill, or a grill pan for direct cooking over high heat. Brush a broiler pan, grill pan, or grill grates with a light coating of oil.

5. In a medium bowl, whisk tamarind paste with hot water to soften. Add chunky peanut butter, coconut milk, the remaining 2 tbsp ginger, the remaining 2 tbsp tamari, and crushed red pepper flakes, and whisk well.

6. Thread seitan onto skewers, and cook, turning once or twice, for 5 to 7 mins, or until browned on all sides.

7. Serve immediately with tamarind-peanut sauce.

Nutritional Values

Calories 271, Fat 9g, Chol 2mg, Sodium 90mg, Potassium 77mg, Carbs 31g, Protein 11g

383. SESAME NOODLES

- Main Course - Prep time: 10 mins, Cook time: 10 mins, Total time: 20 mins, Servings: 8, Grill temp: 300°F

Ingredients

- 2 tsps of kosher salt
- 1 lb. of thin linguine
- ¼ cup of tahini
- ¼ cup of creamy peanut butter
- ¼ cup of hot water
- 2 tbsp of reduced-Sodium tamari or soy sauce
- 2 tbsp of rice vinegar
- 2 tbsp of grated fresh ginger
- 1 tsp of toasted sesame oil
- 1 tsp of chili garlic sauce or Thai chile paste
- 1 medium carrot, julienne cut
- 1 English cucumber, julienne cut
- 3 tbsp of Gomasio
- ¼ cup of thinly sliced scallions, light, and dark green parts

Directions

1. Bring a large pot of water to a boil over medium-high heat. Add kosher salt and

linguine, and cook according to the package directions until pasta is tender. Drain, rinse pasta under cold water, and set aside.

2. In a large bowl, whisk together tahini, peanut butter, hot water, tamari, rice vinegar, ginger, toasted sesame oil, and chili garlic sauce.

3. Add the cooked linguine, carrot, and English cucumber to the sauce. Toss gently, garnish with gomasio and scallions, and serve immediately.

Nutritional Values

Calories 269, Fat 8.9g, Chol 2mg, Sodium 89mg, Potassium 76.7mg, Carbs 32g, Protein 11g

384. SESAME TOFU CUTLETS

- Breakfast - Prep time: 2 hours 30 mins, Cook time: 10 mins, Total time: 2 hours 40 mins, Servings: 3, Grill temp: 300°F

Ingredients

- 1- 16 oz. pkg of firm tofu
- 2 tbsp of reduced-Sodium tamari
- Juice of 1 lemon
- 1 tbsp of toasted sesame oil
- 1 tbsp of grated fresh ginger
- 2 cloves of garlic, finely chopped
- ½ cup of panko breadcrumbs
- ¼ cup of sesame seeds
- ¼ cup of grapeseed oil

Directions

1. Cut tofu horizontally into thirds, and cut each third in ½. Place tofu on several layers of paper towels, top with more paper towels, set a heavy plate on top, and add weight. Set aside to drain for 30 mins.

2. In a large baking dish, whisk together tamari, lemon juice, sesame oil, ginger, and garlic. Add tofu, and refrigerate for 2 hours, turning tofu once or twice.

3. In a small bowl, combine panko breadcrumbs and sesame seeds.

4. Dredge each tofu cutlet in breadcrumb mixture, dip in the marinade again, and dredge in breadcrumb mixture a second time to coat well.

5. In a large frying pan over medium-high heat, heat grapeseed oil until oil begins to shimmer. Add tofu cutlets, and fry, turning once and adjusting heat as necessary to prevent burning, for about 3 mins, per side or until golden and crisp. For Sesame Seitan Cutlets, use seitan instead.

Nutritional Values

Calories 113, Fat 1.8g, Chol 0mg, Sodium 71.4mg, Potassium 67.7mg, Carbs 22g, Protein 2.3g

385. SUMMER SQUASH AND ONION BAKE

- Main Course - Prep time: 15 mins, Cook time: 40 mins, Total time: 55 mins, Servings: 4, Grill temp: 350°F

Ingredients

- 4 tbsp of extra-virgin olive oil
- 2 large sweet onions, such as Vidalia, thinly sliced into rings
- 2 cloves of garlic, finely chopped
- 2 medium zucchinis, thinly sliced
- 2 medium yellow squash, thinly sliced
- 1 tsp of kosher salt
- ¼ tsp of freshly ground black pepper
- 2 tbsp of all-purpose flour
- 1 ½ cups of nondairy milk, such as rice or soy
- ¼ tsp of ground nutmeg
- ½ tsp of finely chopped fresh rosemary
- 1 cup of panko breadcrumbs
- 2 tbsp of finely chopped fresh chives
- 1 tsp of dried thyme

Directions

1. Preheat the oven to 350°F - 180°C. Lightly grease an 8×8-inch- 20×20cm square baking dish.

2. In a wide sauté pan over medium-high heat, heat 2 tbsp of extra-virgin olive oil. Add sweet onions, and cook, stirring, for 5 mins, or until softened.

3. Add garlic, and stir for 1 minute. Remove onions and garlic from the pan, and keep warm.

4. Add 1 tbsp of olive oil, zucchini, and yellow squash, and season with kosher salt and black pepper. Increase heat to high, and cook, stirring every minute or so, for 5

mins, or until vegetables begin to turn golden.

5. Sprinkle with all-purpose flour, reduce heat to medium, and stir for 1 minute to combine well. Return the onion mixture to the pan.
6. Stir in the nondairy milk, nutmeg, and rosemary. Bring to a boil, and cook for about 2 mins, or until thickened. Remove from heat.
7. In a small bowl, combine panko breadcrumbs, chives, thyme, and the remaining 1 tbsp of extra-virgin olive oil.
8. Pour squash mixture into the baking dish, spread gently, and sprinkle evenly with breadcrumb mixture. Bake, uncovered, for 30 mins.
9. Serve immediately.

Nutritional Values

Calories 113, Fat 1.8g, Chol 0mg, Sodium 71.4mg, Potassium 67.7mg, Carbs 22g, Protein 2.3g

386. SWISS CHARD RAVIOLI

- Main Course - Prep time: 30 mins, Cook time: 25 mins, Total time: 55 mins, Servings: 4, Grill temp: 300°F

Ingredients

- ½ cup of raw almonds
- 3 tbsp of extra-virgin olive oil
- 4 cloves of garlic, finely chopped
- 2 bunches of Swiss chard, leaves only, roughly chopped
- 1 tbsp of water
- ½ tsp of kosher salt
- ¼ tsp of freshly ground black pepper
- Juice of a ½ lemon
- 1 tbsp of nutritional yeast
- 1 tsp of water
- 40 wonton wrappers or 1 batch of Fresh Pasta Dough

Directions

1. Soak almonds in cold water for at least 4 hours or overnight.
2. Discard water nuts soaked in, rinse nuts well, and drain.
3. In a large sauté pan over medium-high heat, heat extra-virgin olive oil. Add garlic,

and stir for 30 seconds. Add Swiss chard, with water still clinging to leaves, and cook, frequently stirring, for about 10 mins, or until tender. Add water if Swiss chard begins to dry out. Season with kosher salt and black pepper, and cool slightly.

4. In a food processor fitted with a metal blade, process almonds, Swiss chard, lemon juice, and nutritional yeast in pulses until smooth, adding water if necessary to bring the mixture together. Cool completely.
5. Place wonton wrappers, a few at a time, on a lightly floured surface. Spoon about 1 1 /2 tsps of filling into the center of each wrapper, brush edges of wrappers with water, and pinch edges to seal, pressing out air as you go.- Alternatively, roll Fresh Pasta Dough using a pasta machine or a rolling pin until about 1 /8 -inch [3mm] thick. Use a 3-inch [7.5cm] round cutter to cut pasta rounds and fill as directed.
6. Bring a large pot of salted water to a boil over medium-high heat. Gently drop ravioli into boiling water, and cook for about 3 to 5 mins, or until tender.
7. Serve with your favorite sauce.

Nutritional Values

Calories 113, Fat 1.8g, Chol 0mg, Sodium 71.4mg, Potassium 67.7mg, Carbs 22g, Protein 2.3g

387. TAMALE CASSEROLE

- Main Course - Prep time: 10 mins, Cook time: 1 hour 20 mins, Total time: 1 hour 30 mins, Servings: 6, Grill temp: 350°F

Ingredients

- 4 tbsp of extra-virgin olive oil
- 1 large yellow onion, finely chopped
- 1 medium green bell pepper, ribs, and seeds removed and finely chopped
- 3 cloves of garlic, finely chopped
- 1 tsp of ground cumin
- ½ tsp of dried oregano
- 1 canned chipotle chile in adobo, finely chopped
- 2 tbsp of adobo sauce- from canned chile
- 1 bunch of lacinato kale, tough stems removed and roughly chopped

- 2- 14 oz. can of pinto beans, rinsed and drained
- 1- 14 oz. can of diced tomatoes, with juice
- 1 cup of vegetable stock
- ¼ cup of chopped pimiento-stuffed green olives
- 5 ½ cups of water
- 2 ½ tsps of kosher salt
- ¾ cup of coarse yellow cornmeal
- ½ cup of masa harina
- 1 ½ cups of fresh or frozen corn kernels
- 1 cup of shredded plant-based cheddar-style cheese

Directions

1. Preheat the oven to 375°F - 190°C. Lightly oil a 9×13-inch- 23×33cm baking dish.
2. In a large sauté pan over medium-high heat, heat 3 tbsp of extra-virgin olive oil. Add yellow onion, green bell pepper, and garlic, and cook for 3 mins, adjusting heat as needed to prevent burning.
3. Add cumin, oregano, chipotle chile, adobo sauce, and lacinato kale, and cook, frequently stirring, for 5 mins.
4. Stir in pinto beans, diced tomatoes with juice, vegetable stock, and pimiento-stuffed green olives, and cook for 10 mins, or until all vegetables are tender and the sauce has reduced slightly.
5. Meanwhile, in a large saucepan over high heat, bring water to a boil. Stir in kosher salt, and slowly whisk in yellow cornmeal and masa harina. Reduce heat to medium, and cook, frequently stirring, for 15 mins.
6. Stir in corn and the remaining 1 tbsp of extra-virgin olive oil.
7. Spoon ½ of the cornmeal mixture into the bottom of the prepared baking dish, and spread evenly. Top with vegetables, followed by the remaining cornmeal mixture. Sprinkle cheddar-style cheese over the top, and bake for 40 mins.
8. Serve immediately.

Nutritional Values

Calories 113, Fat 1.8g, Chol 0mg, Sodium 71.4mg, Potassium 67.7mg, Carbs 22g, Protein 2.3g

388. TEMPEH MILANESE

- Main Course - Prep time: 10 mins, Cook time: 60 mins, Total time: 1 hour 10 mins, Servings: 4, Grill temp: 350°F

Ingredients

- 1- 8 oz. pkg. of tempeh
- ½ cup of water
- Juice of 2 lemons
- 2 tbsp of reduced-Sodium tamari
- 4 tbsp of extra-virgin olive oil
- 2 cloves of garlic, finely chopped
- 1 cup of Italian-seasoned panko breadcrumbs
- ½ cup of grapeseed oil
- ½ tsp of kosher salt
- ¼ tsp of freshly ground black pepper
- 4 cups of baby arugula
- 2 cups of grape tomatoes halved
- ½ medium red onion, very thinly sliced
- ¼ cup of pitted kalamata olives

Directions

1. Preheat the oven to 350°F - 180°C.
2. Cut tempeh in ½ horizontally, and cut each piece into 4 equal-size cutlets. Place tempeh in a baking dish large enough to hold it in 1 layer.
3. In a small bowl, whisk together water, 2 tbsp of lemon juice, tamari, 2 tbsp of extra-virgin olive oil, and garlic. Pour over tempeh, cover the dish tightly with aluminum foil, and bake for 50 mins. Remove the foil, drain, and cool tempeh slightly.
4. Place Italian-seasoned panko breadcrumbs in a shallow bowl.
5. In a large frying pan over medium-high heat, heat grapeseed oil until it begins to shimmer.
6. Dredge tempeh cutlets in panko, add to the frying pan, and fry, turning once, for about 2 mins, per side or until golden and crisp.- Adjust heat as necessary to prevent burning.
7. In a large bowl, toss arugula with the remaining 2 tbsp lemon juice and 2 tbsp extra-virgin olive oil, and season with kosher salt and black pepper. 8 Divide arugula among 4 serving plates, and equally divide grape tomatoes and kalamata olives on top.

8. Top each salad with 2 tempeh cutlets, and serve immediately.

Calories 113Kcal, Fat 1.8g, Chol 0mg, Sodium 71.4mg, Potassium 67.7mg, Carbs 22g, Protein 2.3g

389. TOFU AND VEGGIE STIR-FRY

- Main Course - Prep time: 15 mins, Cook time: 10 mins, Total time: 25 mins, Servings: 4, Grill temp: 300°F

Ingredients

- 1 tbsp of soy sauce
- 1 tbsp of toasted sesame oil
- 1 tbsp of rice vinegar
- 1 tbsp of finely chopped fresh ginger
- 2 tbsp of grapeseed oil
- 2 cloves of garlic, finely chopped
- ½ lb. of a firm or extra-firm tofu, cut into ½ -in.- 1.25cm cubes
- 2 cups of thinly sliced bok choy
- 1 cup of small broccoli florets
- 1 medium red bell pepper, diced in ½ -in.- 1.25cm chunks
- 1 medium yellow onion, diced
- 1 cup of sliced shiitake mushrooms
- 1 cup of fresh snow peas
- ¼ cup of water or vegetable stock

Directions

1. In a small bowl, whisk together soy sauce, sesame oil, rice vinegar, and ginger. Set aside.
2. Heat a large wok or cast-iron skillet over medium heat. When hot, add 1 tbsp of grapeseed oil and garlic and cook, stirring, for 30 seconds. Add tofu, and cook, stirring, for about 1 minute or until tofu begins to color slightly.
3. Push tofu to the side, add bok choy and stir for 1 minute.
4. Push bok choy to the side, increase heat to medium-high, and add the remaining 1 tbsp of grapeseed oil. Add broccoli, red bell pepper, yellow onion, and shiitake mushrooms, and cook, stirring, for 2 mins.
5. Add snow peas and water, mix tofu and vegetables, and continue to cook, to stir, for

about 2 mins, or until water is nearly evaporated and vegetables are tender.
6. Add reserved dressing, toss, and serve.

Calories 113Kcal, Fat 1.8g, Chol 0mg, Sodium 71.4mg, Potassium 67.7mg, Carbs 22g, Protein 2.3g

390. TOFU SUMMER ROLLS

- Main Course - Prep time: 15 mins, Cook time: 5 mins, Total time: 20 mins, Servings: 4, Grill temp: 300°F

Ingredients

- 4 oz. of the firm or extra-firm tofu
- 1 tsp of sesame oil
- 4- 8-in. rice paper wrappers
- 4 large leaves of soft green leaf lettuce
- 1 medium carrot, shredded
- ½ cup of shredded napa cabbage
- 5 scallions, thinly sliced
- ½ cup of smooth peanut butter
- 2 tbsp of hoisin sauce
- Juice of 2 limes
- 2 tsps of reduced-Sodium tamari
- 1 tsp of sambal oelek- chili garlic sauce

Directions

1. Place tofu on several layers of paper towels on a cutting board, top with a few more layers of paper towels, place a heavy plate on tofu, and top with a weight such as a large can of tomatoes. Set tofu aside to drain for 30 mins. Blot dry with paper towels, and cut tofu into 1/4 inch-.5cm strips.
2. In a small nonstick sauté pan over medium-high heat, heat sesame oil. Add tofu, and sear, turning once or twice, for about 2 mins, or until browned on all sides. Drain on paper towels.
3. Soak 1 rice paper wrapper in warm water for 30 seconds, remove it from the water, and place it on your work surface. Quickly line the wrapper with 1 lettuce leaf, 2 tbsp carrot, 2 tbsp napa cabbage, and 1 /4 tofu, and sprinkle with 1 tbsp of scallions. Fold short ends of rice paper inward, roll the wrapper like a burrito, and press to seal the seam. Repeat with remaining rice

wrappers and filling. Refrigerate rolls while you make the sauce or overnight.

4. In a small saucepan over medium-low heat, whisk peanut butter, hoisin sauce, lime juice, tamari, and sambal oelek until smooth. Pour into small bowls, and serve hot or cold with rolls.

Nutritional Values

Calories 113, Fat 1.8g, Chol 0mg, Sodium 71.4mg, Potassium 67.7mg, Carbs 22g, Protein 2.3g

391. VEGETABLE ENCHILADAS WITH ROASTED TOMATO SAUCE

- Main Course - Prep time: 45 mins, Cook time: 1 hour 4o mins, Total time: 2 hours 25 mins, Servings: 5 to 6, Grill temp: 375°F

Ingredients

- 2- 10 oz. pkg. of cocktail-size tomatoes, such as Campari
- 4 tbsp extra-virgin olive oil
- 2 medium red bell peppers, ribs, and seeds were removed and cut into 1-in.- 2.5cm strips
- 1 tsp of kosher salt
- ½ tsp of dried oregano
- 2 cups of vegetable stock
- 3 tbsp of dried New Mexico chile powder
- 1 large yellow onion, finely chopped
- 2 poblano chile peppers, seeded and finely chopped
- 2 cloves garlic, finely chopped
- 2 large zucchinis, cut in ½ -in.- 1.25cm dice
- 1- 1 lb. pkg. of roasted corn kernels, or regular frozen corn kernels
- 1- 14 oz. can of black beans, rinsed and drained
- 2 tbsp of finely chopped fresh cilantro
- 6teen- 6-in. handmade-style corn and wheat blend tortillas
- ½ cup of shredded plant-based pepper jack–style cheese- optional

Directions

1. Preheat the oven to 375°F - 190°C. Lightly coat a 9×13-inch- 23×33cm baking pan with a little extra-virgin olive oil.
2. Cut tomatoes in ½, place in the baking pan, and toss with 2 tbsp extra-virgin olive oil,

red bell pepper strips, ½ tsp kosher salt, and oregano. Roast for 1 hour, occasionally stirring, and cool slightly.

3. Purée tomato mixture, vegetable stock, and New Mexico chile powder in batches in a blender or a food processor. Set aside.
4. In a wide sauté pan over medium-high heat, heat the remaining 2 tbsp of extra-virgin olive oil. Add yellow onion and poblano chile peppers, and cook, occasionally stirring, for 4 or 5 mins, adjusting heat as necessary.
5. Add garlic, and stir for 1 minute. Add zucchini, and cook for about 4 or 5 mins, or until vegetables are golden. Stir in roasted corn, and cook another 1 or 2 mins. Stir in black beans, cilantro, remaining ½ tsp kosher salt, and ½ cup of the reserved sauce, and remove from heat.
6. Spread a ½ cup of sauce on the bottom of the prepared baking pan. Spoon about 1 /12 of the filling into the center of 1 tortilla, fill it generously, gently roll, and place in the pan. Repeat with remaining tortillas and filling, fitting them very snugly into the pan.
7. Pour some of the remaining sauce over top of the enchiladas, lightly covering them while leaving edges exposed, and sprinkle with pepper jack–style cheese- if using.
8. Cover with aluminum foil, and bake for about 40 mins, or until hot and bubbly. Serve immediately.
9. For Tortilla Soup, stir 2 cups of sauce into 2 cups of vegetable stock. Heat and stir in 1 cup of lightly crushed tortilla chips and 1 cup of black beans.
10. Serve topped with a spoonful of plant-based sour cream and diced avocado.

Nutritional Values

Calories 222, Fat 17g, Chol 0mg, Sodium 71.4mg, Potassium 67.7mg, Carbs 16g, Protein 3g

392. WHOLE-WHEAT PASTA E CECI- PASTA WITH CHICKPEAS

- Main Course - Prep time: 5 mins, Cook time: 20 mins, Total time: 25 mins, Servings: 4, Grill temp: 300°F

- 8 oz. of tube-shape whole-wheat pasta, such as chocchiole or medium shells
- 3 tbsp of extra-virgin olive oil
- ½ large sweet onion, minced
- ½ tsp of kosher salt
- 2 cloves of garlic, minced
- ¼ tsp of crushed red pepper flakes
- 1 tbsp of tomato paste
- 1- 28 oz. can of peeled Italian plum tomatoes, with juice, lightly crushed by hand
- ½ cup of filtered water or vegetable stock
- 1- 14.5 oz. can chickpeas, rinsed and drained
- ¼ cup of dry white wine
- ¼ tsp of dried oregano

Directions

1. Bring a large pot of salted water to a boil over medium-high heat, and cook whole-wheat pasta according to the package directions until al dente- fully cooked but still firm to the bite. Drain- do not rinse, and set aside.
2. Meanwhile, in a large saucepan over medium-high heat, heat extra-virgin olive oil. Add sweet onion and kosher salt, and cook, frequently stirring, for about 5 mins, or until the onion is softened and translucent.- Adjust heat as necessary.
3. Stir in garlic and crushed red pepper flakes, and stir for 30 seconds. Stir in tomato paste, and add Italian plum tomatoes with juice and filtered water. Bring to a boil, reduce heat to medium, and cook for 5 mins.
4. Stir in chickpeas and pasta, and cook for 2 mins.
5. Stir in white wine and oregano, remove from heat, and serve immediately.

Nutritional Values

Calories 217, Fat 19g, Chol 0mg, Sodium 61.4mg, Potassium 57.7mg, Carbs 5g, Protein 6g

393. WINTER VEGETABLE POT PIE

- Main Course - Prep time: 15 mins, Cook time: 45 mins, Total time: 60 mins, Servings: 6, Grill temp: 400°F

Ingredients

- 4 tbsp of grapeseed oil
- 3 tbsp of all-purpose flour
- 3 cups of Golden Chicken-y Stock
- 1 large yellow onion, cut into small dice
- 4 large stalks of celery, cut into small dice
- 3 medium carrots, cut into small dice
- 1- 10 oz. pkg. of cremini- Baby Bella mushrooms, quartered
- 3 cloves of garlic, minced
- 4 large red-skin potatoes, cut into small dice
- 1 medium sweet potato, cut into small dice
- 2 cups of frozen lima beans
- 1 bay leaf
- 1 tsp of dried thyme
- 1 tsp of kosher salt, plus more to taste
- ½ tsp of freshly ground black pepper
- 1 sheet puff pastry, thawed

Directions

1. Preheat the oven to 400°F - 200°C.
2. In a small saucepan over medium heat, heat 2 tbsp of grapeseed oil. Whisk in all-purpose flour until smooth, and cook, constantly stirring, for about 2 mins, or until flour is lightly golden and smells toasty.
3. Whisk in 2 cups of Golden Chicken-y Stock, and simmer for 5 mins. Remove from heat, and set aside.
4. In a wide sauté pan over medium-high heat, heat the remaining 2 tbsp of grapeseed oil. Add yellow onion, celery, carrots, cremini mushrooms, and garlic, and cook, frequently stirring, for about 10 mins, adjusting heat as necessary, or until vegetables are softened and beginning to color.
5. Stir in the remaining 1 cup of Golden Chicken-y Stock, red-skin potatoes, sweet potatoes, lima beans, bay leaf, thyme, kosher salt, and black pepper. Cover and cook, stirring once or twice and adding a bit of water if the mixture seems dry, for 10 mins.

6. Remove bay leaf, stir in reserved sauce, and pour the vegetable mixture into a 9×13-inch- 23×33cm baking dish.
7. Roll out puff pastry on a floured surface to fit the top of the baking dish with an overhang of ½ inch- 1.25cm. Dock pastry by pricking it all over with a fork, transfer it to the top of the baking dish and lay it gently over vegetables. Tuck overhanging edge down into the inside of the baking dish.
8. Bake for about 30 mins, or until pastry is puffed and filling is hot and bubbly.
9. Serve immediately.

Nutritional Values

Calories 222, Fat 17g, Chol 0mg, Sodium 71.4mg, Potassium 67.7mg, Carbs 16g, Protein 3g

394. TOFU STIR-FRY

- Main Course - Prep time: 10 mins, Cook time: 10 mins, Total time: 20 mins, Servings: 2, Grill temp: 300°F

Ingredients

- ¼ cup of chopped onion
- ¼ cup of chopped button mushrooms
- 8 ounces of chopped extra-firm tofu
- 3 tsps of nutritional yeast
- 1 tsp of Braggs liquid aminos
- 4 cups of baby spinach
- 5 chopped grape tomatoes
- Cooking spray
- Sriracha/another hot sauce for garnishing

Directions

1. Over medium heat, spray a pan with cooking spray and heat. Add the mushrooms and onion and sauté until the onions and mushrooms are translucent and softened- about 4 mins.
2. To the skillet, add tofu. Mix to combine and cook for an extra 2 mins.
3. Add the nutritional yeast and the amino liquids to the pan. Stir until it's all well coated.
4. Add the tomatoes and spinach. Cook for 4 more mins before the spinach begins to wilt a little bit. Plate, top and serve with sriracha.

Nutritional Values

Calories 202, Fat 11g, Chol 0mg, Sodium 71.4mg, Potassium 67.7mg, Carbs 7g, Protein 18g

395. SPINACH & CHICKPEAS WITH 5 INGREDIENT ZITI BAKED

- Prep time: 10 mins, Cook time: 30, Total time: 40 mins, Grill temp: 400°F, Servings: 4

Ingredients

- 16 oz. of ziti pasta
- 4 cups of spaghetti sauce
- 1 can of chickpeas
- 1 ½ cups of shredded cheese
- 2–4 cups of leaves, baby spinach

Directions

1. Preheat the oven to 400 °F- 200°C. In a big saucepan, bring water to a boil. Fill a pot halfway with water and add the ziti noodles. Cook according to the package directions.
2. Drain and add the noodles to the saucepan. Combine the spaghetti sauce, chickpeas, and spinach in a mixing bowl.
3. Pour ½ of the noodle mixture into a large baking dish. ½ of the cheese mixture should be on top. Cover with the remaining cheese and more noodles.
4. Cover with foil and bake for 20 to 25 mins, or until pasta is warm and cheese has melted.

Nutritional Values

Fat 7g, Chol 8mg, Sodium 14mg, Potassium 76mg, Carbs 42g, Calories 240, Protein 12 g

Chapter 11.

Noodles & Pasta Recipes

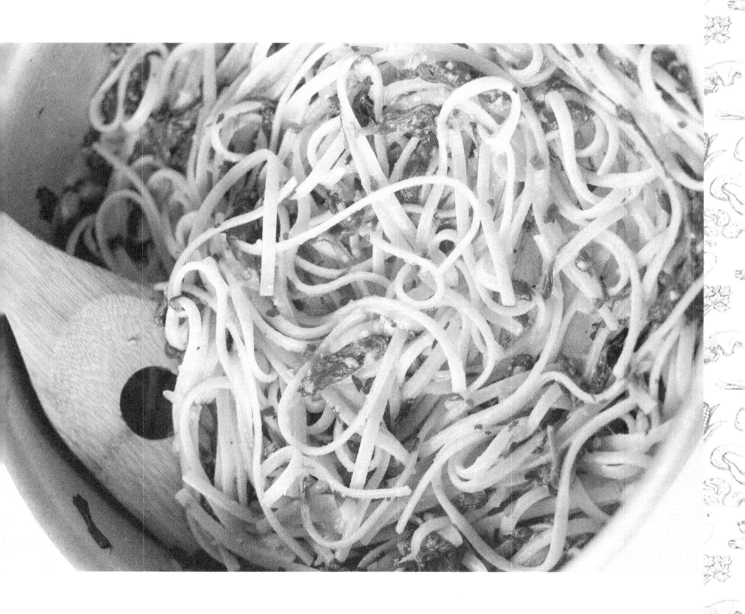

396. SPINACH PARMESAN ZUCCHINI NOODLES

- Prep time: 10 mins, Cook time: 20, Total time: 30 mins, Grill temp: 0, Servings: 4

Ingredients

- 2 cups of packed spinach
- 1 tbsp of butter
- 2 cloves of garlic minced
- Salt and pepper for taste
- ¼ cup of Parmesan cheese
- 3 zucchinis, medium

Directions

1. Spiralize the zucchini and set them to the side.
2. Heat butter & garlic in a large skillet over medium-high heat. Cook for 1–2 mins. In a mixing dish, combine spinach & zucchini noodles. Gently toss.
3. Heat for a couple of mins or until the spinach leaves are wilted. Mix in ¼ cup Parmesan cheese & toss till zucchini noodles are well coated in cheese.
4. Season the dish with salt and black pepper.
5. Remove from the heat & serve.
6. If you overcook the spinach or zucchini noodles, they will get mushy.

Nutritional Values

Fat 3g, Chol 18mg, Sodium 24mg, Potassium 74mg, Carbs 65g, Calories 340, Protein 25 g

397. NO-BOIL VEGETABLE LASAGNA

- Prep time: 40 mins, Cook time: 1 hr. 50 mins, Total time: 2 hr. 30 mins, Grill temp: 350°F, Servings: 4

Ingredients

- 2 packages of frozen mixed vegetables
- 1 can of unsalted crushed tomatoes
- 3 cans of unsalted diced tomatoes
- 1 tbsp ground Italian seasoning
- ½ tsp kosher salt
- ½ tsp garlic powder
- 12 lasagna noodles
- 2 carton ricotta cheese
- 2 packages of frozen spinach
- 2 & ½ cups mozzarella cheese
- ¼ cup of shredded Parmesan cheese.

Directions

1. Preheat your oven to around 350 deg F - 180°C. These frozen mixed vegetables should be rinsed and cooked as directed on the container. Set aside a 3-quart baking dish that has been gently oiled with cooking oil.
2. Add crushed tomatoes, Italian seasoning, tomatoes, garlic powder, and salt to a mixing bowl. 1 cup of sauce that has already been produced should be put into a basin.
3. Place 4 lasagna noodles in a cross on a platter, carefully overlapping them on top of the prepared sauce. 2/3 cup of ricotta cheese spooned over noodles, gently pour over noodles.
4. Place 1/3 of the spinach and 1/3 of the carrots on top. ½ cup mozzarella cheese is sprinkled over the top.
5. Once again, the ½-sauce, spaghetti noodles, ricotta cheese, spinach, vegetables, and mozzarella cheese are layered.
6. Replace the remaining noodles, ricotta cheese, spinach, vegetables, and ½ cup of mozzarella cheese with the remaining ingredients. The remainder of the sauce is poured on top. Place this dish on a baking pan and cover it with foil. Preheat the oven to 400°F and bake for 40 mins.
7. Then reveal it. Over the top, sprinkle the remaining ½ cup of mozzarella and Parmesan cheese. Bake for another 10-15 mins, or until the lasagna is thoroughly cooked and soft noodles. Allow 15 mins for resting time before serving.

Nutritional Values

Fat 6.7g, Chol 6mg, Sodium 14mg, Potassium 73mg, Carbs 55g, Calories 299, Protein 18 g

398. BLT PASTA SALAD

- Prep time: 30 mins, Cook time: 20 mins, Total time: 50 mins, Grill temp: 0, Servings: 4-6

Ingredients

- 12 oz. of farfalle pasta
- Olive oil extra-virgin ¼ cup
- 3 tbsp of red wine vinegar
- Minced garlic cloves 3
- 1 tsp of dried oregano

- 1 tsp of dried parsley
- ¾ tsp of sea salt
- Cherry tomatoes halved 2 cups
- Tempeh Bacon in small pieces
- Dried tomatoes 1/3 cup chopped
- 1 cup sliced cucumber
- ½ cup red onion finely sliced
- 1 avocado, finely sliced
- fresh arugula ½ cups

Directions

1. Bring salted water to a simmer in a large saucepan. Cook the pasta according to the package directions until it's just beyond al dente.
2. Meanwhile, make the salad dressing. Whisk the balsamic vinegar, olive oil, oregano, garlic, parsley, and salt in the bottom of a large mixing bowl.
3. Serve with a side of noodles. Toss in the tempeh bacon, sun-dried tomatoes, tomatoes, cucumber, and onion 1 more time. Gently fold the avocado and arugula into 1 another within the avocado. Serve after seasoning to taste with salt and pepper.

Nutritional Values

Fat 5.4g, Chol 13mg, Sodium 21mg, Potassium 71mg, Carbs 37g, Calories 315, Protein 7 g

399. PESTO PASTA SALAD

- Prep time: 15 mins, Cook time: 12 mins, Total time: 27 mins, Grill temp: 0, Servings: 4-6

Ingredients

- Basil Pesto prepared in ¼ cup of olive oil
- 12 ounces Cellentani, Fusilli or Cavatappi pasta
- ¾ cup water
- 2 small, sliced zucchinis
- 1 small sliced yellow squash
- 1 tbsp lemon juice fresh
- 1 tsp sea salt
- black pepper Freshly ground
- ¼ cup pine nuts toasted
- ½ cup fresh basil
- Red chili flakes

Directions

1. Turn off the heat and set the pesto aside.

2. Bring a large pot of water to a rolling boil. Cook the pasta according to the package directions until it is slightly beyond al dente. Before draining the noodles, scoop 34 cups of starchy spaghetti water and set it aside. Wash the spaghetti and toss it with some olive oil to avoid it from sticking together. Allow the pasta- together with the conserved pasta water, to cool on a room-temperature baking sheet.
3. Toss the spaghetti with the zucchini and pesto. Combine yellow squash, lemon juice, pasta water, salt, and pepper in a large mixing bowl. To taste, season with salt and pepper. Garnish with fresh basil, pine nuts, and chili flakes, if desired. Before serving, allow the salad to cool.

Nutritional Values

Fat 2.4g, Chol 9.4mg, Sodium 6mg, Potassium 95mg, Carbs 39g, Calories 321, Protein 8 g

400. HOW TO MAKE VEGGIE NOODLES

- Prep time: 10 mins, Cook time: 5 mins, Total time: 15 mins, Grill temp: 0, Servings: 2

Ingredients

- Butternut squash
- Cucumber
- Carrot
- Daikon radish
- Sweet potato
- Summer squash
- Zucchini
- Kohlrabi

Directions

1. Select squash with a long neck. By slicing off the plump, seedy bottom of the squash. Slice the squash and spiralize it to make the noodles.
2. What you're searching for is a large beet. Remove the covering and spiralize the zucchini to make noodles.
3. You're searching for a large cucumber. Use a spiralizer or a julienne peeler to make noodles.
4. Consider a carrot with a lot of Fat on it. Clean it well or peel it if it's too unclean. Use a julienne peeler to make noodles.
5. Use a spiralizer to make noodles.

6. You're looking for a large golden squash. Use a julienne peeler to make noodles. Alternatively, produce thick ribbon-shaped noodles using a regular peeler. The squash membrane does not need to be peeled.

7. Remove the greens and keep them aside for later. The kohlrabi bulb's nubby parts should be pulled away. Use a spiralizer to make noodles.

Nutritional Values

Fat 4.8g, Chol 12mg, Sodium 19mg, Potassium 56mg, Carbs 37g, Calories 330, Protein 6 g

401. SPAGHETTI AND MEATBALLS

- Prep time: 20 mins, Cook time: 20 mins, Total time: 40 mins, Grill temp: 0, Servings: 4

Ingredients

- 8 oz. spaghetti
- 2 zucchinis
- Vegan meatballs
- Fresh basil
- Marinara sauce
- Olive oil
- Finely chopped parsley

Directions

1. In a mixing basin, combine the spaghetti and zucchini noodles and divide them into 4 bowls. 2-3 meatballs in each bowl, with plenty of marinaras, herbs, and olive oil drizzled on top.

2. Season to taste with salt and pepper, then garnish with parsley before serving.

Nutritional Values

Fat 8.4g, Chol 14mg, Sodium 19mg, Potassium 54mg, Carbs 40g, Calories 360, Protein 10 g

402. SESAME SOBA NOODLES

- Prep time: 10 mins, Cook time: 10 mins, Total time: 20 mins, Grill temp: 0, Servings: 2-4

Ingredients

Sesame dressing:
- Rice vinegar ¼ cup
- 2 tbsp tamari
- ½ tsp sesame oil toasted
- 1 tsp grated ginger
- 1 grated garlic clove
- ½ tsp honey or maple syrup

For soba noodles:
- 6 oz. soba noodles
- Sesame oil
- 2 sliced avocados
- Juice of lemon
- 2 cups snap peas blanched
- Edamame ¼ cup
- 1 finely sliced watermelon radish
- ¼ cup mint leaves fresh
- Sesame seeds

Directions

1. To prepare the dressing, whisk together all of the ingredients in a large mixing basin.

2. Combine the vinegar, sesame oil, tamari, ginger, garlic, and honey in a small bowl.

3. Bring a pot of water to a boil, then follow the package directions for cooking the noodles.

4. Drain and rinse in cold water completely. This assists in the elimination of Carbs that cause clumping.

5. Toss the noodles in the dressing and divide them into 2 to 4 serving dishes.

6. Squeeze the lemon juice over the avocado slices and toss them in the bowls with the peas, edamame, mint, radish, and sesame seeds.

7. Drizzle with more tamari or sesame oil if preferred.

Nutritional Values

Fat 1.4g, Chol 13mg, Sodium 18mg, Potassium 73mg, Carbs 38g, Calories 230, Protein 7 g

403. ZUCCHINI NOODLES & LEMON /RICOTTA

- Prep time: 15 mins, Cook time: 15 mins, Total time: 30 mins, Grill temp: 0, Servings: 2

Ingredients

- 2-3 large zucchini
- 1 cup sliced cherry
- for drizzling olive oil
- sea salt & black pepper
- microgreens & hemp seeds

Lemon-macadamia ricotta:
- ½ cup macadamia nuts raw
- ¼ cup sunflower seeds raw
- ¼ cup seeds hemp
- 2 Tbsp lemon juice fresh

- 1 Tbsp wine vinegar white
- 1 garlic clove small
- fresh herbs
- ½ tsp sea salt
- ½ cup water

Directions

1. Drain and rinse the macadamia and sunflower seeds after soaking. Except for the water, salt, and pepper, combine everything in your blender. Blend until completely smooth.
2. In a blender, combine hemp seeds and water. Blend until completely smooth. Fill the container halfway with water. Blend until completely smooth. Lubricate your blade with extra virgin olive oil if required.
3. Using a julienne peeler, cut your zucchini into noodle-sized pieces.
4. Toss your zucchini "noodles" with olive oil, ricotta, tomatoes, salt, and pepper to taste. As a final touch, more ricottas might be served on the side.
5. Ricotta may be kept in the refrigerator for up to 1 day if not used immediately away. If it gets runny on the second day, you may mix it until it becomes cohesive again.

Nutritional Values

Fat 1.3g, Chol 9mg, Sodium 14mg, Potassium 89mg, Carbs 36g, Calories 203, Protein 6 g

404. EASY PEANUT NOODLES

- Prep time: 15 mins, Cook time: 15 mins, Total time: 30 mins, Grill temp: 0, Servings: 2-3

Ingredients

- 8 oz. pasta, soba noodles
- Mushroom's shiitake
- Eggplant
- Pepper- red
- Scallions chopped
- Seeds of sesame
- Sauce peanut
- Peanuts crushed

Directions

1. Noodles should be prepared according to the package directions.
2. Heat some oil in a medium-sized skillet. Currently, add the eggplant and

mushrooms and simmer for a few mins or until they are soft. After a few mins, add the red pepper and scallions to the pan and simmer for another few mins. Remove the pan from the heat and add a little quantity of soy sauce.
3. Toss the veggies and peanut sauce with the noodles to incorporate.
4. For a delightful finishing touch, sprinkle sesame seeds and broken peanuts on top. As desired, serve hot or cold.

Nutritional Values

Fat 7.4g, Chol 5mg, Sodium 12mg, Potassium 84mg, Carbs 52g, Calories 394, Protein 17 g

405. COLD CUCUMBER SOBA

- Prep time: 10 mins, Cook time: 20 mins, Total time: 30 mins, Grill temp: 0, Servings: 2

Ingredients

- 4-6 oz. noodles soba
- 1-2 tbsp sesame oil toasted
- 2 cucumbers medium
- ¼ cup scallions chopped
- 1 tbsp soy sauce or tamari
- 2 tbsp vinegar- rice
- 1-2 tbsp sauce ponzu
- Slices avocado
- Seeds sesame

Directions

1. In salted water, cook soba noodles until al dente. Drain and rinse under cold running water after 30 seconds of boiling in ice water to halt the cooking process.
2. Put them in a basin and mix them with sesame oil to keep them from sticking together while preparing the remainder of the dinner.
3. Cucumbers should be finely sliced using a julienne peeler. Slice the avocado around the seeded area in the middle, discarding the skin as you go.
4. Toss the cucumbers and onions with the soba noodles. After that, add the rice vinegar, tamari, and ponzu, and mix it again before serving. After tasting the meal, adjust the seasonings to your preference.
5. To finish, sprinkle sesame seeds and sliced avocado over the top.

6. Serve chilled if possible.

Nutritional Values

Fat 7.2g, Chol 5mg, Sodium 12mg, Potassium 83mg, Carbs 39g, Calories 355, Protein 9 g

406. ZUCCHINI NOODLES & AVOCADO-MISO SAUCE

- Prep time: 10 mins, Cook time: 10 mins, Total time: 20 mins, Grill temp: 0, Servings: 4

Ingredients

- 1 avocado
- 1 cup seeds hemp
- 1 zest & juice lime
- 1 zucchini small
- ½ Tbsp miso
- 1 chopped scallion, white & green parts
- 1 Tbsp ginger minced
- ¼ tsp cumin ground
- ¼ tsp cayenne ground

Directions

1. In a blender, combine all of the ingredients for the miso sauce until smooth. Combine the hemp seeds, lime zest, and juice in a mixing bowl. Combine the zucchini and miso in a mixing bowl. After tasting the meal, adjust the seasonings to your preference.
2. Season zucchini noodles with pepper and salt, then combine with the sauce of your choice. After tasting the meal, adjust the seasonings to your preference.
3. Serve with lime wedges and additional sauce on the side, then top with fresh mango, edamame, and almonds.

Nutritional Values

Fat 7.2g, Chol 3mg, Sodium 5mg, Potassium 84mg, Carbs 58g, Calories 467, Protein 14 g

407. CASHEW BROCCOLI SOBA NOODLES

- Prep time: 10 mins, Cook time: 25 mins, Total time: 35 mins, Grill temp: 400°F, Servings: 3-4

Ingredients

- 2 tbsp of tamari, if desired, more for serving
- 2 tbsp lime juice, fresh
- 2 tbsp orange juice, fresh
- 1 tbsp of sesame oil
- 1 minced garlic clove
- 1 tsp of minced ginger
- 2 tbsp of cashew butter
- 2 tbsp of water, more as required
- 8 oz. soba noodles
- for drizzling sesame seeds
- 1 medium chopped head broccoli, stems thinly sliced
- for drizzling tamari
- 2 sliced scallions
- 1 thinly sliced carrot
- 4- 6 oz. baked tofu, cubed & warmed
- ¼ cup crushed toasted cashews
- sriracha, for serving

Directions

1. Combine the orange juice, tamari, sesame seeds, lime juice, garlic, cashew butter, ginger, and water in a dish to make cashew sauce. If the sauce is too thick to drizzle, thin it up with more water as needed.
2. Cook soba noodles according to package directions in a pot of boiling water. Drain and thoroughly rinse. This assists in the elimination of carbohydrates that cause clumping. After tossing with a drizzle of oil, set aside- sesame oil.
3. Set the steamer basket in a large saucepan filled with 1 inch of boiling water. In a large mixing basin, combine the scallions, broccoli florets and stems, and a couple of dashes of tamari. Heat to a low simmer, cover, and steam the broccoli for 2 to 4 mins, or until tender but bright green.- If you like, you can grill the broccoli. Toss with a splash of tamari and olive oil and roast at 400°F for 15-20 mins.
4. In bowls, combine noodles, steamed broccoli and scallions, carrots, cashews, tofu, and dollops of cashew sauce. Serve with more tamari and sriracha sauce on the side if desired.

Nutritional Values

Fat 1.3g, Chol 9mg, Sodium 16mg, Potassium 67mg, Carbs 34g, Calories 225, Protein 10g

408. GINGER NOODLES WITH KALE & SHIITAKES

- Prep time: 25 mins, Cook time: 45 mins, Total time: 70 mins, Servings: 2, Grill temp: 0

- 2 packs or 7 oz. Miracle shirataki noodles- or any of your choice
- ½ -1 cup shiitake mushrooms, sliced
- 1 cup of kale, thinly chopped
- 1-2 tsp of minced ginger
- 1 minced garlic clove
- 2-3 scallions chopped, white & green parts
- 2-3 cups of vegetable broth, low sodium
- ½ cup of edamame, shelled & thawed
- 1 – 2 tbsp of soy sauce or tamari
- A handful of basil, chopped
- Handful mint, chopped
- lime juice
- Drizzle sesame oil, toasted
- for garnish, sesame seeds
- Olive oil
- red pepper flakes or a splash of sriracha, optional

Directions

1. Prepare the shirataki noodles - they don't need to be cooked, but they need to be drained and washed. They have an off-putting odor. Then drain and rinse again in tepid water. Please keep them in a secure location until you're ready to utilize them.
2. In a skillet, drizzle a little oil. Once the pan is heated, add the mushrooms and a touch of salt. Cook for approximately 5 mins, stirring to mix, or until they've wilted down. In a mixing bowl, combine the kale, scallions, ginger, and garlic. Cook for a few mins or until the kale starts to wilt, but the garlic doesn't burn. Reduce the heat if the ginger and garlic begin to burn.
3. Cook for a few mins with the edamame, broth, and noodles. If the veggies have absorbed all of the broth, add more.
4. Remove the pan from the heat and stir in the lime juice, soy sauce, mint, basil, and red pepper flakes- if using, seasoning to taste with salt and pepper.
5. Serve in bowls with a drizzle of toasted sesame oil and a sprinkling of sesame seeds on top.

Nutritional Values

Fat 1.7g, Chol 9mg, Sodium 16mg, Potassium 87mg, Carbs 37g, Calories 276, Protein 12 g

409. CUCUMBER MANGO MISO NOODLE BOWL

- Prep time: 30 mins, Cook time: 35 mins, Total time: 65 mins, Grill temp: 0, Servings: 4

Ingredients

- 6 oz. rice vermicelli noodles- or any noodle of choice
- 4 thinly sliced Persian cucumbers or 1 large English cucumber,
- ¼ cup scallions, chopped
- 1 diced ripe mango
- ½ thinly sliced or minced jalapeño pepper
- 5 lime slices- 1 for squeezing, 4 for serving
- olive oil- extra-virgin or sesame oil for drizzling
- ⅓ cup toasted cashews, chopped
- ¼ cup of torn mint
- Sea salt
- A Protein of choice or- baked tofu recipe below

Directions

1. In a mixing bowl, combine the ginger, peanut butter, garlic, miso paste, and lime juice to make the peanut-miso sauce. Whisk in the warm water as needed until the sauce reaches a dripping consistency.
2. Combine the mango, cucumbers, jalapeño, and scallions in a mixing bowl with a pinch of salt and a squeeze of lime juice. After tossing, set away.
3. Prepare the rice noodles according to the package directions. Drain and thoroughly rinse with cold water. Drizzle a little sesame or olive oil over your noodles to keep them from sticking together.
4. Toss the noodles with the cucumber mixture, cashews, tofu, mint, and generous drizzles of peanut-miso sauce. Serve with lime wedges and extra sauce, if desired.

Nutritional Values

Fat 2.5g, Chol 8mg, Sodium 17mg, Potassium 95mg, Carbs 42g, Calories 313, Protein 12g

410. TAHINI NOODLE SALAD WITH ROASTED CARROTS & CHICKPEAS

- Prep time: 20 mins, Cook time: 40 mins, Total time: 60 mins, Grill temp: 460°F, Servings: 2-3

Ingredients

- 3 chopped medium carrots
- 1 cup chickpeas- cooked, drained & rinsed
- Olive oil- extra-virgin for drizzling
- 6 oz. whole wheat, soba noodles, or brown rice
- 1 small thinly sliced cucumber
- 6 thinly sliced radishes
- a handful of baby greens- arugula, similar, or spinach
- 1 tbsp of sesame seeds or hemp seeds
- lime wedges for serving
- sea salt
- 1 tbsp of tahini
- 1 tbsp of almond or peanut butter
- 1 tbsp of olive oil, extra-virgin
- 1minced garlic clove
- 1 tbsp of fresh lime juice
- 1 tbsp of rice vinegar
- ¼ tsp of sriracha
- 2 tbsp of warm water, more as needed
- ¼ tsp of honey, optional
- sea salt

Directions

1. Preheat the oven to 460°F and prepare a baking pan with parchment paper.
2. Drizzle oil over the chickpeas and carrots, season with pepper and salt, and place on a baking pan. Roast the carrots for 15-20 mins, or until they are tender but still firm.
3. In a small mixing bowl, add the water, tahini, sriracha, peanut rice vinegar, butter, lime juice, olive oil, salt, and garlic to make the sauce. If the taste is bitter, add honey if required. To taste, season with more sriracha or salt. If necessary, add more water until the sauce has a drizzle-able texture.
4. Bring a medium saucepan ½-filled with salted water to a boil. Cook the noodles according to the package guidelines until all of them are done. After draining, rinse with cold water.
5. In a mixing bowl, toss your noodles with a generous dollop of sauce. Toss the greens,

cucumber, carrots, radishes, hemp seeds, and chickpeas with the remaining sauce. Season to taste with salt and pepper. On the side, lime wedges are offered.

Nutritional Values

Fat 0.1g, Chol 5mg, Sodium 10mg, Potassium 64mg, Carbs 30g, Calories 200, Protein 10 g

411. ROASTED CAULIFLOWER PASTA

- Prep time: 15 mins, Cook time: 45 mins, Total time: 60 mins, Grill temp: 450°F, Servings: 2-3

Ingredients

- 2-3 cups of cauliflower florets
- 2 coarsely chopped shallots
- 2 coarsely chopped garlic cloves
- Olive oil, extra-virgin
- Sea salt & black pepper, fresh
- 6 oz. of spaghetti noodles
- A handful or 2 babies' spinach
- ½ cup pasta water
- Olive oil, extra-virgin
- Lemon juice + lemon zest
- ¼ cup of sun-dried tomatoes, chopped
- ¼ cup of crumbled feta- it's optional
- ¼ cup basil- or any herb if you like, fresh chopped

Directions

1. Preheat the oven to 450°F and roast the garlic, cauliflower, and shallots for 20-30 mins. If the garlic is chopped too finely, it will burn before the cauliflower is completely cooked. When it's golden brown, take it out of the oven. Combine all of the ingredients and give it a taste; it should be nutty and delicious. If it doesn't, add a splash of oil, a little salt, and a pinch of garlic if necessary.
2. Cook for 8 mins, or until the pasta is tender but still firm. Toss the spinach with the spaghetti noodles in a mixing bowl until the spinach begins to wilt. Add a little pasta water to help things along.
3. Add ½ of the roasted veggies, a drizzle of extra-virgin olive oil, a big squeeze of lemon and lemon zest, feta, sun-dried tomatoes, and basil to the bowl. Season to taste with salt and pepper. Add the leftover

roasted cauliflower, almonds, and breadcrumbs to finish- toasted.- Top with poached eggplants if preferred.

Nutritional Values

Fat 1g, Chol 9.5mg, Sodium 15mg, Potassium 90mg, Carbs 30g, Calories 264, Protein 15 g

412. TAHINI ZUCCHINI NOODLES

- Prep time: 10 mins, Cook time: 40 mins, Total time: 50 mins, Grill temp: 400°F, Servings: 2

Ingredients

- 2 cups of chopped kale
- 2 medium zucchinis, spiralized or julienned
- Olive oil, extra virgin for drizzling
- Lemon juice
- Sea salt & black pepper, fresh
- 1 cup tofu, cubed- optional
- 1 tbsp olive oil, extra-virgin
- 5 tbsp of tahini
- 1-2 tbsp of fresh lemon juice
- ½ minced garlic clove
- 4 tbsp of nutritional yeast
- 2 tsp of honey or maple syrup
- 3 tsp of soy sauce or tamari- gluten-free
- ½ tsp of dried turmeric
- ¼ – ½ cup of water; start with less, adding more as needed
- Sea salt & black pepper, fresh
- ¼ cup fresh basil, chopped
- ¼ cup of pine nuts, toasted
- Pinches of red chili flakes
- ¼ cup micro arugula sprouts, optional

Directions

1. When using tofu, preheat the oven to 400°F. On a preheated baking sheet, toss the tofu with a spritz of oil, freshly ground black pepper, and salt. Preheat oven to 350°F and bake for 19–25 mins.
2. In a medium-sized skillet, heat the olive oil and add the lemon juice, kale, salt, and pepper. Cook, stirring periodically until the kale has wilted.
3. To make the sauce, follow these steps: In a blender, blend the turmeric, olive oil, soy sauce, tahini, maple syrup, lemon juice, nutritional yeast, garlic, pepper, and salt until smooth. Blend until completely smooth, adding additional water as needed

to get the desired consistency. Taste and adjust spices as needed, considering that the tastes may dilute- mainly using zucchini noodles.
4. Toss the cooked tofu, zucchini, and kale with the sauce, using as much or as little as you prefer, depending on how thoroughly the veggies are covered.
5. Garnish with chili flakes, basil, microgreens, and pine nuts, if desired. Allow cooling completely before serving.

Nutritional Values

Fat 5.1g, Chol 6mg, Sodium 11mg, Potassium 82mg, Carbs 41g, Calories 320, Protein 16 g

413. ROASTED TOMATO BROWN RICE PASTA

- Prep time: 35 mins, Cook time: 2.5 hr, Total time: 3hr. 5 mins, Grill temp: 0, Servings: 2

Ingredients

- 1 pint of cherry tomatoes
- 6-8 oz. of brown rice pasta
- A few tbsp of olive oil, extra-virgin
- 1-2 cloves garlic, crushed
- handfuls of arugulas
- Lemon juice
- A handful of basil, chopped
- Sea salt & black pepper, fresh
- pine nuts- toasted, optional
- Red pepper flakes, optional
- Dollop pesto, optional
- Shaving parmesan optional

Directions

1. Smitten Kitchen's method of roasting tomatoes is my favorite. Mine took 2 hr, and I pulled them out when they were still damp. Yes, this takes time, but it is really easy since it is all done automatically. It's even feasible to get ahead of time and prepare it.
2. Boil the pasta until it is completely cooked- firm to the bite. Combine the noodles, pepper, olive oil, salt, garlic, basil, arugula, and lemon in a large mixing bowl, saving some starchy pasta water.
3. Taste and adjust the seasonings as required, adding the pasta water to loosen things up if needed. Garnish with pine nuts,

pesto, red pepper flakes, and parmesan cheese, if desired.

Nutritional Values

Fat 0.2g, Chol 9.3mg, Sodium 13mg, Potassium 85mg, Carbs 31g, Calories 206, Protein 11 g

414. CREAMY BUTTERNUT SQUASH PASTA

- Prep time: 35 mins, Cook time: 50 mins, Total time: 85 mins, Grill temp: 425°F, Servings: 4

Ingredients

- ½ small-sized squash of butternut, seeded and cut vertically
- Olive oil
- ½ cup- 2 shallots, finely chopped
- 3 cloves of garlic
- ¾ cup of water
- ½ cup cashews, raw
- 1 tbsp yeast
- 1 tbsp of balsamic vinegar
- 10 sage leaves, fresh
- 1 tbsp thyme, fresh- add more leaves for garnishing
- 12 oz. rotini pasta
- Salt & freshly crushed black pepper
- Broccoli, sautéed- optional for serving

Directions

- Preheat the oven to 425°F and line a baking sheet with parchment paper.
- Drizzle extra virgin olive oil over the squash, season with salt and pepper, and place on a baking sheet, trimmed side down. Wrap the shallot and garlic cloves in foil with a splash of olive oil and a pinch of salt and place them on the baking sheet. Roast the squash until it is soft, about 30 mins.
- In a blender, combine 1 cup squash flesh, peeled garlic, cashews, water, shallot, 2 tbsp olive oil, sage, vinegar, nutritional yeast, thyme, ¾ tsp sea salt, and a few dashes of black pepper. Blend until the mixture is smooth and creamy.
- In a pot, bring water to a boil and season with salt—cook pasta according to package directions. Set aside 1 cup of boiling pasta water.
- Drain the pasta and return it to the pot. Pour the sauce over the noodles, loosening

it if required, with ½ to 1 cup of pasta water, and season with ¼ to ½ tsp of salt. Season with freshly cracked black pepper, thyme leaves, and some sautéed broccoli, if desired.

Nutritional Values

Fat 5.2g, Chol 8mg, Sodium 20mg, Potassium 74mg, Carbs 50g, Calories 347, Protein 15 g

415. ZUCCHINI NOODLES

- Prep time: 15 mins, Cook time: 15 mins, Total time: 30 mins, Grill temp: 0, Servings: 2

Ingredients

- 3 medium-sized zucchinis
- Serving suggestions:
- with parmesan, sea salt, lemon, and olive oil
- marinara sauce
- pesto
- with tomatoes, roasted
- with vegetables, roasted or grilled

Directions

1. Choose the kind of noodle you want to make and follow the directions below for each option.
2. To produce curly "spaghetti" noodles, use a countertop spiralizer: Secure the spiralizer to the counter using a clamp. Remove the zucchini's tip and insert it between the spiralizer's teeth and blades. Turn the handle to create the noodles.
3. To make straight "angel hair" noodles, use a julienne peeler: With 1 hand, hold the zucchini and glide the peeler over it to create strips.
4. Create " fettuccine " noodles using a knife and create "fettuccine" noodles by slicing thin zucchini planks into fettuccine-sized strips.
5. Using an ordinary vegetable peeler, peel tiny zucchini slices to produce "pappardelle" noodles.
6. Serve the zucchini noodles uncooked after tossing them with a heated sauce. Alternatively, brush a pan with olive oil, then add the noodles and simmer for a min, or until barely warm.

7. Remove it from the oven and decorate it with sauces and other toppings.

Nutritional Values

Fat 1.4g, Chol 8mg, Sodium 14mg, Potassium 83mg, Carbs 43g, Calories 242, Protein 12 g

416. SPIRALIZED DAIKON "RICE NOODLE" BOWL

- Prep time: 10 mins, Cook time: 40 mins, Total time: 50 mins, Grill temp: 400°F, Servings: 2

Ingredients

- 8 oz. tofu, cut into small cubes
- 1 daikon
- 1 cucumber, diced
- 2 carrots, skin removed
- 2 radishes, finely diced
- ½ avocado, sliced
- ¼ cup of cilantro
- ¼ cup of mint leaves, fresh
- 2 scallions, diced
- 2 tbsp Cashews, chopped & toasted
- Olive oil
- Salt
- Sriracha
- Lemon wedges
- Sauces: Creamy cashew & Tamari-lime
- 2 tbsp of tamari
- 2 cloves of garlic, crushed
- 4 tsp Lemon juice, fresh
- 4 tsp of rice vinegar
- 1 tbsp maple or cane sugar or agave
- ¼ cup of water
- 1½ tbsp Peanut butter or cashew butter

Directions

1. Preheat the oven to a temp of 400°F. Tofu should be spread out on a baking sheet rimmed with baking paper. Toss with a generous amount of salt and a drizzle of olive oil. Bake for 15-17 mins, or until golden brown around the edges. After removing from the oven, toss with a sriracha spray.
2. Make the sauces ahead of time. Combine the garlic, sugar, rice vinegar, water, tamari, and lime juice in a small bowl. 12 tbsp of sauce should be moved to a separate small bowl. ½ of it should be mixed with creamy cashew butter. Season

to taste with salt and pepper, then set aside.
3. Using a julienne peeler or a spiralizer, cut the cucumber and daikon into noodles. Toss the noodle vegetables with scallions, cashews, cilantro, radish slices, carrot ribbons, radish slices, sliced avocado, mint, and tofu on 2 separate plates.
4. On the side, garnish the dishes with cashew sauces and tamari-lime, as well as lemon wedges.

Nutritional Values

Fat 4.9g, Chol 9mg, Sodium 12mg, Potassium 83mg, Carbs 51g, Calories 342, Protein 14 g

417. SOBA NOODLES WITH SHISHITOS & AVOCADO

- Prep time: 10 mins, Cook time: 40 mins, Total time: 50 mins, Grill temp: 0, Servings: 2

Ingredients

- 6 oz. soba noodles
- Shishito peppers
- 2 tbsp Scallions, finely chopped
- 1 tbsp sesame oil, roasted
- 1 tbsp tamari or soy sauce
- 2 tbsp rice vinegar
- 1 avocado, ripped
- Lime juice- optional
- 1 tbsp sesame seeds

Directions

1. Bring a medium saucepan of water to a boil in a cast iron pan.
2. Cook the soba noodles until they are al dente- firm to the bite- for 8 mins. Before transferring to a large mixing bowl, drain and brush off any excess water.
3. While the soba boils, toast shishito peppers in the preheated cast iron pan- dry or under the broiler. Cook them until they are black and cracked- usually 8 to 10 mins. Remove the pan from the heat and let it cool. Remove the stems and coarsely chop the peppers before adding them to the noodle dish.
4. Combine the scallions, sesame oil, noodles, chopped shishitos, rice vinegar, and soy sauce in a large mixing bowl. Serve with

sesame seeds and chopped avocado. Season to taste with salt and pepper.

5. Add tofu or another Protein of your choice to make this a more substantial supper. Add a touch of sriracha to make it hotter. It may be served warm or at room temp.

Nutritional Values

Fat 0.7g, Chol 12mg, Sodium 23mg, Potassium 75mg, Carbs 36g, Calories 264, Protein 7 g

418. SPICY KOHLRABI NOODLES

- Prep time: 15 mins, Cook time: 40 mins, Total time: 55 mins, Grill temp: 0, Servings: 2-3

Ingredients

- 2-3 kohlrabies
- 4 oz. of rice noodles, cooked & cooled
- ½ jalapeño, diced
- Some Thai chilies, red
- ½ avocado, chopped
- Herbs: mint, basil, or cilantro
- Peanuts, minced
- Sriracha, to taste
- Lemon wedges
- Tofu- optional

Dressing:
- 1 lime juice or zest
- 2 tbsp Of tamari/soy sauce
- 2 tbsp rice wine
- 1 garlic clove, crushed
- 1 tsp ginger, minced

Directions

1. In a mixing basin, combine the dressing ingredients.
2. Peel the kohlrabi if desired. Using a mandolin, slice kohlrabi into planks, then thinly dice the planks into matchsticks. Toss the kohlrabi slices with the chili peppers in the dressing. Allow for the cooling time of 30 mins.
3. Combine the rice noodles, herbs, avocado, marinated kohlrabies, crushed peanuts, and sriracha in a mixing bowl. Season to taste with salt and pepper.
4. Serve chilled or at room temp with more lemon slices on the side.

Nutritional Values

Fat 8.1g, Chol 4mg, Sodium 9mg, Potassium 66mg, Carbs 47g, Calories 329, Protein 9 g

419. COLD SESAME NOODLES WITH KALE & SHIITAKES

- Prep time: 25 mins, Cook time: 40 mins, Total time: 65 mins, Grill temp: 350°F, Servings: 4

Ingredients

- 4-6 oz. of noodles
- Few cups of shiitake mushrooms, diced
- 2 cups of kale, washed & diced
- 1 cup cabbage, finely diced
- 3 carrots, diced
- Radishes, finely diced
- ¼ scallions, diced
- Some tbsp sesame seeds
- ½ package of firm tofu, diced into cubes

Dressing:
- 1 tbsp sesame oil, roasted
- 1 tbsp rice wine
- 1 tbsp of lime juice
- 2 tsp Ginger, crushed
- 2 tsp Tamari or soy sauce
- 1 tsp of sriracha

Directions

1. In a mixing basin, combine the dressing ingredients.
2. Cook the shiitakes in the oven, then thinly slice them and sprinkle with extra virgin olive oil and salt. Preheat the oven to 350°F and bake until crisp and gently browned. Alternatively, you may sauté them in a pan with a little oil, salt, and soy sauce for 10-15 mins. Only stir now and again.
3. Prepare the noodles according to the package directions. After draining, wash with cold water.
4. In a large mixing bowl, combine the noodles, shiitakes, radishes, cabbage, kale, carrots, and the majority of the dressing.- Let everything marinate for a while.
5. Season with salt and pepper after adding the sesame seeds. Add more lime, dressing, soy sauce, and sriracha to taste. Serve at room temp or chilled. Any leftovers should be kept refrigerated. Lunch should be brought to work in to-go containers.

Nutritional Values

Fat 1.4g, Chol 8.3mg, Sodium 13mg, Potassium 78mg, Carbs 35g, Calories 224, Protein 7 g

420. Butternut Squash Noodle Pasta

- Prep time: 20 mins, Cook time: 35 mins, Total time: 55 mins, Grill temp: 0, Servings: 2-3

Ingredients

- 10 sage leaves
- 2 cups butternut squash, spiraled
- 1½ cups of leeks, light green & white parts removed
- 4 oz. brown pasta
- Canola or high-heat oil
- 2 cloves of garlic
- 1 lime juice
- 1 tbsp of unsalted butter
- ¼ cup of walnuts, toasted & chopped
- Some pinches of red chili flakes
- Sea salt & black pepper powder

Directions

1. First, fry the sage. In a big skillet, pour a good quantity of olive oil to coat the bottom fully. Once the oil is hot and shimmering, fry 1 sage leaf to test it. It should become a deeper green, remove and drain the kitchen towel, and it will become crunchy as it dries. Reduce the heat and try again if it burns.- I added 10 sage leaves in the recipe to allow for a few errors. Once your oil has reached the correct temp, fry them all. Drain and set aside the water. Reduce the heat to low and leave the pan aside for a few mins to cool before draining the excess oil and keeping enough to continue cooking.
2. In salted water, cook pasta for 8 mins or until al dente. In the last 2 mins of cooking, toss butternut squash spirals.
3. Reheat your large skillet over medium heat in the meanwhile. Add the leeks and season with salt and pepper to suit. Cook until the onions are translucent and soft, then add the minced garlic. When the pasta and butternut noodles are done, drain and return them to the pan, reserving ¼ to ½ cup of the pasta water for later use.
4. Pepper, salt, and red pepper flakes, as well as a squeeze of lemon and a dollop of butter, are all good additions. Toss everything together to coat. If necessary, loosen the spaghetti by adding ¼ cup of starchy pasta water at a time.
5. When the butternut noodles are done, remove them from the pan. Season with salt and pepper before serving on a platter or in bowls.
6. Serve with walnuts and fried sage leaves as a garnish.
7. Top with shredded pecorino or balsamic vinegar, if preferred.

Nutritional Values

Fat 3.8g, Chol 5mg, Sodium 8mg, Potassium 72mg, Carbs 54g, Calories 268, Protein 9 g

421. Zucchini Coconut Noodles

- Prep time: 10 mins, Cook time: 35 mins, Total time: 45 mins, Grill temp: 0, Servings: 2-3

Ingredients

- 1 tbsp of coconut oil
- 2-3 scallions, diced
- 1 tsp fresh ginger, minced
- 1 cup of coconut milk
- 1 piece of lemongrass- 4 inches
- Splash of tamari
- 1 lemon juice or zest
- A pinch of coconut sugar
- Pepper & salt
- 1 bunch of amaranth greens
- 2 Roma tomatoes, chopped
- 3 zucchinis, thinly diced
- Basil leaves
- Cilantro leaves, fresh
- Peanuts, toasted & crushed
- Chili garlic sauce or sriracha
- Tofu

Directions

1. In a small saucepan over low heat, melt some coconut oil. Add the scallions, ginger, and the full piece of lemongrass- you'll remove it later. Before adding the rest of the ingredients, bring the coconut milk and sauce to a low boil, occasionally stirring. Lemon juice and a pinch of sugar are added to the mix. Taste and make any necessary adjustments. If it becomes too thick, add a few tbsp of water.

2. Before adding the tomatoes to the pan, chop them up and remove the seeds.
3. Put the zucchini noodles in once they've been prepared.
4. In the same pan, add the chopped amaranth leaves. Stir them just until they're wilted.
5. Add the basil and stir until it has softened.
6. Remove the lemongrass from the pan, stir in the zucchini noodles, and serve in bowls right away.
7. Serve with chili sauce, crushed peanuts, and cilantro on the side, as well as crushed peanuts.

Fat 5.1g, Chol 19mg, Sodium 15mg, Potassium 79mg, Carbs 45g, Calories 255, Protein 11 g

422. GINGER MISO NOODLES WITH EGGPLANT

- Prep time: 25 mins, Cook time: 50 mins, Total time: 75 mins, Grill temp: 0, Servings: 3-4

Ingredients

- 10 oz. soba noodles or rice noodles- brown rice
- A few tbsp of olive oil, extra-virgin
- 1 pack or 14 oz. cubed tofu, extra firm
- 1½ cups mushrooms, sliced
- 1½ cups of Japanese or Chinese sliced eggplants
- A few handfuls of greens- spinach, kale
- ½ cup scallions, sliced
- sesame oil for drizzling
- sesame seeds for garnish
- Sea salt & black pepper, fresh
- 2 tbsp of miso paste
- 2 tbsp of honey
- 2 tbsp of mirin- or sake, or rice vinegar
- 1 tsp of minced garlic
- 1 tsp of minced ginger
- ⅔ cup veggie broth, low sodium

Directions

1. Boil the noodles until they are fully cooked, as stated on the package. If the noodles are cooked before the rest of the ingredients, massage them with a little oil before draining to prevent them from sticking together while they rest.

2. Combine the miso, broth, honey, ginger, mirin, and garlic in a mixing bowl to make the sauce. To taste, season with salt and pepper.
3. To prepare the tofu, slice it and dry it on paper towels. Dab the tofu with a paper towel to absorb any excess moisture.
4. To prepare the tofu, follow these steps: Heat the oil in a large skillet. Before adding the tofu, heat the pan to a high temp. Allow everything to settle for 30 seconds to a minute, then toss it all up and continue to stir fry for a few mins, or more until it's nice and golden. After removing the tofu from the pan, set it aside.
5. In the same skillet as the tofu, cook the eggplant and mushrooms- remove any charred parts, add more oil, reheat the pan, and add the eggplant and mushrooms. Just a smidgeon of sauce- the rest will be added later. Stir fry until the mushrooms are golden brown and tender. Depending on the heat of the burner, the time may vary.
6. Reduce the heat to low and add the noodles and the remaining sauce to the pan. You may not need all of it- and it isn't sweet, so start with ½ and add more as required. Return the tofu to the pan, along with a handful of greens and the scallions, and toss to incorporate. If desired, season with more sauce, pepper, and salt.
7. Remove from the heat and top with a drizzle of sesame oil and a sprinkle of sesame seeds.

Fat 7.1g, Chol 12mg, Sodium 21mg, Potassium 91mg, Carbs 43g, Calories 345, Protein 13 g

423. SESAME NOODLE BOWL

- Prep time: 10 mins, Cook time: 15 mins, Total time: 25 mins, Grill temp: 0, Servings: 2-3

Ingredients

Dressing/Sauce

- 2 tbsp white miso paste
- 2 tbsp rice vinegar
- 2 tbsp tamari
- ½ tbsp crisped sesame oil
- orange juice

Bowls

- 1 medium orange
- 2 cups red cabbage, shredded
- 3 oz. cooked soba noodles
- Extra-virgin olive oil
- ⅓ cup scallions, chopped
- 1 cup chopped snap peas
- 8 oz. sliced shiitake mushrooms
- 7 oz. sliced and baked tofu
- Sesame seeds
- A handful of fresh herbs/cilantro/mint
- Sea salt

Directions

1. Whisk together the miso, tamari, rice vinegar, and sesame oil in a bowl until smooth. Slice the orange segments, set them aside, and pour the juice from the orange into the sauce.
2. Divide the red cabbage over 2 or 3 dishes. Apply a little coating of dressing to the cabbage. Arrange the cooked soba next to the cabbage in the bowls.
3. Toss the peas and scallions in the hot oil for about 2 mins, or until just browned but still brilliant green. Place in the bowls.
4. Add more oil to the pan, along with the sliced mushrooms and a pinch of salt, and cook for about 8 mins, or until the mushrooms are tender. In the bowls, combine the mushrooms, tofu, sesame seeds, orange segments, and herbs. Dressing on top and the side.

Nutritional Values

Fat 6.9g, Chol 8mg, Sodium 14mg, Potassium 93mg, Carbs 52g, Calories 421, Protein 12 g

424. GOLDEN TURMERIC NOODLE MISO SOUP

- Prep time: 10 mins, Cook time: 30 mins, Total time: 40 mins, Grill temp: 0, Servings: 4

Ingredients

- 6 cups water
- 1 strip rinsed kombu
- 3 chopped scallions, chopped
- 1 large thinly sliced carrot
- 2 tbsp minced ginger
- 2 minced garlic cloves

- ¼ cup white miso paste
- ½ tsp crushed turmeric
- ½ tsp freshly crushed black pepper
- 2 tbsp lemon juice
- 1 tbsp lime juice
- ½ tbsp coconut oil
- 1 tbsp tamari
- 2 tsp sriracha
- 7 oz. cubed tofu
- 2 ½ oz. rice noodles/zucchini noodles, cooked
- 2 thinly sliced baby Bok choy
- ¼ tsp sea salt
- Fresh mint or cilantro
- Pinch of red pepper flakes

Directions

1. In a medium saucepan, combine the water and kombu. Cook for 10 mins on low heat, occasionally stirring. Remove the kombu. Add the carrots, scallions, garlic, and ginger and cook for 20 mins, or until the vegetables are soft.
2. In a small dish, combine the miso paste and ½ cup broth. Stir everything together in the saucepan until everything is properly combined. Cook for 10 mins on low heat with the coconut oil, turmeric, black pepper, tofu, lemon and lime juice, tamari, noodles, sriracha, and Bok choy.
3. Sprinkle with sea salt and fresh herbs if desired.

Nutritional Values

Fat 6.4g, Chol 10mg, Sodium 16mg, Potassium 93mg, Carbs 56g, Calories 432, Protein 13 g

425. CREAMY VEGAN SHIITAKE & KALE PASTA

- Prep time: 10 mins, Cook time: 20 mins, Total time: 30 mins, Grill temp: 0, Servings: 3-4

Ingredients

- 8 oz. pasta fusilli
- 1 tbsp olive oil, extra virgin
- 8 oz. shiitake mushrooms destemmed & sliced
- ⅓ cup scallions chopped
- ½ a lemon small
- 5-6 sliced kale leaves

- pepper flakes pinch

1. Combine all lemon miso cashew cream sauce in a blender until smooth and creamy- about 30 seconds. Take a step back from the situation.
2. Before washing the pasta, boil salted water and cook according to package directions or al dente in a large pot. Save some starchy water in a separate container.
3. Meanwhile, heat oil in a skillet over medium heat while the pasta cooks. Sauté the shiitake mushrooms in a skillet for 2-3 mins, occasionally stirring. Before adding the scallions, cook for a few more mins until the mushrooms are tender and caramelized. Toss in the kale and a squeeze of fresh lemon juice, then toss everything together thoroughly. Once the kale has wilted a bit further, add some more lemon juice. Return to a boil and simmer for another 8 mins, or until the pasta is al dente. If desired, season with extra salt and pepper, as well as the remaining cream sauce. If the sauce is excessively thick or clumpy, thin it up using some pasta water you saved.
4. If desired, top with parmesan cheese, macadamia nuts, and a pinch of pepper flakes while still hot.

Nutritional Values

Fat 7.3g, Chol 8mg, Sodium 15mg, Potassium 84mg, Carbs 59g, Calories 402, Protein 13 g

426. CREAMY PUMPKIN PASTA SAUCE

- Prep time: 20 mins, Cook time: 50 mins, Total time: 50 mins, Grill temp: 0, Servings: 4

Ingredients

- ½ kabocha squash/small sugar pie pumpkin
- ½ sliced yellow onion
- 2 unpeeled garlic cloves
- 2 tbsp olive oil extra-virgin
- 5 fresh and large sage leaves
- ¾ cup vegetable broth
- ½ cup unsalted and soaked cashews
- 16 oz. penne pasta
- ½ tsp sea salt

- Freshly crushed black pepper

Directions

1. Preheat the oven to 350°F and line a baking sheet with Al foil. Arrange the onions, pumpkin, and garlic on a baking pan. Season with salt and pepper and drizzle with olive oil. Turn the pumpkin over and make a few slits in the skin with a fork. Cover with foil and bake for 35 mins-1 hr, or until the onions are soft and the pumpkin pulp is very tender.
2. Add some sages to the pan in the last few mins of cooking. Remove the baking dish from the oven and cover it with foil to steam for an additional 10-15 mins.
3. In a blender, purée the pumpkin flesh with the vegetable broth, peeled garlic, onion, sage, cashews, salt, and crushed black pepper. Blend the contents until it is smooth and creamy. Add the 2 tbsp olive oil and pulse once more.
4. Boil the pasta in salted water until al dente, or as directed on the box. Save a ½ cup of the pasta water before draining it.
5. Drain the pasta and return it to the pot. Toss ½ of the sauce with the pasta. To make it creamier, add a little additional pasta water at a time. Add the remaining sauce as desired. To taste, add a little salt and pepper. Serve right away.

Nutritional Values

Fat 7.6g, Chol 15mg, Sodium 19mg, Potassium 78mg, Carbs 55g, Calories 432, Protein 13 g

427. BROCCOLI TAHINI PASTA SALAD

- Prep time: 30 mins, Cook time: 10 mins, Total time: 40 mins, Grill temp: o, Servings: 4-6

Ingredients

- 3 cups broccoli, small florets
- 1 cup green beans, cut
- 2 cups gluten-free fusilli pasta, uncooked
- 1 small and thinly sliced zucchini
- 1 cup cherry tomatoes, sliced
- 4 sun-dried and chopped tomatoes
- 8 fresh basil leaves, thinly sliced
- ¼ cup pine nuts
- sea salt & freshly crushed black pepper

Lemon tahini dressing:

- 3 tbsp olive oil- extra-virgin
- 3 tbsp tahini
- 3 tbsp fresh lime juice
- 2 tbsp white wine vinegar
- 1 minced garlic clove
- ½ tsp Dijon mustard
- ½ tsp maple syrup
- ½ tsp sea salt
- 3 tbsp water

Directions

1. Combine the olive oil, lemon juice, garlic, tahini, vinegar, salt, mustard, maple syrup, and water in a small mixing bowl.
2. ½ of a large saucepan should be filled with salted hot water and the other ½ with ice water. Boil the broccoli and green beans in boiling water for 1-2 mins, or until tender but still bright green. To stop the cooking process, turn off the heat and swiftly immerse it in cold water. To chill, soak for at least 15 seconds in cold water. Drain and dry with a kitchen towel after that.
3. In a large pot of lightly salted boiling water, cook the pasta according to package directions until done. After draining, wash with cold water.
4. Combine the boiling broccoli and beans, basil, zucchini, tomatoes, and pasta in a large mixing bowl. Season with salt, pepper, and a squeeze of lemon to taste before tossing with the dressings.
5. After 15 mins, sprinkle the pine nuts over the top.

Nutritional Values

Fat 5.9g, Chol 8mg, Sodium 9mg, Potassium 87mg, Carbs 56g, Calories 443, Protein 13 g

428. CREAMY VEGAN PASTA

- Prep time: 10 mins, Cook time: 20 mins, Total time: 30 mins, Grill temp: 0, Servings: 4

Ingredients

- 2 & ½ cups shell pasta small
- 3 tbsp olive oil extra-virgin
- 1 small chopped yellow onion
- 5 cups chopped stems broccoli florets
- ¼ cup pine nuts toasted
- Lemon wedges

- 1 & ½ cups drained & rinsed white beans, cooked
- ¼ cup broth vegetable
- 3 tbsp lemon juice fresh
- ¼ cup yeast NUTRITIONAL
- 1 minced garlic clove
- ¼ tsp powdered onion
- ½ tsp of sea salt
- Black pepper

Directions

1. In a blender, combine all ingredients except nutritional yeast and mix until smooth. Serve the sauce in a serving dish with arugula on top. Put it on the back burner for now.
2. In a large saucepan, boil salted water. Cook the pasta according to the package guidelines, ensuring it's al dente when it's done. Once you've completed, set the drain aside.
3. In a medium-sized pan, melt some butter over medium heat. Pour in the olive oil. Sauté the onion in olive oil with a pinch of salt for around 5 mins.
4. By adding the shredded broccoli stems, you may add an extra 3-5 mins to the Cook time. Serve with broccoli leaves, vegetarian broth, and water or broccoli florets. Cover the pot and turn off the heat.
5. Steam the broccoli for 2 to 3 mins for a delicate, bright green result. Stir in the noodles and sauce until everything is well combined. If your sauce seems to be too dry, add a splash of broth.
6. Season with salt, pepper, and lemon juice before serving in bowls with the spices. Divide the sauce into the bowls if there is any leftover. Serve with a garnish of lemon wedges and pine nuts.

Nutritional Values

Fat 8.4g, Chol 10mg, Sodium 18mg, Potassium 85mg, Carbs 58g, Calories 475, Protein 15 g

429. ROSEMARY LEMON PASTA

- Prep time: 15 mins, Cook time: 30 mins, Total time: 45 mins, Grill temp: 0, Servings: 2-3

Ingredients

- 4-6 oz. linguini pasta or spaghetti

- Pasta water
- ¼ cup breadcrumbs
- 1 tbsp fresh rosemary, diced
- 2 cups collard greens, chopped and without stems
- ½ -1 clove garlic, minced
- 1-2 lemons
- Few tbsp Of olive oil
- Butter- optional
- Almond, sliced & toasted
- Red chili flakes
- Salt

Directions

1. In salted boiling water, cook your pasta until al dente.
2. In a medium skillet, toast the panko, rosemary, and a pinch of salt while the pasta is cooking. When the panko starts to brown slightly, remove it from the pan and set it aside.
3. Wipe out the pan and toss in the collards with a splash of olive oil, a bit of salt, a sprinkle of garlic, and a generous squeeze of lemon. Cook for approximately 10 mins, or until they're mostly wilted- a few mins. Toss the pasta with a small pat of butter, a squeeze of lime, and enough of the saved pasta water to loosen it, if necessary. Finish with a drizzle of olive oil.
4. Remove the pan from the heat and add the almonds, rosemary-panko mixture, a pinch of red chili flakes, and a squeeze of lemon zest. As required, taste and adjust the seasonings.

Nutritional Values

Fat 6.6g, Chol 12mg, Sodium 19mg, Potassium 80mg, Carbs 60g, Calories 360, Protein 9 g

430. SLOW ROASTED TOMATO PASTA

- Prep time: 10 mins, Cook time: 40 mins, Total time: 50 mins, Grill temp: 400°F, Servings: 4-6

Ingredients

Roast tomatoes:
- 8-10 tomatoes or some cherry tomatoes
- Splash of olive oil
- Sea salt and pepper
- Thyme sprigs, fresh

For pasta:
- 1 lb. brown pasta
- 4 garlic cloves, diced
- Olive oil- ¼ cup or so
- 1 tbsp of anchovy paste
- Lemon zest & juice, fresh
- Some tbsps. of capers
- pine nuts, toasted
- Basil, fresh
- Red chili flakes
- Pepper & salt to taste
- Parmesan cheese- optional

Directions

1. Cut tomatoes in ½ and season with salt and pepper after sprinkling with extra virgin olive oil. Preheat the oven to 200°F and roast the tomatoes. Add fresh thyme leaves towards the end. The time it takes to roast the tomatoes will depend on their size. Cherry tomatoes should be roasted for 2 to 4 hours, while Roma tomatoes should be roasted for 6 to 8 hours.
2. Cook your pasta in salted water until just under al dente, reserving some starchy pasta water.
3. In a large skillet, heat enough olive oil to coat the bottom of the pan. When the oil is hot, add the chopped garlic and anchovy paste. Heat until the combination smells fragrant. Toss in the noodles, and if necessary, add the additional pasta water. Continue to boil the pasta in a pan with a touch of salt and pepper until it is al dente.
4. Remove from the heat and stir in the red chili flakes, capers, basil, pine nuts, salt, pepper, and tomatoes, as well as a few big lemons squeezes and some zest. Season to taste with salt and pepper.
5. Season with salt, olive oil, pepper, and grated parmesan cheese to taste.

Nutritional Values

Fat 4.8g, Chol 13mg, Sodium 17mg, Potassium 93mg, Carbs 56g, Calories 244, Protein 14 g

431. VEGAN SWEET POTATO

- Prep time: 20 mins, Cook time: 35 mins, Total time: 55 mins, Grill temp: 350°F, Servings: 4-6

Ingredients

- 1 sweet potato
- 2 shallots
- 2 cloves of garlic
- 1 cup of cashews, drained & soaked
- 2 tbsp olive oil
- 1 tbsp of balsamic vinegar
- 1 tbsp tomato paste
- Pepper & salt
- 1 tbsp rosemary, chopped
- ⅓ cup of water
- 1 lb. brown fettuccini
- ¼ cup of pine nuts
- ¼ cup of chives
- a few dashes of red chili flakes

Directions

1. Preheat the oven to 350°F - 180°C.
2. After peeling the sweet potato, cut it into quarters. Shallots should be peeled and split in ½. Place the sweet potato and shallot pieces on a foil-lined baking sheet, leaving the garlic wrapped in its paper. With a splash of olive oil and a bit of salt and pepper, toss everything together. Remove the garlic cloves after the first 15 mins of roasting. Roast for 30 mins or until sweet potatoes are mushy and shallots are caramelized on the edges. Allow the pan to cool for a few mins after removing it from the oven.
3. Cook until the pasta is al dente, reserving some of the starchy pasta water.
4. In a high-powered blender, mix the cashews, shallots, peeled garlic, sweet potato, rosemary, olive oil, balsamic vinegar, tomato paste, and a touch of salt and pepper. To get the blade running, puree with a little water. To taste, season with salt and pepper.
5. In a large pan, combine cooked pasta and a portion of the sauce- or a dish. Add pasta water as needed to loosen and adjust the quantity of sauce to your liking. Chop the chives, toast the pine nuts, and add a pinch of red chili flakes to taste. After tasting and adjusting the seasonings, serve.

Nutritional Values

Fat 7.1g, Chol 10mg, Sodium 18mg, Potassium 84mg, Carbs 57g, Calories 379, Protein 15 g

432. CAULIFLOWER MAC & CHEESE

- Prep time: 10 mins, Cook time: 50 mins, Total time: 60 mins, Grill temp: 0, Servings: 4

Ingredients

- 1 big cauliflower, diced
- 12 oz. of elbow pasta
- 1 tbsp of Dijon mustard
- 1 shallot, finely minced
- 3 cloves of garlic
- ½ tsp paprika, smoked
- ¾ - 1 cup of sharp cheddar or cashew cream
- 1 tbsp of vinegar
- Black pepper powder & sea salt to taste
- Reserved pasta water

Cashew cream:
- 1 cup of cashews, soaked for some hr
- ¼ - ½ cup of water
- 1 clove of garlic
- ¼ cup shallot, finely minced
- 2 tbsp lemon juice
- Salt

Directions

1. If you're opting for the vegan option, start with the cashew cream. Combine all of the ingredients in a blender or food processor and blend until smooth. Remove the scooped cream from the mixer and set it aside.
2. Preheat the oven to 400°F or higher.
3. For the pasta, bring a big pot of salted water to a boil. Cook until the cauliflower florets are tender but not mushy, about 8 mins. Drain the cauliflower and use a slotted spoon to set it in a blender. After the cauliflower has been removed, bring the water to a boil, and add the pasta.
4. Prepare the sauce in the meanwhile. Combine 4 cups cauliflower florets, Dijon mustard, salt, smoky paprika, garlic, shallot, and pepper in a blender. Combine ¾ cup cheddar cheese or cashew cream, as well as the sherry vinegar, in a blender. If necessary, thin the sauce with starchy pasta water. Season to taste with salt and

pepper. To make a richer sauce, add more cheese or cashew cream.

5. Remove 1 or 2 of the spaghetti waters when the pasta is al dente, then drain the pasta and water from the large pot. Return the cooked pasta to the pot after mixing in the sauce. To produce a thick sauce, add the remaining pasta water as needed.

6. Put the spaghetti in a large baking dish. Scatter the remaining cauliflower florets over the top. Parmesan cheese, panko, Parmesan cheese, and a dash of olive oil are sprinkled on top.

7. Depending on the size of the dish, bake for 12-20 mins or until the top is golden and crispy.

8. Remove the dish from the oven and top with chives and red chili flakes.

Nutritional Values

Fat 6.2g, Chol 9mg, Sodium 14mg, Potassium 67mg, Carbs 36g, Calories 249, Protein 9 g

433. HAZELNUT TAHINI PASTA

- Prep time: 10 mins, Cook time: 40 mins, Total time: 50 mins, Grill temp: 300°F, Servings: 2-3

Ingredients

For sauce:
- 1 cup hazelnuts, shelled, toasted, and unsalted
- 2 garlic cloves
- ¼ cup of tahini
- 1 lemon juice
- ¼ tbsp extra virgin olive oil
- Salt & pepper
- Water as per requirement

For pasta:
- 8 oz. of pasta and some saved pasta water
- 1 tsp extra virgin olive oil
- 2 cups brussels sprouts, finely chopped
- ¼ cup hazelnuts, toasted & coarsely chopped
- Red chili flakes
- Pepper & salt to taste

Directions

1. Make sure your hazelnuts are well roasted before using.- Preheat the oven to 300°F and bake for 5 mins.

2. Puree the garlic, lemon, olive oil, hazelnuts, and tahini in a high-powered blender to prepare the sauce. To get your blade running, drizzle water on it as required. Season with salt and pepper to taste.

3. Cook the pasta according to the package directions.

4. In a large skillet, heat the olive oil. Place the trimmed brussels sprouts in a single layer in the pan. Season to taste with salt and pepper. Cook for 1 min before turning. Cook for a few more mins, or until golden brown on the sides.

5. Combine the brussels sprouts, pasta, and as much or as little sauce as desired in a mixing bowl. If a creamy sauce is desired, a little amount of pasta water may be added as needed. On top, roasted hazelnuts and a sprinkling of red pepper flakes.

6. To taste, season with salt and pepper.

Nutritional Values

Fat 8g, Chol 5mg, Sodium 7mg, Potassium 95mg, Carbs 39g, Calories 379, Protein 9 g

434. ANNA'S AVOCADO & LEMON ZEST SPAGHETTI

- Prep time: 15 mins, Cook time: 45 mins, Total time: 60 mins, Grill temp: 0, Servings: 4

Ingredients

- Black pepper powder & sea salt
- 400g of spaghetti
- Extra virgin olive oil
- 4 tbsp of capers, coarsely diced
- 1 garlic clove, chopped & peeled
- Lime zest, grated
- ½ lime juice
- Basil leaves, fresh
- Parsley leaves, fresh
- 2 avocados, ripened

Directions:

1. Bring some water to a boil and season liberally with salt. Bring to a boil, then add the pasta and cook for 8-10 mins, or until al dente, as directed on the box.

2. Heat some olive oil in a nonstick frying pan over low heat, add capers and garlic, and gently sizzle until the garlic's edge starts to

brown slightly. Take the pan off the heat and add the lemon zest.

3. Chop the herbs and combine them with the rest of the ingredients in the pan. Make crisscross incisions into the flesh with a knife, cutting it inside the peel, after halves and destoning the avocados. With a spoon, scoop each piece into the pan and swirl to blend all of the flavors.

4. Before draining the noodles, carefully remove ½ a cup of pasta water. Rinse the pasta and toss it in a frying pan with a splash of cooking water and a large squirt of olive oil. Season with pepper, salt, and lime juice as needed.

5. Place the spaghetti in dishes and eat while sitting down.

Nutritional Values

Fat 3.1g, Chol 6mg, Sodium 9mg, Potassium 76mg, Carbs 40g, Calories 330, Protein 9 g

435. SHELLS & ROASTED CAULIFLOWER

- Prep time: 20 mins, Cook time: 35 mins, Total time: 55 mins, Grill temp: 425°F, Servings: 3-4

Ingredients

- 4-5 cups of cauliflower florets, small
- 2 tbsp Extra virgin olive oil; add more for topping
- 1 tbsp unsalted butter
- 1½ tbsp White wine or sherry vinegar
- ½ tsp honey/maple syrup
- ½ tsp red chili flakes or sambal
- 6 oz. pasta, shell-shaped
- ¾ cup pasta water; reserve the water before draining
- 1 shallot, finely sliced
- 2 cloves of garlic, minced
- 4 cups of chard leaves or tatsoi or spinach
- ¼ cup hazelnuts/walnuts, chopped & toasted
- 1 tbsp golden raisins
- ½ cup basil, parsley, or tarragon, chopped
- lime wedges for garnishing
- Black pepper powder & salt

Directions

1. Preheat the oven to 425°F and line a baking sheet with parchment paper. On a baking sheet, toss the cauliflower florets with a splash of olive oil and a sprinkling of salt and pepper. Cook for 25 mins, or until golden brown around the edges.

2. Set aside a small dish containing maple syrup, sherry vinegar, and sambal.

3. For the pasta, bring a big pot of salted water to a boil. Cook the pasta until it is al dente, as directed on the box. Set aside ¾ cup of water before washing the pasta. To keep the spaghetti from sticking together, drizzle it with olive oil and set it aside.

4. In a large skillet, melt the butter and oil. Add the shallot, smashed garlic cloves, and a pinch of salt to taste. Over medium-low heat, cook for 3-5 mins, or until the shallot is soft and the garlic is fragrant. Garlic cloves should be removed before cooking.

5. Cook, occasionally stirring, until the greens are wilted. Cover everything with the vinegar mixture, pasta, and roasted cauliflower. Add ½ to ¾ cup of the saved pasta water to create a light sauce. In a mixing dish, combine the raisins, hazelnuts, and parsley. If necessary, season with pepper, salt, and more sambal.

6. Lemon slices are served on the side.

Nutritional Values

Fat 2.7g, Chol 8mg, Sodium 14mg, Potassium 65mg, Carbs 35g, Calories 241, Protein 11 g

436. TAGLIATELLE WITH TOMATOES AND GREENS

- Prep time: 15 mins, Cook time: 35 mins, Total time: 50 mins, Grill temp: 0, Servings: 4

Ingredients

- 1 tbsp olive oil
- 1 shallot, diced
- 1½ cups carrots, finely chopped
- 3 cloves of garlic, minced
- 1 tsp oregano, dried
- ¼ tsp red chili flakes
- ¼ cup white vinegar, dry
- 1 tbsp balsamic vinegar
- 1 can of tomatoes, chopped
- 4 oz. tagliatelle pasta
- 2 cups kale leaves, diced
- ½ cup of beans, cooked
- ¼ cup of pine nuts

- 2 tsp of capers
- Mixed herbs & chives, chopped
- Black pepper powder & salt to taste
- Shredded Parmesan cheese- if required

Directions

1. In a large pan, heat a couple of tbsp of olive oil over medium heat. Cook, stirring periodically, for about 2 mins, or until the shallot is tender. Combine the red chili flakes, salt, oregano, garlic, and carrots in a large mixing bowl. Allow for a 5-mins, simmer, occasionally stirring, until the vegetables are lightly browned.
2. Fill the glass halfway with white wine. Stir and heat for about 30 seconds or until the wine has virtually evaporated. Combine the diced tomatoes and balsamic vinegar in a mixing bowl. Reduce the heat and cover the pan. Cook for 15 mins or until the carrots are tender.
3. Meanwhile, bring a medium pot of salted water to a boil. Cook the pasta until it is al dente, as directed on the box. Drain and put aside the pasta.
4. Allow about 1 min for the diced kale to wilt in the sauce. Herbs, chives, pine nuts, cannellini beans, pasta, and capers are softly mixed. Season with pepper and salt to taste, and if desired, garnish with grated Parmesan cheese.

Nutritional Values

Fat 4.1g, Chol 6mg, Sodium 13mg, Potassium 74mg, Carbs 33g, Calories 251, Protein 13 g

437. SPAGHETTI BOLOGNESE

- Prep time: 20 mins, Cook time: 50 mins, Total time: 1 hr. 10 mins, Grill temp: 0, Servings: 4

Ingredients

- 2 tbsp Olive oil
- ½ onion, chopped
- 1 carrot, finely diced
- 4 cups mushrooms, diced
- 1 tbsp rosemary, diced
- ½ cup of walnuts, diced
- 2 cloves of garlic, minced
- 1 tbsp of balsamic vinegar

- 1 tbsp tamari
- 1 14 oz. tomatoes, chopped and roasted
- 1 cup brown/green lentils, cooked
- 1 tbsp of tomato paste
- 1 tsp sage, dried
- 1 cup cherry tomatoes, halved
- 8 oz. spaghetti
- 1 cup fresh basil, sliced
- ½ cup peanuts, toasted
- red chili flakes
- Pecorino cheese
- Black pepper & salt

Directions

1. Heat the oil over a low heat setting. Simmer for 3 mins, or until the onion and carrot begin to soften, with a sprinkling of pepper and salt. Cook for another 8 mins, occasionally stirring after adding the mushrooms and another pinch of salt.
2. Mix in the chopped rosemary well. Slide everything to 1 side of the pan to make room for the walnuts. Before mixing everything, toast the crushed walnuts for around 30 seconds. Stir in the minced garlic, then the vinegar and tamari until everything is thoroughly blended. Combine the tomatoes, sage, lentils, tomato paste, and cherry tomatoes in a large mixing bowl.
3. Reduce the heat to low and simmer for another 20-30 mins, or until the sauce has thickened. Season to taste with salt and pepper.
4. In a separate kettle, bring a big container of salted water to a boil. Cook the pasta according to the package directions until it is fully cooked. Drain the pasta and toss it in the pan with the sauce.
5. Peanuts, fresh basil, a sprinkle of chili flakes, and pecorino cheese may be added as a garnish if desired.

Nutritional Values

Fat 3.1g, Chol 7mg, Sodium 13mg, Potassium 82mg, Carbs 37g, Calories 239, Protein 13 g

438. SPRING GREEN LEMON & BASIL PASTA

- Prep time: 20 mins, Cook time: 40 mins, Total time: 60 mins, Grill temp: 0, Servings: 3-4

Ingredients

- ½ pound pasta, homemade or store-bought - whole wheat, or whatever you like
- ¼ cup + 1 tbsp of olive oil.
- 1 finely chopped shallot
- 1 minced garlic clove
- Splash- 1-2 tbsp of white wine
- 1 cup asparagus, chopped, tender parts only
- ½ cup fresh or frozen peas
- 1-2 cups roughly chopped spinach
- a small handful or ¼ cup of basil, chopped
- 1 lemon, juice + zest
- pinches of pepper & salt
- pinch red pepper flakes
- parmesan cheese or pecorino cheese, grated, on top

Directions

1. Pour 1-4th cup olive oil into a dish and add lemon zest to make the lemon oil.
2. Cook until the pasta is nearly done. Save part of the water after straining the pasta.
3. In a large pan, heat the oil, add the chopped garlic and onion, and cook until the shallot is translucent, about 1-2 mins- cautious not to roast the garlic too much. Add the asparagus and peas, along with a splash of white wine- if using - or leave it out entirely. Combine the lemon juice, pepper, and salt in a mixing bowl- from the lemon, which 1 zested earlier. Combine all of the ingredients in a large mixing bowl. Cook for a further 2 mins, or until asparagus is crisp but still crunchy and peas are tender.
4. Toss the cooked pasta with the other ingredients in the pot. Turn off the heat and add the spinach, letting it wilt in the pasta's warmth.
5. Remove the lemon oil's zest and keep it away. Combine the pasta with the lemon oil and toss everything together. If necessary, add more pasta water to get the desired consistency. Add the basil leaves and toss to combine. Taste and adjust spices 1 final time if required.
6. Add a sprinkling of shredded cheese and a pinch of red pepper flakes to finish- both are optional.

Nutritional Values

Fat 1.9g, Chol 10mg, Sodium 14mg, Potassium 64mg, Carbs 45g, Calories 241, Protein 13 g

439. FETTUCCINE & SWEET CORN CREAM

- Prep time: 15 mins, Cook time: 40 mins, Total time: 55 mins, Grill temp: 0, Servings: 4

Ingredients

- 1 & ½ cup of almonds, blanched & skins removed
- 1 & ½ cups frozen or fresh corn kernels- blanched
- 1 cup of water
- 2 tbsp olive oil, extra-virgin
- 1 minced garlic clove
- 2 tbsp onion, chopped
- ½ lemon, juice only
- 1-2 tbsp of agave or honey- according to taste
- Sea salt
- 8 oz. fettuccine- whole grain or gluten-free
- ¾ cup of corn kernels
- 2 cups of arugula or spinach, uncooked
- ½ cup saved pasta water- or more
- ½ – ¾ cup of sweet corn cream sauce- as you like
- ¼ cup of basil, chopped
- ½ lemon juice, to taste
- Sea salt & black pepper, fresh
- Red pepper flakes, optional

Directions

1. In a high-powered blender, puree the lemon, almonds, 1 tbsp agave, corn, onion, water, garlic, pinches of salt, and olive oil to make sweet corn cream- Vitamix works best. Taste and make any necessary adjustments. If you want it to be sweeter, you may add more agave. If you want it to be more acidic, add more lemon or more oil if you want it to be richer. And, of course, season with salt to taste.
2. Boil the pasta in a large saucepan of salted water until it is fully cooked. Save at least ½ a cup of the cooking water after draining and rinsing the pasta.
3. In a large mixing basin, combine the arugula and loose corn kernels. Scoop some of the pasta water that has been kept

aside on top of the cooked spaghetti noodles. Pour in a little at a time the almond cream, along with extra pasta water, to soften the arugula and thin the sauce. If desired, continue to add more sauce, basil, salt, a splash of lime juice, pepper, basil, and red pepper flakes. Taste as you go. It depends on how you're feeling; this might be a light or a hearty lunch.

Nutritional Values

Fat 1.4g, Chol 9mg, Sodium 7mg, Potassium 54mg, Carbs 31g, Calories 231, Protein 11 g

440. SWEET POTATO SURPRISE

- Prep time: 20 mins, Cook time: 45 mins, Total time: 65 mins, Grill temp: 350°F, Servings: 2-3

Ingredients

- 1-2 tbsp olive oil, extra-virgin
- 1 large, chopped shallot
- 1 heaping cup of sweet potatoes, chopped
- 2 minced garlic cloves
- 8 oz. of veggie broth
- ¾ cup of coconut milk, light
- 2 cups pasta- may use Jovial brown rice fusilli, uncooked
- 1 tsp of Dijon mustard
- ¼ cup of nutritional yeast
- 4-5 chopped sage leaves
- 1 tsp of maple syrup
- Salt & pepper
- 2 cups fresh spinach, chopped
- ¼ cup scallions, chopped
- ¼ cup - ½ cup of panko- or breadcrumbs gluten-free
- Pinch of red pepper flakes

Directions

1. In a saucepan, heat the oil. Season the shallots with salt and pepper. Cook until the liquid is clear. In a large mixing basin, combine the coconut milk, sweet potatoes, broth, and garlic. Cover and cook, occasionally stirring, until the potatoes are cooked- approximately 20-25 mins.
2. Cook the pasta according to the package directions, reserving a little amount of the cooked pasta water before filtering.

3. Season with salt and pepper after adding the Dijon mustard, maple syrup, nutritional yeast, and sage to the sweet potato mixture.
4. In a high-powered mixer, blend the ingredients until smooth- Vitamix works best.
5. Taste and make any necessary adjustments. If it's too thick, thin it out with a little pasta water.
6. Combine the spinach and the warm spaghetti noodles- hot pasta heat starts wilting the spinach. Mix in a sweet potato sauce, thinned with more pasta water if necessary.
7. Place it in the baking dish and bake it. On top, scallions, salt, panko, pinches of red pepper flakes, and a spritz of oil are sprinkled.
8. Bake for approximately 20 mins- uncovered at 350 degrees until golden and crusty on top.
9. Turn on the broiler for the last few mins to help with browning.

Nutritional Values

Fat 2.1g, Chol 5mg, Sodium 8mg, Potassium 87mg, Carbs 40g, Calories 270, Protein 15 g

441. CREAMY PASTA POMODORO

- Prep time: 12 mins, Cook time: 40 mins, Total time: 52 mins, Grill temp: 0, Servings: 4

Ingredients

- 1 tbsp olive oil, extra-virgin
- 3 tbsp minced shallot
- 1 large minced garlic clove
- ¼ tsp of sea salt
- Black pepper, freshly ground
- 1 14 oz. can tomato, chopped
- 1 tsp of balsamic vinegar
- ⅛ tsp of cane sugar
- Pinch of oregano, dried
- Pinch of red pepper flakes, crushed
- Marinara recipe- from above
- ¼ cup cashews, raw
- ½ tbsp of tomato paste
- ¼ cup of water
- ¼ cup of pasta water
- ¼ t- ½ tsp sea salt

- 10 oz. rigatoni
- Olive oil for drizzling
- 2 medium sliced zucchinis, thin ½-moons shape
- 2 tbsp thyme leaves, fresh
- 2 14-z drained Mutti Cherry Tomatoes
- 6 cups of spinach or a mix of arugula & spinach
- ¼ cup parsley or basil, chopped
- Sea salt & black pepper, freshly ground

Directions

1. To make the marinara sauce, heat the oil in a saucepan over low heat. With the shallot, a few dashes of pepper, garlic, and salt, cook for 2 mins, stirring often. Combine the tomatoes, cane sugar, juices, balsamic vinegar, oregano, and red pepper flakes in a mixing dish. Cook for 20 mins over low heat, occasionally stirring.
2. In a blender, mix the marinara, tomato paste, cashews, salt, and a 1-4th cup of water to make a creamy sauce. Blend until the mixture is smooth. Keep it in a safe place until you're ready to use it. Before serving, add a 1-4th cup of hot pasta boiling water to soften the spaghetti and evenly coat it.
3. Boil the pasta until al dente according to package directions in a saucepan of lightly salted water.
4. While the pasta is boiling, heat the oil in a skillet over medium heat. In a large mixing basin, combine the zucchini, salt, thyme, and pepper. Cook, stirring regularly, for 3 mins or until lightly browned. Reduce heat to low and continue to cook for another 2-3 mins or until the tomatoes are fully cooked. Toss in the spinach and gently toss until wilted. Season with salt and pepper to taste.
5. Divide the pasta into individual serving bowls, sprinkle with scoops of creamy sauce, and toss to coat. Arrange the vegetables in the bowls and serve with basil or parsley as a garnish.
6. Serve after seasoning with salt and pepper to taste.

Nutritional Values

Fat 2.5g, Chol 6mg, Sodium 14mg, Potassium 97mg, Carbs 33g, Calories 270, Protein 15 g

442. ORECCHIETTE WITH BROCCOLI RABE

- Prep time: 10 mins, Cook time: 40 mins, Total time: 50 mins, Grill temp: 0, Servings: 4

Ingredients

- 3 Italian Sausages, plant-based
- Olive oil, extra-virgin
- 1 & ½ bunch of broccoli rabe
- 8 oz. of dry orecchiette pasta
- 4 sliced garlic cloves
- ¼ cup of dry white wine
- ⅓ cup parmesan cheese, grated
- 1 tbsp of lemon juice + 1 tsp zest
- ¼ - ½ tsp of red pepper flakes
- Sea salt & black pepper, freshly ground
- 2 caramelized onions
- 8 oil-packed chopped tomatoes, sun-dried
- ⅓ cup of pine nuts

Directions

1. Using a sharp knife, cut all of the sausages into small pieces. In a cast-iron pan, brush ½ a tsp of olive oil and fry for 1-2 mins or until beautifully browned. Take the object out of the room and store it away.
2. Trim the ends of the broccoli rabe to ½ an inch. In a saucepan, bring a large pot of salted water to a boil. In a kettle of boiling water, cook the broccoli rabe for 2 mins. Remove the broccoli rabe from the boiling water and put it aside. Drain excess liquid and absorb it with a dry, clean cloth. Before chopping them into 1-inch pieces, make sure they're completely dry.
3. Return the water to a boil, season with salt, and cook the pasta according to the package directions. Remove ½ a cup of the pasta water and set it aside.
4. When the pasta is about a min away from being done, heat 1 tbsp of oil in a large pan over medium heat. After adding the broccoli rabe and garlic, stir for 30 seconds. Pour in the wine and heat for 30 seconds before using the slotted spoon to scoop the pasta directly from the pot onto the pan.

5. With the pasta water preserved, stir in the cheese, lemon zest + lemon juice, ½ salt, flakes of red pepper, and ground pepper. Combine the browned sausage, caramelized onions, pine nuts, and sun-dried tomatoes in a large mixing bowl.
6. Serve after seasoning with salt and pepper to taste.

Nutritional Values

Fat 2g, Chol 9mg, Sodium 4mg, Potassium 76mg, Carbs 38g, Calories 309, Protein 13 g

443. SUMMER SQUASH & CORN ORZO

- Prep time: 10 mins, Cook time: 20 mins, Total time: 30 mins, Grill temp: 0, Servings: 2

Ingredients

- 1-2 Tbsp olive oil extra-virgin
- 1 small chopped red onion
- 1 minced garlic clove
- 2 cups summer squash sliced
- ½ cup of corn
- white wine
- Sea salt & black pepper

Directions

1. In a large saucepan, boil salted water. Cook the orzo according to the package directions until it is al dente. Cook the pasta as directed on the box, drain, and set aside 12 cups of the cooking water.
2. Prepare a squash to sauté as follows: Warm some olive oil in a pan over medium heat. Stir in the onion and cook for 5-7 mins or until softened. In a large mixing bowl, combine the garlic, white wine, and summer squash. Cook for another 10 mins or so until the wine has diminished and the squash has softened. Mix in the corn well. After tasting the meal, adjust the seasonings to your preference.
3. Increase the heat to high and whisk in all of the pasta water accumulated in the pan. Toss in the orzo until everything is well combined. For added heat, garnish with chopped chives and pepper flakes. If desired, season the feta, sun-dried tomatoes, parmesan, and balsamic vinegar.

Nutritional Values

Fat 3.3g, Chol 8mg, Sodium 13mg, Potassium 84mg, Carbs 39g, Calories 273, Protein 11 g

444. 1 POT VEGETABLE PENNE PASTA

- Prep time: 10 mins, Cook time: 10 mins, Total time: 20 mins, Grill temp: 0, Servings: 2

Ingredients

- 6 oz. pasta penne
- 1 & ½ cups cherry tomatoes sliced
- 1 & ½ cups leeks thinly sliced
- 1 cup sliced zucchini
- ½ cup bell pepper thinly sliced
- 3 small, minced garlic cloves
- 2 Tbsp olive oil extra-virgin
- 2 Tbsp lemon juice
- 1 tsp oregano dried
- 1 tsp sea salt
- ½ tsp pepper flakes red
- 1 basil sprig
- 2 ¼ cups of water

Directions

1. In a large pot, combine all of the ingredients and simmer until the pasta is al dente. Season to taste with salt and pepper. Stir in the water until it's well combined. Bring to a boil, then lower to low heat and cover, and cook for 8 mins. Replace the cover after a quick stir at the 5-mins mark to ensure nothing has clung to the pan.
2. After 8 mins of cooking, check the pasta for doneness. After removing the pot from the heat and stirring it, let it thicken for about 2 mins.

Nutritional Values

Fat 6.7g, Chol 9mg, Sodium 14mg, Potassium 78mg, Carbs 43g, Calories 325, Protein 13g

445. EASY PESTO PASTA

- Prep time: 15 mins, Cook time: 10 mins, Total time: 25 mins, Grill temp: 0, Servings: 2

Ingredients

- 6 oz. spaghetti
- 1/3 - ½ cup of vegan p
- Olive oil
- Lemon juice fresh
- 4 cups of arugula
- 2 tbsp of pine nuts

- Red chili flakes
- Sea salt & black pepper freshly ground
- Finely grated Parmesan

Directions

1. Prepare the pasta according to package directions in a large pot of boiling water until al dente. Save ½ cup of cooking liquid before cleaning. Drain the pasta and toss it with a few drops of olive oil.
2. In a skillet over very low heat, combine the pesto and ¼ cup of reserved pasta water. To produce a loose sauce, add the pasta and as much pasta water as needed. You'll need water, depending on the concentration of your pesto.
3. Remove the heat source. Add fresh lemon juice, pepper, and salt to taste. Then add the arugula and stir until it is just wilted. Serve with a garnish of chili flakes and pine nuts.

Nutritional Values

Fat 2.2g, Chol 5mg, Sodium 13mg, Potassium 94mg, Carbs 35g, Calories 215, Protein 11g

446. CREAMY VEGAN PASTA BAKE WITH BRUSSELS SPROUTS

- Prep time: 10 mins, Cook time: 20 mins, Total time: 30 mins, Grill temp: 400*F, Servings: 4-6

Ingredients

White miso sauce:
- 1 cup almonds
- 2 tbsp paste of white miso
- 2 cloves of garlic
- ½ tsp of Dijon mustard
- 1 cup of almond milk
- ¼ cup of lemon juice fresh
- 2 tbsp of olive oil
- ½ tsp of sea salt

For the pasta:
- 10 oz. shell pasta
- 1 tbsp of olive oil
- 3 cups sliced Brussels sprouts
- 2 tbsp of white wine
- 2 sliced scallions
- sea salt & black pepper freshly ground

Bread crumb topping:
- 1 tbsp breadcrumbs

- 1 tbsp of hemp seeds
- ⅛ tsp of sea salt
- Olive oil
- ¼ cup fresh herbs chopped

Directions

1. Preheat the oven to 400°F and oil a baking pan.
2. Follow these procedures to make the white miso sauce: In a high-powered blender, combine the miso paste, almonds, Dijon mustard, garlic, almond milk, olive oil, and salt until smooth.
3. Follow these Directions to make the pasta: Bring a large pot of water to low heat. Unless the pasta is al dente, cook it according to the package recommendations. Wash the spaghetti and toss it with olive oil to keep it from sticking together.
4. 1 tbsp oil, heated in a small pan over medium-high heat. Cook, turning periodically, for 6-8 mins or until the Brussels sprouts are roasted and soft. Remove the saucepan from the heat and whisk the wine within to remove any bits that have adhered to the bottom. Combine the scallions, cooked pasta, and miso sauce in a large pan. After swirling to coat, transfer to the baking tray. Hemp seeds, breadcrumbs, pinches of salt, and cheese are sprinkled on top. To finish, drizzle with oil.
5. Cover and bake for 15 mins or until the Brussels sprouts are tender and the dish is barely warm. Because of the quick Cook time, the filling will not dry out.
6. Before serving, remove the dish from the oven and sprinkle it with herbs.

Nutritional Values

Fat 1.3g, Chol 7mg, Sodium 9mg, Potassium 84mg, Carbs 33g, Calories 205, Protein 10 g

447. SPAGHETTI AGLIO E OLIO

- Prep time: 5 mins, Cook time: 15 mins, Total time: 20 mins, Grill temp: 0, Servings: 4

Ingredients

- 12 oz. spaghetti
- ½ - 1 cup of water

- ¼ cup olive oil
- 4 thinly sliced garlic cloves
- ¼-½ tsp red chili flakes
- 1 bunch of lacinato kale chopped
- ½ tsp sea salt
- Black pepper freshly ground
- 1 tsp lemon zest
- 1 tsp lemon juice
- ⅓ cup chopped parsley
- Parmesan for serving

Directions

1. Place a basin of cold water nearby and bring a large pot to a boil. For a few mins, sauté the asparagus. Cook the pasta until al dente in a pot of boiling water according to package directions. 1 cup of cooking water should be saved before draining the pasta.
2. Heat the oil in a large skillet over medium heat. Now is the time to add the garlic and red chili flakes. Cook for 30 seconds to 1 min, stirring periodically until the garlic is lightly brown around the edges. Cook for 1 min, stirring with fingers until the kale is cooked.
3. Toss in the spaghetti and stir well. ½ cup water, lemon zest, and lemon juice are added. If the pasta seems too dry, add the remaining ½ cup of pasta water to produce a light sauce.
4. To taste, season with salt and pepper.
5. Garnish with parmesan and parsley, if desired.

Nutritional Values

Fat 1.4g, Chol 6mg, Sodium 18mg, Potassium 65mg, Carbs 37g, Calories 213, Protein 7 g

Chapter 12.

Legume Recipes

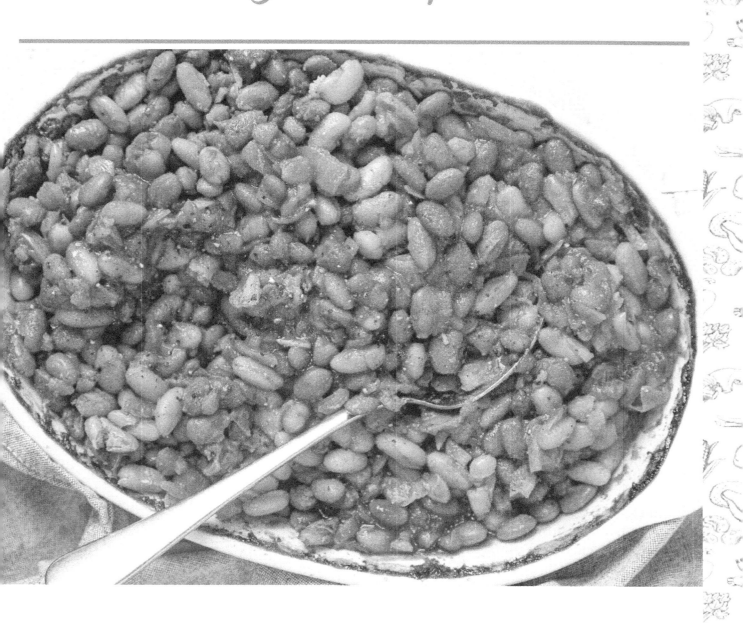

448. SMOKEY TEMPEH BACON

- Prep time: 30 mins, Cook time: 5 mins, Total time: 35 mins, Grill temp: 375°F, Servings: 4 slices

Ingredients

- Tempeh soybeans 1- 8-ounce package
- Marinade
- Low-Sodium tamari ¼ cup
- Date syrup 2 tbsp
- Molasses 1 tbsp
- Liquid smoke 2 tsp
- Onion powder 1 tsp
- Garlic powder ½ tsp
- Black pepper 1/8 tsp freshly ground

Directions

1. Preheat the oven to 375°F - 190°C. Line a baking sheet with parchment paper.
2. Cut the tempeh into ¼-inch strips- about 24 slices and set aside.
3. Optional: In a large, covered saucepan over medium heat, steam the tempeh block for 20 mins. Remove the pan from the heat and put it aside until it is safe to handle. Start slicing after that.
4. Whisk together the marinade ingredients in a container or sealable bag large enough to accommodate the tempeh pieces. Allow the tempeh to marinate for at least 30 mins, but up to overnight.
5. Remove the tempeh from the marinade and put it in a single layer on the parchment paper. Bake for 15
6. mins, or until lightly browned and crispy, rotating halfway through. Overcooking them will cause them to dry out. Alternatively, brown the tempeh in a nonstick pan over medium-high heat for a few mins on each side. Make sure they don't burn by keeping an eye on them.
7. Refrigerate leftovers in an airtight jar for up to 7 days.

Nutritional Values

Fat 2g, Chol 3.5mg, Sodium 4.5mg, Potassium 10mg, Carbs 10g, Calories 94, Protein 8g

449. BURRITO WITH TOFU SCRAMBLE

- Prep time: 30 mins, Cook time: 10 mins, Total time: 40 mins, Grill temp: 300°F, Servings: 4 people

Ingredients

- Tortillas 4 whole grain
- Firm organic tofu 1 container
- Yellow onion chopped ½ cup
- Ground turmeric ½ tsp
- Avocados 2 peel and seed removed
- Refried beans 1 15 oz. can Fat-free
- Green onions sliced 6
- Fresh salsa
- Hot sauce

Directions

1. Sauté the onions in a small amount of water in a nonstick pan over medium heat.
2. Break the tofu and add the turmeric to the pan after the onions are almost cooked. Season to taste with salt and pepper, then whisk to combine. The spices should turn the mixture yellow and make it seem like eggs.
3. Cook the refried beans in a small saucepan over medium heat, frequently stirring to prevent sticking.
4. After wrapping the tortillas in a moist paper towel, microwave them for a few seconds. Alternatively, cover in foil and bake at 300°F for about 10 mins.
5. Assemble: Place 1 tortilla on a plate or cutting board and cover the other tortillas in plastic wrap. Using a spoon or knife, spread refried beans along the center of the tortilla, leaving about an inch on 1 end. Alternatively, fill the center with about ¼ cup of whole beans.
6. Sprinkle ¼ green onion, 1/3 chopped avocado, and a dab of salsa and spicy sauce, to taste on top.
7. Make your vegan sour cream or buy vegan sour cream from the supermarket.
8. Fold the tortilla's bottom first, then the 2 sides in, leaving 1 end open. On the side, serve with additional salsa, spicy sauce, and sour cream.

Nutritional Values

Fat 19.5g, Chol 4.3mg, Sodium 9.2mg, Potassium 10.3mg, Carbs 57g, Calories 483, Protein 24g

450. HUEVOS RANCHEROS CASSEROLE

- Prep time: 15 mins, Cook time: 5 mins, Total time: 20 mins, Grill temp: 350°F, Servings: 6 people

Ingredients

- Corn tortillas - 8 counts, 1 package
- Black beans 2 15 oz. Cans
- Jalapeño- optional 1
- Avocados 2 large halved and cut into slices
- Low salt black olives ½ 6 oz. can

Easy ranchero sauce
- Yellow onion diced ½ large
- Garlic diced 1 clove
- Jalapeño 1- optional
- Ancho chili powder 1 tsp
- Organic tomatoes 1 14.5 oz. can
- Fire-roasted tomatoes 1 14.5 oz. can
- Vegetable broth 2 cups low sodium
- Cilantro chopped ¼ cup

Tofu scramble
- Block firm organic tofu drained 1 12-14 oz
- Onion diced 1/3 cup
- Ground Tumeric 1/3 tsp

Directions

1. Preheat the oven to 350°F - 180°C.
2. In a medium-sized pan, sauté the onions with a little water until they are translucent and nearly done.
3. Toss the tofu into the pan with the turmeric for color. Stir to combine, then boil until the liquid has almost evaporated and the ingredients are well cooked.
4. In a large pan over medium-high heat, cook chopped onion and pepper with a little water. Allow the water to drain and the veggies to gently color before serving. Season with salt and pepper to taste.
5. Reduce the heat to low and simmer, uncovered, for another 30 mins or until the sauce thickened and decreased somewhat.
6. After the sauce has thickened somewhat, remove it from the fire and set it aside to cool. Blend the sauce ingredients until smooth but be careful when combining a spicy sauce since too much heat might cause it to splatter.
7. Apply a little amount of ranchero sauce across the bottom of the baking dish using the back of a spoon. A layer of tortillas is broken up as required to fill the pan, and a sauce drizzle is placed on top.
8. On top of the tortillas, spread ½ of the black beans.
9. On top, ½ of the ranchero sauce, tofu scramble, and more tortilla layers.
10. On top, there's more ranchero sauce, scramble, beans, sauce, and a final layer of tortillas. To keep the tortillas from becoming too crispy in the oven, cover them with sauce.
11. Cover with foil and bake in the oven for 30 mins. After removing the cover, check for liquid in the pan. Return it to the oven for another 5 mins if there is a lot of it.
12. Serve with green onions and sliced olives on top. If desired, add jalapenos and sliced avocado.

Nutritional Values

Fat 18.4g, Chol 2.9mg, Sodium 9.4mg, Potassium 11.6mg, Carbs 54.5g, Calories 455, Protein 18g

451. BURRITO

- Prep time: 15 mins, Cook time: 5 mins, Total time: 20 mins, Grill temp: 0, Servings: 6 burritos

Ingredients

- Dried rice 1 cup- white or brown
- Olive oil 2 tbsp or ¼ cup water
- Onion, diced ½ large
- Green bell pepper, 1 cored and diced
- Fired roasted 1 can- 14oz diced tomatoes, drained
- Diced green chilies, 1 can- 4oz drained
- Cumin 1 tbsp
- Chili powder 1 tsp
- Chipotle powder, 1 tsp optional
- Garlic powder 1 tsp
- - About 1 cup, drained 1 can- 9oz corn
- Black beans 1 can- 14oz- about 1 ½ cups, drained and rinsed
- Cilantro, loosely packed ¼ – ½ cup

- Flour tortillas 6 large
- Shredded lettuce 2 cups

Directions

1. Grain: Prepare your grain according to the package directions and set it aside.
2. Sofrito de Black Beans y Corn: In a large pan or pot, heat the oil/water over medium heat, add the onion or bell pepper, and cook for 5 mins. After adding the tomatoes, green chilies or jalapeno, cumin, chili powder, garlic powder, and salt, cook for another 4–5 mins, occasionally stirring. Cook for a few mins or until the black beans and corn are well warmed. Mix in the cilantro well. To taste, season with salt and pepper.
3. Layer ½ cup black bean mix, shredded lettuce, guacamole, or ½ cup rice on top of tortillas laid flat on a level surface, leaving a few inches at each end. To properly seal the burrito, wrap the edge closest to you up or over, then continue rolling it across from you. Keep the flaps down as you fold each of the end pieces up towards the center.
4. Serve with a side of your choice of condiments.

Nutritional Values

Fat 17.2g, Chol 7.9mg, Sodium 9.8mg, Potassium 13.5mg, Carbs 89g, Calories 584, Protein 21g

452. VEGAN COLLARD GREENS

- Prep time: 10 mins, Cook time: 10 mins, Total time: 20 mins, Grill temp: 0, Servings: 3

Ingredients

- Olive oil 1 tbsp
- Onion 1 cup
- Garlic 2-3 cloves
- diced tomatoes 1 can
- Collard greens 1 bunch
- Beans 14 oz.
- Lemon juice 2-3 tbsp
- Red pepper flakes

Directions

1. In a large wok, heat the oil over medium heat. Add the onions and sauté for 4 mins or until softened. Cook for another min after adding the garlic.

2. After adding the collards, lemon juice, and salt and pepper, cook for another 4 mins.
3. Cook, occasionally stirring, until collards are wilted or beans and tomatoes are fully cooked, then add tomatoes and beans.
4. Serve in separate dishes with a squeeze of lemon. The meal is completed with warm corn tortillas, naan and crusty bread, and a tall drink of lemon water.

Nutritional Values

Fat 1.3g, Chol 2.5mg, Sodium 5mg, Potassium 12mg, Carbs 11g, Calories 63, Protein 1.3 g

453. CHIPOTLE BLACK BEAN AVOCADO TOAST

- **Prep time: 10** mins, **Cook time: 5** mins, **Total time: 15** mins, **Grill temp: 0, Servings:** 4

INGREDIENTS

- Whole-wheat toast 2 pieces
- Black beans 1 can
- Chipotle spice ¼ tsp
- Garlic powder 1 tsp
- Black pepper
- Lime, 1 juiced
- Avocado, 1 diced
- Tomato, ½ diced
- Corn ¼ cup
- Fresh cilantro few tbsp
- Red onion 3 tbsp

DIRECTIONS

1. In a mixing bowl, combine the beans, chipotle spice, garlic powder, a tsp of sea salt, a pinch of pepper, and the juice of 12 limes. Cook until the sauce thickens and becomes starchy.
2. Combine avocado, tomato, red onion, corn, cilantro, lime juice from 12 limes, and pepper in a mixing bowl.
3. 4 pieces of toasted whole-wheat bread with black bean spread on top
4. On top, serve the avocado mixture.

Nutritional Values

Fat 9g, Chol 4.1mg, Sodium 5.2mg, Potassium 11.9mg, Carbs 44g, Calories 290, Protein 12g

454. BAKED BEAN TOAST- 3-INGREDIENT

- Prep time: 5 mins, Cook time: 5 mins, Total time: 10 mins, Grill temp: 0, Servings: 2

Ingredients

- Whole grain bread 2 slices
- Avocado ½
- Mamasezz Baked beans 1 cup

Directions

1. On each slice of whole-grain bread, spread ¼ avocado.
2. On each slice, spread ½ cup of warm MamaSezz Baked Beans.
3. Enjoy a hearty, healthy, and delicious breakfast.

Nutritional Values

Fat 6g, Chol 10mg, Sodium 8mg, Potassium 80mg, Carbs 65g, Calories 340, Protein 14g

455. BLACK BEAN BREAKFAST BURRITOS

- Prep time: 10 mins, Cook time: 10 mins, Total time: 20 mins, Grill temp: 0, Servings: 6 Burritos

Ingredients

- Avocado oil 1 tbsp
- Sweet potato 1 medium cut into 1 cm- ½ inch cubes
- Red onion diced ½ medium
- Black beans 2 14 oz. cans rinsed and drained
- Red bell pepper diced 1 large
- Salsa ½ cup
- Garlic chopped 1 clove
- Ground cumin 1 tsp
- Garlic powder ½ tsp
- Onion powder ½ tsp
- Dried oregano ½ tsp
- Paprika ½ tsp
- Salt ½ tsp
- Baby spinach 4 handfuls
- Tortillas 6 large

Directions

1. Squeeze out as much liquid as you can from the tofu. Wrap the tofu block with a paper towel after removing it from the container. Place something substantial on top of the wrapped tofu, such as a set of cookbooks or textbooks. Allow it to drain while you finish preparing the other ingredients, then crumble it with your hands.
2. To "crumble" the tofu block, place it in a large mixing basin.
3. Then, in a large pan that has been heated over medium-high heat, pour in the cooking oil. Sauté the sliced bell peppers and onions for 7-10 mins- if using.
4. After the peppers have cooked, add the crumbled tofu, garlic powder, curry powder, cumin, and pepper to the pan. Cook for 3 mins, often stirring to distribute the spices evenly throughout the tofu.
5. Finally, add the young spinach and simmer until it wilts, continually stirring. Taste the tofu and adjust the seasonings as required. Serve right away.

Nutritional Values

Fat 8g, Chol 8mg, Sodium 9mg, Potassium 90mg, Carbs 31g, Calories 230, Protein 10g

456. TOFU SCRAMBLE STUFFED BREAKFAST SWEET POTATOES

- Prep time: 15 mins, Cook time: 5 mins, Total time: 20 mins, Grill temp: 0, Servings: 4

Ingredients

- Olive oil 1 tbsp
- Onion, diced ½
- Garlic, minced 2 cloves
- Bell pepper, diced 1
- Tomatoes, diced ½ cup
- Corn ½ cup
- Extra-firm tofu 1 14-ounce package
- Black beans 1 cup
- Salsa ¼ cup
- Chili powder ½ tsp
- Ground turmeric ½ tsp
- Paprika ½ tsp
- Ground cumin ½ tsp
- Black pepper ¼ tsp
- Sweet potatoes 4 baked
- Avocado, sliced 1
- Hot sauce

Directions

1. In a medium skillet over medium heat, warm the oil. Add the onion to the pan once it's hot and cook for 5-7 mins, or until it's lightly browned. Cook for 1 min while

continually stirring. Cook until the bell pepper, tomatoes, and corn are tender, about 5-7 mins.
2. Toss in the tofu, crumble into small pieces, and mix well. Cook for 8-10 mins, or until the tofu is lightly browned.
3. Combine the black beans, salsa, chili powder, paprika, cumin, and pepper in a large mixing bowl. Cook for 2 mins, stirring periodically, until well cooked.
4. Each potato should be packed with tofu scramble. On top, there are avocado slices and a spicy sauce.

Nutritional Values

Fat 14.8g, Chol 15mg, Sodium 7.5mg, Potassium 83mg, Carbs 52.5g, Calories 402, Protein 18g

457. BUTTERNUT SQUASH BLACK BEAN ENCHILADAS WITH JALAPEÑO CASHEW CREMA

- Prep time: 1 hr, Cook time: 30 mins, Total time: 1 hr 30 mins, Grill temp: 350°F, Servings: 6

Ingredients

For cashew cream
- Raw cashews ½ cup
- Garlic 1 cloves
- Jalapeno, ½ seeds removed- reserve the other ½ for topping
- Chopped cilantro 2 tbsp
- Filtered water ⅓ cup
- Salt ¼ tsp

For enchilada sauce
- Tomato sauce 1- 15 ounces can
- Tomato paste 2 tbsp
- Water 2/3 cup
- Apple cider vinegar ½ tsp
- Garlic, minced 3 cloves
- Chili powder 2 ½ tbsp
- Cumin 1 ½ tsp
- Dried oregano 1 tsp
- Cayenne pepper ¼ tsp

For the enchiladas
- Olive oil 1 tbsp
- Garlic, minced 2 cloves
- Red onion, 1 small roughly chopped
- Cubed butternut squash, 4 cups from 1 medium butternut squash
- Chili powder 1 tsp
- Cumin ½ tsp
- Black beans, 1- 15 ounces, can be rinsed and drained
- Corn tortillas 12- 6 inches

To garnish
- Fresh cilantro
- Remaining ½ of jalapeno
- Avocado slices
- Hot sauce

Directions

1. Preheat the oven to 350°F - 180°C. Coat a 9x13 inch baking pan with nonstick cooking spray.
2. In a large mixing bowl, place 12 cups of cashews, then cover with boiling water and soak for 45 mins to an hr while preparing the enchiladas. Alternatively, you may soak your cashews in room temp water overnight and use them in the cashew crème the next day.
3. To make the enchilada sauce, add tomato sauce, apple cider vinegar, chili powder, oregano, garlic, cayenne pepper, and salt in a large mixing bowl. Whisk everything together well to get a smooth mix.
4. Heat the olive oil in a large pan over medium heat. Sauté the garlic and onions in a skillet until the garlic is fragrant- about 30 seconds. After that, put the diced butternut squash, chili powder, cumin, and salt in a mixing bowl. Cover and simmer for about 8 mins, or until fork-tender, often stirring to avoid scorching the squash.
5. Add a few tbsp of water to the pan if necessary to help the squash cook. Transfer the squash to a large mixing bowl after its fork-tender, stir in the black beans, and make the enchilada sauce.
6. Follow these Directions to prepare enchiladas: Cover the bottom of the 9x13 inch pan with about 2/3 cup enchilada sauce. Warm tortillas in the microwave for 20-30 seconds, wrapped in a damp paper towel, to help roll them easier.
7. Each tortilla should be filled with the butternut squash and black bean mixture. Each tortilla should be folded up and put in the baking pan seam-side down. Pour the

leftover enchilada sauce on the top. Preheat the oven to 350°F and bake for around 25 to 30 mins.

8. Make the cashew crema while your enchiladas are still baking: Combine the drained cashews, cilantro, water, garlic, jalapeno, and salt in a blender. Blend unless a chunky sauce emerges, adjusting the consistency with a tbsp or 2 of water as required.

9. Fill a Ziploc bag halfway with cashew sauce, snip a piece off, and squeeze the sauce all over the enchiladas. 2 enchiladas per person, for a total of 6 people.

Nutritional Values

Fat 7.5g, Chol 5mg, Sodium 9.5mg, Potassium 72mg, Carbs 62g, Calories 396, Protein 19g

458. VEGETARIAN CHILI

- Prep time: 15 mins, Cook time: 5 mins, Total time: 20 mins, Grill temp: 0, Servings: 10

Ingredients

- Olive oil 2 tbsp
- Yellow onion, diced 1 Large
- Green bell pepper, diced 1
- Red bell pepper, diced 1
- Sweet potatoes 2
- Garlic 4 cloves
- Black beans 1- 15 oz. can
- Kidney beans 1- 15 oz. can
- Pinto beans, 1- 15 oz. can drain, rinsed
- Diced tomatoes 1- 28 oz. can
- Red enchilada sauce 1- 20 oz. can
- Chili powder 1/3 cup
- Cumin 2 tsp
- Bay leaves 2
- Cilantro
- Avocado
- Green onions

Directions

1. Heat the oil in a large oven or soup pot. For about 4-5 mins, or until the onions soften, sauté onions, bell peppers, and sweet potatoes in a skillet. After adding the garlic, cook for another 2 mins.

2. Combine the beans, tomatoes, chili powder, enchilada sauce, cumin, bay leaves, and salt in a large mixing bowl. Just cover the beans

with enough water to keep them submerged.

3. Bring the water to a boil in a large pot. Reduce to low heat and cook uncovered, for 1 hr, often stirring to ensure nothing sticks to the bottom.

4. Avocado, cilantro, and green onions should be placed on top of the dish.

Nutritional Values

Fat 7g, Chol 12mg, Sodium 8mg, Potassium 56mg, Carbs 88g, Calories 503, Protein 23g

459. BLACK BEAN CHILI

- Prep time: 10 mins, Cook time: 10 mins, Total time: 20 mins, Grill temp: 0, Servings: 6

Ingredients

- Olive oil 1 tbsp
- White onion, chopped 1 medium
- Red bell pepper, diced 1
- Garlic 3 cloves, minced
- Chili powder 3 tbsp
- Cooked black beans 3 cups
- Fire-roasted tomatoes 1 14-ounce can dice
- Green chiles 1 4-ounce can
- Maple syrup 1 tsp
- Fresh lime juice 1 tbsp
- Cayenne, optional ¼ tsp

Directions

1. Heat the oil in a saucepan over medium heat. Cook, occasionally stirring, for 5 to 8 mins, or until the onion is translucent, adding the bell pepper, onion, and salt. Cook for 30 seconds, stirring regularly until the garlic and chili powder is fragrant.

2. In a large mixing bowl, combine the beans, bean liquid, maple syrup, tomatoes, green chiles, and a few grinds of pepper. Reduce the heat to low and simmer for 20 mins, occasionally stirring, or until the chili thickens.

3. If desired, after adding the lime juice, season with more salt, pepper, chili powder, and cayenne. Serve with toppings of your choice.

Nutritional Values

Fat 3.5g, Chol 18mg, Sodium 8.5mg, Potassium 72mg, Carbs 49g, Calories 264, Protein 14g

460. INSTANT POT BLACK BEANS

- Prep time: 5 mins, Cook time: 5 mins, Total time: 10 mins, Grill temp: 0, Servings: 8

Ingredients

- Dried black beans 2 cups
- Water 6 cups
- Diced white onion heaping ½ cup
- Garlic cloves, chopped 2 large
- Chili powder 1 tsp
- Cumin 1 tsp
- Oregano 1 tsp

Directions

1. Remove and discard any stones or rubbish from the beans in a large colander.
2. After washing the beans, place them in the Instant Pot. In a large mixing basin, combine the water, onion, garlic, salt, oregano, chili powder, cumin, and several grinds of black pepper. Set the Instant Pot's pressure to high and close the cover. Cook on high for 25 mins.
3. Allow the Instant Pot to release pressure naturally. It will take between 20 and 30 mins to complete this task. Once the float valve has been lowered, remove the lid.
4. To serve, use black beans.

Nutritional Values

Fat 6g, Chol 15mg, Sodium 9.4mg, Potassium 95mg, Carbs 27g, Calories 194, Protein 9g

461. CREAMY POTATO SOUP

- Prep time: 10 mins, Cook time: 5 mins, Total time: 15 mins, Grill temp: 0, Servings: 6

Ingredients

- Olive oil divided into 3 tbsp
- White onion, chopped 1 large
- Garlic 4 cloves, chopped
- White wine vinegar 1 tbsp
- Vegetable broth 4 cups
- Yukon gold potatoes 1½ pounds
- Cooked white beans, 1½ cups drained and rinsed
- Dijon mustard ½ tsp
- Fresh lemon juice 1 tbsp
- Smoked paprika ¼ tsp
- Black pepper freshly ground

Directions

1. Heat the olive oil in a large saucepan or Dutch oven over medium heat. In a mixing dish, combine the onion, salt, and a few grinds of pepper. Cook, occasionally stirring, for 6 to 8 mins, or until the vegetables are softened.
2. Cook for another 2 mins after adding the garlic. After 30 seconds of cooking, while tossing in the white wine vinegar, add the broth, potatoes, and white beans. Bring to a boil, then reduce to a low heat setting and cook for another 30 mins.
3. Allow ½ of the soup to cool before mixing with the remaining olive oil, mustard, lemon juice, and paprika. After mixing until smooth, return the pureed soup to the stove.
4. Using a potato masher, gently smash the potato pieces and beans. Season to taste with salt and pepper and serve with desired toppings.

Nutritional Values

Fat 6.4g, Chol 19mg, Sodium 15mg, Potassium 74mg, Carbs 17g, Calories 149, Protein 6g

462. SMOKY-SWEET POTATOES WITH BLACK BEANS & CORN

- Prep time: 30 mins, Cook time: 10 mins, Total time: 40 mins, Grill temp: 0, Servings: 4

Ingredients

- Chipotle Vinaigrette ¼ cup
- Mango Salsa ½ cup
- Cooked Black Beans ½ cup
- Corn kernels 1 ear fresh raw
- Crumbled quark, ⅓ cup cotija, or feta cheese
- Pickled Red Onions ¼ cup
- Serrano pepper, thinly sliced 1
- Cilantro leaves 2 tbsp

Directions

1. On a plate, drizzle the chipotle dressing over the roasted sweet potato rounds.
2. On top, evenly layer the mango salsa, cheese, onions, black beans, corn, serrano peppers, and cilantro. Drizzle some more chipotle dressing on top.
3. Serve with a pinch of black pepper to taste.

Fat 6.5g, Chol 14mg, Sodium 14mg, Potassium 82mg, Carbs 58g, Calories 317, Protein 13g

463. SANTA FE BLACK BEAN BURGER

- Prep time: 10 mins, Cook time: 10 mins, Total time: 20 mins, Grill temp: 0, Servings: 2

Ingredients

- Organic black beans, 1 can- 14 oz. drained and rinsed
- Oats- rolled or quick ¼ cup
- Flax meal or flour ¼ cup
- Cumin 1 tsp
- Cayenne or chipotle powder ½ tsp
- Garlic powder ½ tsp
- Pink salt ½ tsp
- Chunky salsa ¼ cup
- Olive oil, for pan-frying, 1 tbsp
- Cornmeal, for dusting- optional

Directions

1. In a medium-sized mixing bowl, mash black beans with a fork or a potato masher, leaving some lumps for texture if preferred.
2. In a mixing dish, combine all of the ingredients for the patty mixture. Mix the oats, flour, spices, salt, and salsa until well incorporated, using your hands if necessary. If the mixture is too wet, add more flax meal/flour. Otherwise, it should be OK.
3. Taste it to see whether it's delicious.
4. Make patties out of the ingredients and shape them into whichever size you choose. I like 2 burger patties, but 3 to 4 smaller ones will suffice.
5. Sprinkle some cornmeal on top if you have some on hand. It will give the meal a terrific crunch, flavor, and crispiness.

Nutritional Values

Fat 1g, Chol 4mg, Sodium 7mg, Potassium 87mg, Carbs 39g, Calories 247, Protein 15g

464. CAESAR SALAD

- Prep time: 10 mins, Cook time: 5 mins, Total time: 15 mins, Grill temp: 400°F, Servings: 4

Ingredients

- Romaine lettuce, chopped 3 heads
- Avocado, 1 sliced- optional
- Chickpea croutons
- Almond parmesan
- Chickpeas- garbanzo beans, 1 can- 15oz drained and rinsed
- Olive oil 1 tbsp
- Garlic powder ¾ tsp

Caesar dressing

- raw cashews ¾ cup
- Water ½ cup
- Garlic 2 cloves
- Capers 2 tsp
- vegan Worcestershire 1 tbsp
- Dijon mustard 2 tsp
- Lemon juice of 1 medium

Directions

1. Preheat the oven to 400°F - 200°C. Line a rimmed baking sheet with parchment paper or Silpat.
2. Chickpea Croutons: To make chickpea croutons, gently massage cleaned chickpeas between 2 clean dishcloths to dry them, eliminating loose skins. Drizzle chickpeas with oil on a preheated baking sheet, toss to coat, then season with garlic powder. With chickpeas and garlic cloves in a single layer, bake for 40–45 mins, stirring every 10 mins. If the garlic cloves seem to be overdone, remove them. After you've done it, put everything away.
3. Dressing Caesar Salad: After 5 mins of soaking in hot water, drain the cashews- not boiling. In a high-powered or personal blender, combine the cashews, water, capers, Worcestershire, roasted garlic cloves, Dijon, lemon juice, and pepper until velvety smooth. This recipe generates around 1 cup of the finished product.
4. To create the Caesar Salad, combine the chopped romaine with as much or as little dressing as you want- you may have some leftover in a medium mixing dish. Chickpea croutons, avocado, and Almond Parmesan cheese are sprinkled on top.

Nutritional Values

Fat 40g, Chol 2.9mg, Sodium 5.6mg, Potassium 92mg, Carbs 23g, Calories 481, Protein 10g

465. CURRIED CHICKPEA SALAD

- Prep time: 15 mins, Cook time: 5 mins, Total time: 20 mins, Grill temp: 0, Servings: 6

Ingredients

- Cooked chickpeas 3 cups- garbanzo beans
- Carrots 2 – 3- about 1 cup, diced
- Scallions/green onions 3 – 4- about 1 cup, sliced
- Raisins, dried currants, ½ cup of chopped dates
- Cashews ½ cup
- Vegan mayo ½ – 2/3 cup
- Juice of 1 lemon
- Curry powder 1 tbsp
- Garlic powder ¾ tsp

Directions

1. Curry Dressing: In a small bowl, whisk together vegan mayonnaise, curry powder, garlic powder, and a generous pinch of salt. Blend until completely smooth.- If using vinegar or maple syrup, stir it into the hummus at this point, as directed in the Directions below.
2. Place chickpeas in a medium mixing bowl and mash about ½ to 2-thirds of them with the back of a strong fork or a potato masher. When mashed potatoes are used as a sandwich filler, they help to hold the sandwich together.
3. Toss the carrots, raisins, scallions, and cashews in a large mixing bowl with the dressing and a squeeze of lemon, and toss well to combine. Season to taste with salt and pepper, if necessary.
4. Serve with sliced red bell peppers and crackers on a bed of fresh greens.

Nutritional Values

Fat 12.9g, Chol 14mg, Sodium 9.5mg, Potassium 84mg, Carbs 71g, Calories 441, Protein 18g

466. GREEK QUINOA SALAD

- Prep time: 15 mins, Cook time: 20 mins, Total time: 35 mins, Grill temp: 0, Servings: 6

Ingredients

- Dried quinoa, rinsed 1 cup
- Water 1 ¾ cups
- Garlic powder 1 tsp
- Chickpeas- garbanzo beans, 1 can- 14 oz. drained and rinsed
- Grape tomatoes, 1 cup sliced in ½
- English cucumber, diced 1 cup
- Red onion, diced ½
- Kalamata olives- about 1 cup, 1 jar- 7 oz. pitted and sliced
- Loosely packed ¼ cup fresh parsley, chopped
- Fresh dill, 3 tbsp chopped
- Lemon juice of 1 large

Directions

1. Quinoa: Rinse the quinoa in a fine-mesh sieve. In a medium-sized saucepan, bring the water, quinoa, and garlic powder to a boil. Cook for 15 mins on low heat, covered. Remove the pan from the heat and set it aside for 10–15 mins, covered. Fluff the mixture with a fork. This Quinoa can also be made in an Instant Pot.
2. After the quinoa is done, add chickpeas, cucumber, onion, tomatoes, olives, and parsley. Make a thorough mix. Salt freshly cracked pepper and 1 large lemon juice to taste.
3. Serve on its own or with arugula. It's delicious with pepperoncini and a squeeze of lemon juice on top. Drizzle with extra virgin olive oil if desired. To taste, season with salt and pepper.
4. This meal can be served at room temp, cold, or hot.

Nutritional Values

Fat 8.1g, Chol 14mg, Sodium 17mg, Potassium 99mg, Carbs 30g, Calories 221, Protein 7.1g

467. BLACK BEAN, CORN & AVOCADO SALAD

- Prep time: 15 mins, Cook time: 10 mins, Total time: 25 mins, Grill temp: 0, Servings: 6-8

Ingredients

- Black beans, 2 cans- 14 oz. drained and rinsed
- Corn, cut off cobs 2 ears- about 1 ½ cups
- Grape tomatoes dry pint- or about 1 ½ cups, quartered
- Jalapeno, 1 large

- Red onion, finely diced ½ small
- Avocado- firm but ripe, 1 finely diced
- Cilantro, loosely packed ½ cup chopped

Dressing
- Olive oil 2 – 3 tbsp
- Juicy lime 1 large- about 2 tbsp
- Apple cider vinegar, 1 tbsp optional
- Garlic, minced 2 cloves
- Cumin + chili powder ½ tsp

Directions

1. In a small bowl, whisk together the oil, lime juice, garlic, cumin, apple cider vinegar, chili powder, and a pinch of salt.
2. Combine the black beans, tomatoes, corn, jalapeno, red onion, avocado, and cilantro in a large mixing bowl. Toss the salad with the dressing to coat it evenly. To taste, season with salt and pepper.
3. Serve chilled or at room temp.

Nutritional Values

Fat 5.3g, Chol 12mg, Sodium 15mg, Potassium 94mg, Carbs 29g, Calories 181, Protein 9g

468. POZOLE- POSOLE VERDE

- Prep time: 10 mins, Cook time: 20 mins, Total time: 30 mins, Grill temp: 0, Servings: 6

Ingredients

- Olive oil 1 tbsp
- Onion, diced 1 large
- Jalapeno, diced 1 large
- Garlic 3 – 4 cloves, minced
- Cumin 1 heaping tsp
- Oregano 1 heaping tsp
- Hominy drained and rinsed 1 can- 25 – 28 oz.
- Pinto beans, 2 cans drained and rinsed
- Tomatillos- about 1 lb., 6 medium husks removed
- Vegetable broth 4 cups low Sodium
- 1 – 2 juicy limes

Directions

1. Heat the oil/water, add the onion, and cook for 5 mins in the Instant Pot. After adding the garlic, jalapeno, cumin, oregano, salt, and pepper, cook for 1 min, more, or until aromatic. In a large mixing bowl, combine pinto beans, tomatillos, hominy, and

vegetable broth. Place the lid on top and secure it. Set the SEALED position on a valve.

2. Set the pressure cooker to HIGH and manually set the timer for 20 mins. Allow 10 mins for natural release before switching the valve to VENTING to remove any remaining steam. Toss with lime juice and season with salt and pepper to taste.

Nutritional Values

Fat 14g, Chol 13mg, Sodium 9mg, Potassium 78mg, Carbs 16g, Calories 313, Protein 30g

469. LEMON ROSEMARY WHITE BEAN SOUP

- Prep time: 5 mins, Cook time: 10 mins, Total time: 15 mins, Grill temp: 0, Servings: 6

Ingredients

- Olive oil 2 tbsp
- Onion, diced 1 small
- Carrots, 3 large sliced or diced
- Celery, sliced 2 stalks
- Garlic, minced 2 cloves
- Dried thyme + rosemary ½ tsp each
- White beans, 3 cans- 15oz drained and rinsed
- Vegetable broth 4 – 5 cups low Sodium
- Tahini 2 tbsp
- Lemons, juice of 1-2

Directions

1. Sauté: In a large saucepan over medium heat, heat the oil or water, then add the carrots, onion, and celery and simmer for 7 mins. After adding the garlic, thyme, and rosemary, cook for another min.
2. Simmer: In a large mixing bowl, combine the white beans, tahini, vegetable broth, and pepper, stir well, bring to a boil, reduce heat to low, cover, and stew for 10 mins, occasionally stirring.
3. Remove from the fire, stir in the lemon juice, and cool slightly before serving. The soup thickens as it rests for a bit. Season with more salt, pepper, or herbs if desired.

Nutritional Values

Fat 8g, Chol 19mg, Sodium 6mg, Potassium 74mg, Carbs 46g, Calories 309, Protein 16g

470. GREEN BEANS ALMONDINE- AMANDINE

- Prep time: 5 mins, Cook time: 10 mins, Total time: 15 mins, Grill temp: 0, Servings: 6

Ingredients

- Green beans 12 oz. French
- Vegan butter 2 tbsp
- Slivered almonds ½ cup
- 1 – 2 lemons

Directions

1. Green Beans: Combine 1–2 cups water and a generous quantity of salt in a heavy-bottomed pot, then add green beans and bring to a boil. Reduce heat to medium-low and cook for 4–5 mins, uncovered, or until green beans have brightened in color. Green beans should be served on a dish or in a casserole. Cover to keep warm.
2. Almonds: In the same saucepan, melt the butter, add the almonds, and cook, often stirring, until golden, about 5–6 mins.
3. Season with salt and a squeeze of lemon before spreading the almonds on top of the green beans. Mix the ingredients in a serving dish rather than heaping them.

Nutritional Values

Fat 13g, Chol 19mg, Sodium 9.5mg, Potassium 87mg, Carbs 12.7g, Calories 168, Protein 4.3g

471. HEARTY LENTIL SOUP

- Prep time: 10 mins, Cook time: 40 mins, Total time: 50 mins, Grill temp: 0, Servings: 6

Ingredients

- Olive oil ¼ cup
- Onion, diced 1 medium
- Carrots- about 1 cup, 2 – 3 diced
- Celery ribs, diced 2
- Garlic, minced 3 cloves
- Green beans, 1 cup- 6oz.
- Diced tomatoes with juices 1 can- 14oz
- Baby potatoes, diced 1 lb.
- Dried brown 1 ½ cups
- Paprika 1 ½ tsp
- Cumin ½ tsp
- Curry ½ tsp
- Water 6 cups
- Baby spinach or kale 2 handfuls
- Lemon juice of 2 small

- Parsley chopped ½ cup

Directions

1. In an oven or saucepan, heat the water and olive oil over medium heat. Cook the carrots, celery, onions, and garlic for 5 mins.
2. Bring the green beans, lentils, paprika, curry, tomatoes, potatoes, cumin, and liquids to a boil, then lower the heat to low, cover, and simmer for 30–35 mins, occasionally stirring.
3. Add the greens 5 mins before the soup is done. If required, add up to 1 cup more water. Salt, pepper, and lemon juice to taste.
4. Top soup bowls with a dusting of fresh chopped parsley and a squeeze of lemon juice for added brightness. With vegan cornbread, vegan naan, or artisan bread, it's fantastic.

Nutritional Values

Fat 3g, Chol 16mg, Sodium 4.5mg, Potassium 73mg, Carbs 45g, Calories 270, Protein 18g

472. CHICKPEA TIKKA MASALA

- Prep time: 10 mins, Cook time: 40 mins, Total time: 50 mins, Grill temp: 0, Servings: 6

Ingredients

- Olive oil 2 tbsp
- Onion, diced 1 large
- Cumin seeds 1 tsp
- Garlic 3 – 4 cloves, minced
- Ginger 2-inch piece
- Ground coriander, 1 tbsp optional
- Turmeric 1 ½ tsp
- Garam masala 1 heaping tsp
- Cayenne ½ – 1 tsp
- Diced tomatoes, 2 cans- 14oz with juices
- Tomato paste 2 tbsp
- Chickpeas- garbanzo beans, 2 cans- 14oz drained and rinsed
- Coconut milk 1 can- 15oz.

Directions

1. Heat the oil or water in a large saucepan over medium heat, add the onions and cumin seeds, and cook for 5–7 mins, or

until the onions are brown around the edges.

2. After adding the ginger and garlic, cook for another 1 to 2 mins. With the garam masala, garam masala, turmeric, and cayenne, cook for 1–2 mins, or until fragrant.

3. Cook for 4 mins, or until the tomatoes are somewhat broken down. Reduce to low heat, occasionally stirring, and add the tomato paste, chickpeas, and coconut milk. Cook, covered, for 25 to 30 mins over low heat, occasionally stirring. To taste, season with salt and pepper.

4. Serve with quinoa, cilantro-lime rice, couscous, or vegan naan bread and rice.

Nutritional Values

Fat 9.4g, Chol 7mg, Sodium 9mg, Potassium 80mg, Carbs 34g, Calories 249, Protein 10.3g

473. 1 POT CHILI MAC

- Prep time: 10 mins, Cook time: 20 mins, Total time: 30 mins, Grill temp: 0, Servings: 6-8

Ingredients

- Olive oil 1 tbsp
- Onion, diced 1 large
- Garlic, minced 4 cloves
- Peppers- bell or poblano, 1 – 2 seeds removed and diced
- Tempeh crumbled 1 package- 8oz.
- Chili powder 1 – 2 tbsp
- Cumin 1 tsp
- Oregano 1 tsp
- Paprika- smoked or regular 1 tsp
- Red kidney beans, 1 can- 15oz. Drained and rinsed
- Sweet corn drained 1 can - 15oz.
- diced tomatoes 1 can- 28oz
- Vegetable broth 4 cups
- Dark beer- Modelo Negra 1 bottle
- Elbow pasta, about 2 ½ cups

Directions

1. Sauté: In an oven or saucepan, heat the oil/water over medium heat, then sauté the onion, peppers, garlic, and tempeh for 5 mins. Add the chili powder, cumin, paprika,

oregano, and salt and cook for 1 min, or until fragrant.

2. Simmer and boil: Toss in the tomatoes, beans, pasta, and corn, then add the liquids and stir to combine. Bring to a boil, then reduce to low heat and simmer for 10 mins, or until pasta is tender. Season with salt and pepper to taste. A sprinkle of cayenne pepper may be added to make it spicier.

Nutritional Values

Fat 9.8g, Chol 7mg, Sodium 7mg, Potassium 65mg, Carbs 65g, Calories 457, Protein 35g

474. BEAN CHILI

- Prep time: 5 mins, Cook time: 25 mins, Total time: 30 mins, Grill temp: 0, Servings: 4

Ingredients

- Olive oil 1 tbsp
- Onion, diced 1 large
- Garlic, minced 3 cloves
- Jalapenos, 2 seeds removed and diced
- Chili powder 3 tbsp
- Chipotle powder 1 tsp
- Black beans, 1 can- 15 oz. drained and rinsed
- Kidney beans, 1 can- 15 oz. drained and rinsed
- Pinto beans, 1 can- 15 oz. drained and rinsed
- Diced tomatoes, 1 can- 28oz with juices
- Cocoa powder, 1 tbsp optional
- Vegetable broth 1 ½ cups

Directions

1. Sauté: Heat the olive oil in a large saucepan over medium heat and sauté the onion for 7 mins, or until tender and translucent. After adding the garlic, jalapeno, chili, and chipotle powder, cook for 1 minute or until fragrant.

2. Simmer: Bring the beans, chocolate, tomatoes, and liquids to a boil, then reduce to low heat, cover, and simmer for 15–20 mins, occasionally to stir. Add more water as needed. Season with salt and pepper, as well as anything else you think it requires.

3. Serve with sweet chia cornbread or jalapeno cornbread muffins, sour cashew cream, and chopped green onions.

Fat 1.3g, Chol 7mg, Sodium 10mg, Potassium 23mg, Carbs 49g, Calories 243, Protein 1.4g

475. COLLARD GREENS

- Prep time: 10 mins, Cook time: 10 mins, Total time: 20 mins, Grill temp: 0, Servings: 3

Ingredients

- Olive oil 1 tbsp
- Diced onion 1 cup- shallot or onion
- Garlic 2 – 3 cloves, minced
- Diced tomatoes, diced 1 can- 14oz.
- Collard greens 1 bunch- 12 – 16 oz.
- Beans- chickpeas, cannellini, or pinto, 1 can- 14oz. Drained and rinsed
- Lemon juice 2 – 3 tbsp- 1 large or 2 small lemons
- Red pepper flakes- optional

Directions

1. In a large wok, heat the oil over medium heat. Add the onions and sauté for 4 mins or until softened. Cook for another min after adding the garlic.
2. After adding the collards, lemon juice, and salt and pepper, cook for another 4 mins.
3. Cook, occasionally stirring, until collards are wilted or beans and tomatoes are fully cooked, then add tomatoes and beans. The ultimate Cook time may vary depending on how tender you want your collards.
4. Serve in separate dishes with a squeeze of lemon. The meal is completed with warm corn tortillas, naan and crusty bread, and a tall drink of lemon water.

Nutritional Values

Fat 6.8g, Chol 5mg, Sodium 15mg, Potassium 32mg, Carbs 27.7g, Calories 192, Protein 8.5g

476. RUSTIC CABBAGE, POTATO & WHITE BEAN SOUP

- Prep time: 10 mins, Cook time: 40 mins, Total time: 50 mins, Grill temp: 0, Servings: 6

Ingredients

- Water ¼ cup
- Leeks sliced and rinsed 2
- Carrots, diced 2
- Celery, diced 2 stalks
- Garlic, minced 2 – 3 cloves
- Herbs de Provence 1 tbsp
- diced tomatoes 1 can- 15 oz.
- Vegetable broth 5 – 6 cups low-Sodium
- Gold potatoes, diced 3 medium- 1 lb.
- Cabbage- about 4 cups, ½ head large sliced- savoy or green
- Cooked white beans 3 cups
- Parsley, to garnish ¼ cup chopped

Directions

1. Leeks should be cleaned by slicing off the dark green parts as well as the root end. Cut in ½ lengthwise with a sharp knife. Run under cold running water to remove debris between the leaf sheaths, breaking up the layers as you rinse. Cut into thin horizontal slices on a flat surface- widthwise.
2. Sauté: In an oven or stockpot, heat the water/oil until it boils, then add the leeks, carrots, and celery and simmer for 5 mins. It already smells fantastic! Cook for another min or until the garlic and spices are aromatic.
3. Combine the remaining ingredients: tomatoes, beans, potatoes, cabbage, and vegetable broth in a large mixing bowl.
4. Cook, occasionally stirring, for 20–30 mins, or until potatoes and cabbage are tender. Bring to a boil, then reduce to a low heat setting. Season with salt and pepper to taste, if needed.
5. Serve with gluten-free socca, crusty artisan bread, and parsley on the side. Enjoy.

Nutritional Values

Fat 2g, Chol 3mg, Sodium 5mg, Potassium 12mg, Carbs 49g, Calories 247, Protein 10.3g

477. BARLEY BOWL

- Prep time: 10 mins, Cook time: 50 mins, Total time: 10 mins, Grill temp: 0, Servings: 3

Ingredients

- Dried pearl barley 1 cup
- Water 2 ¾ cups
- Olive oil divided into 2 tbsp

- Butternut squash 1 small- about 2 ½ cups, diced
- Onion, sliced ½ small
- Great northern, 1 can- 15 oz. Drained and rinsed
- Baby spinach 2 – 3 handfuls
- Garlic powder generous dash
- Dried thyme ½ tsp
- Avocado, to serve

Directions

1. Preheat the oven to 400°F - 200°C.
2. In a medium-sized pot, combine barley and water and bring to a boil. Cover, reduce to low heat, and cook for 45 mins. Before fluffing with a fork, remove the cover and let it rest for 5–10 mins. Any leftover beverages should be emptied.
3. While your barley is cooking, cube your butternut squash into ¾ to 1-inch chunks. Place in a roasting pan coated with parchment, Silpat, or gently oiled. In a mixing dish, combine the squash, 1 tbsp olive oil, thyme, and salt. Place on the middle rake for 25–30 mins, stirring once. It's done when a fork easily pierces the squash.
4. **Beans**: In a medium-sized pan, heat the remaining olive oil over medium heat, add the onions, and cook for about 5 mins. Cook until the spinach has wilted- covering the pan will help the spinach wilt faster; then stir in the beans and a splash of garlic powder.
5. Divide the barley, beans, and butternut squash into separate bowls to serve. On the side, serve with sliced avocado.
6. Season with pepper to taste and serve with avocado.

Nutritional Values

Fat 2.3g, Chol 5mg, Sodium 16mg, Potassium 26mg, Carbs 73.5g, Calories 354, Protein 12.5g

478. KALE + BLACK BEAN BURRITO BOWL

- Prep time: 5 mins, Cook time: 15 mins, Total time: 20 mins, Grill temp: 0, Servings: 3

Ingredients

- Dry quinoa 1 cup
- Water 1 ¾ cups
- Garlic powder ½ tsp
- Onion Powder ½ tsp
- Red pepper flakes ½ tsp

Kale
- Kale ½ bunch
- Limes 1 – 2

Chipotle tahini sauce
- Tahini 3 tbsp
- Water 2 – 3 tbsp
- Juice of ½ lime
- Chipotle powder 1/8 – ¼ tsp
- Dash garlic + onion powder

To serve
- Black beans 1 can- 15 oz.
- Pico de Gallo 1 batch
- Avocado, sliced 1
- Lime wedges
- Cilantro, chopped

Directions

1. **Quinoa**: In a medium saucepan, bring quinoa, water, garlic and onion powder, and red pepper flakes to a boil. Cover, reduce to low heat, and cook for 15 mins. Before fluffing with a fork, remove the cover and let it rest for 10 mins. Almost sure there will be some leftovers.
2. After removing the core stem, rinse the kale and julienne it. 1–2 limes, squeezed over the top, stirred to coat, and set aside to allow the kale to marinate.
3. To prepare the chipotle dressing, whisk together all of the ingredients in a small bowl. Taste for flavor and make any necessary adjustments. Add a bit more tahini if you want it thicker and a little more water if you want it thinner. Allow for flavor melding by setting it away for a few mins.
4. Whether or not to cook the beans is entirely up to you. If you're reheating the beans, combine them with the liquids in a small saucepan and heat over medium heat until they're warm. If the beans haven't been heated, drain, and rinse them well.
5. In a serving dish, combine the cooked quinoa, beans, and greens. On top, there's pico de Gallo, avocado, and chipotle tahini sauce. Put a few broken tortilla chips or

pepitas over the top for a crunchy accent. Combine all of the ingredients in a mixing bowl and serve.

Nutritional Values

Fat 12g, Chol 7mg, Sodium 9mg, Potassium 30mg, Carbs 58g, Calories 424, Protein 24g

479. ROASTED POBLANO TACOS

- Prep time: 10 mins, Cook time: 10 mins, Total time: 20 mins, Grill temp: 0, Servings: 3

Ingredients

- Poblano chiles 2 medium
- Pinto, black beans 1 can- 15 oz.
- Scallions, sliced 2
- Cabbage, shredded purple or green
- Cilantro
- Avocado, sliced
- Corn tortillas 6
- Lime wedges to serve

Directions

1. Preheat the broiler to high and arrange the poblanos on a baking sheet. Broil for 7–10 mins, turning every few mins to ensure equal sear and browning on both sides. Poblanos will crackle and pop as they cook, and when a fork is put against their side, they will be burned and softened. Fill a bowl halfway with poblanos and steam for a few mins, covered with a plate or plastic wrap. Remove the skin, lay the peeled poblano on a flat surface, make a slit across the center, and scoop out the seeds. Cut the lengthwise slices into ½ " strips using a sharp knife.
2. In a small saucepan, cook the beans over medium heat, occasionally stirring, until they are warm. Add a dash or 2 of garlic powder to give pinto or black beans a bit extra flavor. Drain and rinse canned whole beans before using them if you don't want to cook them.
3. Chop the scallions, purple cabbage, and avocado for the veggies. On a gas/electric burner, heat the tortillas until they are slightly charred.
4. Layer beans, poblanos, avocado, cabbage, scallions, cilantro, a pinch of pink salt, and

a dollop of cashew cream or sriracha on top of your tacos.

Nutritional Values

Fat 9.2g, Chol 6mg, Sodium 5mg, Potassium 37mg, Carbs 58g, Calories 345, Protein 13.1g

480. CREAMY DILL POTATO SALAD

- Prep time: 10 mins, Cook time: 20 mins, Total time: 30 mins, Grill temp: 0, Servings: 8

Ingredients

- Potatoes- red or gold 2 ½ lbs.
- Chickpeas- garbanzo beans, 1 can- 14 oz. Drained and rinsed- optional
- Celery, diced ½ cup
- Red onion, ¾ cup finely diced
- Fresh dill, chopped ¼ – 1/3 cup

Dressing

- Tahini 4 heaping tbsp
- Dijon mustard 2 tbsp
- Lemon, juice of 1 juicy

Directions

1. **Potatoes**: Place potatoes in a large saucepan with enough water to cover them and a fair amount of salt. Bring to a boil, then reduce to low heat and continue to cook for 13–15 mins, or until fork-tender. Drain and put the potatoes aside to cool. After the skin has cooled, gently remove it. Pinch the skin between your thumb and index finger, and it will move; the skin should simply slip off. Potatoes should be chopped into ½-inch to 3/4-inch chunks.
2. While the potatoes are cooking and cooling, prepare the onion, celery, dill, and chickpeas.
3. Whisk together the tahini/mayo, mustard, lemon juice, and pepper in a small bowl to prepare the dressing. Make a thorough mix. If using tahini, gradually add water until you get the desired consistency. Thin the dressing with a bit more water and lemon juice if it's too thick.
4. Mix the following materials: In a large mixing basin, combine the potatoes, chickpeas, onion, celery, and dill- or the saucepan you used to boil the potatoes in. Pour the dressing over the top and

thoroughly mix it in. To taste, season with mineral salt and freshly cracked pepper.
5. As an appetizer or a Sides, this dish is delicious.

Nutritional Values

Fat 10.2g, Chol 8mg, Sodium 14mg, Potassium 30mg, Carbs 29.8g, Calories 221.9, Protein 4.8g

481. BALELA SALAD

- Prep time: 10 mins, Cook time: 5 mins, Total time: 15 mins, Grill temp: 0, Servings: 6

Ingredients

- Chickpeas- garbanzo beans, 2 cans- 14 oz. Drained and rinsed
- Black beans, 1 can- 14 oz. Drained and rinsed
- Roma tomatoes, 2 firm seeds removed and diced
- Red onion, diced ½
- English cucumber, diced ½
- Garlic, minced 3 cloves
- Fresh mint, chopped 2 tbsp
- Fresh parsley, chopped ¼ cup
- Sumac 1 tsp
- Olive oil 3 – 4 tbsp
- Lemon juice of 1 large

Directions

1. Combine the chickpeas, onion, cucumber, black beans, tomatoes, garlic, mint, and parsley in a large mixing bowl. Toss in the sumac, olive oil, lemon juice, and pepper to taste. Whisk everything together well to get a smooth mix.
2. Refrigerate or serve at room temp. Refrigerate leftovers in an airtight jar for up to 5 days.
3. This salad is wonderful when served with hummus and arugula on pita bread. Toss in a large handful of arugulas and serve with pita bread and hummus on the side.

Nutritional Values

Fat 10.3g, Chol 9mg, Sodium 14mg, Potassium 22mg, Carbs 38g, Calories 281, Protein 12.6g

482. BLACK BEAN + QUINOA BURRITOS

- Prep time: 15 mins, Cook time: 55 mins, Total time: 1 hr 10 mins, Grill temp: 375°F, Servings: 6-8

Ingredients

- Dried quinoa ½ cup
- Water ¾ cup + 1
- Olive oil 1 tbsp
- Red onion diced ½ large
- Orange bell pepper, 1 seed removed and diced
- Diced tomatoes, 1 can- 14oz drained
- Zucchini, diced 1 medium
- Black beans, 2 cans- 14 oz. drained and rinsed
- Corn drained 1 can- 14 oz.
- Cilantro, roughly chopped ¼ – ½ cup
- Cumin 2 tsp
- Chili powder 1 tsp
- Chipotle powder ¾ – 1 tsp
- Garlic powder 1 tsp
- Onion Powder ½ tsp
- Tortillas 6 – 8 medium/large

Directions

1. Quinoa: In a small/medium saucepan, combine the quinoa and water, bring to a boil, cover, reduce heat to low, and cook for 13 mins. Before fluffing with a fork, remove the cover and set it aside for 10 mins.
2. Filling: In a large skillet or pot, heat the oil/water over medium heat, add the onion and cook for 4 mins; add the bell pepper, and cook for another 2 mins. After adding the tomatoes, zucchini, and corn, cook for another 3 mins or so. Continue to cook until the black beans, chipotle, garlic, quinoa, cilantro, cumin, and onion powder, as well as the salt, are fully cooked.
3. Place the tortillas on a flat surface, top with a mound of filling, leaving enough room all the way around, fold it in ½, fold up every end, and roll the burrito away from you to seal it fully.
4. Wrap in Saran wrap, Freeze using foil, freezer paper, or whatever freezing method you're used to. If using paper sandwich bags, consume them within a few weeks to avoid freezer burn. They're not going to last very long!

5. Warm for 10 mins in a toaster oven at 375°F or 30 seconds in the microwave if room temp. If frozen, reheat for 30 mins in a 375°F oven or 1: 30–2 mins in the microwave.
6. Serve with sliced avocado and your favorite salsa.

483. REFRIED BEANS

- Prep time: 10 mins, Cook time: 10 hr, Total time: 10 hr 10 mins, Grill temp: 0, Servings: 8

Ingredients

- Dried pinto beans 1 lb.
- Onion, chopped 1 small
- Garlic, chopped 2 – 3 cloves
- Cumin 1 tsp
- Chili powder 1 tsp
- Jalapeno, optional 1
- Bay leaves 2
- Black pepper 1 – 2 tsp
- Vegetable broth 9 cups

Directions

1. Begin by washing the beans completely. Place the beans in a colander and rinse them under cold running water. Remove any beans that have a strange shape or are unappealing.
2. In a slow cooker, combine all of the ingredients. Add the beans, cumin, chili powder, jalapeño, onions, garlic, bay leaves, salt, pepper, and liquids to the slow cooker's bowl.
3. Low heat is used for cooking the beans. Cook for 8–10 hr on HIGH in the slow cooker.
4. It is necessary to drain the beans. Allow the beans to cool for a few mins before draining the liquid and storing up to 2 cups.
5. The beans should be pureed or mashed. Using a potato masher, mash and puree the beans until smooth. Thin with as much of the liquids you've stored as you need.

Alternatively, leave all beans as it is for charro or ranchero style beans.
6. Taste it to see whether it's delicious. Season to taste, then season with more salt and pepper if necessary.

484. HEALTHY BAKED BEANS

- Prep time: 10 mins, Cook time: 30 mins, Total time: 40 mins, Grill temp: 0, Servings: 6-8

Ingredients

- Water ¼ cup
- Onion, diced 1 medium
- Smoked paprika 2 tsp
- Garlic powder 1 heaping tsp
- Dried white beans 1 1b. Small
- Vegetable broth 4 cups low Sodium
- Pure maple syrup 1/3 cup
- Tomato paste ¼ cup
- Apple cider vinegar ¼ cup
- Mustard 2 tbsp
- Fresh ground pepper ½ tsp
- Bay leaves 2

Optional add-ins
- Jalapeno
- Green bell pepper
- Unsulfured blackstrap molasses 2 – 4 tbsp

Directions

1. Use the sauté option on your Instant Pot to add ¼ cup of water. Add the onion to the pan once it is hot and cook for 4 mins. After adding the smoked paprika and garlic powder, cook for 1 min, or until fragrant, stirring frequently.
2. Then, mix the beans, broth, apple cider vinegar, tomato paste, maple syrup, mustard, bay leaves, and pepper until the tomato paste is completely dissolved and everything is well combined.
3. Make sure the vent is adjusted to seal before putting the lid on top. After pushing the pressure cooker button, manually set the pressure cooker HIGH for 75 mins. Allow the steam to vent for 20 mins. If there is still steam present, move the vent to the open position, careful not to burn

yourself. Remove the lid and set it aside to cool somewhat before seasoning to taste with salt. After removing the bay leaves, transfer the beans to a serving dish.

4. The beans will thicken after they have cooled. If the mixture is too thick, add a little water until the desired consistency is reached, stirring thoroughly after each addition.

Nutritional Values

Fat 0.5g, Chol 3.6mg, Sodium 15.8mg, Potassium 19mg, Carbs 27g, Calories 119, Protein 6g

485. CHICKPEA NOODLE SOUP

- Prep time: 10 mins, Cook time: 20 mins, Total time: 30 mins, Grill temp: 0, Servings: 6-8

Ingredients

- Olive oil 1 tbsp
- Onion, diced 1
- Carrots, peeled and diced 3 large
- Ribs celery, 3 sliced
- Dried thyme, 1 tsp each basil, and oregano
- Chickpeas 2 cans- garbanzo beans
- Rotini pasta 12 – 16 ounces
- Water 10 – 12 cups
- Fresh chopped parsley ¼ cup
- Lemon wedges to serve

Directions

1. Sauté: In a stockpot or oven, heat the oil over medium heat, add the onion, carrots, celery, and herbs, and cook for 5–6 mins, stirring often.
2. Simmer: Combine the pasta, chickpeas, and liquids in a large pot, bring to a boil, then reduce to low heat and simmer for 6–7 mins, or until pasta is al dente.
3. After tossing in the chopped parsley, season to taste with salt and pepper.
4. Serve with lemon wedges for squeezing and pour into individual bowls.

Nutritional Values

Fat 8.3g, Chol 10mg, Sodium 19mg, Potassium 79mg, Carbs 53g, Calories 319, Protein 8.4g

486. CRISPY CHICKPEAS

- Prep time: 10 mins, Cook time: 45 mins, Total time: 55 mins, Grill temp: 400°F, Servings: 3

Ingredients

- Chickpeas- garbanzo beans 1 can- 15oz
- Olive oil 1 – 2 tsp
- Flavor seasoning – 1 tsp garlic salt

Directions

1. Preheat the oven to 400°F.
2. Drain and rinse canned chickpeas in a colander under cold running water if using canned chickpeas.
3. Place the chickpeas between the 2 sides of a large dish towel and flour sack to dry. Roll the chickpeas with your hands flat on the counter, moving towards the garbanzo beans with your palm and extended fingers. Make every effort to get rid of as much moisture as possible.
4. Remove any loose skins by gently pressing the chickpeas between your thumb and index finger after they have dried to remove any skins that have become detached or loosened. Roll the chickpeas 1 more time for good measure.
5. Spread the chickpeas out on a rimmed baking sheet that has been lightly oiled or covered with parchment paper or Silpat. Toss with a drizzle of olive oil and a pinch of salt and pepper to coat. Arrange the chickpeas on the baking sheet in a single layer. Preheat the oven to 400°F and bake for 40–45 mins, stirring every 10 mins. Allow it cool for a few mins before using or storing.

Nutritional Values

Fat 3.9g, Chol 7mg, Sodium 13mg, Potassium 65mg, Carbs 16g, Calories 119, Protein 6g

487. BLACK BEANS

- Prep time: 10 mins, Cook time: 40 mins, Total time: 50 mins, Grill temp: 0, Servings: 5

Ingredients

- Dried black beans, 1 lb. Rinsed, and odd beans removed
- White onion, diced 1 small
- Garlic, diced 3 cloves
- Jalapeno, 1 seed removed and diced
- Cumin 1 tsp

- Oregano, optional 1 tsp
- Pepper 1 tsp
- Bay leaves 2
- Water or vegetable broth 4 cups

1. Cleaning the beans is the first step. Rinse the beans in a colander under cold running water. Remove any beans that are strangely shaped and discard them.
2. In the instant pot, combine all of the ingredients. Before adding the liquids, put the black beans, onions, garlic, cumin, and jalapeno- if using bay leaves, salt, and pepper in the instant pot's bowl.
3. In a pressure cooker, cook the beans. Manually set the Instant Pot to Increased pressure for 35 mins after closing the vent to sealing. After the pressure cooker has completed normally, allow it to vent for around 25 mins.
4. Taste it to see whether it's delicious. Season the beans with lime juice, salt, and pepper to taste.
5. The beans will absorb any remaining liquids as they cool. Remove the bay leaves before serving.

Nutritional Values

Fat 0.4g, Chol 9mg, Sodium 18mg, Potassium 78mg, Carbs 21g, Calories 114, Protein 8g

488. RED BEANS & RICE

- Prep time: 10 mins, Cook time: 50 mins, Total time: 60 mins, Grill temp: 0, Servings: 6

Ingredients

- Dried red beans 1 lb.
- Yellow onion, diced 1 large
- Garlic, minced 5 cloves
- Green bell pepper, 1 large cored and diced
- Celery, sliced 3 – 4 stalks
- Cajun or creole seasoning 1 tbsp
- Oregano, 1 tsp each thyme, and smoked paprika
- Hot sauce, 1 tsp tabasco or sriracha
- Bay leaves 2 – 3
- Vegetable broth 4 cups
- Vegan sausage, optional
- Fresh parsley, chopped ¼ cup

Directions

1. Cleaning the beans is the first step. Rinse the beans in a colander under cold running water. Remove any beans that are strangely shaped and discard them- no soaking required.
2. In the instant pot, combine all of the ingredients. In the instant pot's bowl, combine the red beans, onions, bell pepper, oregano, bell pepper, garlic, spice, bay leaves, salt, pepper, and liquids.
3. In a pressure cooker, cook the beans. Manually set the Instant Pot to Increased pressure for 50 mins and close the vent to SEAL- or 60 mins if using kidney beans. When you're done, let for 20–25 mins of natural pressure cooker steam venting.
4. Season with salt and pepper to taste after adding the sausage. Remove the bay leaves from the dish and set them aside. Add the sausage and parsley if desired. Season with as much black pepper as required after tasting for seasoning. The beans will absorb any remaining liquids as they cool. To produce a thicker sauce that resembles gravy, mash some of the beans against the bowel wall with the back of a fork.
5. Make the rice ahead of time. While the beans are pressure cooking, make the rice according to package directions, using at least 1 cup of rice.

Nutritional Values

Fat 11g, Chol 14mg, Sodium 9mg, Potassium 98mg, Carbs 41g, Calories 314, Protein 15g

489. PEANUT BUTTER PLUS RICE CRISPY CACAO NIBS TREATS

- Prep time: 5 mins, Cook time: 30 mins, Total time: 35 mins, Grill temp: 0, Servings: 9

Ingredients

- Brown rice syrup 1 cup
- Natural peanut butter 1 cup
- Rice crispy cereal 5 cups
- Cacao nibs 1/3 cup

Directions

1. Line a 9 × 9 square pan with parchment paper. Alternatively, lightly coat the pan with coconut oil and non-dairy butter.

2. In a large saucepan or skillet, warm peanut butter and rice syrup on low heat, stirring often. Remove the pan from the heat and stir in the rice crispy cereal until almost all of it has been integrated. Mix in the cacao nibs until they're evenly distributed.
3. Place the ingredients in the prepared pan/dish and gently but firmly press them down until they are evenly distributed and crushed.
4. Cut into squares and serve right away, or chill for 30 mins to harden the pan/dish.

Nutritional Values

Fat 17.9g, Chol 17mg, Sodium 23mg, Potassium 83mg, Carbs 46g, Calories 359, Protein 17g

490. TERIYAKI TOFU-TEMPEH CASSEROLE

- Prep time: 10 mins, Cook time: 30 mins, Total time: 40 mins, Grill temp: 400 °F, Servings: 6

Ingredients

- Organic tofu cubed 10 oz.
- Tempeh, cubed 8 oz.
- Combo of snow peas 12 oz.
- Long grain rice 1 cup

Teriyaki sauce
- Tamari ¾ cup
- Water ¾ cup
- Pure maple syrup ½ cup
- Ground ginger ½ tsp
- Garlic powder, minced ½ tsp
- Cornstarch 2 tbsp

Directions

1. Preheat the oven to 400°F.
2. Begin by preparing the tofu for the tofu tempeh. Drain the tofu and place it between 2 clean folded dish towels, then place a medium saucepan on top to absorb the excess liquid for about 10 mins. If you're using extra-firm tofu, you may skip this step. Cube the final product into 3/4- to 1-inch cubes. Also, cut the tempeh into cubes.
3. Follow these Directions to prepare the teriyaki sauce: In a small saucepan, bring the tamari, maple syrup/sugar, water, ginger, and garlic to a boil, then reduce to low and cook for 1 min. In a small bowl, whisk together the cornstarch/tapioca powder and the water until smooth. Before adding the mixture to the teriyaki sauce, cook for another min or until the sauce thickens. Turn off the heat, cover the pan, and set it aside. Taste it to see whether it's delicious. Add a tbsp or 2 of your chosen sweeteners if you want a sweeter teriyaki sauce.
4. Place tofu and tempeh in a 9x13 casserole or baking dish, pour in 1 cup teriyaki sauce, and gently toss to coat. On the middle shelf of the oven, bake for 20–25 mins. Preheat the oven to 350°F.
5. Follow the package directions for cooking the rice. Rice Cook times vary, with some reaching up to 40 mins. If you're making longer-cooking rice, get started as soon as possible.
6. Use a bamboo steamer, microwave, or any other method to steam the veggies.
7. Toss everything together: set aside the tofu and tempeh in the cooked dish, then add the cooked rice and steamed vegetables. Toss with the remaining teriyaki sauce, reserving a small portion for serving. If required, go to the next step to warm up completely.
8. Serve with a drizzle of the remaining sauce on separate plates. On top, a dusting of toasted sesame seeds would be great.

Nutritional Values

Fat 7.2g, Chol 6mg, Sodium 14mg, Potassium 78mg, Carbs 123g, Calories 692, Protein 35g

491. SPANISH VEGAN PAELLA

- Prep time: 20 mins, Cook time: 25 mins, Total time: 45 mins, Grill temp: 0, Servings: 6

Ingredients

- Saffron or turmeric ½ heaping tsp
- Olive oil 2 tbsp
- Yellow onion, 1 large thinly sliced
- Bell peppers 2- red, orange, or yellow
- Garlic, minced 4 cloves
- Green beans 1 ½ cups
- Tomatoes, 1 lb.- 16 oz.
- Smoked paprika 1 ½ tsp
- Red pepper flakes, 1 tsp optional
- Bay leaves 2 – 3

- Short grain rice 1 ½ cups
- Vegetable broth 3 ½ cups low sodium
- Artichoke hearts in water, 1 can/jar- 14 oz. drained and quartered
- Green peas 1 cup- fresh or frozen, thawed
- Parsley leaves, chopped to garnish
- Lemon wedges to serve

Directions

1. Saffron steeping: Soak the saffron threads in warm water for 10 mins.
2. Heat some olive oil/broth in a paella pan over medium heat. Cook, occasionally turning, until the onions & bell peppers are tender, about 5 mins. With the garlic, green beans, red pepper flakes, tomatoes, smoked paprika, and bay leaves, cook for another 3 mins, stirring often. Cook for another 7 mins or so for softer veggies after adding the remaining ingredients, for a total of 10 mins.
3. In a large saucepan, combine the rice, broth, saffron mixture/turmeric, and salt. Move the vegetables around gently so that the rice falls to the pan's bottom as much as possible.
4. Bring to a boil, then reduce to low heat and simmer, uncovered, for 15 mins at a steady, moderate boil. It's not a good idea to stir the rice. If you're using a large paella pan- 15 inches or more, periodically rotate it over the heat to let the rice cook evenly. Stay in the kitchen and tidy up so you can adjust the pan quickly if needed. If liquids seem to be boiling off too quickly, add a little extra warm water/broth.
5. Cook for a further 5 mins after adding the peas and artichoke hearts after 15 mins of boiling.
6. Cover to steam: Turn off the heat and cover for 10 mins with a kitchen towel or similar appropriate cover. The rice will absorb the remaining liquid while boiling the peas and warming the artichoke hearts and other optional ingredients specified below. When the rice is done, fluff it lightly with a fork before serving. Remove the bay leaves before eating. Season with salt, pepper, or more paprika to taste.

7. Garnish with chopped parsley before serving. This meal is perfect with a side of fresh greens and a squeeze of lemon on top. Serve right away from the pan or in individual dishes.

Nutritional Values

Fat 8.7g, Chol 7mg, Sodium 15mg, Potassium 65mg, Carbs 51g, Calories 332, Protein 9g

492. LEMON CHICKPEA ORZO SOUP

- Prep time: 10 mins, Cook time: 20 mins, Total time: 30 mins, Grill temp: 0, Servings: 4

Ingredients

- Olive oil 1 tbsp
- Onion, diced ½
- Carrots, 3 peeled and diced
- Garlic, minced 3 cloves
- Vegetable broth 7 – 8 cups
- Whole wheat orzo 1 cup
- Chickpeas- garbanzo beans, 2 cans- 15oz. Drained and rinsed
- Tahini 1/3 cup
- Lemon juice ¼ – ½ cup- about 2 – 4 large lemons
- Fresh baby kale or spinach, a large handful
- Chopped fresh dill to taste

Directions

1. Heat the oil or water over medium heat, add the onion and carrot, sauté for 5–7 mins, add the garlic, and cook for 1 min more.
2. Bring the broth or water to a boil, then add the orzo or chickpeas, reduce to medium-low heat, and cook for 8 to 9 mins, or until the orzo is tender.
3. Take the pan off the heat and mix in the tahini and lemon juice- start with a tiny quantity of juice and add more to the taste. Toss in the young kale or spinach, and the greens will soften and wilt in just a few mins. Season to taste with salt and pepper, as well as a lot of dills as you want. Because the soup will thicken after sitting for a bit, add more liquids as needed.
4. To scoop up all of the luscious juices, serve in separate dishes with crusty artisan bread.

Nutritional Values

Fat 3.9g, Chol 13mg, Sodium 23mg, Potassium 83mg, Carbs 35g, Calories 196, Protein 7g

493. ROSEMARY BREAD

- Prep time: 20 mins, Cook time: 1 hr 40 mins, Total time: 2 hr, Grill temp: 0, Servings: 8 – 10

Ingredients

- 1 & ¾ cups water warm
- 1 package dry yeast active
- 1 tbsp sugar cane
- 3 & ½ cups flour all-purpose
- 1 & ½ cups flour whole wheat
- 1 bulb Garlic Roasted
- 2 tbsp rosemary chopped
- ½ tsp pepper flakes red

Directions

1. In a medium basin, combine the yeast, sugar, and water. Allow 5 mins for the yeast to froth up in a warm location.
2. In the stand mixer bowl with the dough hook connected, combine the salt, flours, olive oil, and yeast mixture. Mix for 5-6 mins or until the dough forms a spherical around the hook.
3. Place on a floured surface and roll into a ball. Knead your dough many times, adding more flour as needed. Brush your dough with olive oil and place it in a basin. Cover and set aside for 40-50 mins to double in size.
4. Coat a baking sheet that measures 10 inches by 15 inches with the remaining 14 cups of olive oil and flour. After the dough has been pounded down, knead it several times. The dough will be spread to the pan's edges by pushing the dough firmly into the pan's edges. With your fingers, make indentations in the dough at few-inch intervals. Cover the baking sheet with plastic wrap and let the dough rise for about 40 mins, or until it doubles in size.
5. Preheat the oven to 425°F - 200°C. Remove the plastic wrap and throw it away. To use roasted garlic, split each clove in ½ and rub the garlic paste into the dough with your fingers.
6. Bake for 20 mins, stirring regularly, until the cheese has melted and the topping has become brown.

Fat 6.3g, Chol 9mg, Sodium 16mg, Potassium 94mg, Carbs 58g, Calories 453, Protein 14g

494. VEGETABLE CHILI

- Prep time: 10 mins, Cook time: 1 hr 40 mins, Total time: 1 hr 50 mins, Grill temp: 0, Servings: 6

Ingredients

- Red onion, diced 1
- Carrots- about 1 cup, 2 large peeled and diced
- Celery 2 sticks- about 1 cup, diced
- Diced green chilis 1 can- 4oz.
- Diced tomatoes, 1 can- 14 oz. With juices
- Sweet corn drained 1 can - 14 oz.
- Tempeh crumbled 8 oz. Package
- Kidney beans, 1 can- 14 oz. drained and rinsed
- Black beans, 1 can- 14 oz. drained and rinsed
- Tomato paste 1 can- 6 oz.
- Chili powder 2 tbsp
- Cumin 1 tbsp
- Coriander 1 tsp
- Garlic powder 1 tsp
- Chipotle powder ½ tsp
- Water 2 cups
- Dried quinoa, optional ½ cup

Directions

1. Combine all of the ingredients in an oven or pot, stir well, come to a boil, reduce to low heat and simmer for 1 to 1 ½ hr, occasionally stirring.
2. To serve, garnish with your preferred toppings.

Nutritional Values

Fat 6.6g, Chol 2mg, Sodium 22mg, Potassium 34mg, Carbs 35g, Calories 230, Protein 11g

Chapter 13.

Grains Recipes

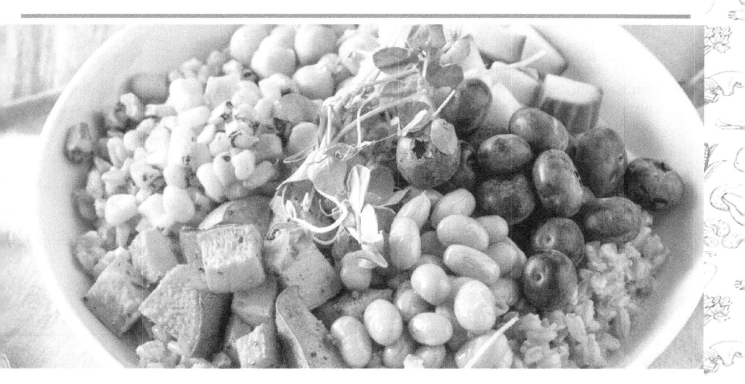

495. INGREDIENTS MEXICAN QUINOA

- Prep time: 20 mins, Cook time: 15 mins, Total time: 35 mins, Grill temp: 0, Servings: 4

Ingredients

- 1 cup fresh or frozen corn kernels
- 3 cups of cooked white quinoa or 1 cup of uncooked
- 1- 15 oz. can of organic black beans
- 1 cup jarred salsa
- 1 tbsp ground cumin
- Cilantro to garnish optional

Directions

1. Heat the oil in a large skillet over medium heat. Cook, occasionally stirring, until the corn is tender, about 3 mins.
2. In a mixing bowl, combine the cumin and quinoa. Continue to cook the quinoa until it becomes somewhat crunchy and heated. It takes around 3 mins to complete.
3. Add the salsa and continue to cook for another 2 mins, or until everything is well combined and the quinoa begins to dry up.
4. Remove from the heat and let it cool for 5–10 mins before fluffing with a fork.
5. If desired, garnish with chopped cilantro.

Nutritional Values

Fat 6g, Chol 3mg, Sodium 5mg, Potassium 12mg, Carbs 70g, Calories 348, Protein 23g

496. HEALTHY HUEVOS RANCHEROS TACOS

- Prep time: 5 mins, Cook time: 10 mins, Total time: 15 mins, Grill temp: 0, Servings: 2

Ingredients

- 1 tsp coconut oil
- 6 tortilla shells, small corns
- 1 cup organic can of black beans
- 1 cup eggplant whites
- 2 eggplants
- 1 cup salsa, prepared
- ½ cup mashed avocado or prepared guacamole
- Salt and pepper- to taste
- 1 lemon
- ½ cup cilantro, chopped

Directions

1. In a frying pan over medium heat, melt the oil.
2. Mix in the beans and ½ a cup of salsa.
3. Make holes in the bean mixture, then break the eggplants into them and swirl the whites in.
4. Season to taste with salt and pepper.
5. Reduce the heat to low and cover for 5 mins while the eggplants cook.
6. Warm the tortilla shells in a separate small skillet and divide them between 2 plates.
7. Add the leftover salsa, mashed avocado, or guacamole with fresh lime and cilantro on the top.

Nutritional Values

Fat 2g, Chol 5mg, Sodium 10mg, Potassium 15mg, Carbs 54g, Calories 198, Protein 3g

497. VANILLA VEGAN BUCKWHEAT PANCAKES

- Prep time: 5 mins, Cook time: 25 mins, Total time: 30 mins, Grill temp: 0, Servings: 4

Ingredients

- 1 ¼ cups flour- buckwheat
- ¼ cup tapioca flour
- 1 ½ tsp baking powder
- 2 tbsp coconut sugar
- 1 tbsp apple cider vinegar
- 2 tsp vanilla essence
- 1 ½ cups almond milk/drinking coconut/cashew milk

Directions

1. In a large mixing bowl, combine the flours- buckwheat and tapioca. Stir in the coconut sugar to combine.
2. Sift the flour into a well, then sprinkle the baking powder on top.
3. Pour the apple cider vinegar over it and wait for it to bubble. As a consequence, the baking powder becomes activated.
4. Using a whisk, combine the milk and vanilla essence- avoid over-mixing the ingredients.
5. In a frying pan, heat a tiny amount of coconut oil over medium heat. Start by pouring pancake batter into the pan and cooking 3 at a time.
6. Cook for 2 mins on each side.

7. Place a clean tea towel on a plate, then transfer the first stack of pancakes to the platter and cover with the tea towel. To make the remaining pancakes, repeat the procedure.

Fat 8.3g, Chol 5mg, Sodium 7mg, Potassium 10mg, Carbs 43g, Calories 307, Protein 10g

498. CHOCOLATE CHIP, APRICOT, AND ORANGE SCONES

- Prep time: 10 mins, Cook time: 25 mins, Total time: 35 mins, Grill temp: 435°F, Servings: 2

Ingredients

- cup of whole flour wheat, white
- tsp baking powder
- ½ tsp salt
- 1 orange zest
- 1 tbsp eggplant replacer + 3 tbsp water- whisk until frothy, & put it aside for 1-2min
- ¼ cup vegan butter
- oz of unsweetened applesauce
- ¼ cup pure maple syrup
- ¼ to ½ C. of soy milk
- ½ cup vegan chocolate chips or chunks
- ½ cup chopped apricots, dried
- 2 tbsp soy milk to brush scones tops
- For sprinkling, demerara sugar

Directions

1. Preheat the oven to 435°F and prepare 2 baking sheets with parchment paper.
2. Combine the flour, baking soda, salt, and orange zest in a large mixing basin. In tiny bits, blend in the butter until the batter resembles coarse grain.
3. Whisk together the soy milk, eggplant replacer, applesauce, and maple syrup in a separate bowl. Combine the dry ingredients and, if required, add more soy milk. The chocolate chips and dried apricots should only be stirred in until the dough is completely incorporated.
4. Form the batter into a ball and roll it out on a floured board. From the puff pastry, cut a ½ -inch-diameter round. After splitting the circle into 8-12 pieces, place it on the baking pan. Brush the tops of the triangles

with soy milk and sugar after gently dividing them.
5. Preheat oven to 350°F and bake for 15 to 20 mins, or until golden brown. Allow for a min of cooling before moving the scones to a cooling rack. Eat dinner while it's still warm!

Nutritional Values

Fat 7.2g, Chol 4mg, Sodium 4mg, Potassium 13mg, Carbs 47g, Calories 378, Protein 13g

499. ENCHILADA RICE

- Prep time: 10 mins, Cook time: 10 mins, Total time: 20 mins, Grill temp: 0, Servings: 6

Ingredients

- Olive oil 1 tbsp
- Onion 1 medium- any color, diced
- Garlic, minced 3 – 4 cloves
- Green bell pepper, diced 1 large
- White rice 1 ½ cups long-grain
- Vegetable broth 1 ¾ cups low Sodium
- Black beans, 1 can- 14oz drained and rinsed
- Corn drained 1 can- 14oz
- Fire-roasted 1 can- 14oz diced tomatoes, with juices
- Cumin 1 tsp
- Chili powder 1 tsp
- Dried oregano ½ tsp
- Enchilada sauce 1 ½ cups

Directions

1. Sauté: Combine the oil/water, bell pepper, onion, and garlic in the Instant Pot insert, press the sauté button, and cook for 5 mins, stirring regularly.
2. Cook: In a saucepan, mix the rice, water, spices, tomatoes, corn, black beans, and enchilada sauce. Manually set the pressure to high for 5 mins after closing the lid and turning the valve to sealing. Let go of the tension when you're done.
3. Remove the lid and whisk well to allow the sauce to thicken. It will seem liquid at first, but it will thicken after a few mins. To taste, season with salt and pepper.

Nutritional Values

Fat 10g, Chol 2mg, Sodium 8mg, Potassium 13.5mg, Carbs 24g, Calories 267, Protein 20g

500. HEALTHY CARROT CAKE COOKIES

- Prep time: 10 mins, Cook time: 25 mins, Total time: 35 mins, Grill temp: 370°F, Servings: 16

ingredients

- 1 cup of rolled oats
- 1 cup pastry flour, whole wheat
- 1 tsp of baking powder
- ½ tsp of salt
- ½ tsp of ginger
- ¼ tsp of cinnamon
- 1 lemon, zest only
- 1 cup carrots, grated
- ½ cup walnuts, chopped
- ¼ cup golden raisins, chopped
- 3 tbsp coconut oil, melted
- ¼ cup of apple butter
- ¼ cup of maple syrup
- 1 oz. cream cheese- reduced Fat, room temp
- 1 tbsp creamy almond butter
- Almond milk- enough to thin, unsweetened
- 4-5 drops of liquid stevia

Directions

1. Preheat the oven to 370°F and line a baking pan or Silpat with parchment paper.
2. Combine the dry ingredients in a mixing bowl and whisk well.
3. In a small mixing bowl, combine the coconut oil, maple syrup, and apple butter. Combine all of the ingredients in a large mixing bowl and whisk until totally smooth.
4. In the big mixing basin, thoroughly combine the wet materials using a spatula.
5. Form THE DOUGH into golf ball-sized balls and place THEM on a baking pan, gently pressing down to form a disc shape. When cookies are cooked, they do not spread or flatten out much.
6. Preheat the oven to 350°F and bake for approximately 10 mins. Allow cooling on the baking sheet for a few mins before transferring it to a wire rack to cool completely.

Nutritional Values

Fat 3.2g, Chol 4mg, Sodium 8mg, Potassium 15mg, Carbs 47g, Calories 265, Protein 6g

501. CARROT MUFFINS

- Prep time: 10 mins, Cook time: 35 mins, Total time: 45 mins, Grill temp: 375°F, Servings: 5

Ingredients

- 2 cups whole-wheat flour
- 1 cup oats or wheat bran
- 1 tbsp cornstarch
- 3 tbsp baking powder
- 1 tsp allspice
- ½ tsp cinnamon, ground
- ½ tsp salt
- 1 cup raw carrots, grated
- 1 cup water
- 1/3 cup sugar or maple syrup
- ¼ cup of oil or melted vegan butter

Directions

1. Preheat the oven to 375°F - 190°C.
2. Combine rice, oats or bran, cinnamon, baking powder, salt, cornstarch, and allspice in a large mixing basin. In a large mixing bowl, thoroughly combine the shredded carrots. Combine the water, sugar or maple syrup, and oil or butter in a small mixing dish.
3. Fill each muffin tray 2/3 full of batter using a flour-lined or lightly oiled muffin pan. Preheat the oven to 350°F and bake for 25 mins, or until a wooden skewer inserted in the center comes out clean. Allow for 5 mins of chili ng time before transferring it to a cooling rack.

Nutritional Values

Fat 6.2g, Chol 6mg, Sodium 10mg, Potassium 10mg, Carbs 53g, Calories 259, Protein 6g

502. PUMPKIN SPICE OVERNIGHT OATS RECIPE

- Prep time: 25 mins, Cook time: 3 hr. 5 mins, Total time: 3 hr. 30 mins, Grill temp: 0, Servings: 1

Ingredients

- ½ cup of rolled oats- gluten-free
- 1 tbsp of buckwheat groats
- 1 tbsp of chia seeds
- 2 tbsp of pumpkin puree- pure
- ¼ cup of coconut yogurt- plain
- 1 tbsp of maple syrup- pure
- 1 tsp of pumpkin pie- spice mix
- ½ cup of unsweetened milk

Optional toppings:
- 1 tbsp of almond butter
- 1 tsp of jam
- ½ tbsp of pumpkin seeds
- Sprinkle your preferred granola

Directions

1. Mix all ingredients- excluding the chosen toppings, until well combined in the jar or dish.
2. Refrigerate for a minimum of 3 hr and up to 24 hr.
3. Combine almond butter, jam, granola, and pumpkin seeds- if used in the morning and microwave or enjoy cold.

Nutritional Values

Fat 6g, Chol 2mg, Sodium 9mg, Potassium 17mg, Carbs 54g, Calories 154, Protein 10g

503. HEALTHY CHAI-SPICED CARROT BANANA BREAD WITH CREAM CHEESE FROSTING

- Prep time: 25 mins, Cook time: 1 hr 20 mins, Total time: 1 hr 45 mins, Grill temp: 350°F, Servings: 12

Ingredients

For the bread:
- 2 tbsp of ground flax
- 6 tbsp of water
- ¼ cup of coconut oil
- 1 cup of grated carrots
- 2 cups of pastry flour- whole wheat
- 1 tsp of baking soda
- 1 ½ tsp of cinnamon
- 1 tsp of cardamom
- ½ tsp of ground ginger
- ½ tsp of allspice
- ½ tsp of sea salt
- 1 ½ cups of mashed banana
- ½ cup of coconut sugar
- 2 tbsp of almond milk

- 1 tsp vanilla extract
- ⅓ cup of chopped pecans

For the cream cheese frosting:
- ⅓ cup of cream cheese
- ⅓ cup of powdered sugar- organic
- ½ tsp of vanilla extract

Directions

1. Preheat the oven to 350°F - 180°C. Oil a - 5x9 inch loaf pan with butter.
2. In a small mixing bowl, combine flax and water. Allow for the thickening of the sauce. Melt the coconut oil in the small dish and leave it aside to cool. Set the shredded carrots aside.
3. In a large mixing bowl, combine flour, salt, spices, and baking soda.
4. Combine the mashed bananas, shredded carrot, flax mix, coconut oil, sugar, vanilla extract, and milk in a medium mixing bowl.
5. Pour the marinade components into the dry ingredients, constantly whisking to avoid overmixing. Gently fold in pecans. Bake for 1 hr and 10 mins in the baking dish, and cover with foil after 50 mins.
6. Meanwhile, make the frosting by whisking together cream cheese, vanilla, and powdered sugar in a medium mixing bowl until smooth.
7. Remove the bread from the oven and allow it to cool in the pan for approximately 15 mins.
8. Remove the pan from the oven and set it on a wire rack to cool completely.
9. Cover the bread with icing and a sprinkling of nuts when it has fully cooled.
10. After that, cut and serve!

Nutritional Values

Fat 14g, Chol 4mg, Sodium 7mg, Potassium 10mg, Carbs 40g, Calories 391, Protein 16g

504. PEANUT BUTTER CINNAMON TOAST

- Prep time: 10 mins, Cook time: 15 mins, Total time: 25 mins, Grill temp: 0, Servings: 2

Ingredients

- 2 slices of toasted wheat bread
- 2 small, sliced bananas
- 2 tbsp of peanut butter
- Cinnamon for taste

1. Spread the peanut butter on the toast and add banana slices on top.
2. Toss in a pinch of cinnamon to taste.

Nutritional Values

Fat 3.2g, Chol 1mg, Sodium 4mg, Potassium 9mg, Carbs 55g, Calories 330, Protein 20 g

505. QUINOA & CHIA OATMEAL MIX

- Prep time: 5 mins, Cook time: 25 mins, Total time: 30 mins, Grill temp: 0, Servings: 12

Ingredients

- 2 cups rolled oats
- 1 cup of rolled wheat or barley flakes
- 1 cup quinoa
- 1 cup of dried fruit, like raisins, cranberries, and chopped apricots
- ½ cup of chia or hemp seeds
- 1 tsp ground cinnamon
- ¾ tsp salt

Directions

1. To prepare the hot cereal dry mix, combine the following ingredients in a mixing bowl.
2. Combine the oats, wheat or barley flakes, dried fruits, quinoa, almonds, cinnamon, and salt in an airtight dish. To make 1 serving of hot cereal, put the following ingredients in a mixing bowl.
3. Combine 1/3 cup Quinoa and Chia Oatmeal with ¼ cup water- or milk in a small pan. Bring the water to a boil over high heat.
4. Reduce heat to low, partially cover, and cook, occasionally stirring, for 12 to 15 mins or until thickened.
5. Cover and set aside for 5 mins. Finish with a sweetener of your choice, nuts, and extra-dried fruit if desired. The result from this recipe makes 1 cup.

Nutritional Values

Fat 3.5g, Chol 5mg, Sodium 8mg, Potassium 11mg, Carbs 45g, Calories 366, Protein 17g

506. SAVORY VEGAN BREAKFAST BOWL

- Prep time: 5 mins, Cook time: 20 mins, Total time: 25 mins, Grill temp: 0, Servings: 1

Ingredients

- 1 serving medium or firm tofu, crumbled
- 1 cup sliced mushrooms
- 9½ an avocado
- ½ cup diced white onions
- ½ cup cooked brown rice

Directions

1. In a small dish, combine the tofu scramble ingredients and set them aside. It is recommended that it be mixed before cooking for 1 serving. When using a complete tofu box, it's simple to combine all ingredients in 1 dish.
2. Cook the onions, greens, and mushrooms together. Cook in a pan with ½ tsp avocado or olive oil or a splash of water over medium-high heat. Cook for 5-8 mins, or until the veggies are tender and browned on the outside. Don't stir them too much if you want them to brown. After they've done cooking, scoop them onto a bowl.
3. Cook for another 5 mins or until the tofu is cooked through and colored in the pan. Alternatively, while the mushrooms and kale are cooking, stir the tofu and scramble in with them. Mix everything before serving.
4. Combine the tofu scramble with the kale mixture in a mixing bowl, then top with avocado, brown rice, and salsa to form the breakfast bowls.
5. Serve right now or freeze for later.

Nutritional Values

Fat 12g, Chol 3mg, Sodium 5mg, Potassium 12mg, Carbs 50g, Calories 135, Protein 21g

507. EASY OIL-FREE GRANOLA- WITH LOTS OF CRUNCHY CLUSTERS!

- Prep time: 10 mins, Cook time: 15 mins, Total time: 25 mins, Grill temp: 375°F, Servings: 3

Ingredients

- ¼ cup of whatever dry ingredient- nuts, seeds, nuts, cereal, quinoa, coconut, buckwheat, etc.
- 1 cup crispy brown rice cereal
- 1 ¾ cup rolled oats
- ½ cup maple syrup- 1 more tbsp for extra clusters

Directions

1. Preheat the oven to 375°F.
2. Mix all of the ingredients in a mixing bowl.
3. Evenly coat all of the dry ingredients.
4. Spread out on a baking sheet lined with parchment paper.
5. Cut it into a ¼-inch-thick rectangle.
6. Bake at 375°F for at least 10 mins, or until the edges start to brown. It shouldn't be stirred frequently.
7. Preheat the oven to 350°F. Remove the baking sheet from the oven. Before stirring, moving, or touching it, let it cool for 30 mins.
8. After that, cut it into pieces.
9. Keep it in an airtight jar for 5 days.

Nutritional Values

Fat 2g, Chol 3.5mg, Sodium 4mg, Potassium 9.5mg, Carbs 43g, Calories 312, Protein 10 g

508. INSTANT POT BUCKWHEAT PORRIDGE

- Prep time: 20 mins, Cook time: 30 mins, Total time: 50 mins, Grill temp: 0, Servings: 4

Ingredients

- 1 cup raw buckwheat groats
- 1 banana- sliced
- 3 cups rice milk
- ½ tsp vanilla
- ¼ cup raisins
- 1 tsp ground cinnamon
- Chopped nuts optional

Directions

1. Buckwheat should be washed and added to the Instant Pot.
2. In a container, combine the banana, rice milk, raisins, vanilla, and cinnamon. Cover the container with a lid.
3. Close the steam release valve and set the high-pressure Cook timer to 6 mins manually.
4. Switch the cooker off when the timer beeps after the cooking cycle has finished. Allow the pressure to dissipate naturally. It takes roughly 20 mins to complete.
5. Open the lid with care. After the pressure is released, stir the porridge using a long-handled spoon.

6. Add more rice milk to each serving to get the appropriate consistency. Top with chopped nuts if desired.

Nutritional Values

Fat 8g, Chol 7mg, Sodium 10mg, Potassium 20mg, Carbs 56g, Calories 397, Protein 16 g

509. CREAMY TOMATO, BASIL & RICE SOUP

- Prep time: 10 mins, Cook time: 15 mins, Total time: 25 mins, Grill temp: 0, Servings: 2

Ingredients

- ½ cup brown rice, cooked
- 1 can of crushed tomatoes
- ½ cup coconut milk- full of Fat
- 2 cup basil
- 3 tbsp nutritional yeast- for a cheesier flavor

Directions

1. Combine all ingredients, except the rice, in a food processor or blender and pulse until smooth.
2. Season with salt and pepper to taste. Heat the mixture in a saucepan over medium-high heat until the liquid begins to simmer.
3. Divide the rice into 2 bowls and top with the soup. To combine, keep stirring.

Nutritional Values

Fat 7.2g, Chol 2mg, Sodium 6mg, Potassium 13mg, Carbs 65g, Calories 350, Protein 17 g

510. VEGAN COCONUT RICE PUDDING

- Prep time: 5 mins, Cook time: 20 mins, Total time: 25 mins, Grill temp: 0, Servings: 4

Ingredients

- 1 can of coconut milk
- ½ tsp crushed cardamom or 12 whole pods
- ½ tsp cinnamon
- ¼ tsp vanilla extract
- 2 tbsp maple syrup
- 1 ½ cups rice, cooked
- 2 tsp orange zest

Directions

1. 1 min, over medium heat, simmer the coconut milk with cardamom pods in a small saucepan. To absorb the taste, reduce

the heat to low and simmer the milk for 10 mins.

2. Using a spoon, remove the cardamom pods.
3. In a glass of milk, combine the cinnamon, vanilla extract, and maple syrup.
4. Cook, occasionally stirring, for 10 mins over medium heat, or until the rice is beautiful and creamy.
5. Mix in the orange zest well.
6. Sprinkle shredded coconut, fresh berries, maple syrup, or whatever else you desire on top of the pudding.

511. EASY LOW FODMAP SHAKSHUKA

- Prep time: 10 mins, Cook time: 20 mins, Total time: 30 mins, Grill temp: 0, Servings: 4

Ingredients

- 1 tbsp olive oil- garlic-infused
- ½ cup leek leaves, chopped
- 1 cup chopped red bell pepper
- 2 cups Arrabbiata Sauce
- 1 tbsp crushed cumin
- 4 large whole eggplants
- 2 cups cooked white or brown rice
- Optional Garnishes
- 2 tbsp fresh parsley, chopped
- ¼ cup shredded feta cheese

Directions

1. After the olive oil has heated up, add the leek leaves and bell pepper. Stir occasionally while cooking until the pepper slices are tender and the leek leaves are bright green, soft, and fragrant.
2. Reduce to a medium setting. Add in the crushed cumin and low-FODMAP arrabbiata. Cook, occasionally stirring, until the gravy is almost boiling.
3. Make a well in each 4th of the mixture using a spatula. Carefully place 1 eggplant in each well.
4. Cook until the eggplants are tender, covered with a lid. Remove the heat from the room.

5. Serve immediately with shredded feta cheese and chopped parsley on top of cooked rice.

512. PINA COLADA GRANOLA- VEGAN & CAN BE GF

- Prep time: 10 mins, Cook time: 40 mins, Total time: 50 mins, Grill temp: 350°F, Servings: 10

Ingredients

- 1 & ½ cups of rolled oats
- 1 & ½ cups of puffed brown rice cereal- certified GF if required
- ¼ cup of ground flaxseed
- 2-3 packets of stevia
- ¼ cup applesauce, unsweetened
- 3 tbsp of agave nectar or honey- raw
- 2 tbsp melted coconut oil
- ½ tsp cinnamon, ground
- ¼ tsp ginger, ground
- ¼ tsp of salt
- ¼ cup macadamia nuts, chopped
- ¼ cup pineapple, diced- unsweetened & unsulphured
- ¼ cup coconut flakes, unsweetened

Directions

1. Preheat the oven to 350°F.
2. Wax paper should be used to line a baking pan.
3. Combine the oats, flaxseed, and rice cereal in a mixing basin and set aside.
4. Combine the applesauce, coconut oil, agave nectar, cinnamon, stevia, ginger, and salt in a separate bowl.
5. Combine the wet and dry ingredients by pouring the wet over the dry. In a mixing dish, combine the coconut flakes and macadamia nuts.
6. Spread the batter evenly on the baking pan that has been prepared.
7. Bake for 35 mins, or until the granola is lightly browned and crisp- to achieve even crisping, stir the granola every 10 mins during baking!

8. Remove the granola from the oven and set it aside to cool completely.
9. Maintain the container's airtightness.
10. Enjoy!

Fat 2g, Chol 7mg, Sodium 9mg, Potassium 13mg, Carbs 43g, Calories 245, Protein 5g

513. CAULIFLOWER RICE KIMCHI BOWLS

- Prep time: 15 mins, Cook time: 35 mins, Total time: 50 mins, Grill temp: 0, Servings: 3

Ingredients

Coconut sauce:
- ⅓ cup of coconut milk
- 2 tbsp Miso paste
- 1 tbsp rice vine or fresh lemon juice
- 1 tsp ginger, crushed
- A pinch of salt

For bowls:
- 1 small top of the cauliflower, washed
- ½ cup scallions, diced
- ½ clove of garlic, minced
- 7 oz. mushrooms, diced
- ½ tsp of rice vine
- ½ tsp of tamari
- 6 leaves of kale, cut & stemmed
- 14 oz. baked tofu
- 1 avocado, sliced
- ½ cup of kimchi
- ¼ cup of microgreens
- Sesame seeds, if required
- Olive oil
- Salt
- Lemon wedges for serving

Directions

1. In a small mixing bowl, whisk together miso paste, coconut milk, rice vinegar or lime juice, salt, and ginger to make the coconut sauce. Set it to the side.
2. In a large nonstick skillet, heat a dash of olive oil over low heat. Cook for 3 mins, occasionally turning, to eliminate the cauliflower's raw flavor. Add the riced cauliflower, garlic, a pinch of salt, scallions, and garlic. Remove the pan from the heat and add ½ tbsp of coconut sauce, whisking constantly. Cauliflower florets should be divided into 4 dishes.
3. Using a paper towel, wipe any residual cauliflower bits from the pan. Return the pan to moderate heat with a few sprays of olive oil. Cook, occasionally turning, until the diced mushrooms and salt are mushy, about 5 mins. Reduce the heat to low and add the rice vinegar and tamari. Place the mushrooms on the cauliflower plates.
4. Wipe the pan clean, then add a splash of water and the kale to boil. Cover for 1 min or until the kale has wilted somewhat.
5. Pour extra coconut sauce atop each cauliflower piece to finish assembling the bowls. Combine the kimchi, tofu, kale, and avocado, as well as the microgreens and sesame seeds, in the bowls. Serve with lime wedges and any sauce leftover on the side.

Fat 6.2g, Chol 10mg, Sodium 15mg, Potassium 20mg, Carbs 56g, Calories 380, Protein 17g

514. STUFFED YELLOW PEPPERS

- Prep time: 10 mins, Cook time: 20 mins, Total time: 30 mins, Grill temp: 350°F, Servings: 6

Ingredients

- 1 large-size yellow/green peppers
- 2 lb of uncooked minced turkey
- ¼ cup of chopped onion.
- 1 ½ cups of brown rice- cooked
- ½ cup frozen peppers & onion. stir-fry these vegetables.
- ½ cup of mild salsa
- 1 ½ tsp of garlic & herb, unsalted blend.
- 2 tsp of poultry seasoning
- ¼ tsp of kosher salt
- ½ cup of water
- ⅓ cup of breadcrumbs
- 2 tbsp of vegetable oil melted spread
- ½ tsp of paprika

Directions

1. Preheat the oven to 350°F - 180°C.
2. To remove the seeds and membranes from sweet peppers, cut them in ½. Cook the pepper halves in enough boiling water in a large Dutch oven for about 2 mins.
3. Drain the pepper halves and set them cut side up on a baking dish. Combine the minced turkey and onion in a large skillet

and sauté until the turkey is no longer pink, breaking it up as it cooks. Get rid of some additional Fat if at all possible.

4. Combine the rice, vegetables, spice blend, salsa, chicken seasoning, and salt in a skillet. ½-fill the pepper halves with the filling. Once the peppers have been filled, fill them with water. Combine breadcrumbs, paprika, and molten vegetable spread in a small mixing bowl.

5. Serve with stuffed peppers and salt and pepper seasoning. Bake for about 30 mins with the lid on. After removing the cover, bake for another 5 mins.

Nutritional Values

Fat 3.5g, Chol 9mg, Sodium 12mg, Potassium 14mg, Carbs 49g, Calories 367, Protein 16 g

515. ROASTED VEGGIE BROWN RICE BUDDHA BOWL

- Prep time: 10 mins, Cook time: 15 mins, Total time: 25 mins, Grill temp: 0, Servings: 1

Ingredients

- ½ cup brown rice- cooked
- 1 cup of roasted vegetables
- ½ cup of roasted tofu
- ¼ tbsp sliced scallions
- 2 tbsp diced fresh cilantro
- 2 tbsp Creamed Vegan Cashew Sauce

Directions

1. Combine rice, vegetables, and tofu in a bowl or 4-cup sealable container, then top with scallions and cilantro.
2. Serve with a dab of cashew sauce on top.

Nutritional Values

Fat 4.5g, Chol 6mg, Sodium 14mg, Potassium 20mg, Carbs 44g, Calories 266, Protein 14g

516. SPINACH, FETA & RICE CASSEROLE

- Prep time: 30 mins, Cook time: 1 hr 15 mins, Total time: 1 hr 45 mins, Grill temp: 400°F, Servings: 6

Ingredients

- 1 tbsp of olive oil
- ½ cup of chopped onion
- 1 package of chopped spinach- thawed & dried

- 2 chopped cloves of garlic.
- 3 cups of brown rice- cooked
- ¾ cup of grated feta cheese
- ¼ cup of chopped dill
- ½ tsp of crushed pepper
- ¼ tsp of salt
- 1 large size eggs
- ¼ cup of sour cream
- 3 tbsp of lemon zest

Directions

1. Preheat the oven to 400°F - 200°C. In a large ovenproof skillet, heat the oil over medium heat.
2. Cook, stirring periodically, for approximately 4 mins, or until the onion begins to brown.
3. Cook, constantly stirring, for 1-2 mins after adding the spinach and garlic. Allow the pan to cool after removing it from the heat.
4. Combine the rice, feta, pepper, salt, and dill in a mixing bowl. In a mixing bowl, whisk together the eggs and sour cream.
5. Stir it into the rice mixture to incorporate it. Using a spatula, smooth the surface. Bake for 25 mins, or until lightly browned.
6. Before serving, allow for a 5-mins rest time.

Nutritional Values

Fat 5.2g, Chol 9mg, Sodium 13mg, Potassium 20mg, Carbs 45g, Calories 330, Protein 18 g

517. COOKED BROWN RICE

- Prep time: 5 mins, Cook time: 55 mins, Total time: 60 mins, Grill temp: 0, Servings: 4

Ingredients

- 2 cups well-rinsed brown rice uncooked
- 2 cups of water
- 2 tsp olive oil extra-virgin

Directions

1. In a saucepan, bring the washed rice, water, and olive oil to a boil. Cook for 45 mins with the cover on and the heat down to low.
2. After removing it from the heat, let it sit for another 10 mins, covered. Fluff the mixture with a fork.

Nutritional Values

Fat 3g, Chol 2.9mg, Sodium 4mg, Potassium 9mg, Carbs 34g, Calories 220, Protein 9 g

518. CHANA MASALA

- Prep time: 10 mins, Cook time: 20 mins, Total time: 30 mins, Grill temp: 0, Servings: 4

Ingredients

- 1 & ½ tbsp olive oil extra-virgin
- 1 large diced yellow onion
- 1 tsp cumin seed, whole
- 1 tsp coriander, ground
- 1 tsp turmeric, ground
- 3 minced cardamom pods
- 3 minced garlic cloves
- 1 tsp of garam masala
- 1 tsp ginger, fresh
- ¼ tsp of cayenne pepper
- 1 can of diced tomatoes
- 2 cans chickpeas
- 5-8 oz. spinach fresh
- 1 Tbsp lemon juice
- 1 cup chopped fresh cilantro
- Sea salt & black pepper

Directions

1. In a large skillet, melt the butter and oil over low heat. Add some onion and season heavily with salt and pepper, then cook for 8-10 mins, occasionally stirring, until tender and caramelized. Stir in the cumin seeds halfway through.
2. Heat the cayenne pepper and coriander, if using, for 30-60 seconds until fragrant. Combine the turmeric and cardamom in a bowl. Scratch the bottom of the pan and pour in the water, scraping as you go. Cook for another 5 mins after adding the tomatoes and salt. Cook, constantly stirring, over low heat until it barely starts to boil. To thicken the sauce, cook for 6 mins at a moderate temp.
3. Cook, occasionally stirring, for 10-12 mins after adding the chickpeas, water, and salt, or until the liquid has decreased and the stew has thickened.
4. Cook for approximately 2 mins or until the spinach has wilted. Remove the saucepan from the burner and set it aside.

5. 1 lemon or lime juice should be added. Toss well to mix, then taste. Extra lime or lemon juice may be added if desired. Sprinkle the chopped cilantro over the top just before serving. If desired, serve with steamed rice and naan bread.

Nutritional Values

Fat 7.2g, Chol 10mg, Sodium 15mg, Potassium 22mg, Carbs 40g, Calories 270, Protein 6 g

519. KIMCHI BROWN RICE BLISS BOWLS

- Prep time: 20 mins, Cook time: 40 mins, Total time: 60 mins, Grill temp: 0, Servings: 2

Ingredients

- 1 cup of cooked brown rice
- ¼ cup kimchi, heaping
- 1 peeled Persian cucumber
- ½ cup red cabbage, thinly sliced
- ½ sliced avocado
- 8 oz. grilled or baked, Marinated Tempe
- ½ recipe of Peanut Sauce
- ½ tsp of sesame seeds
- 2 sliced Thai chiles
- Lemon slices for serving
- Microgreens, for garnish- optional

Directions

1. In the bowls, combine the rice, cabbage, kimchi, avocado, cucumber, and tempeh.
2. Top with a generous amount of sesame seeds, peanut sauce, and, if desired, Thai chilies.
3. Serve with a side of leftover peanut sauce and lemon wedges. Microgreens may be added if desired.

Nutritional Values

Fat 7g, Chol 9mg, Sodium 14mg, Potassium 19mg, Carbs 55g, Calories 395, Protein 17 g

520. POMEGRANATE RICE SALAD

- Prep time: 20 mins, Cook time: 40 mins, Total time: 60 mins, Grill temp: 0, Servings: 4

Ingredients

- 4 cups long-grain rice, any kind -cooked
- 2 tsp olive oil, extra-virgin
- 1 bunch of chopped scallions, white & green parts
- 3minced cloves garlic

- ⅓ cup toasted pistachios, chopped
- ½ cup parsley, chopped
- ½ cup of pomegranate arils
- ⅓ cup mint leaves, fresh
- Sea salt & black pepper, freshly ground
- Roasted Chickpeas- optional
- 2 tbsp olive oil, extra-virgin
- 2 tbsp of white wine vinegar
- 1 tbsp of fresh orange juice + 1 tsp zest
- 1 tbsp lemon juice, fresh
- ½ tsp of maple syrup
- ½ tsp of ground cumin
- ½ tsp of ground coriander
- ¼ tsp of cinnamon
- ½ tsp of sea salt
- Black pepper, freshly ground

Directions

1. In a small mixing bowl, whisk together the orange juice, olive oil, lemon juice + zest, vinegar, maple syrup, cinnamon, cumin, pepper, coriander, and salt.
2. Heat the olive oil in a pan over medium heat. Cook for 1 min, or until the scallions and garlic are soft, seasoning with salt and pepper. Reduce the heat to low and add the boiled rice, stirring to break up any clumps with a wooden spoon. Heat until well warmed. After turning off the heat, add the dressing, pistachios, pomegranates, and parsley.
3. Garnish with roasted chickpeas and mint leaves, if desired. Serve after seasoning with salt and pepper to taste.

Nutritional Values

Fat 2g, Chol 13mg, Sodium 17mg, Potassium 23mg, Carbs 53g, Calories 360, Protein 14 g

521. STUFFED POBLANO PEPPERS

- Prep time: 20 mins, Cook time: 40 mins, Total time: 60 mins, Grill temp: 410°F, Servings: 4

Ingredients

- 4 poblano peppers, medium
- Olive oil for drizzling
- 1/3 cup of red onion, sliced or chopped scallions
- 1 heaping cup of cauliflower florets, sliced into small pieces
- ½ cup red bell pepper, diced

- ½ tsp of cumin
- ½ tsp of coriander
- ½ tsp of oregano
- 1 minced garlic clove
- 1 cup black beans- cooked, drained & rinsed
- 1 cup white or brown rice, cooked
- 3 cups spinach, fresh
- 2 tbsp of lime juice + slices for serving
- ¼ cup tomatillo salsa or store-bought
- Sea salt & black pepper, freshly ground

Directions

1. Preheat the oven to 410°F and prepare a baking pan with parchment paper.
2. By slicing the peppers in ½, you can remove the seeds and ribs. Spray the baking pan with oil and season with salt and pepper. Slices side up, roast for 15 mins.
3. In a medium-sized pan, heat 1 tbsp olive oil. In a large mixing bowl, combine the cumin, onion, red pepper, cauliflower, coriander, ½ tsp salt, oregano, garlic, and a few pinches of pepper. Cook for 5 to 8 mins, or until onion is soft and cauliflower is lightly browned.
4. After removing the skillet from the heat, stir in the rice, black beans, spinach, tomatillo salsa, and lime juice. Season to taste with salt and pepper.
5. Bake for 15 mins after filling the peppers with the filling.
6. Serve avocado slices with cilantro, salsa, tomatillo, creamy green chili cashews, and lime wedges on the side.

Nutritional Values

Fat 4.1g, Chol 4mg, Sodium 12mg, Potassium 15mg, Carbs 50g, Calories 315, Protein 13 g

522. VEGAN SUSHI

- Prep time: 25 mins, Cook time: 1 hr 25 mins, Total time: I hr 50 mins, Grill temp: 400°F, Servings: 5

Ingredients

- 2 Chioggia beets, pink
- Olive oil to drizzle
- 1 tbsp of rice vinegar
- 1 tbsp tamari

- ½ tbsp sesame oil
- ½ tsp ginger, chopped
- Salt to taste

For rice
- 1 cup of rice, short-grained and not cooked
- 2 tbsp rice vinegar
- 1 tbsp brown sugar
- 1 tsp salt

For rolls
- 4 sheets of nori
- 1 cucumber, diced
- 1 avocado, sliced into strips
- Sesame seeds
- Tamari, to serving
- Ginger, pickled
- Sriracha & vegan mayo- optional

Directions

1. To prepare the beets, preheat the oven to 400°F. Drizzle olive oil and a sprinkle of salt over the beets on a foil-lined baking sheet. Wrap the beets in foil and roast them on a baking sheet for 45-60 mins or until soft and fork-tender. The length of time needed depends on the freshness and size of the beets. Remove the beets from the oven after removing the foil. When the skins are chilly to the touch, peel them. Remove their skin with your hands. Cut the beets lengthwise into ¼-inch strips.
2. In a flat basin or baking dish, combine sesame oil, tamari, rice vinegar, and ginger. Toss the beets in the dressing to coat them, then put them aside to marinate. To ensure a homogeneous coating, toss again after 15 mins.
3. Prepare the rice as follows: To make the rice, follow the directions on this page. In a mixing dish, combine the sugar, salt, cooked rice, and vinegar.
4. Putting the rolls together: Place a nori sheet, shiny side down, on a bamboo mat and squish a generous quantity of rice into the bottom 2/3 of the sheet. At the bottom of the rice, arrange a row of avocado, beets, and cucumber. Rolling will be more difficult if the container is overfilled. Use the bamboo mat to tuck and roll the nori. Simply shape the rolls with a bamboo mat and gently press them after they've been

transferred. Roll the cut side down to the side. Carry on with the rest of the rolls.
5. Sushi should be cut with a sharp knife. Using a damp rag or tissue, wipe the blade clean.
6. Add a liberal quantity of sesame seeds on the top. Top with vegan mayo, tamari, and pickled ginger with a dash of sriracha if desired.

Nutritional Values

Fat 0.8g, Chol 2mg, Sodium 4mg, Potassium 8mg, Carbs 47g, Calories 264, Protein 16 g

523. VEGAN BURRITO BOWL

- Prep time: 20 mins, Cook time: 50 mins, Total time: 1 hr 10 mins, Grill temp: 0, Servings: 2

Ingredients

- 1 cup of beans, washed, drained, and cooked
- 1-2 diced chipotle peppers
- ½ tsp olive oil
- 1 cup rice, cooked- white or brown
- 2 cups of arugula, diced
- ½ cup of guacamole
- ½ cup of pineapple salsa
- ¼ cup cilantro, diced
- Black pepper powder & sea salt
- Veggies
- 2 mushroom caps
- Olive oil for sprinkling
- Adobo sauce
- Black pepper & salt
- 1 bell pepper, red & sliced
- 1 green bell pepper, cut into strips
- 1 jalapeño, cut into strips

Directions

1. In a small bowl, combine the cooked beans, olive oil, chipotle peppers, lemon juice, 14 tsp salt, and several pinches of pepper.
2. Prepare the vegetables: Preheat a cast-iron skillet over medium heat inside the house. The mushrooms will be cooked directly on the grill, while the chopped peppers will be roasted in a cast-iron skillet.
3. Over the mushroom caps, drizzle some olive oil and a couple of tsp of adobo sauce. Use as much space as possible to completely cover the mushrooms on all

sides. Season with pepper and salt to taste. Grill the portobello mushrooms for 4-5 mins on each side, or until golden and soft. Slice just before arranging the bowls.

4. Season the pepper strips with salt and pepper after drizzling olive oil over them. In a cast-iron skillet or grill pan, cook for 8-10 mins, occasionally rotating, until browned and soft.

5. Combine the beans, peppers, cilantro, rice, arugula, pineapple salsa, sliced mushrooms, guacamole, and cilantro in a large mixing bowl. Serve with extra salsa and lemon wedges on the side.

Nutritional Values

Fat 4g, Chol 1mg, Sodium 7mg, Potassium 17mg, Carbs 39g, Calories 249, Protein 12 g

524. MANGO GINGER RICE BOWL

- Prep time: 5 mins, Cook time: 25 mins, Total time: 30 mins, Grill temp: 0, Servings: 2

Ingredients

- 2 handfuls of snap peas
- 1-2 cups rice, cooked & short-grained
- 2 cups of grated green cabbage
- 1 carrot, thinly diced into coins
- ½ cucumber, thinly diced into coins
- 1 mango, sliced and ripened
- ½ cup beans, washed, drained, and cooked
- 2 tbsp Ginger, pickled
- ¼ cup basil, finely diced & fresh
- ¼ cup peanuts, toasted
- Sesame seeds- optional
- ¼ - ½ avocado- optional

Dressing
- 2 tbsp of tamari
- 2 tbsp rice vine
- 2 tbsp fresh lemon juice
- 2 cloves of garlic, crushed
- 2 tsp of cane sugar
- ½ tsp sriracha

Directions

1. Whisk together sriracha, garlic, vinegar, tamari, lemon juice, and cane sugar to prepare the dressing in a small bowl.

2. Boil water in a large pot and have an ice water dish nearby. Cook the snap peas for 2 mins in boiling water, then remove them and drop them in cold water to stop the cooking. After rinsing, patting dry, and letting to cool, cut.

3. Arrange the carrots, mango, ginger, black beans, rice, shredded cabbage, cucumber, and basil in the bowls. Top with avocado, roasted peanuts, and sesame seeds, if desired. ½ of the dressing should be poured into the bowls, with the rest served on the side with tamari and sriracha if desired.

Nutritional Values

Fat 8g, Chol 7mg, Sodium 9mg, Potassium 15mg, Carbs 56g, Calories 399, Protein 20g

525. AVOCADO CUCUMBER SUSHI ROLL

- Prep time: 40 mins, Cook time: 1 hr 15 mins, Total time: 1 hr 55 mins, Grill temp: 0, Servings: 4

Ingredients

- Sushi rice
- 1 cup rice, short-grained & rinsed
- 2 cups of water
- 2 tbsp Of rice vinegar
- 1 tbsp brown sugar
- 1 tsp sea salt

For rolls:
- 1 cucumber, diced into long strips
- 1 mango, diced into long strips
- 1 avocado, diced
- ⅓ cup of microgreens- optional
- 2 tbsp sesame seeds- optional
- 4 sheets of nori
- Serve with Ponzu or tamari sauce

Directions

1. In a medium saucepan, combine the water, olive oil, and rice and bring to a boil. Reduce the heat to low and cook for 45 mins. Remove the rice from the heat and leave it aside, covered, for another 10 mins. After fluffing with a fork, add the salt, sugar, and rice vinegar. Cover and keep warm until ready to use.

2. Arrange the sushi rolls in the following order: Place 1 nori sheet, shiny side down, on a bamboo mat and press a scoop of rice into the bottom 2/3 of the sheet. Toppings should be placed at the

bottom of the rice. Rolling will be more difficult if the container is overfilled. Use a bamboo mat to fold and roll the nori. Set aside the section of the roll that has been sliced. Carry on with the rest of the rolls.

3. Sushi should be cut with a sharp chef's knife. Clean the blade with a moist towel in between cuts.
4. Toss with ponzu or tamari sauce, as well as coconut peanut sauce if desired.

Nutritional Values

Fat 5.2g, Chol 9mg, Sodium 16mg, Potassium 18mg, Carbs 57g, Calories 371, Protein 15g

526. BUTTERNUT SQUASH BURRITO BOWLS

- Prep time: 20 mins, Cook time: 45 mins, Total time: 1 hr 5 mins, Grill temp: 400°F, Servings: 4

Ingredients

- Tomato-corn Pico de Gallo
- 1 cup tomatoes, diced
- ½ cup corn kernels, fresh
- ¼ cup red onion, thinly diced
- 1 clove of garlic, minced
- 1 lime juice
- ½ serrano, sliced
- Cilantro, chopped
- Black pepper powder & sea salt

For bowls:
- 1 butternut squash, cut into cubes & peeled
- Olive oil
- Black pepper powder & sea salt
- ½ tsp of chili powder
- 2 cups brown rice, cooked
- 1 black bean, drained and washed
- Some kale leaves lightly brushed with olive oil
- ¼ cup pepitas, toasted

Avocado crema:
- 1 avocado, ripened
- ¼ cup of yogurt
- ½ lime juice
- 1 clove of garlic
- 1 tbsp onion, minced
- ½ tsp cumin, ground
- ½ tsp coriander, ground
- ¼ cup of cilantro, diced

- Black pepper powder & sea salt
- Water

Directions

1. Preheat the oven to 400°F or higher.
2. In a mixing bowl, add corn, garlic, onion, lime juice, tomatoes, garlic, serrano, and coriander, along with a pinch of pepper and salt, to make Pico de Gallo. Allow it to cool for 30 mins before serving, then taste and adjust the seasonings.
3. Drizzle the butternut squash with extra virgin olive oil, salt, and pepper. Bake for 30 mins, then flip and roast until gently browned- for 10 mins. Remove the pan from the heat and season with red chili powder.
4. Avocado crema is made by blending avocados, yogurt, lime juice, pepper, salt, coriander, onion, garlic, and cumin in a blender. Blend until the mixture is smooth. Season with salt and pepper to taste. Refrigerate until you're ready to use it.
5. In bowls, combine butternut squash, Pico de Gallo, beans, brown rice, and kale.
6. On top, serve with avocado crema and toasted pepitas.

Nutritional Values

Fat 6.7g, Chol 5.5mg, Sodium 11mg, Potassium 16mg, Carbs 38g, Calories 370, Protein 12g

527. TOASTED OATS CEREAL- CAMPING BREAKFAST

- Prep time: 5 mins, Cook time: 10 mins, Total time: 15 mins, Grill temp: 0, Servings: 2

Ingredients

- 1 tbsp olive oil
- cup rolled oats- Use gluten-free
- ¼ cup chopped nuts- seeds
- tbsp maple syrup- sub agave or honey can also be used
- ¼ cup dried fruit- dried cranberries or raisins
- To serve: milk or non-dairy milk substitute

Directions

1. It's easy to make at home on the stovetop. At the campground, a propane camp burner may be used to prepare it.

2. Heat the oil in a large, heavy skillet over medium-high heat. Toss in the nuts and oats with the hot oil.
3. Cook for 5-7 mins, stirring often. Cook until the oats are golden brown. Stir often to avoid burning the nuts.
4. As soon as the color becomes golden, remove the pan from the heat. Combine the maple syrup and the water. Stir everything together until it's completely smooth.
5. Mix in the dried fruit well.
6. Serve with warm or cold milk on top of the cereal.
7. Serve right away or store for up to a week in an airtight container.

Nutritional Values

Fat 12g, Chol 12mg, Sodium 10mg, Potassium 23mg, Carbs 49g, Calories 313, Protein 12g

528. CHIA OVERNIGHT OATS 2 WAYS!

- Prep time: 5 mins, Cook time: 5 mins, Total time: 10 mins, Grill temp: 0, Servings: 1

Ingredients

- ½ cup or 60g rolled oats
- 1 cup or 240g of non-dairy milk
- 2 tbsp or 16g chia seeds
- 1 tbsp or to taste maple syrup
- 1 tbsp of cashew butter
- 1 tsp of cinnamon- optional
- pinch of salt- optional
- For the creamy texture: ½ cup of fruit you like, frozen
- Toppings: fruit, seeds, nuts, toasted coconut, yogurt, cereal, etc.

Directions

1. In a jar, combine all of the ingredients.
2. Stir or shake the ingredients together.
3. Allow at least 1 night in the refrigerator.
4. The following day, add toppings and eat as is. Alternatively, blend ½ a cup of frozen fruit- of your choice until smooth and creamy, then top with whipped cream and enjoy!

Nutritional Values

Fat 2g, Chol 12mg, Sodium 18mg, Potassium 28mg, Carbs 43g, Calories 145, Protein 8 g

Chapter 14.

Salad Recipes

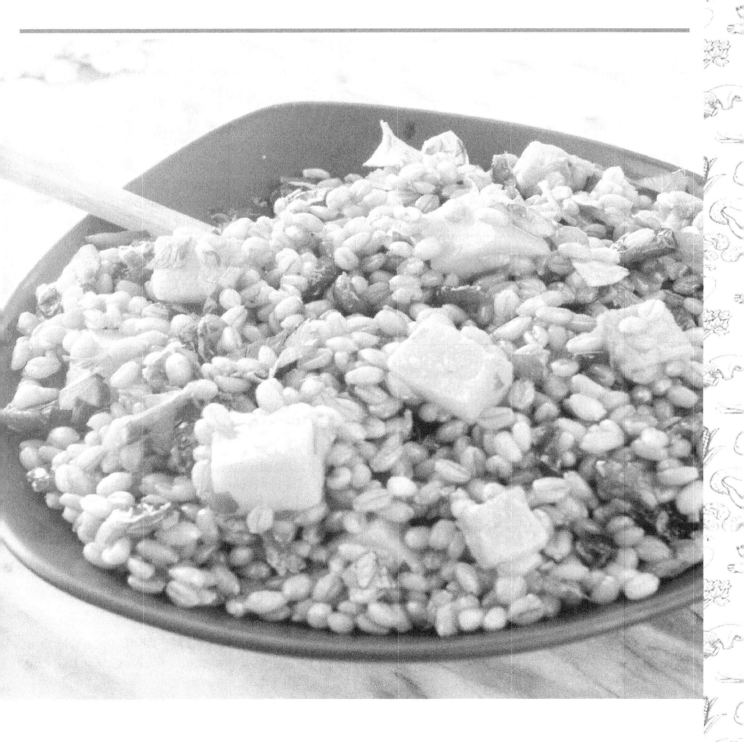

529. Autumn Wheat Berry Salad

- Lunch - Prep time: 25 mins, Cook time: 2 hours, Total time: 30 mins, Servings: 4, Grill temp: 300°F

Ingredients

- 2 ½ cups of wheat berries, soaked overnight
- ¼ cup of plus
- 2 tbsp of apple cider vinegar
- ¼ cup of brown rice syrup
- 2 celery stalks, thinly sliced
- ½ cup of chopped green onion- white and green parts
- 2 tbsp of minced tarragon
- 1 Bosc pear, cored and diced
- ½ cup of fruit-sweetened dried cranberries
- Salt and freshly ground black pepper to taste

Directions

1. Bring 5 cups of water to a boil in a medium saucepan and add the wheat berries.
2. Return to a boil over high heat, reduce the heat to medium, cover, and cook until the wheat berries are tender, about 1¾ hours.
3. Drain the excess water from the pan and rinse the berries until cool.
4. Combine all the other ingredients in a large bowl.
5. Add the cooled wheat berries and mix well. Chill for 1 hour before serving.

Nutritional Values

Calories 113, Fat 1.8g, Chol 0mg, Sodium 71.4mg, Potassium 67.7mg, Carbs 22g, Protein 2.3g

530. Baby Bok Choy Salad With Sesame Dressing

- Lunch - Prep time: 5 mins, Cook time: 25 mins, Total time: 30 mins, Servings: 8, Grill temp: 300°F

Ingredients

Sesame dressing
- ¼ cup of brown sugar
- ¼ cup of olive oil
- 2 tbsp of red wine vinegar
- 2 tbsp of sesame seeds- toasted
- 1 tbsp of soy sauce

Salad
- 2 tbsp of olive oil
- 1 package of ramen noodles
- ¼ cup of sliced almonds
- 1 bunch of baby boy choy sliced
- 5 chopped scallions

Directions

To make the dressing
1. Combine the olive oil, brown sugar, sesame seeds, vinegar, & soy sauce in a tiny jar/bowl with a tight-fitting cover.
2. Let the flavors mix at room temp as the rest of the salad is being prepared.

To make the salad
1. In a wide saucepan, heat the olive oil till it shimmers, on med heat. Lower the heat.
2. Add the ramen noodles & almonds, sauté for around 10 mins, till toasted, stirring regularly to prevent scorching.
3. Combine the baby bok choy, the scallions, and the crunchy mix in a wide bowl. Sprinkle salad dressing on the top & toss till evenly mixed. At room temperature, serve.

For toasting sesame seeds
1. Warm the sesame seeds in a med pan on med heat till they are golden brown & fragrant, often stirring, for around 3 to 5 mins.
2. Take it from heat & move it to a plate instantly to cool fully. Place in an airtight jar in the pantry for 6 months or up to 1 year in a freezer.

To make ahead
1. Mix the sesame dressing and store it in the fridge.
2. Scallions & Baby bok choy can be minced & kept separately in the fridge within the containers.
3. The crunchy combination can be toasted in advance, cooled, and kept at room temp.

Nutritional Values

Calories 222, Fat 17g, Chol 0mg, Sodium 71.4mg, Potassium 67.7mg, Carbs 16g, Protein 3g

531. Baby Lima Bean And Quinoa Salad

- Lunch - Prep time: 5 mins, Cook time: 25 mins, Total time: 30 mins, Servings: 4, Grill temp: 300°F

Ingredients

- 2 tbsp of brown rice syrup
- ¼ cup of brown rice vinegar
- Zest of 1 lime and juice of 2 limes
- 4 cups of cooked quinoa
- 2 cups of cooked baby lima beans or 1 15-ounce can drain and rinse
- 1 cup of shredded red cabbage
- 1 carrot, peeled and grated
- ½ cup of chopped cilantro
- Salt and freshly ground black pepper to taste

Directions

1. Place the brown rice syrup, brown rice vinegar, lime zest, and juice in a large bowl and whisk to combine.
2. Add the quinoa, baby lima beans, red cabbage, carrot, cilantro, and salt and pepper, and toss until well mixed. Refrigerate before serving.

Nutritional Values

Calories 113, Fat 1.8g, Chol 0mg, Sodium 81.4mg, Potassium 61mg, Carbs 22g, Protein 2.3g

532. BULGUR, CUCUMBER, AND TOMATO SALAD

- Lunch - Prep time: 5 mins, Cook time: 25 mins, Total time: 30 mins, Servings: 4, Grill temp: 300°F

Ingredients

- 1 ½ cups of bulgur
- 1 cup of cherry tomatoes halved
- 1 medium cucumber halved, seeded, and diced
- 3 cloves garlic, peeled and minced
- 4 green onions- white and green parts, sliced
- Zest and juice of 2 lemons
- 2 tbsp of red wine vinegar
- 1 tsp of crushed red pepper flakes, or to taste
- ¼ cup of minced tarragon
- Salt and freshly ground black pepper to taste

Directions

1. Bring 3 cups of water to a boil in a medium pot and add the bulgur. Remove the pot from the heat, cover with a tight-fitting lid, and let it sit until the water is absorbed and the bulgur is tender for about 15 mins. Spread the bulgur on a baking sheet and let cool to room temperature.
2. Transfer the cooled bulgur to a bowl, add all the remaining ingredients, and mix well to combine. Chill for 1 hour before serving.

Nutritional Values

Calories 211, Fat 1.8g, Chol 0mg, Sodium 71.4mg, Potassium 67.7mg, Carbs 32g, Protein 3.3g

533. BUTTERY GARLIC GREEN BEANS

- Lunch - Prep time: 10 mins, Cook time: 10 mins, Total time: 20 mins, Servings: 4, Grill temp: 300°F

Ingredients

- 1 lb. of green beans
- 3 tbsp of butter
- 3 chopped garlic cloves
- Lemon pepper to taste
- Salt

Directions

1. In a big pan, put the green beans & fill them with water, and carry them to a simmer. Lower the heat to med-low & boil for around 5 mins before the beans begin to soften. Drain the water. Put the butter to the green beans, mix & cook for 2 - 3 mins, till the butter is melted.
2. Cook & mix garlic only with green beans for 3-4 mins, till garlic is soft & fragrant.
3. Garnish with lemon pepper & salt.

Nutritional Values

Calories 116, Fat 8.8g, Chol 0mg, Sodium 71.4mg, Potassium 67.7mg, Carbs 9g, Protein 13g

534. CITRUS GREEN BEANS WITH PINE NUTS

- Lunch - Prep time: 5 mins, Cook time: 20 mins, Total time: 25 mins, Servings: 4, Grill temp: 300°F

Ingredients

- 1 lb. of trimmed green beans
- 1 tsp of grated orange rind
- 2 tsps of olive oil
- ¾ cup of sliced shallots
- 1 tbsp of orange juice fresh
- 1 tbsp of toasted pine nuts
- ¼ tsp of black pepper
- 1/8 tsp of the coarse salt sea

Directions

1. Cook the green beans for 2 mins in boiling water. Drain under cold running water. Drain well.
2. Over medium-high heat, heat a nonstick skillet. In a pan, add oil, and swirl to coat. Add shallots, and sauté for 2 mins or until soft. Garnish with green beans, and stir well.
3. Add juices, rind, salt, pepper, and sauté for 2 mins. Spoon it into a dish; and sprinkle it with nuts.

Nutritional Values

Calories 186, Fat 3.8g, Chol 0mg, Sodium 71.4mg, Potassium 67.7mg, Carbs 12g, Protein 12g

535. CURRIED RICE SALAD

- Lunch - Prep time: 5 mins, Cook time: 50 mins, Total time: 55 mins, Servings: 4, Grill temp: 300°F

Ingredients

- 2 cups of brown basmati rice
- Zest and juice of 2 limes
- ¼ cup of brown rice vinegar
- ¼ cup of brown rice syrup
- ½ cup of currants
- 6 green onions, finely chopped
- ½ small red onion, peeled and minced
- 1 jalapeño pepper, minced
- 1 tbsp of curry powder
- ¼ cup of chopped cilantro
- Salt and freshly ground black pepper to taste

Directions

1. Rinse the rice under cold water and drain. Add it to a pot with 4 cups of cold water. Bring it to a boil over high heat, reduce the heat to medium, and cook, covered, for 45 to 50 mins, or until the rice is tender.
2. While the rice is cooking, combine the lime zest and juice, brown rice vinegar, brown rice syrup, currants, green onion, red onion, jalapeño pepper, curry powder, cilantro, and salt and pepper in a large bowl and mix well. When the rice is finished cooking, drain off the excess water, add the rice to the bowl, and mix well.

Nutritional Values

Calories 136, Fat 1.8g, Chol 0mg, Sodium 61.4mg, Potassium 37.7mg, Carbs 23g, Protein 2.3g

536. FRUITED MILLET SALAD

- Lunch - Prep time: 10 mins, Cook time: 15 mins, Total time: 20 mins, Servings: 4, Grill temp: 300°F

Ingredients

- 1 cup of millet
- Zest and juice of 1 orange
- Juice of 1 lemon
- 3 tbsp of brown rice syrup
- ½ cup of dried unsulfured apricots, chopped
- ½ cup of currants
- ½ cup of golden raisins
- 1 Gala apple, cored and diced
- 2 tbsp of finely chopped mint

Directions

1. Bring 2 quarts of lightly salted water to a boil over high heat and add the millet. Return to a boil, reduce the heat to medium, cover, and cook for 12 to 14 mins. Drain the water from the millet, rinse it until cool, and set it aside.
2. Place the orange juice and zest, lemon juice, and brown rice syrup in a large bowl. Whisk to combine. Add the apricots, currants, raisins, apple, and mint and mix well. Add the cooked millet and toss to coat. Refrigerate before serving.

Nutritional Values

Calories 213, Fat 1.8g, Chol 0mg, Sodium 71.4mg, Potassium 67.7mg, Carbs 52g, Protein 2.3g

537. GREEK BROCCOLI SALAD

- Lunch - Prep time: 15 mins, Cook time: 0 mins, Total time: 15 mins, Servings: 4, Grill temp: 0

Ingredients

Broccoli salad

- ¼ cup of sliced almonds
- 1 and ¼ lb. of chopped to bite-sized broccolis
- ¼ cup of chopped shallot/red onion
- ⅓ cup of sun-dried tomatoes chopped
- ¼ cup of crumbled feta cheese/thinly sliced Kalamata olives

Dressing

- ½ tsp of Dijon mustard
- ¼ cup of olive oil
- 1 tsp of honey or maple syrup, or agave nectar
- Pinch red pepper flakes
- 1 clove of garlic, pressed or minced
- 2 tbsp of lemon juice
- ½ tsp of dried oregano
- ¼ tsp of salt, more to taste

Directions

1. Toss the broccoli, red onion, sun-dried tomatoes, olives, and almonds in a serving bowl.
2. Whisk together all of the ingredients in a bowl until blended. Drizzle over the salad with the dressing and toss well.
3. Let the salad rest for 30 mins before serving the best flavor so that the broccoli marinates in the lemony dressing.

Nutritional Values

Calories 272, Fat 2g, Chol 0mg, Sodium 51.4mg, Potassium 47.7mg, Carbs 17g, Protein 8g

538. ISRAELI QUINOA SALAD

- Lunch - Prep time: 5 mins, Cook time: 25 mins, Total time: 30 mins, Servings: 4, Grill temp: 300°F

Ingredients

- 4 ½ cups of quinoa
- ¼ tsp of ground cumin
- ¼ tsp of turmeric
- 1 cup of finely chopped tomatoes
- 1 cup of finely chopped cucumber
- ½ cup of finely chopped roasted red bell pepper
- 1 tbsp of basil, finely chopped
- Juice of 1 lemon
- Salt and freshly ground black pepper to taste

Directions

1. Rinse the quinoa under cold water and drain. Bring 1 and ¼ cups of water to a boil in a medium saucepan over high heat. Add the quinoa, cumin, and turmeric and bring to a boil over medium-high heat.
2. Reduce the heat to low, cover, and cook for 10 to 15 mins, or until all the water is absorbed, occasionally stirring. Remove the pan from the heat, fluff the quinoa with a fork, and allow it to cool for 5 mins.
3. While the quinoa cools, combine the tomato, cucumber, red pepper, basil, and lemon juice in a medium bowl. Stir in the cooled quinoa and season with salt and pepper.

Nutritional Values

Calories 223, Fat 3.8g, Chol 0mg, Sodium 71.4mg, Potassium 67.7mg, Carbs 32g, Protein 2.3g

539. QUINOA ARUGULA SALAD

- Lunch - Prep time: 5 mins, Cook time: 25 mins, Total time: 30 mins, Servings: 4, Grill temp: 300°F

Ingredients

- 1 ½ cups of quinoa
- Zest and juice of 2 oranges
- Zest and juice of 1 lime
- ¼ cup of brown rice vinegar
- 4 cups of arugula
- 1 small red onion, peeled and thinly sliced
- 1 red bell pepper, seeded and cut into ½-inch cubes
- 2 tbsp of pine nuts, toasted
- Salt and freshly ground black pepper to taste

Directions

1. Rinse the quinoa under cold water and drain. Bring 3 cups of water to a boil in a pot. Add the quinoa and bring the pot back to a boil over high heat. Reduce the heat to medium, cover, and cook for 15 to 20 mins, or until the quinoa is tender. Drain any excess water, spread the quinoa on a baking sheet, and refrigerate until cool.
2. While the quinoa cools, combine the orange zest and juice, lime zest and juice, brown rice vinegar, arugula, onion, red pepper, pine nuts, and salt and pepper in a large bowl. Add the cooled quinoa and chill for 1 hour before serving.

Nutritional Values

Calories 233, Fat 1.8g, Chol 0mg, Sodium 71.4mg, Potassium 67.7mg, Carbs 35g, Protein 7.3g

540. QUINOA TABBOULEH

- Breakfast/Lunch - Prep time: 15 mins, Cook time: 0 mins, Total time: 5 mins, Servings: 4, Grill temp: 300°F

Ingredients

- 2 ½ cups of quinoa, cooked and cooled to room temperature
- Zest of 1 lemon and juice of 2 lemons, or to taste
- 3 Roma tomatoes, diced
- 1 cucumber, peeled, halved, seeded, and diced
- 2 cups of cooked chickpeas or 1 15-ounce can of chickpeas, drained and rinsed
- 8 green onions- white and green parts, thinly sliced
- 1 cup of chopped parsley
- 3 tbsp of chopped mint
- Salt and freshly ground black pepper to taste

Directions

1. Combine all ingredients in a large bowl. Chill for 1 hour before serving.

Nutritional Values

Calories 226, Fat 1.8g, Chol 0mg, Sodium 71.4mg, Potassium 67.7mg, Carbs 32g, Protein 9.3g

541. QUINOA, CORN, AND BLACK BEAN SALAD

- Breakfast/Lunch - Prep time: 5 mins, Cook time: 25 mins, Total time: 30 mins, Servings: 4, Grill temp: 300°F

Ingredients

- 2 ½ cups of cooked quinoa
- 3 ears of corn, kernels removed
- 1 red bell pepper, roasted, seeded, and diced
- ½ small red onion, peeled and diced
- 2 cups of cooked black beans or 1 15-ounce can drain and rinse
- 1 cup of finely chopped cilantro
- 6 green onions- white and green parts, thinly sliced
- 1 jalapeño pepper, minced- for less heat, remove the seeds
- Zest of 1 lime and juice of 2 limes
- 1 tbsp of cumin seeds, toasted and ground
- Salt to taste

Directions

1. Combine all ingredients in a large bowl and mix well.
2. Chill for 1 hour before serving.

Nutritional Values

Calories 178, Fat 2.8g, Chol 0mg, Sodium 54mg, Potassium 77mg, Carbs 26g, Protein 5.3g

542. RICE SALAD WITH FENNEL, CHICKPEAS, AND ORANGE

- Lunch - Prep time: 5 mins, Cook time: 25 mins, Total time: 30 mins, Servings: 4, Grill temp: 300°F

Ingredients

- 2 cups of cooked chickpeas
- 1 orange, peeled, zested, and segmented
- ½ tsp of crushed red pepper flakes
- 1 ½ cups of brown basmati rice
- 1 fennel bulb, diced and trimmed
- ¼ cup plus 2 tbsp of white wine vinegar
- ¼ cup of finely chopped parsley

Directions

1. Combine the rice with 3 cups of cold water in a pot.

2. Bring to a boil over high heat, then reduce the heat and cook for around 50 mins.
3. Mix the chickpeas, orange zest fennel, segments, crushed red pepper flakes, white wine vinegar, and parsley in a large mixing bowl while the rice boils.
4. When the rice is done, pour it into the mixing dish and stir well.

Nutritional Values

Calories 222, Fat 1.8g, Chol 0mg, Sodium 36.4mg, Potassium 73.7mg, Carbs 32g, Protein 2.3g

543. SPICY ASIAN QUINOA SALAD

- Breakfast/Lunch - Prep time: 5 mins, Cook time: 25 mins, Total time: 30 mins, Servings: 4 to 6, Grill temp: 300°F

Ingredients

- ¼ cup plus 2 tbsp of brown rice vinegar
- 4 cloves garlic, peeled and minced
- Zest and juice of 2 limes
- 1 ½ tbsp of grated ginger
- 1 ½ tsps of crushed red pepper flakes
- 4 cups of cooked quinoa
- 2 cups of cooked adzuki beans or 1 15-ounce can drain and rinse
- ¾ cup of mung bean sprouts
- ½ cup of finely chopped cilantro
- 6 green onions- white and green parts, thinly sliced
- Salt to taste
- 4 cups of spinach

Directions

1. Combine the brown rice vinegar, ginger, lime zest and juice, garlic, and crushed red pepper flakes in a large bowl and mix well.
2. Add the quinoa, green onions, mung bean sprouts, adzuki beans, cilantro, and salt and toss to coat. Refrigerate for 30 mins before serving on top of the spinach.

Nutritional Values

Calories 223, Fat 3.8g, Chol 0mg, Sodium 71.4mg, Potassium 67.7mg, Carbs 32g, Protein 2.3g

544. SPRING ASPARAGUS SALAD WITH LEMON VINAIGRETTE

- Lunch/Sides - Prep time: 35 mins, Cook time: 0 mins, Total time: 35 mins, Servings: 4, Grill temp: 0

Ingredients

- ½ lemon juiced & zested
- 2 scallions chopped
- 1 ½ lb. of asparagus spears
- 3 tsps of white wine vinegar
- Black pepper
- 1 ½ tsps of mint finely diced
- 1/3 cup of sliced almonds toasted
- 1 cup of grape tomatoes quartered
- 4 tbsp of olive oil
- Sea salt
- ½ cup of shaved Parmesan/Manchego cheese

Directions

1. In a bowl, combine the lemon zest and scallions, vinegar, lemon zest & juice, and salt and pepper to taste. Stir and let sit for 15 mins.
2. In a frying pan, toast the sliced almonds over medium-low heat for 5 mins, often stirring, until golden brown. Remove and cool from the stovetop.
3. To thinly slice the asparagus into strips, use a vegetable peeler. Pace the sliced spears with the quartered tomatoes in a large bowl.
4. Drizzle the oil in a thin and steady stream into the lemon-vinegar mixture, whisking constantly. Season with salt and pepper to taste.
5. Toss ½ of the cheese, asparagus, almonds, mint, and tomatoes in the dressing. If desired, season with pepper and salt again. Allow the salad to sit before serving for 10 mins, then top with the remaining cheese.

Nutritional Values

Calories 288, Fat 23g, Chol 0mg, Sodium 71.4mg, Potassium 67.7mg, Carbs 12g, Protein 11g

545. WARM RICE AND BEAN SALAD

- Lunch - Prep time: 5 mins, Cook time: 25 mins, Total time: 30 mins, Servings: 4, Grill temp: 300°F

Ingredients

- 1 ½ cups of brown basmati rice, toasted in a dry skillet over low heat for 2 to 3 mins,
- 2 cups of cooked navy beans or 1 15-ounce can, drained and rinsed
- ¼ cup plus 2 tbsp of balsamic vinegar
- ¼ cup of brown rice syrup
- Zest and juice of 1 lemon
- 1 cup of thinly sliced green onion- white and green parts
- 2 tbsp of minced tarragon
- ¼ cup of minced basil
- Salt and freshly ground black pepper to taste
- 4 cups of packed baby spinach

Directions

1. Rinse the toasted rice under cold water and drain. Add it to a pot with 3 cups of cold water. Bring it to a boil over high heat, reduce the heat to medium, and cook, covered, for 45 to 50 mins, or until the rice is tender.
2. While the rice is cooking, add the beans, balsamic vinegar, brown rice syrup, lemon zest and juice, green onion, tarragon, basil, and salt and pepper to a large bowl and mix well. When the rice is finished cooking, drain off the excess water, add it to the bowl and mix well. Divide the spinach between 4 plates and spoon the salad on top.

Nutritional Values

Calories 218, Fat 1.8g, Chol 0mg, Sodium 71.4mg, Potassium 67.7mg, Carbs 27g, Protein 5.3g

546. WINTER GREENS SALAD WITH POMEGRANATE & KUMQUATS

- Lunch/Sides - Prep time: 5 mins, Cook time: 35 mins, Total time: 35 mins, Servings: 12, Grill temp: 300°F

Ingredients

- 6 tbsp of pomegranate juice
- 1 ½ tsps of cornstarch
- 1 ½ tsps of sugar
- ⅛ tsp of garlic salt
- 1 cup pomegranate arils/raspberries
- ¼ cup of extra-virgin olive oil
- 1 ½ tbsp of orange juice

- 2 heads of Belgian endive without
- ¼ cup of toasted walnuts
- 5 cups of bitter baby greens
- ½ cup of kumquats, thinly sliced/orange segments
- 1 small head-torn radicchio
- ½ tsp of orange zest
- ¼ cup of toasted pepitas/pistachios

Directions

1. In a small saucepan, combine the orange zest, sugar, pomegranate juice, orange juice, cornstarch, and garlic salt, and whisk well. Heat over medium-high heat, constantly stirring, before the mixture starts to boil, darkens, and becomes cooler, around 5 mins. Remove from the heat and leave to cool for 20 mins at room temperature. Whisk the oil in.
2. On a plate, arrange radicchio, endive, and baby greens. Cover with oranges and raspberries and drizzle with the dressing. Sprinkle with pistachios and walnuts.

Nutritional Values

Calories 337, Fat 13g, Chol 0mg, Sodium 71.4mg, Potassium 67.7mg, Carbs 28g, Protein 28g

547. ZUCCHINI AND AVOCADO SALAD WITH GARLIC HERB DRESSING

- Lunch/Sides - Prep time: 20 mins, Cook time: 25 mins, Total time: 45 mins, Servings: 4, Grill temp: 400°F

Ingredients

Chickpeas
- Fifteen ounces of chickpeas
- Salt to taste
- 1 tbsp of olive oil
- Black pepper to taste

Salad
- 4 medium zucchinis
- 1 jicama
- 2 large avocados
- Kale
- Arugula
- Basil
- Microgreens
- Chopped parsley
- ½ cup of chopped green onion

Dressing

- ½ cup of tahini
- ½ cup of cilantro
- 1 lemon juiced
- 1 and ¼ cups of parsley without stem
- Pepper to taste
- 1 tbsp of apple cider vinegar
- 1 tbsp of honey
- Salt to taste
- Water

Directions

Chickpeas

1. Preheat the oven to 400 ° F. Toss the dried and rinsed chickpeas with salt, pepper, and olive oil in a medium bowl. Spread the chickpeas over the baking sheet evenly and roast for around 30 mins or until crispy. Remove from the oven and cool aside.
2. Meanwhile, shave the zucchini thinly while the chickpeas are roasting. Slice the jicama and cube the avocado into thin matchsticks. Just set aside.
3. Arrange the greens in a large salad bowl — arugula, kale, microgreens- if required, chopped green onions, and fresh herbs. To combine, toss. On top of the greens, arrange the zucchini ribbons, jicama, and avocado, and top it with cooled roasted chickpeas.

Dressing

1. In a blender, add all ingredients and process until creamy and smooth. Add water if required and any necessary seasoning.
2. Drizzle and serve with your preferred amount of dressing garlic herb. The dressing will last up to 3-4 days in the refrigerator.

Nutritional Values

Calories 775, Fat 49g, Chol 0mg, Sodium 71.4mg, Potassium 67.7mg, Carbs 74g, Protein 21g

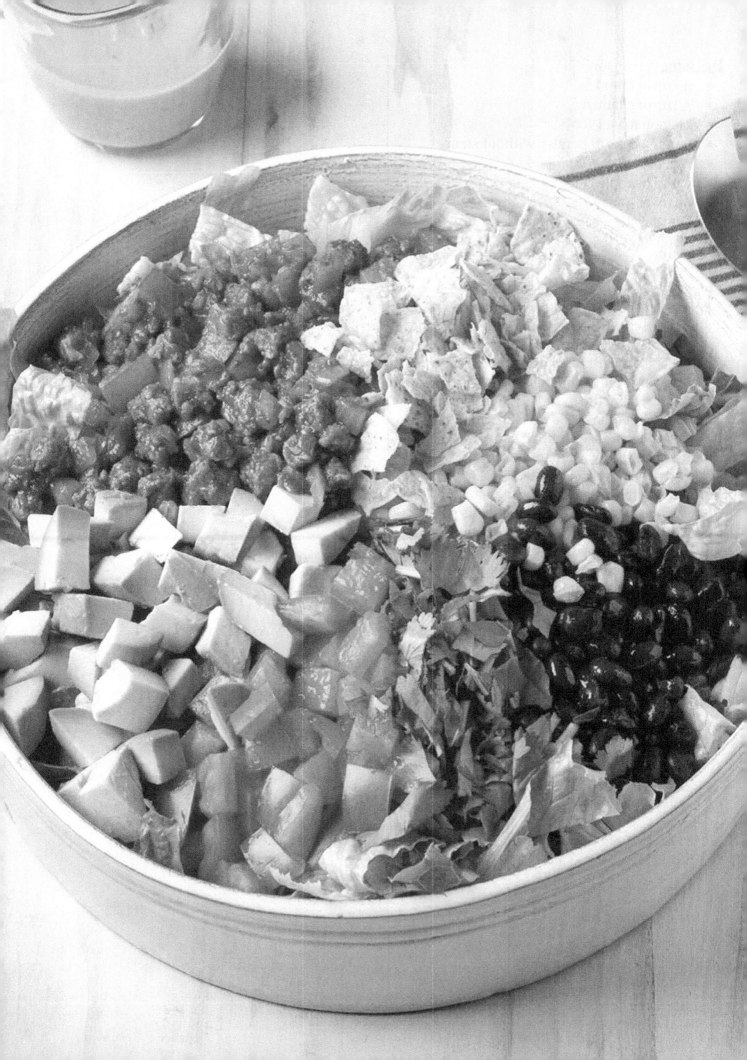

Chapter 15.

Vegan Recipes

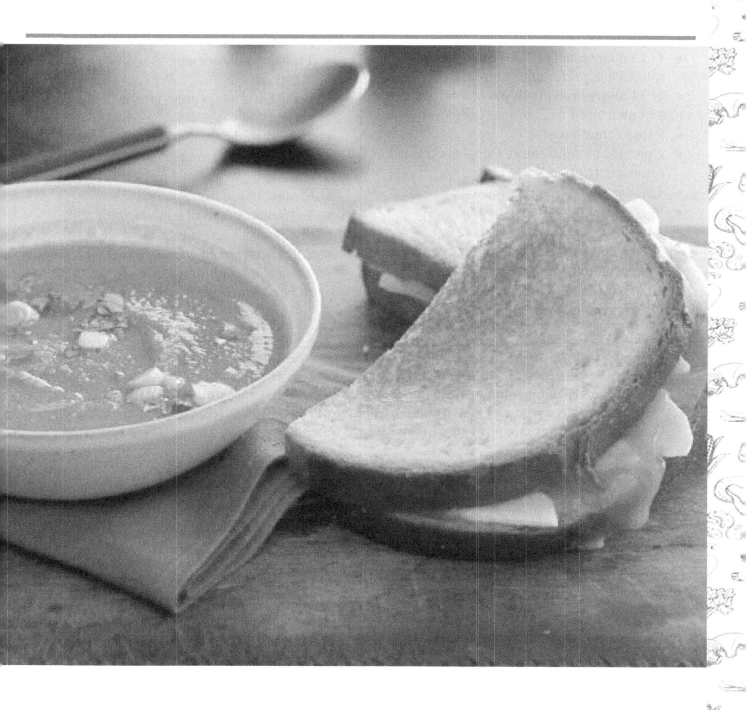

548. SLOW-COOKER CHICKEN & CHICKPEA SOUP

- Prep time: 20 mins, Cook time: 4 hrs, Total time: 4 hrs 20 mins, Servings: 6

Ingredients

- 4 cups water
- 1 ½ cups chickpeas, dried-soaked overnight
- ½ tsp salt
- 1 big yellow onion, chopped finely
- ¼ cup halved pitted oil-cured olives
- 1- 15 ounces can of diced tomatoes, no-salt-added, preferably fire-roasted
- 1- 14 ounces can artichoke hearts, drained and quartered
- 2 tbsp tomato paste
- 2 pounds bone-in chicken thighs, skin removed, trimmed
- 4 cloves garlic, finely chopped
- ¼ tsp ground pepper
- 1 bay leaf
- ¼ cup chopped fresh parsley or cilantro
- 4 tsp ground cumin
- 4 tsp paprika
- ¼ tsp cayenne pepper

Directions

1. Place chickpeas in a 6-quart /larger slow cooker, drained. Stir together 4 cups water, onion, tomatoes and juice, tomato paste, garlic, bay leaf, cumin, paprika, cayenne, and ground pepper. Toss in the chicken.
2. Cook on low for about 8 hrs or high for 4 hrs, covered.
3. Allow the chicken to cool slightly on a clean chopping board. Bay leaf should be discarded. Stir together the artichokes, olives, and salt in the slow cooker. Remove the bones from the chicken and shred them. Add the chicken to the broth and mix well.
4. Serve with parsley on top or cilantro.

Nutritional Values

Calories 447kcal, Carbohydrates-43g, Protein 33.6g, Fat 15g, Sodium 761.8mg

549. BUTTERNUT SQUASH SOUP WITH APPLE GRILLED CHEESE SANDWICHES

- Prep time: 30 mins, Cook time: 15 mins, Total time: 45 mins, Servings: 4

Ingredients

- 1 cup chopped onion
- 1 cup shredded smoked Gouda or Cheddar cheese
- 2 tbsp minced fresh ginger
- 4 slices of whole-wheat country bread
- 1 tsp ground cumin
- 1 tbsp lime juice
- 1 tsp ground turmeric
- ¾ tsp salt
- ¼ tsp cayenne pepper, plus more for garnish
- 1 small apple, thinly sliced, divided
- 5 cups cubed- 1-inch peeled butternut squash
- Ground pepper for garnish
- 1- 15 ounces can of light coconut milk, divided
- 2 tbsp grapeseed oil or coconut oil divided
- 2 cups low-Sodium no-chicken broth or chicken broth

Directions

1. Take a large saucepan and heat 1 tbsp oil over medium heat. Cook, occasionally stirring, until the onion and ginger begin to soften, approximately 3 mins. Cook, constantly stirring, for 30 seconds after adding cumin, turmeric, and cayenne. Combine the squash, broth, ½ of the apple pieces, and coconut milk- save 4 tbsp for decoration, if wanted, and salt in a large mixing bowl. Bring the water to a boil. Reduce the heat to a low simmer & cook, occasionally stirring, for approximately 20 mins or until the squash is soft. Add the lime juice and mix well. Remove the pan from the heat.
2. Using an immersion blender or batches in a blender, puree the soup in the pan.- When combining hot liquids, use care.
3. Split ½ a cup of cheese between 2 pieces of bread. Add the remaining apple pieces, cheese, and bread to the top. In a large non-

stick skillet, heat the rest of the 1 tbsp oil over medium heat.

4. Cook for approximately 2 mins on each side until the sandwiches are gently browned on both edges and the cheese is melted. Slice in ½. If preferred, top the soup with the saved coconut milk, more cayenne, and ground pepper.

Nutritional Values

Calories   419kcal,   Carbohydrates-43.3g, Protein 11g, Fat 10.6g, Sodium 826.9mg

550. WHEAT BERRY SALAD WITH ROASTED BEETS & CURRY CASHEW DRESSING

- Prep time: 15 mins, Cook time: 1 hr, Total time: 1 hr 15 mins, Servings: 6

Ingredients

- 1 ½ cups wheat berries- soaked overnight
- ¼ cup parsley- chopped
- ½ cup pecans- lightly roasted
- ½ cup kalamata olives- optional
- ¼ cup cranberries
- 6 beets
- 2 tbsp golden raisins

For the curry cashew dressing:

- ½ cup cashews- soaked for 30 mins, then drained
- Salt to taste
- 1 tsp curry powder
- Juice of 1 lemon
- ¼ tsp turmeric
- 1 tsp Sriracha sauce

Directions

1. The wheat berries should be cooked. Rinse the berries & combine them with 4 cups water and 1 tsp salt in a saucepan. Bring to a boil, then reduce to low heat and cook for an hour, or until the berries are soft but still chewy. Add 4 cups of water to a pressure cooker and cook for 3 whistles. Before using, drain the cooked wheat berries.
2. Preheat the oven to 400°F before beginning to roast the beets. You may peel the beets before or after roasting. Because the skins peel off more readily after the procedure, on a baking sheet, roast the beets for 35-40 mins; halfway through the

Cook time, flip the chicken. When you can easily pierce the middle of the beets with a fork, they're tender. Transfer the beets from the oven and cool them before cutting them into 12-inch chunks.

3. To make the dressing, combine all of the ingredients with ½ cup of water in a blender. Blend until the mixture is completely smooth.
4. In a large mixing bowl, combine the raisins, cranberries, wheat berries, and olives- if using pecans and parsley. Add the beets next since they will turn everything a deep red. Serve with the dressing drizzled on top.

Nutritional Values

Calories 354kcal, Carbohydrates-53g, Protein 11g, Fat 13g, Sodium 260mg

551. CARROT AND GINGER SOUP RECIPE

- Prep time: 10 mins, Cook time: 0 mins, Total time: 10 mins, Servings: 4

Ingredients

For The Soup:

- 2 medium onions, peeled and chopped
- 600g of carrots, peeled and chopped
- Sea salt and black pepper
- 1 clove of garlic, peeled and crushed
- 1 ½ liters of good stock, chicken or vegetable
- 3tbsp olive oil
- The pared rind of 1 lemon
- 1tsp powdered ginger
- 1tsp medium curry powder

For The Lemon Herb Cream, For Serving:

- 2 tsp parsley, chopped
- The rind of 1 lemon, finely grated
- 2 tsp chives, chopped
- 1- 200g crème fraîche

Directions

1. Take a saucepan and heat olive oil, then add the carrots & onions, simmer for several mins, occasionally stirring. The veggies should not be browned.
2. Cook for another minute after adding the ginger, garlic, and curry powder. Add the lemon strips & stock to the saucepan, cover

halfway with the lid, and cook for 20 mins or until carrots are soft.

3. Allow cooling somewhat before pureeing the soup until smooth. Sprinkle with salt and pepper to taste. To serve, reheat the dish.
4. To make the lemon herb cream, combine the following ingredients in a mixing bowl. Combine all of the ingredients and pour a tsp on top of the soup.

Nutritional Values

Calories 148kcal, Carbohydrates-33g, Protein 4g, Fat 1g, Sodium 1209mg

552. WARM BROCCOLI AND CHICKEN SALAD RECIPE

- Prep time: 10 mins, Cook time: 15 mins, Total time: 25 mins, Servings: 4

Ingredients

- A small handful of fresh tarragon leaves, roughly chopped
- 200g- 7oz Tenderstem broccoli
- 150g- 5oz mixed salad leaves
- 1 clove of garlic, crushed
- 150g- 5oz cherry tomatoes, halved
- 1tbsp sunflower oil
- 4 boneless, skinless chicken breasts cut into chunky strips
- Salt and pepper
- 25g- 1oz pine nuts, toasted
- Grated zest of 1 lemon
- 6 spring onions, sliced

Directions

1. To create this superfood dish, combine the chicken strips, tarragon, lemon zest, salt, and pepper in a mixing bowl and toss thoroughly. Allow marinating for several hours in the refrigerator.
2. In a small dish, combine the dressing ingredients and leave them aside.
3. Put the salad greens, tomatoes, & spring onions in a serving dish and add salt and pepper when ready to dine.
4. In a heavy-bottomed frying pan, heat the oil and cook the chicken for 8-10 mins, regularly flipping, until golden brown & cooked through. Last-minute, add the garlic. Remove the pan from the heat and

whisk in the dressing, covering the chicken and removing any pieces from the pan's bottom.

5. Meanwhile, simmer the broccoli for 4-5 mins in boiling, salted water or until just tender.
6. Add the broccoli & chicken to the salad, then top with toasted pine nuts.

Nutritional Values

Calories 237kcal, Carbohydrates-33.1g, Protein 6.9g, Fat 1g, Sodium 431mg

553. CHEESY GROUND BEEF & CAULIFLOWER CASSEROLE

- Prep time: 15 mins, Cook time: 15 mins, Total time: 30 mins, Servings: 6

Ingredients

- ½ cup chopped onion
- 1- 15 ounces can petite-diced tomatoes, no-salt-added
- 1 pound lean ground beef
- ¼ tsp ground chipotle
- 3 cups bite-size cauliflower florets
- ½ tsp salt
- 3 cloves garlic, minced
- 1 tsp dried oregano
- 1 tbsp olive oil- extra-virgin
- 2 tsp ground cumin
- 2 cups extra-sharp Cheddar cheese, shredded
- ⅓ cup pickled jalapeños, sliced
- 1 medium green bell pepper, chopped
- 2 tbsp chili powder

Directions

1. Place the rack in the top third of the oven. Preheat the broiler to its highest setting.
2. In a big oven-safe skillet, heat the oil over medium heat. Cook, occasionally turning, until the onion & bell pepper is softened, approximately 5 mins. Cook, tossing occasionally and breaking up the meat into tiny pieces, until no longer pink, 5 to 7 mins.
3. Stir in the garlic, chili powder, cumin, oregano, salt, and chipotle, and simmer for 1 minute, or until fragrant. Bring the tomatoes & their juices to a simmer, then cook, stirring periodically, for another 3

mins, or until the liquid has reduced & the cauliflower is soft. Remove the pan from the heat.

4. Cheese should be sprinkled over the meat mixture, and sliced jalapenos should be placed on top. Broil for 2 to 3 mins, or until the cheese is melted & browned in places.

Nutritional Values

Calories 351kcal, Carbohydrates-11g, Protein 26g, Fat 23g, Sodium 672mg

554. EASY ITALIAN WEDDING SOUP

- Prep time: 10 mins, Cook time: 10 mins, Total time: 20 mins, Servings: 6

Ingredients

- 1 ⅓ cup chopped yellow onion
- ⅔ cup chopped carrot
- 24 cooked chicken meatballs- 12 ounces
- ⅔ cup chopped celery
- ½ tsp kosher salt
- 2 tbsp minced garlic
- 1 ½ tbsp chopped fresh oregano
- 6 cups unsalted chicken broth
- ¼ cup grated Parmesan cheese
- 4 tbsp extra-virgin olive oil, divided
- 4 cups of baby spinach
- 6 ounces orzo, preferably whole-wheat

Directions

1. Take a big saucepan and heat 1 tbsp oil over medium-high heat. Add the onion, carrot, celery, and garlic and simmer, occasionally stirring, for 4 to 5 mins, or until the onion are transparent. Bring the broth to a boil, covered. Add the orzo, oregano, and salt, cover, and simmer, occasionally stirring, for approximately 9 mins, or until the orzo are just soft.

2. Cook, occasionally stirring, until the meatballs are cooked through and spinach has wilted for about 2 to 4 mins. Serve with the remaining 3 tbsp oil drizzled over top and cheese sprinkled on top.

Nutritional Values

Calories 415kcal, Carbohydrates-36.1g, Protein 25.8g, Fat 4.7g, Sodium 738mg

555. SLOW-COOKER CHICKEN & WHITE BEAN STEW

- Prep time: 15 mins, Cook time: 7 hrs 35 mins, Total time: 7 hrs 40 mins, Servings: 6

Ingredients

- 6 cups unsalted chicken broth
- 2 bone-in chicken breasts- 1 pound each
- 1 pound dried cannellini beans, soaked overnight, and drained
- 2 tbsp extra-virgin olive oil
- 1 cup chopped yellow onion
- ½ tsp ground pepper
- 1 cup sliced carrots
- ½ tsp kosher salt
- 1 tsp finely chopped fresh rosemary
- 1 tbsp lemon juice
- 1- 4 ounces Parmesan cheese rind plus 2/3 cup grated Parmesan, divided
- ¼ cup flat-leaf parsley leaves
- 4 cups chopped kale

Directions

1. In a 6-quart slow cooker, combine the broth, beans, onion, rosemary, carrots, and Parmesan rind. Serve with chicken on top. Cover and simmer on low for 7 to 8 hours, or until the beans & veggies are cooked.

2. Move the chicken to a clean chopping board and set aside for 10 mins, or until cool enough to handle. Remove the bones from the chicken and shred them.

3. Stir in the greens and transfer the chicken to the slow cooker. Cook on high for 20 to 30 mins, or until the kale is soft.

4. Remove the Parmesan rind and add lemon juice, salt, and pepper to taste.

5. Serve the stew with a drizzle of oil and a sprinkling of Parmesan and parsley on top.

Nutritional Values

Calories 493kcal, Carbs 53.8g, Protein 44.2g, Fat 10.9g, Sodium 518mg

556. SPINACH & ARTICHOKE CASSEROLE WITH CHICKEN AND CAULIFLOWER RICE

- Prep time: 20 mins, Cook time: 25 mins, Total time: 45 mins, Servings: 4

Ingredients

- 1 pound boneless, skinless chicken breasts cut into 1-inch pieces
- 1 ½ cups low-fat plain Greek yogurt

- ¼ tsp salt
- 3 cups coarsely chopped fresh spinach
- ¼ tsp ground pepper
- 1 cup shredded part-skim mozzarella, divided
- 2 cloves garlic, minced
- 1- 14 ounces can quarter artichoke hearts, drained and chopped
- ½ cup unsalted chicken broth
- 1 tbsp extra-virgin olive oil
- 4 cups cauliflower rice

Directions

1. Preheat the oven to 375°F. Spray a baking dish lightly with cooking spray.
2. In a big saucepan over medium heat, heat the oil. Add the chicken, season with salt and pepper, and cook, occasionally tossing, for 4 mins, or until opaque on both sides. Cook for 1 minute, constantly stirring. Cook, constantly stirring, until the liquid is reduced & the chicken is cooked through about 3 to 4 mins. Remove the pan from the heat and add the cauliflower rice, spinach, yogurt, and ½ cup of mozzarella cheese.
3. Sprinkle the leftover ½ cup cheese over the top of the mixture in the prepared baking dish. Bake for 20 to 25 mins, or until the cheese melt & begins to color in areas. Allow for at least 5 mins of resting time before serving.

Nutritional Values

Calories 396kcal, Carbohydrates-19g, Protein 47g, Fat 14g, Sodium 543mg

557. Spicy Weight-Loss Cabbage Soup

- Prep time: 0 mins, Cook time: 20 mins, Total time: 20 mins, Servings: 8

Ingredients

- 2 cups chopped onions
- 1 tsp ground cumin
- ½ tsp ground coriander
- 2 tbsp extra-virgin olive oil
- 2 tbsp lime juice
- 1 cup carrot, chopped
- ½ cup chopped fresh cilantro, plus more for serving
- 1 cup celery, chopped

- ¾ tsp salt
- 1 cup poblano or green bell pepper, chopped
- 2- 15 ounces cans of low-Sodium pinto or black beans, rinsed
- 4 large cloves of garlic, minced
- 4 cups water
- 8 cups sliced cabbage
- Crumbled queso fresco, nonfat plain Greek yogurt, and diced avocado for garnish
- 1 tbsp tomato paste
- 1 tbsp minced chipotle chiles in adobo sauce
- 4 cups low-sodium vegetable broth or chicken broth

Directions

1. In a big soup pot- 8 quarts or bigger, heat the oil over medium heat. Cook, turning regularly, until carrot, onions, poblano- or bell pepper, celery, and garlic are cooked for about 10 to 12 mins. Cook, occasionally stirring, for another 10 mins or until the cabbage is somewhat softened. Cook, constantly stirring, for 1 minute longer after adding the tomato paste, chipotle, cumin, and coriander.
2. Add the broth, water, beans, and salt to the pot. Bring to a boil, covered, over high heat. Reduce heat to low and cook, partly covered, for approximately 10 mins, or until the soft veggies.
3. Take the pan off the heat and add the cilantro & lime juice. If preferred, garnish with cheese, yogurt, and avocado.

Nutritional Values

Calories 167kcal, Carbohydrates-27.1g, Protein 6.5g, Fat 3.8g, Sodium 408mg

558. Chicken Cutlets With Sun-Dried Tomato Cream Sauce

- Prep time: 10 mins, Cook time: 20 mins, Total time: 30 mins, Servings: 4

Ingredients

- ¼ tsp salt, divided
- 1 pound of chicken cutlets
- ½ cup heavy cream
- ¼ tsp ground pepper, divided
- 2 tbsp chopped fresh parsley

- ½ cup slivered oil-packed tomatoes- sun-dried, plus 1 tbsp oil from the jar
- ½ cup shallots, finely chopped
- ½ cup white wine, dry

Directions

1. 1/8 tsp each of salt and pepper on the chicken. In a large pan, heat the sun-dried tomato oil over medium heat. Cook, rotating once until the chicken is golden brown and a thermometer put into the thickest section registers 165°F, approximately 6 mins, total. Place on a platter to cool.
2. Toss in the sun-dried tomatoes & shallots in a pan. Cook for 1 minute, constantly stirring. Increase the heat to high & pour in the wine. Cook for about 2 mins, or until the liquid has very much evaporated. Reduce heat to medium-low and mix in the cream, residual chicken juices, and the leftover 1/8 tsp salt and pepper; cook for 2 mins. Return the chicken to a pan and toss it around in the sauce to coat it. Serve the chicken with the sauce & parsley on the side.

Nutritional Values

Calories 324kcal, Carbohydrates-8.4g, Protein 25g, Fat 18.9g, Sodium 249mg

559. AMERICAN GOULASH

- Prep time: 25 mins, Cook time: 5 mins, Total time: 30 mins, Servings: 4

Ingredients

- 1 ½ cups chopped onion
- 1 pound lean ground beef
- 1 cup low-Sodium beef or chicken broth
- 2 large cloves of garlic, minced
- 1- 8 ounces can of no-salt-added tomato sauce
- 2 tsp paprika
- 1- 14 ounces can of no-salt-added diced tomatoes, undrained
- 1 tsp Italian seasoning
- ¼ tsp ground pepper
- 1 tbsp extra-virgin olive oil
- 2 tbsp grated Parmesan cheese
- 1 ¼ cups whole-wheat elbow macaroni
- 1 tsp salt

Directions

1. In a large saucepan, heat the oil over medium-high heat. Cook, breaking up the meat with a spoon until it is no longer pink, approximately 5 mins. Cook, constantly stirring, for 1 minute after adding the paprika, garlic, salt, Italian seasoning, and pepper. Toss in the tomatoes, their juices, the tomato sauce, and the broth. Bring the water to a boil. Reduce the heat to medium-low & cook for 5 mins, covered.
2. Cook, uncovered, for 6 to 9 mins, or until macaroni is cooked, occasionally stirring. Before serving, remove from the heat and set aside for 5 mins. If preferred, top with Parmesan cheese.

Nutritional Values

Calories 418kcal, Carbohydrates-39.9g, Protein 31.1g, Fat 16g, Sodium 725mg

560. 1-POT CHICKEN & CABBAGE SOUP

- Prep time: 20 mins, Cook time: 20 mins, Total time: 40 mins, Servings: 4

Ingredients

- 1 cup chopped sweet onion
- 3 tbsp extra-virgin olive oil
- 4 tbsp grated Parmesan cheese
- 4 cups shredded cabbage
- 2 tbsp sherry vinegar
- 2 cloves garlic, minced
- 2 cups shredded cooked chicken
- 4 cups of low-Sodium chicken broth
- ¼ tsp ground pepper
- 2 medium Yukon Gold potatoes, peeled and chopped
- Chopped fresh flat-leaf parsley leaves for garnish
- 1 medium turnip, peeled and chopped
- ¼ tsp salt

Directions

1. In a big Dutch oven or saucepan, heat the oil over medium heat. Cook, often turning, until onion is translucent, approximately 6 mins. Cook, often stirring, for approximately 6 mins or until the cabbage softens.
2. Add the broth, potatoes, turnip, and salt and pepper to taste. Bring to a boil at

medium-high heat, lower to medium-low heat and continue to cook for 15 mins. Stir in the chicken and simmer for another 5 mins or until the potatoes & turnips are soft. Remove from the heat and add the vinegar. If preferred, sprinkle Parmesan on top of each plate and garnish with parsley.

Nutritional Values

Calories 359kcal, Carbohydrates-25g, Protein 31g, Fat 16g, Sodium 395mg

561. CABBAGE ROLL CASSEROLE

- Prep time: 35 mins, Cook time: 25 mins, Total time: 60 mins, Servings: 8

Ingredients

- 1 pound lean ground beef
- ¼ tsp crushed red pepper
- 1 cup chopped onion
- 2 tsp dried dill
- 3 cloves garlic, minced
- 8 cups chopped green cabbage- 1 ¼ pound
- 2 cups low-sodium chicken or beef broth
- ½ tsp ground pepper, divided
- 1- 15 ounces can of no-salt-added tomato sauce
- 1 ½ cups shredded Cheddar cheese
- 1 cup long-grain white rice
- 3 tbsp extra-virgin olive oil, divided
- ½ tsp salt, divided

Directions

1. Preheat the oven to 360°F. Spray a baking dish lightly with spray.
2. Take a large saucepan and heat 1 tbsp oil over medium heat. Cook, occasionally stirring, until the ground beef is no longer pink, approximately 5 mins. Cook for 1 minute or until garlic is aromatic. Bring to a boil with the broth, rice, tomato sauce, ¼ tsp salt, and ¼ tsp pepper.
3. Cover, decrease the heat to maintain a low simmer, and cook, whisking once or twice, for approximately 17 mins or until the rice is cooked. Remove the top and turn off the heat.
4. In a large pan, heat the remaining 2 tbsp oil over medium heat. Combine the cabbage, dill, crushed red pepper, and the remaining ¼ tsp salt and pepper in a mixing bowl.

Cook, occasionally turning, for 5 to 7 mins or until the cabbage is tender. Remove the pan from the heat.
5. In the bottom of the baking dish, spread ½ of the cabbage. ½ of the meat mixture should be on top, followed by ½ of the cheese. Using the leftover cabbage, meat mixture, and cheese, repeat the process.
6. Bake for approximately 25 mins or until the cheese has melted & begun to color.

Nutritional Values

Calories 309kcal, Carbohydrates-16g, Protein 20g, Fat 18g, Sodium 362mg

562. VEGAN ALMOND FLOUR SHORTBREAD COOKIES

- Prep time: 5 mins, Cook time: 13 mins, Total time: 18 mins, Servings: 4

Ingredients

- 1 cup superfine almond flour
- A pinch of sea salt or pink salt
- ½ cup deglet noor dates, about 12. Soak in water for 30 mins and drain
- 1 tsp pure vanilla extract
- 3 tbsp extra virgin olive oil
- ¼ tsp cardamon powder- from green cardamoms

Directions

1. Preheat the oven to 350°F.
2. Place the dates in a food processor dish and purée until they are very minute bits.
3. In a food processor, combine the other ingredients and pulse until the dough mixes.
4. Make 12 balls out of the dough by dividing them into 12 pieces.
5. Place the dough balls approximately an inch apart on a baking sheet. Then, using the prongs of a fork, draw a crosshatch pattern by pressing down on every ball once and then again at a right angle.
6. Put the cookies inside the oven to bake for 13-14 mins, or until the edges and top are faintly brown. Remove the cookies from the baking pan and set them aside to cool.

Nutritional Values

Calories 65kcal, Carbohydrates-6.1g, Protein 0.7g, Fat 4.7g, Sodium 67mg

563. VEGAN CARROT ALMOND BREAKFAST PUDDING

- Prep time: 10 mins, Cook time: 35 mins, Total time: 45 mins, Servings: 3

Ingredients

- 3 large carrots, grated
- A handful of raisins and cashews for garnish- optional
- 2 ½ cups vanilla almond milk, unsweetened
- 2 tsp coconut oil divided
- ½ cup pitted Medjool dates
- ½ cup ground almonds or almond flour
- 1 tsp green cardamom powder
- ½ tsp pure vanilla extract

Directions

1. Take a big non-stick wok or broad saucepan and heat 1 tbsp of oil. Add the shredded carrots and a bit of salt to taste. Stir everything up well, then seal with a tight lid which can keep some water on top. It allows the carrots to steam without burning & cook more quickly. Allow the carrots to cook for 15 mins, occasionally stirring to prevent them from adhering to the bottom.
2. Combine the dates, 1 cup almond milk, and almond flour in a blender, and add carrots. Mix in the cardamom well. Cover the pot with a cover, add a few drops of water to the top, and simmer the carrots for a further 15 mins, occasionally stirring.
3. The carrots should have soaked all of the almond milk and be rather dry at this point. Cook uncovered for several mins until any visible liquid has evaporated. Stir in the remainder 1 tsp of oil until the carrots are well coated. Cook, uncovered, for a further 10 mins, stirring often. By this time, the carrots should be considerably deeper in color, extremely soft, and have lost their earthy taste.
4. Cook until warmed through, then add the vanilla as well as the remaining ½ cup almond milk. Add extra almond milk if you want the pudding to be a bit runnier.
5. If used as a garnish, spray the bottom of a small pan with cooking spray & toast the cashews & raisins until the raisins swell up and the cashews become brown.
6. Before serving, sprinkle over the pudding.

Nutritional Values

Calories 304kcal, Carbohydrates-35g, Protein 7.1g, Fat 2g, Sodium 489mg

564. WILD RICE MASON JAR SALAD WITH BASIL PESTO

- Prep time: 0 mins, Cook time: 45 mins, Total time: 45 mins, Servings: 4

Ingredients

Wild rice salad

- 2 corn cobs, husked
- 1 cup uncooked Lundberg Farms Organic WildBlend Rice
- 2 cups watercress
- 2 tbsp olive oil
- ¼ cup shelled pistachios
- 1 cup cherry tomatoes, halved
- 2 medium zucchini, cut into ½" strips

Basil pesto dressing

- ¼ cup pine nuts
- juice of 1 lemon
- ½ cup packed fresh basil leaves
- ½ cup extra-virgin olive oil
- 3 clove garlic
- ¼ tsp salt

Directions

1. 1 cup wild rice and 1-third cup water in a 4-quart saucepan. Bring to a boil, covered. Reduce heat to a low simmer and cook for 45 mins or until all the liquid has evaporated. Remove the pan from the heat, stir with a fork, and set it aside to cool.
2. Preheat the oven to broil and transfer the baking tray to the top of the oven while the rice is cooking. Brush olive oil on corn cobs & zucchini slices. Broil corn for 15 mins, turning halfway through. Remove the dish from the oven and set it aside to cool.
3. Mix the ingredients for basil pesto inside a blender and put aside while the corn and zucchini cook.
4. Refrigerate until you're ready to use it.

Nutritional Values

Calories 439kcal, Carbohydrates-16g, Protein 5g, Fat 41g, Sodium 172mg

565. THAI SALAD WITH GINGER PEANUT SAUCE

- Prep time: 25 mins, Cook time: 0 mins, Total time: 25 mins, Servings: 4

Ingredients

- ½ cup uncooked quinoa
- 3-4 green onions diced
- 1 large carrot shaved or sliced thin
- 2 tbsp cilantro
- 1 cup fresh pineapple chopped
- ¼ cup chopped basil
- 2 cup kale, loosely packed
- 1 batch of Thai Peanut Sauce
- ¾ cup edamame
- ½ large red bell pepper sliced thin
- ½ cup roasted cashews

Directions

1. Bring 1 cup of water and quinoa to a boil. Cover and cook for 15-20 mins. Cooked quinoa should be fluffed with a fork & put in the fridge to chill.
2. Prepare all of the salad ingredients while the quinoa is cooking. All of the veggies should be sliced, and the kale should be rubbed.
3. Whisk together the Thai Peanut Sauce Ingredients in a small bowl until smooth.
4. Mix all salad ingredients after the quinoa has cooled. Serve with a dollop of Thai Peanut Sauce on top.

Nutritional Values

Calories 478kcal, Carbohydrates-29g, Protein 13g, Fat 36g, Sodium 656mg

566. THE ULTIMATE DETOX SALAD WITH LEMON GINGER DRESSING

- Prep time: 10 mins, Cook time: 0 mins, Total time: 10 mins, Servings: 2

Ingredients

Lemon ginger dressing
- ¼ tsp salt
- 2 tbsp fresh lemon juice
- 1 tsp turmeric
- 2 cloves garlic, crushed
- 1 tsp maple syrup
- 1 tbsp freshly grated ginger
- pepper, to taste
- 4 tbsp olive oil
- 1 tbsp apple cider vinegar

Detox Salad
- 1 tsp olive oil
- 2 tbsp fresh mint, minced
- pinch of salt
- 2 tbsp fresh cilantro, minced
- 2 cups red cabbage, thinly chopped
- 1 small avocado, cubed
- 1 medium carrot, peeled into thin strips
- ¼ cup roasted sunflower seeds
- 2 green onions, chopped
- 2 radishes, thinly sliced
- 4 large leaves of curly kale, de-stemmed
- 1 rounded cup of broccolini, chopped

Directions

1. In a small blender, combine all of the dressing ingredients and put them aside.
2. Finely chop the kale and combine it with 1 tbsp olive oil and salt in a big salad bowl. Rub the kale with your fingers for a couple of mins until it's darker, soft, and glossy.
3. Toss in the rest of the salad ingredients with Lemon-Ginger Dressing.
4. Serve immediately or keep refrigerated for up to 2 days in an airtight jar.

Nutritional Values

Calories 428kcal, Carbohydrates-21g, Protein 5g, Fat 37g, Sodium 346mg

567. ZUCCHINI NOODLES WITH PESTO

- Prep time: 10 mins, Cook time: 0 mins, Total time: 10 mins, Servings: 2

Ingredients

- about 12 cherry tomatoes, halved
- 1 large zucchini
- red pepper flakes
- 1 batch of vegan pesto
- 1 tbsp olive or coconut oil
- 1 tbsp fresh basil, thinly sliced

Directions

1. Zucchini should be cut off at ½ " spacing. Spiralize the zucchini according to the spiralizer's Directions.
2. In a pan, heat the coconut oil and softly sauté the noodles for 3-4 mins. Take the pan from the heat and put it aside to cool.

3. Follow these Directions to make a vegan pesto.
4. Toss the zucchini noodles with pesto after they've cooled. Add cherry tomatoes that have been halved.
5. Serve the salad on 2 plates with fresh basil & red pepper flakes on top.

Nutritional Values
Calories 93kcal, Carbohydrates-5g, Protein 2g, Fat 8g, Sodium 17mg

568. VEGAN QUINOA SALAD

- Prep time: 15 mins, Cook time: 20 mins, Total time: 35 mins, Servings: 8

Ingredients

Quinoa salad
- about 10 stalks of asparagus, sliced into 1" pieces
- 1 ½ cup quinoa, uncooked
- ¼ cup toasted pine nuts
- 1 cup cherry tomatoes, halved
- 1 cup frozen peas
- ¼ cup fresh basil, chopped

Lemony vinaigrette
- juice of 1 large lemon
- 2 tbsp olive oil
- ¼ tsp pepper
- 2 tbsp white wine vinegar
- ½ tsp salt

Directions

1. Quinoa should be cooked according to the package directions. Prepare the remainder of the salad while the quinoa is cooking.
2. Boil the peas and asparagus in a small saucepan of water for 3 mins. Prepare an ice bucket while the veggies are cooking. When the veggies are soft, drain them through a strainer and immediately lay them in an ice bath to stop them from cooking any more.
3. Mix the ingredients for the lemon vinaigrette in a small blender.
4. Remove the quinoa from the pan & fluff with a fork after it is done. To chill the quinoa, place it in a large mixing dish & refrigerate for 30 mins.
5. After the quinoa has cooled, combine the other ingredients. Mix with the dressing &

serve right away, or keep refrigerated until ready to be served.

Nutritional Values
Calories 195kcal, Carbohydrates-24g, Protein 6g, Fat 8g, Sodium 150mg

569. VEGAN TACO SALAD

- Prep time: 20 mins, Cook time: 30 mins, Total time: 50 mins, Servings: 4

Ingredients

- taco salad
- 3 small corn tortillas
- 1 batch of walnut/taco meat
- water, as needed
- 2 heads of romaine lettuce, chopped
- ½ -1 tsp salt
- 1 ½ cups black beans
- 1 lime, juiced
- 1 cup cherry tomatoes, halved
- ¼ cup salsa
- 2 small avocados divided
- 1 tbsp coconut oil
- walnut/taco meat
- 1 tbsp coconut oil
- 3-4 cloves of garlic
- 1 tsp chili powder
- ½ cup walnuts, chopped into small pieces
- ½ tsp cumin
- ¼ cup white onion, minced
- ½ cup green lentils
- 1 tsp salt

Directions

1. Cook the lentils as directed on the packet.
2. Heat 1 tbsp coconut oil in a medium cast-iron pan over medium heat while lentils are cooking. When the oil is heated, add the garlic and onions and cook, occasionally stirring, for 5 mins, or until the onions are transparent and aromatic.
3. Stir in the salt, chili, and cumin to coat. Stir in the walnuts and cook for another 5 mins, or until they are gently browned. In a food processor, combine the walnuts and onions. Pulse the cooked lentils a few times till they have a beef-like texture. Remove from the equation.
4. In a blender, combine 1 avocado, salsa, ½ tsp salt, and lime juice to produce the

avocado salsa dressing. Blend until completely smooth. If it's too thick, thin it out with a little water, 1 tbsp at a time, until it's creamy and pourable. Adjust the salt & lime as required.

5. Heat the remaining 1 tbsp coconut oil in a small frying pan. When the pan is heated, add the corn tortillas and cook for 3 mins, on each side or golden and crispy. Remove from the fire, wipe away any leftover oil using a paper towel, and slice into thin strips.

Nutritional Values

Calories 401kcal, Carbohydrates-47g, Protein 18g, Fat 18g, Sodium 449mg

570. SOUTHWEST QUINOA SALAD

- Prep time: 10 mins, Cook time: 20 mins, Total time: 20 mins, Servings: 6

Ingredients

Quinoa salad
- 1 red bell pepper, diced
- 1 ½ cups dried quinoa
- 1 jalapeño, seeded and sliced
- 1 cup of fresh corn
- 1 cup black beans, drained and rinsed
- 1 cup red onions, diced

Dressing
- juice of 2 limes
- ¼ cup olive oil
- 1 tsp salt, to taste
- ¼ cup cilantro, minced
- 2 tsp cumin

Directions

1. Set aside quinoa after rinsing it. Bring 2 ½ cups of water to a boil. Reduce the heat to a low and add the quinoa. Cook for 20 mins or until the water has drained and the quinoa is tender. Mix with a fork in a large mixing bowl. Allow it to chill for at least 20 mins in the refrigerator.
2. Cut the bell peppers, onions, and jalapeno pepper into small pieces. Clean the black beans & corn by rinsing them.
3. While the quinoa is cooking, combine the salad dressing ingredients in a mixing bowl. Mix in the salad dressing until the

quinoa is well covered and no longer warm to the touch.

4. Combine the veggies, black beans, & corn in a large mixing bowl. Season with salt and pepper to taste. Place in the fridge until ready to be served.

Nutritional Values

Calories 314kcal, Carbohydrates-42g, Protein 9g, Fat 12g, Sodium 9mg

571. MEDITERRANEAN QUINOA SALAD

- Prep time: 15 mins, Cook time: 30 mins, Total time: 45 mins, Servings: 4

Ingredients

Quinoa salad
- 1 medium cucumber, chopped
- ½ cup quinoa, uncooked
- ⅓ cup Kalamata olives pitted and halved
- 2 cups Italian parsley, chopped
- ½ avocado, cubed
- 1 cup cherry tomatoes, halved
- ½ cup red onion, thinly sliced

Lemon-pepper dressing
- 2 tsp maple syrup
- 3 tbsp olive oil
- ½ tsp pepper
- juice of 1 large lemon
- ½ tsp salt

Directions

1. Prepare the quinoa as per the package directions.
2. Cut the cucumber, parsley, onions, tomatoes, and olives while the quinoa is cooking.
3. To make the Lemon Pepper Dressing, combine all of the ingredients and put them aside.
4. Remove the quinoa from the heat and set it aside to cool for 30 mins. Mix with the prepped veggies and toss with the lemon pepper dressing after it has cooled.
5. Keep it refrigerated until you're ready to use it.

Nutritional Values

Calories 264kcal, Carbohydrates-23g, Protein 5g, Fat 17g, Sodium 491mg

572. VEGAN SPRING ROLLS WITH SWEET POTATO NOODLES

- Prep time: 20 mins, Cook time: 0 mins, Total time: 20 mins, Servings: 6

Ingredients

- 1 small sweet potato
- ¼ cup loosely packed fresh mint
- 2 tbsp sesame oil, divided
- ¼ cup loosely packed fresh basil
- 4 oz. tempeh
- ½ red bell pepper, cut into 2-3" matchsticks
- 2 tbsp soy sauce
- 1 batch of Thai Peanut Sauce
- 1 tbsp maple syrup
- ½ small carrot, cut into 2-3" matchsticks
- 6 spring roll rice paper wrappers
- ½ small cucumber, cut into 2-3" matchsticks

Directions

1. The sweet potato should be peeled. Then, using the smallest blade on your spiralizer, spiralize the potato into noodles.
2. 1 tbsp sesame oil, heated in a large pan over medium heat. Lightly sauté the sweet potato noodles for 3-4 mins, or until they are deep orange and pliable enough to bite into. Remove the pan from the heat and put it aside.
3. Clean the skillet with a paper towel and heat the leftover sesame oil in it over medium heat. Slice the tempeh into 12"x12" rectangles while the oil is heated. Cook for 4-5 mins, turning regularly until tempeh is brown in hot oil- it should crackle when they drop. Continue to cook until all of the liquid has been absorbed, then add the soy sauce & maple syrup. Take the pan from the heat and put it aside to cool.
4. Get your veggies ready. Remove the stems from the mint & basil but leave them intact.
5. Fill a deep pie dish halfway with heated water to prepare the rice noodles. Put 1 rice paper sheet in the water for 20 seconds, or until it is malleable but not rippable.
6. On a dry surface, place the pliable wrapping. Put 1 small handful of potato noodles on the bottom 1/3 of the wrapper, leaving 1" on either side. Top with 2-3 pieces of tempeh, veggies, and herbs that have been sautéed.
7. Over the filling, fold in the sides and bottom. Then, without tearing the spring roll, wrap it as firmly as possible. Set aside the other 5 spring rolls and proceed with the other 5 spring rolls.
8. Serve right away with Thai Peanut Sauce.

Nutritional Values

Calories 152kcal, Carbohydrates-16g, Protein 6g, Fat 7g, Sodium 449mg

573. EASY GUACAMOLE

- Prep time: 5 mins, Cook time: 0 mins, Total time: 5 mins, Servings: 6

Ingredients

- 2 ripe avocados
- ¾ tsp cumin
- 2-3 cloves garlic, minced
- juice of 1 lime
- ½ jalapeno, diced
- salt, to taste
- ¼ cup red onion, diced
- ⅓ cup cilantro, chopped

Directions

1. In a medium-sized mixing bowl, combine all of the ingredients. Season with salt and pepper to taste.
2. Serve immediately with tortilla or chips.

Nutritional Values

Calories 110kcal, Carbohydrates-6g, Protein 1g, Fat 9g, Sodium 5mg

574. VEGAN CHEDDAR CHEESE WITH JALAPEÑO

- Prep time: 20 mins, Cook time: 0 mins, Total time: 20 mins, Servings: 12

Ingredients

- 1 ½ cups raw cashews- soaked for almost 6 hrs
- ½ cup coconut oil, melted

- 3 tbsp sun-dried tomatoes- soaked for almost 60 mins,
- ½ tsp smoked paprika
- ¼ cup nutritional yeast
- ½ tsp turmeric
- 1 tsp white wine vinegar
- 1 tsp salt
- 1 tsp spicy mustard
- 1 jalapeno, minced
- 1 tbsp tahini paste
- 1 tsp onion powder

Directions

1. The cashews should be drained and rinsed. Blend them with tomatoes, tahini, nutritional yeast, mustard, vinegar, and spices in a food processor until smooth. Slowly drizzle in the coconut oil while the engine is running until it is thoroughly integrated.
2. Place in a large mixing basin. Mix in the diced jalapenos by hand until fully blended. Refrigerate for 4 hours, or until the cheese is solid enough to mold, in an airtight container.
3. Shape the cheese into a wheel or ball once it's moldable, then top with sliced jalapenos and serve with fruit and crackers.

Nutritional Values

Calories 183kcal, Carbohydrates-6g, Protein 3g, Fat 16g, Sodium 204mg

575. 4 INGREDIENT COOKIES

- Prep time: 5 mins, Cook time: 10 mins, Total time: 15 mins, Servings: 3

Ingredients

- ⅓ cup peanut butter
- 2 very ripe bananas, mashed
- 1 ½ cups old-fashioned oats
- ¼ cup chocolate chips or mix-ins of choice

Directions

1. Preheat the oven to 350°F. Set aside a baking sheet lined with parchment paper.
2. In a large bowl, mash the bananas & mix them with oats & peanut butter. Mix thoroughly. Chocolate chunks should be folded in.

3. Bake for 10-12 mins in bite-sized spoonfuls on the prepared baking sheet. Until a light brown color appears, allow 5 mins for the cookies to cool on the baking sheet, then move to a wire rack to cool.
4. Cooking that hasn't been consumed should be stored airtight at room temperature for 5 days.

Nutritional Values

Calories 77kcal, Carbohydrates-10g, Protein 2g, Fat 3g, Sodium 23mg

576. ROASTED GARLIC HUMMUS

- Prep time: 30 mins, Cook time: 0 mins, Total time: 30 mins, Servings: 8

Ingredients

- 2 tbsp olive oil
- salt to taste
- 2 cups canned chickpea, drained & liquid reserved
- ¾ tsp cumin
- ¼ cup tahini paste
- ¼ cup reserved chickpea liquid
- juice of 2 lemons
- roasted garlic hummus
- 10-12 cloves of roasted garlic
- toppings- optional

Directions

1. Combine chickpeas, tahini, 2 tbsp olive oil, roasted garlic, lemon juice, cumin, saved chickpea liquid, & salt in a food processor. Scrape down the sides of the blender as required until it's completely smooth.
2. Serve with crackers, pita, or veggies and desired toppings.
3. Refrigerate for up to 5 days if stored in an airtight container.

Nutritional Values

Calories 117kcal, Carbohydrates-8g, Protein 3g, Fat 8g, Sodium 117mg

577. VEGAN QUESO

- Prep time: 10 mins, Cook time: 20 mins, Total time: 30 mins, Servings: 6

Ingredients

- ¼ tsp turmeric

- 2-3 garlic cloves minced
- ½ tsp chili powder
- 2 jalapeños, seeded & minced
- ½ tsp cumin
- 4 cups cauliflower florets
- ½ cup Nutritional yeast
- ½ cup vegetable broth
- ¼ cup raw cashews, soaked in hot water for at least 1 hr
- ⅓ cup unsweetened non-dairy milk
- salt, to taste
- 1 small yellow onion, diced
- 2 tbsp vegan butter or coconut oil
- 2 sundried tomatoes

Directions

1. Before creating the queso, soak the cashews in boiling water for 1 hour. Drain and rinse after soaking. Remove from the equation.
2. Heat oil or vegan butter in a large cast-iron pan over medium heat. Sauté for 5-7 mins, turning periodically, until onions, garlic, and jalapenos are lightly golden and aromatic. ½ of the onion/jalapeno combination should be left aside.
3. Stir in cauliflower & vegetable broth with the remaining ½ of the onions/jalapenos in the pan. Reduce the heat to low and cover. Cook, occasionally stirring, for approximately 15 mins, or until cauliflower is soft and liquid has been absorbed.
4. Add the other ingredients, including the cashews, to a high-powered blender. Blend until the mixture is smooth. If required, add more milk, 1 tbsp at a time.
5. Serve in a serving dish. Top with fresh jalapenos and the leftover onions and jalapenos. Serve with raw carrots or chips.

Nutritional Values

Calories 119kcal, Carbohydrates-9g, Protein 4g, Fat 7g, Sodium 111mg

578. MEXICAN-STYLE STUFFED ZUCCHINI BOATS

- Prep time: 15 mins, Cook time: 40 mins, Total time: 55 mins, Servings: 4

Ingredients

- ¼ cup fresh cilantro stems removed

- 3 tbsp olive oil, divided
- ⅓ cup black olives
- ½ large red onion, diced
- 1 Roma tomato, diced
- 12 oz. tempeh
- ½ large avocado, peeled & diced
- 3 tbsp taco seasoning
- ¼ cup cauliflower queso
- 4 small or 2 large zucchini
- toppings
- ½ cup tomato sauce
- salt and pepper, to taste
- stuffed zucchini boats
- ½ cup water

Directions

1. Preheat the oven to 400°F. Set aside a 9x12 baking dish lined with tin foil.
2. Cut the zucchinis lengthwise in ½. Scoop out the interior pulp of the zucchini with a grapefruit spoon, leaving approximately 14" around the sides. Set aside in the baking dish after brushing with 1 tbsp olive oil.
3. In a big cast-iron skillet, heat the oil over medium heat. Add the diced onions and cook for 5 mins, or until fragrant and translucent. Crumble the tempeh with your fingers until it looks like ground beef while the onions are frying.
4. Stir in the crumbled tempeh & taco seasoning to coat the onion. Cook for a further 3-5 mins, or until the tempeh is golden brown. Combine tomato sauce & water in a mixing bowl. Allow simmering, stirring regularly, until most of the water has evaporated. It takes around 3 mins.
5. Fill the zucchini holes halfway with taco tempeh filling, forming a rounded top. Cover and bake for 35 mins. Remove the tin foil and continue baking for another 10-15 mins, or until the zucchini is easily punctured with a fork.
6. Prepare your toppings while the zucchini boats are baking.
7. Remove the zucchini boats from the oven and set them aside for 10 mins to cool. Serve immediately after sprinkling with toppings.

Nutritional Values

Calories 277kcal, Carbohydrates-16g, Protein 16g, Fat 18g, Sodium 1240mg

579. VEGAN ENCHILADAS SKILLET

- Prep time: 15 mins, Cook time: 15 mins, Total time: 30 mins, Servings: 4

Ingredients

- 10 small corn tortillas cut into strips
- ½ tsp salt
- 1 can of black beans, drained and rinsed
- 2 tbsp oil divided
- 2 green onions diced
- ½ large red onion diced
- 1 jalapeño diced
- 2-3 cloves minced garlic
- a few springs of cilantro chopped
- 1 small butternut squash peeled & cut into ½" cubes
- salt and pepper to taste
- 1 ½ tsp chili powder
- 4 large kale leaves chopped small
- 10 ounces enchiladas sauce
- 1 cup crushed tomatoes
- 1 avocado
- ½ tsp cumin
- ½ tsp paprika
- ½ cup corn frozen or canned

Directions

1. 1 tbsp oil, heated in a big cast skillet cook, often tossing, for 5 mins, or until tortilla strips are lightly crispy & browned. Place on a paper towel to absorb excess liquid.
2. Add the rest of the oil and cook, stirring regularly, for 5 mins, or until onions are transparent and fragrant. Sauté for another 30 seconds after adding the garlic.
3. Combine the chili powder, butternut squash, paprika, cumin, and salt in a large mixing bowl. Reduce heat to low & cover after stirring to coat. Cook until the squash is soft, about 15 mins. It takes around 5 mins.
4. Combine the corn, black beans, enchiladas sauce, tomatoes, and kale in a large mixing bowl. Cook for another 3 mins, or until the kale has wilted. Salt & pepper to taste.
5. Stir in the corn tortillas & bring to a boil, then reduce to low heat for approximately

10 mins, or until the liquid has reduced. Remove the enchiladas from the pan and put them aside for another 10 mins before serving.
6. Add cilantro, jalapeno, and green onions to the top.

Nutritional Values

Calories 447kcal, Carbs 71g, Protein 11g, Fat 17g, Sodium 448mg

580. EGGPLANT CHICKPEA CURRY

- Prep time: 20 mins, Cook time: 20 mins, Total time: 40 mins, Servings: 4

Ingredients

- 1 tbsp coconut oil
- ¼ tsp cayenne pepper
- ½ tsp salt
- 1 medium eggplant, chopped into 1" cubes
- 3-4 cloves garlic, minced
- ¼ fresh cilantro for garnish
- 1 medium onion, thinly sliced
- 1 ½ cup vegetable broth
- 1 tbsp fresh ginger, minced
- 1 can chickpeas, drained & rinsed
- 1 tbsp curry powder
- 1 cup uncooked rice
- 1 tsp cumin
- ½ tsp turmeric
- 4 cups cherry tomatoes, halved

Directions

1. Cook the rice as directed on the packet. Depending on the kind of rice you use, this may vary.
2. In a big soup pot, heat the oil over medium heat. Add the onions and cook for 5-7 mins, stirring periodically, until aromatic and transparent. Cook for another minute with the garlic and ginger.
3. Stir in the cumin, curry powder, cayenne pepper, turmeric, and salt until the garlic/onion combination is well coated.
4. Mix the tomatoes, eggplant, vegetable broth, and chickpeas in a large mixing bowl. Bring to a low boil, then reduce to low heat and cook, uncovered, for 20-25 mins, or until the tomatoes and eggplant are tender and approximately a third of the liquid has been absorbed.

5. Serve with fresh cilantro on top of rice.

Nutritional Values

Calories 257kcal, Carbohydrates-48g, Protein 5g, Fat 5g, Sodium 665mg

581. VEGAN BOLOGNESE SAUCE WITH MUSHROOMS

- Prep time: 15 mins, Cook time: 30 mins, Total time: 45 mins, Servings: 6

Ingredients

- 1 pound button mushrooms
- 12 ounces Fettuccine Pasta
- ¼ cup fresh basil minced
- 1 yellow onion roughly chopped
- ¼ cup fresh parsley minced
- 2 celery stalks roughly chopped
- ¼ cup tomato paste
- 1 cup dry red wine
- 1 cup unsweetened non-dairy milk
- 28 ounces crushed tomatoes
- 2 tbsp olive oil, divided
- 2 carrots peeled and roughly chopped
- 1 cup raw walnuts
- 4 cloves of garlic roughly chopped
- 1 pound shiitake mushrooms
- salt and pepper to taste

Directions

1. Begin by boiling the pasta in salted water in a big saucepan. Make sure the pot is big enough to prevent the pasta from sticking together as it cooks. Cook for 12 mins, occasionally stirring. Drain the pasta in a strainer and mix it with 1 tbsp of olive oil after it's done. As the pasta cools, this keeps it from sticking together.
2. 2 tbsp oil, heated in a wide sauté pan over medium heat Pulse celery, onions, garlic, carrots, and walnuts a few times in a food processor until finely minced. Transfer to a saucepan and cook, stirring periodically, for 3-4 mins. Clean the food processor before adding the mushrooms. Pulse a few times to break down the mushrooms until they resemble minced meat. Add them to the vegetables and simmer for 3-4 mins, more, or until mushrooms have shrunk in size.
3. Bring the wine to a low simmer. Simmer for 5-7 mins, or until the wine has completely evaporated. Cook for another 5-6 mins, or until the non-dairy milk has evaporated, after stirring in the non-dairy milk.
4. Add the tomato paste, tomatoes, salt, fresh herbs, and pepper when the milk has simmered down. Cook until the sauce is rich & thick, uncovered. Remove the pan from the heat.
5. Serve.

Nutritional Values

Calories 392kcal, Carbohydrates-35g, Protein 13g, Fat 23g, Sodium 310mg

582. PORTOBELLO STEAKS

- Prep time: 5 mins, Cook time: 25 mins, Total time: 30 mins, Servings: 4

Ingredients

- 4 large portobello mushrooms, destemmed
- 2 tbsp balsamic vinegar
- ¼ cup olive oil
- 2 tbsp steak seasoning, salt-free

Directions

1. Preheat the oven to 400°F.
2. Combine balsamic vinegar, olive oil, and steak seasoning in a big shallow dish. Brush the marinade liberally on the tops & bottoms of every mushroom using a pastry brush.
3. Place the mushrooms, top side down, in the leftover marinade and bake for 20 mins, uncovered. Remove from oven, turn, and bake for a further 5-10 mins, or until mushrooms are fully cooked. Serve with grilled veggies and baked potatoes.
4. Optional: Heat a cast iron pan at medium-high heat after the mushrooms have completed baking. Place mushrooms in a heated pan, top side down, and cook for 2-3 mins, or until steak is slightly browned.

Nutritional Values

Calories 132kcal, Carbohydrates-2g, Protein 11g, Fat 13g, Sodium 2mg

583. VEGAN ZUCCHINI NOODLE LASAGNA

- Prep time: 35 mins, Cook time: 50 mins, Total time: 1 hr 25 mins, Servings: 2

- herbed ricotta
- 2 tbsp water
- tempeh "beef"
- 2 tbsp fresh parsley, chopped
- ½ tsp dried sage
- 1 tbsp fresh chives, chopped
- 12 ounces tempeh
- 1 tbsp fresh oregano
- 1 tbsp soy sauce
- 1 batch of cashew ricotta
- ⅛ tsp pepper
- ¼ cup vegan parmesan
- ½ tsp dried oregano
- 2 big zucchinis
- ½ tsp dried parsley
- 2 cloves garlic, minced
- ¼ tsp smoked paprika
- ½ small yellow onion, diced
- ⅕ tsp pepper
- 1 jar - 24 ounces of marinara sauce
- 1 tbsp cooking oil

Directions

1. Preheat the oven to 375°F.
2. Make the cashew ricotta first. Add the rest of the herbed ricotta ingredients and mix until completely combined when it looks like ricotta. Keep it aside until you're ready to utilize it.
3. In a dish, crumble the tempeh into tiny pieces. Mix the soy sauce, spices, herbs, and pepper in a mixing bowl. In a heavy bottom pan, heat the cooking oil over medium heat. Add the garlic and onions and cook, turning regularly, for 5 mins, or until the onions are fragrant & transparent. Sauté the seasoned tempeh until it is lightly browned. Remove the pan from the heat and put it aside.
4. Remove 1" of zucchini from either end. Cut the zucchini lengthwise.
5. 12 cup marinara sauce is layered in a 7x11 pan. Add 1 layer of zucchini on top. In that sequence, layer herbed ricotta, tempeh meat, and marinara sauce. Rep with the marinara sauce in the end. A layer of

zucchini & marinara sauce should be added. Add vegan parmesan cheese on top.
6. Bake for 35 mins, covered with foil. Uncover and bake for another 15 mins, or until the Parmesan is brown and the sauce underneath is boiling.
7. Allow 10 mins to rest before serving.

Nutritional Values

Calories 175kcal, Carbohydrates-10g, Protein 14g, Fat 10g, Sodium 247mg

584. VEGAN SUSHI BOWL

- Prep time: 30 mins, Cook time: 0 mins, Total time: 30 mins, Servings: 4

Ingredients

Sushi bowls
- 1 avocado, cubed
- 1 medium carrot, peeled into strips
- 1 cup cooked Jasmine Rice
- 1 cucumber, thinly sliced
- 1 red bell pepper, seeded and thinly sliced
- 1 cup frozen edamame, thawed

Additional toppings
- quick pickle sauce
- pickled sushi ginger
- ¼ tbsp rice vinegar
- black sesame seeds
- pinch of salt
- roasted seaweed, optional
- ½ cup water

Sesame soy dressing
- 1 tbsp rice vinegar
- 2 tbsp soy sauce
- 1 tbsp sesame oil
- ⅛ tsp wasabi, optional

Directions

1. In a small bowl, mix the ingredients for pickle sauce. Make sure the carrots and cucumbers are well soaked in the liquid before adding them. Cover and chill while you finish the remainder of the dinner.
2. Cook the rice as directed on the packet.
3. Prepare the red bell pepper, edamame, and avocado.
4. To make the sesame soy dressing, combine all of the ingredients and put them aside.
5. Divide the rice into 4 bowls and assemble the bowls. Divide the red bell pepper,

pickled veggies, and edamame into equal portions. Sesame seeds & pickled ginger are sprinkled on top.

6. Serve with Sesame Soy Sauce right away.

Nutritional Values

Calories 240kcal, Carbohydrates-24g, Protein 8g, Fat 13g, Sodium 523mg

585. LEMON PEPPER CAULIFLOWER STEAKS

- Prep time: 15 mins, Cook time: 45 mins, Total time: 1 hr, Servings: 2

Ingredients

- 2 tbsp pine nuts
- 1 medium head of cauliflower
- freshly ground pepper
- 3 cloves garlic, minced
- salt, to taste
- 2 tbsp olive oil
- Juice of 1 lemon
- 1 tbsp fresh parsley, minced

Directions

1. Preheat the oven to 400°F. Set aside a baking sheet lined with parchment paper.
2. Remove the stems from the cauliflower and discard the leaves. Cut directly through the middle of the cauliflower, holding it with its bottom on the cutting surface to make 2 halves. Cut a 1-inch thick steak from each side large; you'll have 2 1's in the end. Steaks are a popular choice. The leftover cauliflower ends may be cooked alongside the steak or used in other cauliflower dishes.
3. Brush the cauliflower with oil and place it on the baking pan. Bake for 30 mins after adding the garlic. Flip the steaks after 30 mins, and brush the undersides with oil. Bring to the oven & bake for another 10-15 mins, or until the steaks are cooked and browned on the edges.
4. Dry roast the pine nuts over the skillet while the cauliflower steaks bake. It takes around 3-4 mins of continual shaking. Remove the pan from the heat and put it aside.
5. Remove the dish from the oven. If used, quickly shred vegan Parmesan over the heated steaks to melt it. Sprinkle the lemon

juice evenly over the 2 steaks, then season with freshly ground pepper.

6. Serve with spaghetti or a big caesar salad, topped with pine nuts & parsley.

Nutritional Values

Calories 205kcal, Carbs 2g, Protein 1g, Fat 21g, Sodium 2mg

586. TOFU STIR FRY WITH BROCCOLI AND BELL PEPPERS

- Prep time: 20 mins, Cook time: 20 mins, Total time: 40 mins, Servings: 4

Ingredients

- 1 cup uncooked rice
- ¼ cup dry-roasted peanuts
- 1 tbsp peanut
- a few sprigs of cilantro
- ½ red onion, thinly sliced
- 2 green onions
- 1 red bell pepper, seeded & chopped
- 1 medium head of broccoli, chopped
- 8 ounces extra-firm tofu, pressed
- 2 batches of Thai Peanut Sauce

Directions

1. Cook the rice as directed on the packet. Prepare the remainder of the stir-fry while the rice is cooking.
2. Preheat the oven to 400°F. Set aside a baking sheet lined with parchment paper.
3. Prepare and put aside the Thai Peanut Sauce. Place the tofu on a shallow plate and cut it into 12" pieces. Stir in ¼ cup of Thai Peanut Sauce to coat the tofu.
4. Bake the tofu for 20 mins, turning it after 10 mins, on the prepared baking sheet.
5. In a cast-iron skillet, heat the peanut oil over medium heat. Add the onions and cook for 5 mins, or until they are transparent. Add the bell peppers & broccoli & cook for another 5 mins, or until the veggies are soft. Remove from heat and stir in the leftover peanut sauce.
6. To serve, divide the rice equally among 4 plates. Stir in the broccoli and peppers, as well as the cooked tofu. Green onions, peanuts, and cilantro go on top.
7. Serve right away.

Nutritional Values

Calories 329kcal, Carbs 51g, Protein 10g, Fat 10g, Sodium 125mg

587. BLACK BEANS AND RICE

- Prep time: 0 mins, Cook time: 30 mins, Total time: 30 mins, Servings: 4

Ingredients

- 1 cup brown rice, uncooked
- 1 can of black beans, drained & rinsed
- 1 small red onion, diced
- juice of 1 lime
- 2-3 cloves garlic, minced
- ½ - 1 tsp salt
- ½ red bell pepper, chopped
- ¼ tsp cayenne
- 1 small jalapeño, seeded & thinly sliced
- 1 tsp oil
- 1 tsp cumin

Directions

1. Cook the rice as directed on the packet. Prepare the beans while the rice is cooking.
2. In a big cast-iron skillet, heat the oil over medium heat. Sauté for 7 mins, or until onions and garlic are transparent and fragrant.
3. Stir in the bell peppers and jalapenos until everything is well combined.
4. Mix cumin, salt, cayenne, and lime juice in a mixing bowl.
5. Stir in the black beans until fully blended, then bring to a low boil. Cook for 5 mins while the rice is still cooking. Remove the pan from the heat.
6. Stir in the cooked rice and garnish with fresh cilantro & lime juice right away.

Nutritional Values

Calories 312kcal, Carbohydrates-62g, Protein 9g, Fat 1g, Sodium 4mg

588. RAW CHOCOLATE CHIA PUDDING

- Prep time: 5 mins, Cook time: 0 mins, Total time: 5 mins, Servings: 4

Ingredients

Chocolate chia pudding
- 2 cups Oat Milk
- ¼ tsp salt
- 8 large Medjool dates, pitted
- ¼ cup raw cacao powder
- ½ cup chia seeds
- 1 tsp vanilla extract

Toppings- optional
- Cacao Nibs
- Coconut whipped cream
- Fresh berries

Directions

1. Combine all of the ingredients for Chocolate Chia Pudding in a blender and mix until smooth. Swap the dates with 2 tbsp maple syrup and mix the chia pudding aggressively by hand for a more textured dessert.
2. Freeze for at least 2 hours after pouring the chia pudding into 4- 5 oz. custard cups. Allow chia pudding to set overnight for optimal results.
3. Breakfast, a noon snack, or dessert are all good options. Top with cacao nibs, fresh berries, & coconut whipped cream before serving.

Nutritional Values

Calories 315kcal, Carbohydrates-60g, Protein 7g, Fat 8g, Sodium 207mg

589. VEGAN CHOCOLATE CHEESECAKE BARS

- Prep time: 30 mins, Cook time: 0 mins, Total time: 30 mins, Servings: 9

Ingredients

- pinch of salt
- 2 cups raw cashews, soaked for almost 6 hours & rinsed
- chocolate hazelnut crust
- ½ tsp salt
- 1 ½ cups hazelnut meal
- ½ cup raw cacao powder
- ¼ cup maple syrup
- ½ cup water
- ¼ cup raw cacao powder
- ½ cup maple syrup
- cheesecake filling
- ½ cup coconut oil, melted
- ¼ cup hazelnut butter
- ganache topping
- ¼ cup maple syrup
- chopped hazelnuts

- ¼ cup raw cacao powder
- cacao nibs
- ⅓ cup coconut oil, melted
- 1 tsp vanilla extract
- toppings- optional

Directions

1. Set aside a small 8x8 baking dish lined with parchment paper.
2. To prepare the crust, mix all ingredients in a food processor and process until smooth and sticky when pushed between fingers. Press the dough into the pan's bottom. Remove from the equation.
3. To create the cheesecake filling, combine the ingredients in a mixing bowl. Cashews, water, maple syrup, salt, and coconut oil should be combined in a food processor or strong blender. Scrape down the edges of the processor as needed to ensure complete smoothness. Blend in the cocoa powder & hazelnut butter until the mixture is equally combined.
4. Spread the filling evenly on top of the crust.
5. Place the cheesecake in the fridge until it is completely firm- at least 2 hours.
6. To prepare the Ganache Topping, whisk together all of the ingredients using a fork. Pour evenly over the frozen cheesecake. Return to the freezer for another 2-3 mins. Return to freezer for a further 10 mins, after adding chopped hazelnuts & cacao nibs.
7. Pull the edges of the parchment paper to release the cheesecake from the pan. Serve soon after cutting into 9 even pieces.

Nutritional Values

Calories 591kcal, Carbohydrates-42g, Protein 10g, Fat 47g, Sodium 138mg

590. RAW CARROT CAKE BITES

- Prep time: 20 mins, Cook time: 0 mins, Total time: 20 mins, Servings: 4

Ingredients

- 1 ½ cups raw walnuts
- carrot cake
- 3 tbsp maple syrup
- carrot cake
- ¼ cup water

- 2 ½ cups shredded carrots, about 4 large carrots
- 1 cup raw cashews
- 1 cup Medjool dates, pitted
- cashew cream frosting
- 1 cup unsweetened shredded coconut
- walnuts and extra cinnamon for finish
- ½ tsp ground ginger
- pinch of salt
- 1 tsp ground cinnamon
- juice of ½ lemon
- ¼ tsp ground nutmeg
- 1 tsp vanilla extract
- ⅓ cup coconut oil, melted

Directions

1. Prepare an 8x8 baking dish- or another pan of similar size with parchment paper, allowing the edges to hang over the sides.
2. Shred the carrots by hand or in a food processor with a grating attachment. Set them aside in a large mixing dish. Mix the walnuts and dates until they make a homogenous crumb that adheres together when squeezed between your fingers. Blend in the carrots, coconut, spices, and salt until the carrots are well mixed, scraping down the sides as required.
3. While creating the cream cheese frosting, press the cake into the prepared pan, level over the top, and set it in the freezer.
4. In a high-powered blender, mix water, cashews, maple syrup, or agave nectar, salt, vanilla, and lemon juice to produce the cream cheese frosting. Blend until the mixture is very smooth. Blend in the coconut oil until smooth. Smooth the top of the cold cake with a spatula. Refrigerate for at least 2 hours after wrapping in plastic wrap.
5. Remove the cake from the freezer when ready to serve. Pull up the edges of the paper to remove it from the pan. Sprinkle with walnuts and cinnamon. Allow 10 mins for it to defrost at room temperature.
6. Cut the cake into 2 x 2-inch slices with a warm, sharp knife. Allow an extra 15 mins for the cake to defrost if it is frozen.

Nutritional Values

Calories 239kcal, Carbohydrates-16g, Protein 3g, Fat 19g, Sodium 17mg

591. RAW CHUNKY MONKEY ICE CREAM

- Prep time: 30 mins, Cook time: 0 mins, Total time: 30 mins, Servings: 6

Ingredients

- 1 tsp vanilla extract
- ⅓ cup walnuts
- 6 very ripe bananas
- mix-ins
- 1 cup almond milk
- ½ tsp vanilla extract
- raw chocolate
- 1 tbsp raw agave
- ¼ cup raw cacao powder
- ice cream base
- 3 tbsp coconut oil melted
- 2 tbsp maple syrup

Directions

1. Combine vanilla extract, almond milk, bananas, and sweetener of choice in a blender and process until smooth. Refrigerate for at least 2 hours after transferring to a small bowl and covering it with plastic wrap. Alternatively, throw it in the fridge for 30 mins or until completely cooled.
2. In the meanwhile, create the chocolate by whisking together all of the ingredients in a mixing dish. Place in a small container and place in the freezer. Remove the chocolate from the freezer and chop it into tiny bits.
3. Fill your ice cream maker halfway with an ice cream base and process according to the manufacturer's directions. Place the ice cream in a dish and, by hand, mix in the walnuts and chocolate bits. Place in a sealed jar and place back in the freezer. Allow ice cream to solidify for 4-5 hours.
4. Remove from the fridge 10 mins before serving to allow for thawing.

Nutritional Values

Calories 361kcal, Carbs 52g, Protein 4g, Fat 18g, Sodium 85mg

592. VEGAN CHOCOLATE BANANA CREAM PIE

- Prep time: 30 mins, Cook time: 10 mins, Total time: 40 mins, Servings: 12

Ingredients

- 2 tbsp coconut oil, melted
- ½ cup creamed coconut
- walnut crust
- ¼ cup raw cacao powder
- 1 ½ cups raw walnuts
- 3 tbsp maple syrup
- 1 - 2 tbsp maple syrup
- coconut banana custard
- chocolate banana custard
- 1 ½ cups shredded coconut, unsweetened
- pinch of salt
- 1 cup raw cashews, soaked for almost 2 hours
- 1 tsp pure vanilla extract
- juice of 1 lemon
- 2 very ripe bananas
- extras
- ¼ cup coconut oil, melted
- 1 tsp vanilla extract
- 1 cup cashews, soaked for 2 hours
- pinch of salt
- 3 very ripe bananas
- 3 bananas, sliced

Directions

1. Preheat the oven to 350°F. Combine walnuts and coconut in a food processor and pulse until smooth. Blend in the maple syrup until a crumbly mixture forms that stay together when pushed. Move the walnut mix to a 9" pie pan & press the crust into the pan's bottom and edges to make it approximately 14" thick. Bake for 10-12 mins, or until the crust is gently browned and toasted around the edges. Remove from the oven and set aside to cool. Place a layer of banana slices on the bottom & refrigerate after it has cooled.
2. Drain and rinse 1 cup of raw cashews before making the coconut banana custard. Blend them with the lemon juice & coconut oil in a high-powered blender until perfectly smooth. Combine the coconut cream, bananas, vanilla essence, and salt in

a mixing bowl. Blend until everything is properly incorporated. Spread the contents evenly in the chilled pie shell. Place the pie in the fridge to cool while you prepare the chocolate banana pudding.

3. Remove the blades from the blender. Blend the leftover cashews with the maple syrup until very smooth to produce the chocolate banana custard. Blend in the vanilla extract, bananas, cacao powder, and salt until smooth. Slowly drizzle in the coconut oil while the engine is running. Place the mousse on top of the cold banana custard and refrigerate for 2 hours to allow the custards to solidify.

4. Garnish with fresh bananas when ready to serve. It's best to serve the pie refrigerated.

Nutritional Values
Calories 420kcal, Carbohydrates-25g, Protein 8g, Fat 40g, Sodium 12mg

593. RAW CHOCOLATE PEANUT BUTTER CUPS

- Prep time: 20 mins, Cook time: 30 mins, Total time: 50 mins, Servings: 16

Ingredients
- Coarse Sea Salt
- ¾ cup Cacao Powder
- Cacao Nibs
- ¾ cup Coconut Oil, melted
- toppings- optional
- ¼ + 2 tbsp Maple Syrup
- 1-2 tbsp Maple Syrup or Agave Nectar
- nut butter filling
- raw dark chocolate
- ¾ cup Raw Almond Butter

Directions
1. Place 16 baking cups in a small muffin tray and put them aside.
2. To make the dark chocolate, whisk together all of the ingredients until smooth. Apply a generous coating of chocolate to the interior of each baking cup.
3. Allow the chocolate to settle at room temperature for 10-20 mins before brushing if it is too thin. To firm the chocolate cups, please place them in the freezer.

4. Mix the almond butter with your preferred sweetener. Fill each chocolate cup with roughly 2 tbsp Sweetened almond butter. Finish with the leftover chocolate and any other toppings if desired.
5. Place in the freezer for approximately 30 mins, or until completely frozen. Remove the cake wrapper from the chocolate cups after they've frozen and served.

Nutritional Values
Calories 173kcal, Carbohydrates-5g, Protein 3g, Fat 17g, Sodium 1mg

594. BLUEBERRY OVERNIGHT OATS

- Prep time: 10 mins, Cook time: 4 hrs, Total time: 4 hrs 10 mins, Servings: 2

Ingredients
- 1 cup rolled oats
- ½ cup almond milk
- 1 cup fresh blueberries
- 1-2 tbsp maple syrup
- pinch of salt
- overnight oats
- shredded coconut
- fresh blueberries
- 1 tsp vanilla extract
- ½ cup coconut milk
- chia seeds
- 1 tbsp chia seeds

Directions
1. Combine the milk, oats, chia seeds, salt, vanilla essence, and maple syrup in a large mixing bowl. Stir everything together until it's completely smooth. In a large mixing bowl, combine the fresh blueberries with the rest of the ingredients.
2. Cover and chill for at least 4 hrs or overnight in 2 8-ounce mason jars. When everything is done, top with your favorite toppings and enjoy!

Nutritional Values
Calories 377kcal, Carbohydrates-49g, Protein 8g, Fat 17g, Sodium 93mg

595. PROTEIN PACKED CHIA PUDDING

- Prep time: 5 mins, Cook time: 2 hrs 5 mins, Total time: 10 mins, Servings: 2

- 1 tsp vanilla extract
- 1 cup non-dairy milk
- 2 tbsp cacao nibs, optional
- ¼ cup chia seeds
- 2 tbsp peanut flour
- 2 tsp maple syrup
- ½ tsp ground cinnamon

Directions

1. Whisk together all of the ingredients in a tiny mixing bowl.
2. Fill- 2 6-ounce mason jars with chia pudding. They should be roughly ½-full at this point. To set the pudding, cover it and store it in the fridge for 2 hours.
3. You may serve the pudding right away after it has thickened. Any leftover chia pudding may be kept in the fridge for up to 3 days.

Nutritional Values

Calories 330kcal, Carbohydrates-25g, Protein 14g, Fat 19g, Sodium 65mg

596. MATCHA CHIA PUDDING

- Prep time: 10 mins, Cook time: 0 mins, Total time: 10 mins, Servings: 4

Ingredients

- Matcha chia pudding
- 2 tbsp cacao nibs
- ½ cup chia seeds
- 2-3 tbsp goji berries
- 2 ½ cups macadamia or cashew milk
- 1 kiwi, peeled and sliced
- 2 ½ tsp matcha green tea
- 1 tsp almond extract
- ½ tsp vanilla extract
- 1 tbsp maple syrup

Directions

1. Combine all of the ingredients for the green tea pudding in a small bowl.
2. Fill 4 4-ounce mason jars with the mixture. Refrigerate for 4 hours after securing the lids.
3. The chia pudding is rich and creamy after 4 hours. Serve immediately or keep in the fridge for up to 3 days.

Nutritional Values

Calories 231kcal, Carbohydrates-21g, Protein 9g, Fat 11g, Sodium 80mg

597. GLUTEN-FREE, VEGAN BREAKFAST COOKIES

- Prep time: 15 mins, Cook time: 15 mins, Total time: 30 mins, Servings: 12

Ingredients

- 1 cup gluten-free rolled oats
- ¼ cup mini chocolate chips
- ½ cup unsweetened shredded coconut
- ¼ cup cranberries or raisins
- 1 tsp ground cinnamon
- ¼ cup pumpkin seeds
- ½ tsp baking powder
- 1 tsp vanilla extract
- ½ tsp baking soda
- ¼ cup chopped walnut
- ½ cup almond meal
- ⅓ cup pure maple syrup
- ½ tsp salt
- ⅓ cup natural peanut butter
- 2 chia eggs
- ¼ cup melted coconut oil

Directions

1. Preheat the oven to 350°F. Set aside a baking sheet lined with parchment paper.
2. Make the chia eggs first. 6 tbsp water and 2 tbsp chia seeds, whisked together in a small basin. Allow for 10 mins for the mixture to thicken.
3. Combine oats, shredded coconut, almond meal, baking powder, cinnamon, soda, & salt in a medium mixing basin.
4. Combine the coconut oil, chia eggs, maple syrup, peanut butter, & vanilla extract in a small mixing dish. Incorporate the wet and dry ingredients in a mixing bowl and whisk to combine.
5. Combine the cranberries, pumpkin seeds, chia seeds, and walnuts in a mixing bowl.
6. Form a ball out of 14 cups of the dough and set it on a baking sheet. Rep till all of the dough is gone. Bake for 12-15 mins, or until gently browned, pressing down lightly.

7. Remove cookies from the oven and cool them on a baking sheet for 10 mins before fully transferring them to a cooling rack.
8. Keep for up to 5 days in an airtight container.

Nutritional Values

Calories 235kcal, Carbohydrates-18g, Protein 5g, Fat 16g, Sodium 180mg

598. CHOCOLATE PEANUT BUTTER OATMEAL

- Prep time: 5 mins, Cook time: 20 mins, Total time: 25 mins, Servings: 2

Ingredients

- almond or soy milk
- 1 tbsp cacao powder
- hemp seeds
- 3 tbsp maple syrup
- cacao nibs
- 1 tsp vanilla extract
- raw cashews or peanuts
- ¼ tsp salt
- 2-3 tbsp natural peanut butter
- 1 cup steel-cut oats
- shredded coconut, unsweetened
- 3 cups water
- chocolate steel-cut oats
- mix-ins and add-ons- optional

Directions

1. Bring salt, water, maple syrup, cacao powder, and vanilla extract to a boil in a medium saucepan. Reduce to low heat, toss in the oats, and cook for 20 mins until the water is drained and the oats are tender.
2. Remove from the heat and divide into 2 bowls.
3. Combine the peanut butter and desired toppings in a mixing bowl.
4. Serve right away.

Nutritional Values

Calories 495kcal, Carbohydrates-77g, Protein 17g, Fat 14g, Sodium 386mg

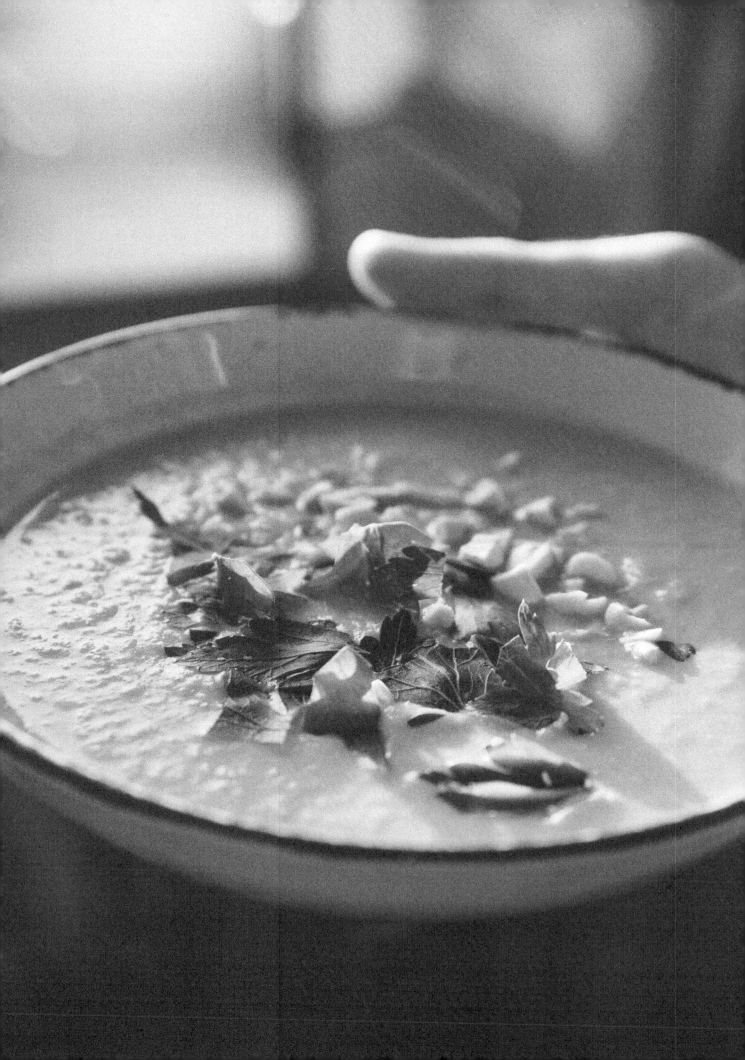

Chapter 16.

Vegetable Recipes

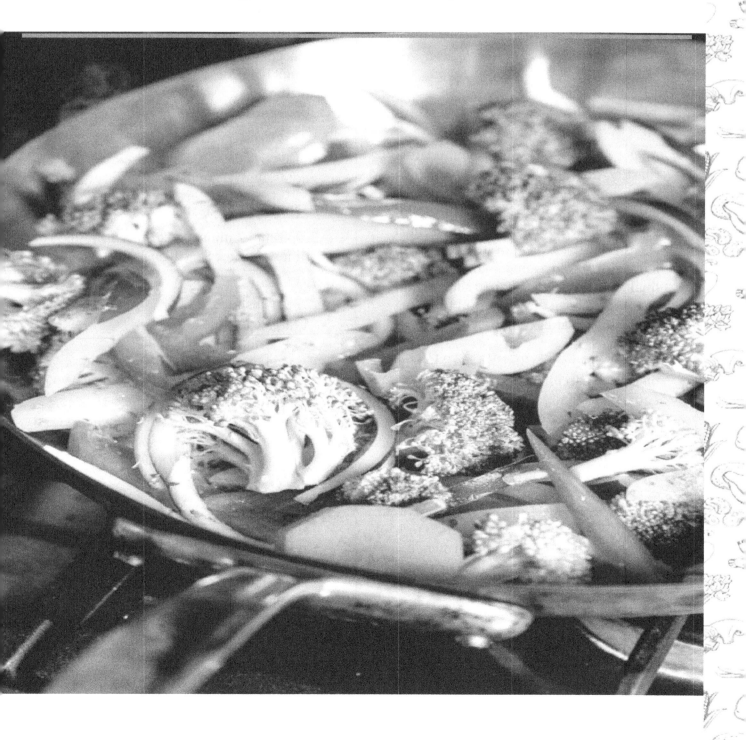

599. BEST ROASTED VEGETABLES- PERFECTLY SEASONED!

- Prep time: 15 mins, Cook time: 30 mins, Total time: 45 mins, Servings: 8

Ingredients

- 1 crown broccoli- ½ pound
- 1 medium head cauliflower- 2 pounds
- 2 tsp Old Bay seasoning
- 1 medium red onion
- 2 tsp garlic powder
- 2 medium sweet potatoes- 1 ½ pound
- 1 tsp kosher salt
- 1 red pepper
- 1 yellow pepper
- 4 tbsp olive oil

Directions

1. Adjust the oven racks to accommodate 2 roasting trays. Preheat the oven to 455°F.
2. Chop the veggies as follows: Make florets out of the cauliflower and broccoli. Using a ½ -inch slicer, cut the onion into ½ -inch slices. Slice the sweet potato in 2 lengthwise, then again lengthwise, and finally into small pie-shaped slices from each quarter see the photo. Cut the peppers in ½ after chopping them into ½ - inch slices.
3. Preheat the oven to 350°F. Line 2 baking pans with parchment paper. On each sheet, equally distribute the veggies. Drizzle ½ of the olive oil over each tray, followed by ½ of the spices. Mix everything with your hands until it's uniformly covered.
4. Place in the oven for 20 mins- without stirring!
5. Remove the plates from the oven, flip them, and roast for another 10 mins- for a total of 30 mins, until soft and gently browned. Immediately transfer to a bowl or platter and serve.

Nutritional Values

Calories 160kcal, Carbohydrates-26.8g, Protein 4.6g, Fat 7.5g, Sodium 300mg

600. DIPPING SAUCE

- Sides - Prep time: 15 mins, Cook time: 0 mins, Total time: 15 mins, Servings: 2 cups, Grill temp: 0

Ingredients

- 2 tbsp of minced or grated ginger
- 2 tbsp of minced or pressed garlic
- 2 tsps of chili-garlic sauce- or more to taste
- 6 tbsp of soy sauce
- ½ cup of rice vinegar
- ½ cup of hoisin sauce
- ½ cup of low-Sodium vegetable stock

Directions

1. Merge together all the ingredients in a small bowl, or place in a jar with a tight-fitting lid and shake until well mixed.
2. Use immediately.

Nutritional Values

Calories 51, Fat 2g, Chol 0mg, Sodium 66mg, Potassium 42.7mg, Carbs 8g, Protein 0.3g

601. ULTIMATE SAUTEED VEGETABLES

- Prep time: 7 mins, Cook time: 13 mins, Total time: 20 mins, Servings: 4

Ingredients

- ½ tsp kosher salt
- 1 large carrot
- 1 tsp dried oregano
- 1 head broccoli- 8 ounces, stem on
- 2 tbsp olive oil, divided
- 1 medium red onion
- 2 multi-colored bell peppers- we used red and yellow
- Fresh ground black pepper

Directions

1. Peppers should be thinly sliced. Cut the onion into thin pieces. Carrots should be cut into thin rounds on the bias. Broccoli should be cut into tiny florets.
2. Toss the veggies with 1 tbsp olive oil, oregano, kosher salt, and lots of freshly ground black pepper in a large mixing dish.
3. Heat the rest of the 1 tbsp olive oil in a large pan over medium-high heat. Cook, occasionally turning, for 10 - 12 mins, or until tender and faintly charred.
4. Taste and season with a few pinches of salt to taste. Serve right away.

Nutritional Values

Calories 220kcal, Carbohydrates-10.3g, Protein 1.8g, Fat 7.4g, Sodium 279mg

602. FAT-FREE CROCK POT CHILI

- Prep time: 0 mins, Cook time: 7 hrs mins, Total time: 7 hrs, Servings: 2

Ingredients

- 1 cup fresh or frozen corn kernels
- 2 garlic cloves, minced
- ½ tsp oregano
- 1 green bell pepper, chopped
- 2 tsp cumin
- 1 zucchini, diced
- ½ cup water
- 8 ounces mushrooms, sliced
- 2 tbsp chili powder
- 1 onion, diced
- 3 cups cooked kidney
- Dash of cayenne pepper or to taste
- 3 cups diced tomatoes, fresh or packaged in BPA-free cartons

Directions

1. Mix all ingredients in a pot.
2. Cover and cook on low heat for almost 7 hours.

Nutritional Values

Calories 286kcal, Carbohydrates-55g, Protein 21g, Fat 2.5g, Sodium 151mg

603. VEGAN APPLE CINNAMON OATMEAL

- Prep time: 15 mins, Cook time: 15 mins, Total time: 30 mins, Servings: 2

Ingredients

- 1-2 tbsp maple syrup
- ½ tsp cinnamon- more for sprinkling
- 1 cup rolled oats
- 2 tbsp walnuts- chopped
- 1 cup vanilla almond milk- or any non-dairy milk
- 1 large apple- cored, peeled, and cut into a ¼-inch dice
- 2 cups water
- ⅛ tsp salt

Directions

1. In a heavy-bottomed saucepan, bring the oats, salt, and water to a boil, then add the sliced apples and ½ of the almond milk. To combine, stir thoroughly.
2. When the oatmeal comes to a boil, reduce the heat to a low degree, cover the bowl, and cook for about 15 mins, stirring often. Add additional almond milk or water if the oats become too dry.
3. Remove the oats from the heat when it is smooth and creamy. Combine the maple syrup, cinnamon, and the rest of the almond milk in a mixing bowl.
4. Ladle into bowls, top with additional cinnamon and walnuts, and serve right away.

Nutritional Values

Calories 323kcal, Carbohydrates-52g, Protein 8g, Fat 11g, Sodium 325mg

604. CURRIED TEMPEH QUINOA BREAKFAST HASH

- Prep time: 15 mins, Cook time: 15 mins, Total time: 30 mins, Servings: 2

Ingredients

- 1 red onion- finely diced
- Salt and ground black pepper to taste
- 8 oz. tempeh- cut into 1-cm cubes
- 2 level tbsp curry powder
- 1 cup cooked quinoa
- Juice of 1 lemon
- 1 large sweet potato- cut into ¼-inch cubes
- 1 tsp dry basil- or 1 tbsp fresh basil
- 15 oz. canned white beans
- 4 cloves garlic- smashed and minced
- 1 tsp cayenne

Directions

1. Add 2 tbsp of water to a big pot or wok. Over medium-high heat, add the onions and garlic, along with a sprinkle of salt & ground black pepper, and sauté until the onions are transparent.
2. Add the potatoes, cover, & cook for 8-10 mins, until they are tender. Stir occasionally to avoid sticking and, if necessary, add additional water.
3. Stir in the cayenne, curry powder, and basil after the sweet potatoes are cooked.

4. Stir in the beans, quinoa, & tempeh until everything is completely combined. Warm well before serving.

Nutritional Values

Calories 189kcal, Carbohydrates-29g, Protein 11g, Fat 4g, Sodium 313mg

605. DETOX TURMERIC GINGER MISO SOUP

- Prep time: 10 mins, Cook time: 12 mins, Total time: 22 mins, Servings: 2

Ingredients

- ½ tsp turmeric
- 4 cups water
- 2 tbsp scallions
- 2 4- inch pieces of kombu
- ½ oz. block of firm tofu cut into small cubes, 6
- 4 tbsp mellow or white miso
- 1 tsp finely grated ginger; peel the ginger first
- 1 medium carrot grated

Directions

1. Start the dashi the day before by soaking the seaweed in 4 cups of water overnight.
2. Heat water with dashi in it the next morning. Remove the bits of dashi when the water starts to boil. Set aside the stock.
3. 1 tbsp dashi stock, ginger, turmeric, and carrots, heated in a medium pot, cook for a few mins, constantly stirring, or until the liquid has evaporated.
4. Measure out a cup of dashi stock and stir in the miso paste until it has completely dissolved. Remove from the equation.
5. Add the rest of the dashi into the saucepan with the ginger, turmeric, and carrots, stir, then bring to a boil and simmer for 8 mins.
6. Bring the water back to a boil with the tofu chunks.
7. Turn off the heat and add the scallion leaves.
8. Add the miso paste and mix well.
9. Serve immediately.

Nutritional Values

Calories 158kcal, Carbohydrates-186g, Protein 9g, Fat 5g, Sodium 725mg

606. SMOKY ROASTED EGGPLANT SOUP WITH ZA'ATAR- FAT-FREE

- Prep time: 10 mins, Cook time: 20 mins, Total time: 30 mins, Servings: 4

Ingredients

- ¼ tsp cayenne
- 1 large eggplant- halved
- 2 tbsp cashews- optional
- 6 large cloves of garlic- peeled
- Salt and ground black pepper to taste
- 2 medium onions- either white or yellow, chopped
- 1 tbsp parsley- chopped
- ¼ tsp roasted cumin seeds
- 1 tbsp za'atar
- 3-6 cups vegetable stock- or water
- Juice of 1 lemon

Directions

1. Cut the eggplant lengthwise and set it cut side down on an aluminum foil or parchment paper-lined baking pan. Roast for 30 mins at 425°F, or until a fork pierces completely through the middle of the pumpkin without resistance.
2. To get a smooth paste, mix the cashews with ¼ cup of water. Remove from the mix.
3. In a large saucepan, combine the onions and garlic with ¼ cup of vegetable stock or water.
4. Bring to a boil, covered. Reduce the heat to low and cook for 10 mins.
5. Using a spoon, scrape the eggplant flesh from the peel and slice it into smaller pieces. When the eggplant has been roasted, this should be a breeze. 2 cups of water or stock should be added to the garlic and onions.
6. Stir in the cumin, cayenne, salt, & ground black pepper to taste.
7. Turn the heat off. Place the soup in a blender and puree until completely smooth. If necessary, add more water or stock, and adjust the soup's thickness to your desire. When working with extremely hot liquids, exercise extreme caution. If you like, leave the soup to cook a bit longer.

8. Return the pureed soup to the pot and add the lemon juice, za'atar, and parsley to taste. Bring to a boil.
9. Pour into bowls and, if desired, add a dollop of cashew cream to each.
10. Serve immediately.

Nutritional Values

Calories 97kcal, Carbohydrates-18g, Protein 3g, Fat 3g, Sodium 279mg

607. MIXED BEANS BOWL WITH SWEET POTATOES & TURMERIC RICE

- Prep time: 15 mins, Cook time: 30 mins, Total time: 45 mins, Servings: 8

Ingredients

For Mixed Beans Masala:
- 1 ½ cups dry kidney beans
- Salt to taste
- 3-4 cups vegetable stock
- Cilantro, chopped, for garnish
- 1 medium onion- finely chopped
- 1 tbsp garam masala
- 4 cloves garlic- crushed or minced
- ½ tsp cayenne
- 1-inch piece ginger-grated
- ½ tsp turmeric
- 1 cup tomato puree
- 1 tsp paprika

For Sweet Potato Stir-Fry:
- ½ cup orange juice
- 2 large sweet potatoes- diced
- Ground black pepper and salt to taste
- ¼ cup vegetable stock
- ½ tsp garam masala

For Turmeric Rice:
- 2 dry bay leaves
- 1 ½ cups long-grain rice- rinsed
- Salt to taste
- 3 cups vegetable stock
- ¼ tsp turmeric
- 3 cloves
- 3 green cardamom pods
- 1 tsp cumin seeds

Directions

1. Place 14 cups of vegetable stock in a large pot and heat to a boil. Add the onions, ginger, & garlic, season with salt and pepper, and cook, often turning, over medium-low heat until the onions are tender.
2. Combine the turmeric, tomatoes, cayenne, paprika, and garam masala in a mixing bowl. Allow the mixture to come to a boil while constantly stirring. Allow it to simmer for another 5 mins, occasionally stirring.
3. Add the beans and, if you have any, around 2 cups of the cooking liquid. If not, add vegetable stock or broth. Bring to a boil, then reduce to low heat and continue to cook the beans masala for another 10 mins. Add extra stock if it begins to dry out.
4. If necessary, season with salt. Remove the pan from the heat and scatter the coriander leaves on top.
5. Place the sweet potatoes and vegetable stock in a wok or a wide pan. Set the heat to low and allow the liquid to come to a simmer.
6. Add the garam masala, orange juice, and black pepper to taste. Over medium heat, stir in the sweet potatoes, cover, and simmer for 8-10 mins or until cooked. To avoid mashing the sweet potatoes, gently stir them. Check them once or twice throughout cooking to assure they aren't clinging to the bottom; if they are, add a tbsp of stock at a time until they are no longer sticking.
7. As required, season with salt.
8. In a medium-high-heat saucepan, place the stock. Combine the cumin seeds, turmeric, cloves, bay leaves, and cardamom in a large mixing bowl- use the whole pods.
9. Once the water has to a boil, add the rice. Bring the rice back to a boil, cover, & cook for 15 mins on low heat. After turning off the heat, let it be alone for at least another 10 mins. Then, before serving, open & fluff with a fork.
10. While the sweet potatoes, rice, and beans masala are still hot, layer them in a bowl and enjoy!

Nutritional Values

Calories 340kcal, Carbohydrates-76g, Protein 13g, Fat 1g, Sodium 446mg

608. SWEET POTATO & BLACK BEAN CHILI

- Prep time: 20 mins, Cook time: 20 mins, Total time: 40 mins, Servings: 4

Ingredients

- 1 medium-large sweet potato, peeled and diced
- 4 tsp lime juice
- 1 large onion, diced
- 1 14-ounce can of diced tomatoes
- 4 cloves garlic, minced
- 2 15-ounce cans of black beans, rinsed
- 2 tbsp chili powder
- 2 ½ cups water
- 4 tsp ground cumin
- ½ cup chopped fresh cilantro
- ½ tsp ground chipotle chile
- 1 tbsp plus 2 tsp extra-virgin olive oil
- ¼ tsp salt

Directions

1. In a Dutch oven, heat the oil over medium-high heat. Cook, often turning, until the sweet potato & onion are starting to soften, approximately 4 mins. Cook, frequently stirring, for 30 seconds after adding the garlic, chipotle, cumin, chili powder, and salt. Bring the water to a low boil, then reduce to low heat. Cover, decrease the heat to maintain a slow simmer, and cook for 10 to 12 mins until the potato is cooked.
2. Increase the heat to high and bring to a simmer, often whisking, with the beans, tomatoes, and lime juice. Reduce heat to low and cook for 5 mins or until somewhat reduced. Remove the pan from the heat and add the cilantro.

Nutritional Values

Calories 323kcal, Carbohydrates-54.7g, Protein 12.5g, Fat 7.6g, Sodium 573.3mg

609. CORN PAKORA, BAKED, NO OIL

- Prep time: 10 mins, Cook time: 25 mins, Total time: 35 mins, Servings: 4

Ingredients

- 2 cups corn kernels; use fresh or frozen
- Salt to taste
- 10 tbsp chickpea flour or besan
- 2 tbsp crushed kasoori methi- dry fenugreek leaves, optional
- ½ cup cornmeal
- 2 tbsp coriander leaves, finely chopped
- 1 tsp cumin seeds, coarsely powdered
- 1 tsp cayenne pepper
- ½ tsp turmeric

Directions

1. Preheat the oven to 370°F.
2. In a mixing dish, combine all ingredients and add enough water to form a thick batter.
3. With a whisk, thoroughly combine all ingredients, ensuring no pieces of chickpea flour are left.
4. Spray a baking sheet with cooking spray and line it with parchment paper. Drop dollops of mixture on the baking sheet, approximately ½ inch apart, using a tbsp measure.
5. Preheat the oven to 350°F and bake for 30 mins, turning halfway through.
6. If cooking in a pan, use a nice non-stick skillet or gently coat a cast iron pan with cooking spray. Drop a 12-inch apart dollop after a dab of batter onto the pan. Cook until the sides are brown & dry, then flip & cook for another couple of mins.

Nutritional Values

Calories 60kcal, Carbohydrates-12g, Protein 2.5g, Fat 2g, Sodium 432mg

610. SLOW COOKER BUTTERNUT SQUASH DAL

- Prep time: 10 mins, Cook time: 2 hrs, Total time: 2 hrs 10 mins, Servings: 6

Ingredients

- ½ to 1 tsp cayenne
- 1 medium onion, chopped
- 2 tbsp cashew yogurt
- 4 cloves garlic, smashed and minced
- 3 spring onions, green and white parts chopped, optional
- 2 tbsp finely chopped coriander leaves or cilantro
- Salt and ground black pepper to taste
- 1 tbsp grated ginger
- 2 tbsp garam masala

- 1 cup French lentils, washed
- 3 cups ½-inch butternut squash cubes
- 3 medium potatoes, cut into ½-inch cubes
- ½ tsp turmeric

Directions

1. Add the garlic, ginger, onions, and coriander leaves to the crockpot and turns it on high. Stir to combine, season with salt & ground black pepper, cover, and set aside to simmer for a few mins while preparing the rest of your meal. Ingredients.
2. In a large mixing bowl, combine the butternut squash, lentils, potatoes, turmeric, cayenne pepper, and garam masala. 3 cups of water/vegetable stock should be added.
3. Stir thoroughly, season with salt, and simmer for 2 hours, covered. Check once or again, and if necessary, add a cup of water. Don't make the dal too dry since it will thicken as it sits.
4. Remove the pan from the heat and add the cashew yogurt. If using, garnish with spring onions.
5. Serve with roti/rice when still hot.

Nutritional Values

Calories 134kcal, Carbohydrates-21g, Protein 4.9g, Fat 1.1, Sodium 325mg

611. SLOW COOKER CHANA MASALA

- Prep time: 10 mins, Cook time: 6 hrs, Total time: 6 hrs 10 mins, Servings: 8

Ingredients

- Salt to taste
- 1 medium onion
- ¼ cup cilantro
- 2 large tomatoes
- 1 tsp cayenne
- 2 large potatoes- cut into small dice
- 1 tsp chaat masala
- 4 cloves garlic
- ¼ tsp turmeric
- 1-inch knob of ginger- finely chopped
- 1 tsp paprika
- 2 tbsp tomato paste
- 1 tbsp chana masala powder- or garam masala
- 2 bay leaves

- 1 tbsp coriander seeds- powdered
- 29 oz. chickpeas
- ½ tsp cumin seeds- powdered

Directions

1. Combine the onions, tomatoes, garlic, and ginger in a blender and puree until smooth.
2. Place all of the ingredients in the crockpot, except the salt & coriander leaves, in the crockpot.
3. Set the slow cooker to high and add 3 cups of water.- It's critical to set this too high.
4. Allow 6 hours for the chana masala to simmer. Check on it from time to time and, if necessary, add more water.
5. Add salt & coriander leaves after 6 hours and stir thoroughly.
6. Serve with Rotis or rice.

Nutritional Values

Calories 263kcal, Carbohydrates-49g, Protein 12g, Fat 3g, Sodium 545mg

612. VEGAN LENTIL TACOS

- Prep time: 20 mins, Cook time: 35 mins, Total time: 55 mins, Servings: 4

Ingredients

- 1 jalapeno pepper- minced
- 2 tsp ground cumin
- 1 cup brown lentils
- 8 flour tortillas
- 1 onion- finely chopped
- ½ cup cilantro- minced
- 2 medium tomatoes- diced
- ¼ cup chives- optional, minced
- 4-6 cloves of garlic- minced
- 2 tsp thyme- minced

For serving
- Guacamole
- Salsa

Directions

1. Using medium-high heat, heat a pan.
2. With 2 tbsp of water and ¼ tsp of salt, add the sliced onions to the pan.
3. Cook, often stirring, for approximately 5 mins or until the onions soften. If the onions get dry and stick, add 2 tbsp of water at a time.

4. Sauté for another minute after adding the minced garlic.
5. Combine the cumin powder, tomatoes, cilantro, habanero pepper, and thyme in a large mixing bowl.
6. Stir thoroughly, cover with a lid, and cook until tomatoes have broken down, occasionally stirring. It should take around 7-8 mins to complete this task.
7. Stir in the rinsed lentils well. Cover the lentils with enough water to cover them.
8. Put the lentils to a boil, then reduce to low heat and cook until the lentils are very soft but still maintain their form. If the mixture dries out before the lentils are entirely cooked, add extra water, no more than ½ cup at a time. However, don't overdo it since you want the lentil center to be dry.
9. When the lentils are done, continue to simmer them over medium heat till the mixture is completely dry, and no liquid is visible.
10.   Mix in the salt well.
11.   Transfer to a bowl and top with chives.
12.   Place a couple of tbsp of the filling in the middle of a tortilla, then top with salsa & guacamole.

Calories 192kcal, Carbohydrates-33g, Protein 9g, Fat 2g, Sodium 211mg

613. VEGAN GUMBO

- Prep time: 15 mins, Cook time: 30 mins, Total time: 45 mins, Servings: 8

Ingredients

- 1 large onion- finely diced
- Water or vegetable stock
- 6 cloves garlic- finely minced
- 2 tbsp tamari
- 1 green bell pepper- finely diced
- 1 chipotle chili- minced, with 1 tsp of the adobo sauce
- 2 carrots- cut into rounds
- 1 tbsp Cajun seasoning
- 2 cups button mushrooms or crimini mushrooms- sliced
- 1 tbsp thyme
- 2 cups frozen or fresh okra- cut into rings
- 1 tbsp dry sage
- 1 cup pureed tomatoes
- Salt and ground black pepper to taste
- 2 tbsp brown rice flour
- 3 cups canned red beans

Directions

1. Brown rice flour is added to a big saucepan that has been heated. Over medium-low heat, roast, stirring regularly, until the roux is darker. Transfer to a bowl right away.
2. Add the onions, carrots, and garlic to the same saucepan, along with ½ cup of water/vegetable stock. Salt & pepper to taste. Cook until the onions are softened, and the liquid has evaporated, constantly stirring.
3. Cook, occasionally stirring, for another 5 mins, after adding the tomatoes, bell peppers, and mushrooms. Mix the chipotle chile and adobo sauce, herbs, tamari, and Cajun spice until everything is thoroughly combined.
4. Stir in the beans and okra until everything is fully combined. Return the brown rice flour to the saucepan and whisk to combine. Allow 2 cups of vegetable stock to come to a boil in the gumbo over medium-high heat. Add extra water or stock if the gumbo is too thick. Reduce the heat to a low level and continue to cook for a further 10 mins.
5. If necessary, season with additional salt. Turn the heat off. If you like, you may also add some vegan sausage, which should be chopped into rounds. It will increase the Protein composition of the gumbo while also adding a modest amount of Fat.
6. Enjoy!

Nutritional Values

Calories 122kcal, Carbohydrates-23.6g, Protein 7.1g, Fat 2.2g, Sodium 356mg

614. QUICK SAUTEED PEPPERS AND ONIONS

- Prep time: 10 mins, Cook time: 15 mins, Total time: 25 mins, Servings: 4

Ingredients

- 1 medium yellow onion
- 3 multi-colored bell peppers

- ½ tsp kosher salt
- 1 medium red onion
- Fresh ground pepper
- 2 tbsp olive oil, divided
- 1 tsp dried oregano

Directions

1. Peppers should be thinly sliced. Slice the onions very thinly. Toss them with 1 tbsp olive oil, oregano, salt, and pepper in a mixing dish.
2. Heat the remaining 1 tbsp olive oil in a large pan over medium-high heat. Cook, occasionally turning, until the peppers are cooked and a little charred, approximately 10 to 12 mins for crisp-tender or around 15 mins, for tender. Taste and season with more salt if necessary.
3. Serve right away.

Nutritional Values

Calories 210kcal, Carbs 11.9g, Protein 1.7g, Fat 1.5g, Sodium 315g

615. SIMPLE SAUTEED BROCCOLI

- Prep time: 3 mins, Cook time: 7 mins, Total time: 10 mins, Servings: 4

Ingredients

- 2 tbsp olive oil
- ⅛ tsp garlic powder
- 2 green onions
- Optional: 1 tsp lemon zest
- 1 ½ pounds- 2 large heads of broccoli
- 2 tsp Italian seasoning
- ½ tsp kosher salt, plus more to taste

Directions

1. Broccoli should be chopped into medium-sized florets. Green onions should be thinly sliced.
2. Heat the olive oil in a large pan over medium heat. Cook for 5 mins, stirring regularly, after adding the broccoli florets. Combine the garlic powder, Italian seasoning, green onion, and kosher salt in a large mixing bowl.
3. Cook for 3 mins, longer, covered, until crispy tender but still brilliant green. Taste and season with a sprinkle of salt and freshly ground pepper, if desired. Transfer

the broccoli to a serving dish and serve right away. If using, finish with a sprinkling of lemon zest.

Nutritional Values

Calories 245kcal, Carbohydrates-6.2g, Protein 2.6g, Fat 7.4g, Sodium 292mg

616. SAUTEED SPINACH- THAT TASTES AMAZING

- Prep time: 5 mins, Cook time: 5 mins, Total time: 10 mins, Servings: 4

Ingredients

- 2 tbsp olive oil
- 3 bunches of spinach- about 1 ¼ pound total with stems
- 1 ½ tbsp fresh lemon juice
- 3 large garlic cloves, peeled and smashed
- ¼ tsp salt plus 2 pinches

Directions

1. Remove the stems and coarsely slice the leaves if the spinach is in a bunch.
2. In a large pan, heat the olive oil at medium-high heat for about 2 mins, occasionally tossing until the entire garlic cloves are browned. Then gently add the spinach & cover the pan. Although the pile of leaves seems to have a large volume, it will rapidly wilt down to a very tiny size. Simmer for 1 minute covered, then uncover and toss for a few seconds to combine cooked and raw spinach, then cook for another 1 minute covered.
3. Take off the cover. Cook for another 30 seconds, constantly stirring, until the spinach is totally wilted but still brilliant green. Remove from the fire after adding the kosher salt & fresh lemon juice.
4. Taste and season with a few more grains of salt if necessary.- Spinach is sensitive to salt, so only use small amounts at a time! The taste should be noticeable but not salty. Remove the spinach to a dish right away; if you keep it in the pan any longer, it will brown. Warm the dish before serving.

Nutritional Values

Calories 210kcal, Carbohydrates-3.7g, Protein 2.2g, Fat 1g, Sodium 410mg

617. PERFECT SAUTEED CARROTS

- Prep time: 3 mins, Cook time: 7 mins, Total time: 10 mins, Servings: 4

Ingredients

- 2 tbsp olive oil
- 8 medium carrots- 1 pound
- ¼ tsp plus 1 kosher pinch salt
- 1 tbsp chopped fresh thyme- or other fresh herbs

Directions

1. Peel the carrots & cut them into rounds diagonally- on the bias.
2. In a large pan, heat the olive oil over medium-high heat. Cover with carrots. Cook for 4 mins, occasionally stirring.
3. Remove the cover, mix in the 14 tsp kosher salt, and serve. Cook, tossing regularly, for another 3 to 4 mins, uncovered, until golden. Remove the pan from the heat and add the fresh herbs and a pinch of kosher salt to taste. Serve right away.

Nutritional Values

Calories 161kcal, Carbohydrates-10.9g, Protein 1.1g, Fat 7.3g, Sodium 355mg

618. SAUTEED RAINBOW CHARD

- Prep time: 5 mins, Cook time: 5 mins, Total time: 10 mins, Servings: 4

Ingredients

- 2 garlic cloves
- 2 tbsp shredded Parmesan cheese- optional
- 2 tbsp olive oil
- Fresh ground black pepper
- ¼ tsp kosher salt
- 2 tbsp toasted pine nuts- optional
- 1 bunch- 12 ounces rainbow chard
- 1 pinch of red pepper flakes

Directions

1. The chard leaves should be washed and dried. Remove the stems and cut the chard coarsely. Thinly slice the delicate section of the stems and add to the mix if desired.
2. Garlic cloves should be smashed and peeled.
3. In a large pan, heat the olive oil over medium-high heat. Cook for 4 mins, turning regularly until the chard has wilted and become brilliant green.
4. Remove the pan from the heat and season with kosher salt, red pepper flakes, and a few pinches of freshly ground pepper.
5. Remove the garlic cloves & serve right away.
6. Serve with grated Parmesan & toasted pine nuts, if preferred.

Nutritional Values

Calories 239kcal, Carbohydrates-3.9g, Protein 1.7g, Fat 7.3g, Sodium 337mg

619. EASY SAUTEED CABBAGE

- Prep time: 5 mins, Cook time: 10 mins, Total time: 15 mins, Servings: 4

Ingredients

- 2 tbsp olive oil
- Fresh ground black pepper
- 1 tbsp butter- optional
- 2 to 3 tsp fresh lemon juice- ¼ lemon or 2 wedges
- ¼ tsp garlic powder
- 10 cups green cabbage- about 1 ¼ to 1 ½ pounds of cabbage
- 1 tsp kosher salt

Directions

1. Cut the cabbage into thin slices and measure out approximately 10 cups.
2. Heat the olive oil & butter in a big pan. Combine the kosher salt, garlic powder, cabbage, and lots of black pepper in a large mixing bowl. Cook for 8 to 10 mins or until the spinach is wilted and soft.
3. Toss in the juice from 2 lemon wedges after it's done. Taste and make any required adjustments to the taste.

Nutritional Values

Calories 111kcal, Carbohydrates-12.9g, Protein 2.9g, Fat 10.1g, Sodium 390mg

620. PERFECT SAUTEED ZUCCHINI

- Prep time: 5 mins, Cook time: 10 mins, Total time: 15 mins, Servings: 4

Ingredients

- 2 tbsp olive oil or butter
- 2 tbsp grated Parmesan cheese- optional

- ½ tsp garlic powder
- ½ tsp kosher salt
- ½ tsp onion powder
- Finely chopped fresh basil, if desired-optional
- 1 ¾ pound zucchini- 2 medium-large or 3 to 4 small
- 1 tsp oregano

Directions

1. Zucchini should be sliced into ¼-inch thin rounds.
2. Heat the olive oil or butter in your biggest skillet over medium-high heat. Stir in the oregano, garlic powder, and salt, then add the zucchini slices, turning and tossing to coat all of them.
3. Cook for 1 min with the lid off, then uncover & stir. Cover for another minute, then uncover and stir, sliding slices to the lower side as needed to brown them.
4. Continue to rotate the zucchini and transfer them to the lower side so they cook evenly, keeping the skillet uncovered for another 6 to 8 mins when most of the zucchini is soft and browned.
5. If preferred, add Parmesan cheese & fresh basil before serving.

Nutritional Values

Calories 321kcal, Carbohydrates-1g, Protein 1.3g, Fat 7.7g, Sodium 421mg

621. SAUTEED MUSHROOMS

- Prep time: 2 mins, Cook time: 7 mins, Total time: 9 mins, Servings: 4

Ingredients

- ⅓ cup chopped fresh thyme and oregano
- 16 ounces baby Bella- aka cremini mushrooms
- Fresh ground pepper
- 3 tbsp olive oil- or butter
- 2 tbsp fresh lemon juice
- ½ tsp kosher salt

Directions

1. After cleaning the mushrooms, slice them. Chop the thyme and oregano leaves.
2. Heat the olive oil in a saute pan/skillet over medium-high heat. Cook, often stirring, for 2 mins, after adding the mushrooms.
3. Cook for another 4 to 5 mins, stirring periodically, until most of the liquid has evaporated and the mushrooms are soft, add the herbs, kosher salt, and pepper as needed.- Taste to see if it's done.
4. Remove the pan from the heat and mix in the lemon juice. If required, season with another pinch of salt.

Nutritional Values

Calories 211kcal, Carbohydrates-3.7g, Protein 3.5g, Fat 10.9g, Sodium 370mg

622. BEST EVER SAUTEED KALE

- Prep time: 5 mins, Cook time: 3 mins, Total time: 8 mins, Servings: 4

Ingredients

- 2 garlic cloves
- 1 pound or 2 bunches of Tuscan kale
- Optional: Lemon wedges, shredded Parmesan cheese
- 2 tbsp olive oil
- ¼ tsp kosher salt
- Fresh ground pepper

Directions

1. The kale leaves should be washed and dried before being destemmed and coarsely chopped.
2. Garlic cloves should be smashed and peeled.
3. In a large pan, heat the olive oil over medium-high heat. Cook for 3 mins, often turning, until the kale has wilted and become brilliant green.
4. Remove the pan from the heat & season with kosher salt and freshly ground pepper. Remove the garlic cloves & serve right away.- You may add lemon juice or Parmesan cheese, but neither is essential with Tuscan kale's delicious taste! If you're using curly kale, you might want to think about them.

Nutritional Values

Calories 199kal, Carbohydrates-10.4g, Protein 4.9g, Fat 8.1g, Sodium 300mg

623. PERFECT SAUTEED GREEN BEANS

- Prep time: 5 mins, Cook time: 10 mins, Total time: 15 mins, Servings: 4

Ingredients

- 1 shallot- optional but recommended
- ½ tsp kosher salt
- 1 pound of fresh green beans
- Fresh ground black pepper
- 1 tbsp olive oil or butter
- 2 tbsp fresh lemon juice- and zest of ½ lemon if desired

Directions

1. Green beans should be trimmed. Chop the shallot finely.
2. In a large pan, combine the beans and 1/3 cup of water. Heat to a medium-high temperature. Cover the pan and cook the beans for 4 mins after the water begins to boil. Then cover and simmer for 1 minute or until the water has completely evaporated.
3. Add the olive oil or butter, chopped shallot, and kosher salt after the water has evaporated. Cook for another 2 mins, stirring regularly until the vegetables are soft.
4. Remove the beans to a dish and turn off the heat. Add the lemon juice and, if desired, the grated lemon zest. Taste, then season with a generous amount of freshly ground pepper and a couple of pinches of kosher salt. Eat as soon as possible. Leftovers last for 2 to 3 days in the refrigerator, and while the vibrant green color fades, they still taste great.

Nutritional Values

Calories 130kcal, Carbohydrates-8.8g, Protein 2.2g, Fat 3.8g, Sodium 320mg

624. SIMPLE SAUTEED ONIONS

- Prep time: 5 mins, Cook time: 10 mins, Total time: 15 mins, Servings: 4

Ingredients

- 2 tbsp olive oil or butter- or 1 tbsp of each
- 3 medium yellow onions- or sweet onions
- Optional adder: Add 1 tbsp balsamic vinegar with the kosher salt

- ½ tsp kosher salt
- Fresh ground black pepper

Directions

1. Cut the onions into thin slices.
2. Heat the olive oil/butter in a big sauté pan or skillet over medium-high heat. Cook, stirring periodically, for 4 mins, after adding the onion.
3. Cook for another 4-5 mins, stirring regularly, after adding the kosher salt and freshly ground black pepper. Taste to see whether it's done, then season with a few pinches of salt until the flavor bursts.

Nutritional Values

Calories 121kcal, Carbohydrates-11.2g, Protein 1.3g, Fat 1.1g, Sodium 155mg

625. QUINOA SALAD

- Prep time: 5 mins, Cook time: 10 mins, Total time: 15 mins, Servings: 4

Ingredients

- 1 cup sliced grape tomatoes
- 1- 15 ounces can of white beans
- 1 lemon
- 2 cups of water- to cook with quinoa
- ½ cup chopped parsley
- 1 cup- of dry quinoa
- ¼ cup diced sweet onion
- ¼ cup olive oil
- 1 cup sliced black olives
- Sea salt- optional

Directions

1. Cook the quinoa according to the package directions and set it aside to cool.
2. White beans should be drained and rinsed.
3. Stir together the tomatoes, beans, onion, olives, lemon juice, parsley, and olive oil in a large food storage container.
4. Mix in the quinoa and optional sea salt, then cover and chill.
5. Within 3-4 days, you should be able to enjoy it.

Nutritional Values

Calories 211kcal, Carbohydrates-11.2g, Protein 1.3g, Fat 1.1g, Sodium 175mg

626. SUPER CRUNCH SALAD

- Prep time: 5 mins, Cook time: 10 mins, Total time: 15 mins, Servings: 6

Ingredients

- ½ head cauliflower
- 3 tbsp olive oil
- 1 red bell pepper
- 1 tbsp of crushed garlic
- 2 large carrots
- Juice from 1 lemon
- ¼ a head of purple cabbage
- ½ cup parsley
- 2 cups baby kale
- Sea salt & black pepper
- ¾ cup currants
- ½ head broccoli
- ½ cup hemp hearts

Directions

1. All veggies should be finely chopped and placed in a large mixing bowl. You may chop the vegetables by hand or in a food processor.
2. Garlic, hemp hearts, currants, olive oil, lemon juice, and salt and pepper to taste
3. Combine all ingredients, serve, and enjoy!

Nutritional Values

Calories 131kcal, Carbohydrates-11.2g, Protein 1.3g, Fat 1.1g, Sodium 188mg

627. TURMERIC NOODLE SOUP

- Prep time: 5 mins, Cook time: 10 mins, Total time: 15 mins, Servings: 6

Ingredients

- 1 small broccoli
- 4 oz. brown rice pad Thai noodles
- 2 carrots
- pinch of sea salt
- 1 cup red onion
- 1 tbsp coconut oil
- 1-inch fresh ginger
- 2 cups vegetable broth
- 1-inch fresh turmeric
- Fresh cilantro and lime
- 1 large bok choy
- 1 can of full-Fat coconut milk

Directions

1. Carrots, broccoli, and bok choy should be washed, peeled, and chopped.
2. Next, finely slice the red onion and peel & slice the turmeric & ginger.
3. In a blender jar, combine the ginger, vegetable broth, turmeric, and coconut milk and mix on high for 1 minute.
4. In a deep skillet over medium heat, add 1 tbsp coconut oil and red onions, and sauté for 5 mins.
5. After that, pour in the turmeric ginger broth and cook for 20 mins.
6. Finally, add all veggies & brown rice noodles to the pan, ensuring they are thoroughly coated in liquid. Simmer for 15 mins, then serve with fresh cilantro and just a squeeze of lime!

Nutritional Values

Calories 170kal, Carbohydrates-11.2g, Protein 1.3g, Fat 1.1g, Sodium 121mg

628. MILLET MEDLEY NOURISH BOWL

- Prep time: 5 mins, Cook time: 10 mins, Total time: 15 mins, Servings: 4

Ingredients

- ½ cup white beans- cooked, drained & rinsed
- 2 oz. pea greens- shoots
- 2 servings of Hilary's Eat Well Traditional Herb Millet Medley
- 2 tbsp tahini
- 1 avocado
- 1 lemon, juiced
- 2 endive
- 2 tbsp hemp hearts- seeds
- 6 radish
- 3 tbsp olive oil

Directions

1. In a small bowl, mix the lemon juice, olive oil, and tahini.
2. Endives and radishes should be washed and sliced. The avocado should be peeled, pitted, and sliced.
3. Prepare Millet Medley as directed on the packet. Divide the millet medley into 2 serving dishes after it has been sufficiently cooked.

4. Add the salad with white beans, radish, endive, avocado, lemon tahini sauce, and hemp hearts.
5. Enjoy!

Nutritional Values

Calories 159kcal, Carbs 11.2g, Protein 1.3g, Fat 1.1g, Sodium 333mg

629. ROOT BOWL WITH MEYER GARLIC SAUCE RECIPE

- Prep time: 5 mins, Cook time: 10 mins, Total time: 15 mins, Servings: 4

Ingredients

- ¼ cup extra virgin olive oil
- 1-2 parsnips
- 1 garlic head
- 1 purple sweet potato
- 2 cups baby greens
- 1 golden beet
- 1 Limoneira Meyer lemon
- 2-3 large carrots

Directions

1. Preheat the oven to 350°F.
2. All root vegetables should be peeled and chopped. Cut off the tip of the garlic and remove the paper peel.
3. Brush a big pan with olive oil and add the vegetables and garlic head.
4. Preheat oven to 350°F and bake for 45 mins. After 30 mins, remove the garlic.
5. Combine the roasted cloves, olive oil, lemon juice, and a pinch of salt in a blender.
6. Blend until completely smooth.
7. Toss greens with roasted root vegetables in a large mixing basin, then sprinkle with sauce.

Nutritional Values

Calories 250kcal, Carbs11g, Protein 3g, Fat 1.1g, Sodium 338mg

630. COCONUT LEMONGRASS NOODLE SOUP

- Prep time: 5 mins, Cook time: 10 mins, Total time: 15 mins, Servings: 4

Ingredients

- ½ Limoneira lime
- 1- 15-ounce can of full-fat coconut milk
- 1 tbsp lemongrass paste
- 10-12 basil leaves
- 1 cup vegetable stock
- 1 green onion
- 1 tbsp coconut oil
- 1 red bell pepper
- 1- 15-ounce can of chickpeas
- ½ pound sliced mushrooms
- 2 tbsp maple syrup
- 1 tsp Thai chili paste
- 4-ounce brown rice noodles

Directions

1. Soak brown rice noodles for 20 mins in water.
2. Slice red bell pepper using a mandolin slicer. The green onion should be chopped.
3. In a big soup pot, melt the coconut oil over medium heat.
4. Lemon juice, maple syrup, lime juice, Thai chili paste, lemongrass paste, and sliced mushrooms should all be added at this point. Combine all ingredients in a mixing bowl.
5. Red bell pepper, vegetable stock, green onion, chickpeas, coconut milk, basil leaves, and brown rice noodles should all be added at this point.
6. Cook for 20 mins before serving.

Nutritional Values

Calories 636kcal, Carbs 76g, Protein 16.2g, Fat 32.6g, Sodium 1560mg

631. MIXED SPICE MUESLI RECIPE

- Prep time: 10 mins, Cook time: 0 mins, Total time: 10 mins, Servings: 3

Ingredients

- 30g bran flakes
- 25g pomegranate seeds
- 25g raspberries
- 25g blackberries
- 1 tbsp pistachio nuts, chopped
- 2 tbsp dried cranberries
- 75g sultanas
- ½ tsp mixed spice
- 50g flaked almonds- toasted
- 125g jumbo oats
- 25g sunflower seeds

- Milk to serve
- 1 tbsp pumpkin seeds

1. To create the muesli, place the ingredients in a mixing dish and stir thoroughly. Keep the container sealed.
2. To serve, add 1/3 of the muesli into a bowl, pour enough milk to taste, then top with the toppings of your preference.

Nutritional Values

Calories 421kcal, Carbs 43g, Protein 11g, Fat 1g, Sodium 444mg

632. CUCUMBER AND PRAWN STIR-FRY RECIPE

- Prep time: 20 mins, Cook time: 3 mins, Total time: 23 mins, Servings: 2

Ingredients

- 2 tsp salt
- 1 cucumber
- 1 tbsp sweet chili sauce
- 4 tsp oil- groundnut or sunflower
- 2 tbsp Chinese wine or dry sherry
- 1-2 cloves garlic, peeled and finely chopped
- 1 tbsp sesame oil
- 1 tsp freshly grated root ginger
- 2 spring onions, trimmed and chopped
- About 400g- 14oz mixed fish and prawns
- 2 tbsp light soy sauce

Directions

1. Using a tsp, peel the cucumber, divide it lengthwise, and remove the seeds. Slice the cucumber halves into ½ " slices, season with salt. Place them in a colander and set aside for 20 mins to drain.
2. Quickly wash the cucumber slices under running water and wipe dry with a tea towel or kitchen paper.
3. Heat a wok or a big frying pan to high temperatures. When the oil is heated, add the cucumber & stir-fry for several mins until it browns. Place in a serving dish to keep warm.
4. Stir-fry for 30 seconds with the remaining oil, garlic, ginger, and spring onions, then add the fish & prawns & stir-fry for a minute. Cook for a minute, stirring slowly to prevent breaking up the fish, before

adding the soy sauce, chili sauce, wine, and sesame oil. Toss in with the cooked cucumber.
5. Serve with noodles and a sprinkle of coriander, if desired.

Nutritional Values

Calories 462kcal, Carbs 54g, Protein 21g, Fat 7g, Sodium 467mg

633. SOY-CURED TUNA NOODLES RECIPE

- Prep time: 10 mins, Cook time: 2 mins, Total time: 12 mins, Servings: 4

Ingredients

- Finely grated zest and juice of ½ a lime
- 1 tsp coriander seeds, lightly crushed
- 4 spring onions, trimmed and sliced
- 3 tbsp soft brown sugar
- 2 tbsp sesame oil
- 1 tbsp soy sauce
- 300g pack of fresh egg noodles
- 3 tbsp balsamic vinegar
- A handful of fresh coriander leaves
- 500g- 1lb tuna steak, cut in 2
- 200g- 7oz broccoli, cut into small florets

Directions

1. In a small bowl, whisk the soy sauce, coriander seeds, sugar, lime zest, and vinegar until the sugar dissolves. Pour ½ of the marinade over the tuna in a shallow dish. Allow 15 mins to pass.
2. Blanch the broccoli florets for 1-2 mins in boiling water, drain, rinse, and chill in cold water. Cook the noodles as directed on the package.
3. 1 tbsp sesame oil, 1 tbsp sesame oil, 1 tbsp sesame oil, 1 tbsp sesame oil, 1 tbsp sesame oil, 1 tbsp sesame oil, 1 tbsp sesame oil. Remove the tuna from the pan and set it aside to rest.
4. Reheat the pan and gently sauté the spring onions for 2 mins before adding the broccoli and heating through. Mix the cooked noodles, the remaining sesame oil, & some coriander leaves in a heated bowl. Distribute the noodles into 4 bowls. Place the fish on top, broken into bits.
5. Pour the remaining marinade over the fish & serve in dishes with lime juice.

Calories 587kcal, Carbs 35g, Protein 11g, Fat 17g, Sodium 435mg

634. ROAST TOMATO AND ORANGE SOUP RECIPE

- Prep time: 20 mins, Cook time: 1 hr 25 mins, Total time: 1 hr 45 mins, Servings: 4

Ingredients

- 2 garlic cloves, finely chopped
- 900g tomatoes, halved
- The zest of 1 small orange to serve
- 4 tbsp olive oil
- 100ml orange juice
- 2 onions, diced
- Edible flowers to serve- optional
- 2 carrots, peeled or scrubbed and diced
- 1 celery stick, diced
- 560ml hot vegetable stock

Directions

1. Preheat the oven to 350°F.
2. Sprinkle the chopped garlic over the tomatoes on a big baking dish. Season with salt & a grind or 2 of black pepper and sprinkle with 2 tbsp olive oil. Preheat the oven to 350°F and roast the tomatoes for 45 mins, stirring halfway through.
3. After the tomatoes have been stirred, heat the rest of the olive oil in a wide, deep-sided skillet and sauté the onions, carrots, and celery for 20 mins over low heat. Add the roasted tomatoes & garlic to the pan, along with the stock and orange juice, and give everything a thorough stir.
4. Bring the soup to a low simmer for a min, or 2, then remove from the heat and set aside to cool somewhat before blending. Return the stew to the pan and season to taste with additional salt and ground black pepper. If you're serving it right away, make sure it's well hot.
5. If you want to serve the soup chilled, let it cool fully before pouring it into a big container and chilling it for a few hours.
6. Serve with a touch of orange zest and, if desired.

Nutritional Values

Calories 173kcal, Carbs 8.7g, Protein 1g, Fat 14.8g, Sodium 551mg

635. AVOCADO COUSCOUS SALAD RECIPE

- Prep time: 10 mins, Cook time: 25 mins, Total time: 35 mins, Servings: 6

Ingredients

- 500g couscous
- 1tbsp flat-leaf parsley, chopped
- 1tbsp lemon juice
- 2tbsp mint, chopped
- 1 x 220g can chickpeas, drained
- 2tbsp virgin olive oil
- 1 red pepper, finely chopped
- 100g pine nuts, toasted
- 1 pomegranate
- 2 avocados
- 4tbsp orange juice

Directions

1. Boiling water should be used to cover the couscous. Allow it to soak for 20 mins, covered with a moist tea cloth. To loosen the grains, use a fork.
2. Cut the avocado into pieces after peeling. Add the lemon juice and mix well.
3. Add the avocado, chickpeas, and pepper to the couscous and mix well.
4. Remove the seeds from the pomegranate by splitting them in ½. To catch any fluids, do this over a dish. Toss the couscous with the seeds.
5. Combine the orange juice and lemon juice in a mixing bowl with the oil. Toss the couscous with the dressing & herbs and toss well. With a dusting of pine nuts on top, serve.

Nutritional Values

Calories 442kcal, Carbs 58g, Protein 13g, Fat 17g, Sodium 237mg

636. CHUNKY ENGLISH GARDEN SALAD RECIPE

- Prep time: 10 mins, Cook time: 0 mins, Total time: 10 mins, Servings: 4

Ingredients

- 2 small cos/romaine lettuces
- 1 cucumber

- Lemon juice
- 8 radishes, halved
- Sea salt and freshly ground black pepper
- A few small mint leaves
- Olive oil

Directions

1. Slice the cucumber into 4 sections, then cut each section into 4 or 6 wedges.
2. Place the lettuce pieces, cucumber wedges, radish, and torn mint leave on a tray.
3. Drizzle with a generous amount of olive oil and a squeeze of lemon. Season with a pinch of salt and pepper.

Nutritional Values

Calories 54kcal, Carbohydrates-34g, Protein 11g, Fat 6g, Sodium 421mg

637. THAI QUINOA SALAD

- Prep time: 15 mins, Cook time: 10 mins, Total time: 25 mins, Servings: 4

Ingredients

- ¼ cup cilantro
- Thai peanut salad
- 1 tsp maple syrup
- 2 cups red cabbage, shredded
- 1-2 cloves garlic, minced
- 1 ½ cups broccoli florets, chopped
- 2 tsp fresh ginger, chopped
- ½ large red bell pepper, thinly sliced
- 2 tbsp soy sauce; use tamari for a gluten-free option
- sesame peanut sauce
- ¼ cup natural peanut butter
- 2 tbsp sesame oil
- 1 large carrot, chopped
- 3 green onions, chopped
- 1 bag of Quinoa
- 1 batch of Sesame Peanut Sauce
- ¼ cup roasted peanuts
- 1 tbsp rice vinegar

Directions

1. Quinoa should be cooked according to the package directions.
2. Cut the carrots, cabbage, broccoli, bell peppers, green onions, and cilantro while the quinoa is cooking. Set aside.

3. In a small blender, combine all of the peanut sauce ingredients and mix until smooth.
4. Remove the quinoa from the boiling water using tongs or a slotted spoon. Allow 10 mins for the bag to cool after cutting it open.
5. In a large mixing basin, combine the quinoa and the prepared veggies. Toss with roasted peanuts and peanut sauce.
6. Serve immediately or keep refrigerated for up to 3 days in an airtight jar.

Nutritional Values

Calories 262kcal, Carbs 15g, Protein 9g, Fat 19g, Sodium 653mg

638. CREAMY PEA AND WATERCRESS SOUP RECIPE

- Prep time: 5 mins, Cook time: 20 mins, Total time: 25 mins, Servings: 4

Ingredients

- 1 onion, finely chopped
- 1-liter vegetable stock
- 25g butter
- 60g natural bio yogurt
- 300g fresh or frozen peas, reserve 100g
- Fresh mint, chopped to serve, optional
- 100g or 2 bags of watercress
- Salt & Black Pepper
- 1 large potato, peeled and cubed
- A handful of fresh mint

Directions

1. In a saucepan, melt the butter and add the onion; simmer until translucent and tender.
2. Cook until the peas, watercress, and potato are soft and wilted, then add the remaining 200g peas, watercress, and potato.
3. Add the veggie stock and cook for 15-20 mins before adding the remainder of the peas to give the soup a brighter color.
4. Blend in the mint and spices until completely smooth.
5. Pour into heated bowls, top with yogurt, and garnish with fresh mint.

Nutritional Values

Calories 208kcal, Carbs 54g, Protein 14g, Fat 10.4g, Sodium 557mg

639. ANTHONY WORRALL THOMPSON'S HERBY FRUIT SALAD RECIPE

- Prep time: 10 mins, Cook time: 10 mins, Total time: 20 mins, Servings: 4

Ingredients

- 1 tbsp liquid honey
- 1 small mango, peeled and diced
- Lemon or lime juice, to taste
- 1 banana, peeled and sliced
- 2 blood oranges or small pink grapefruit, peeled and sliced
- 2 tbsp chopped coriander leaves
- 1 small pineapple, peeled and diced
- 4 tbsp reduced-fat coconut milk
- 1 pink-skinned apple, cored and diced

Directions

1. Combine the coconut milk, honey, and lemon juice in a mixing bowl.
2. Toss the fruits with the coriander in the dressing and serve.

Nutritional Values

Calories 141kcal, Carbs 18g, Protein 5g, Fat 0.5g, Sodium 224g

640. 7-VEG STIR-FRY RECIPE

- Prep time: 15 mins, Cook time: 10 mins, Total time: 25 mins, Servings: 6

Ingredients

- 1-2 tbsp groundnut oil
- 4-6 spring onions, trimmed and thinly sliced
- 2.5cm- 1in piece fresh root ginger, peeled and cut into slivers
- 100g or 150g pack of fresh beansprouts, depending on the pack size available
- 8 baby sweetcorn, halved lengthways
- 2 heads pak choi, quartered lengthways
- 2 medium carrots, peeled and cut into batons
- 1 red chili, deseeded and finely chopped, optional
- 8 asparagus tips
- 4tbsp sweet chili dipping sauce or hoisin sauce
- Thai rice noodles- 250g pack
- Soy sauce to serve

- Handful each of mint and coriander leaves, roughly chopped
- 1 red pepper, deseeded & sliced into thumb-length pieces
- 100g- 3½ oz. mini sugar-snap peas or mangetout, or normal-sized ones, halved lengthways

Directions

1. Pour sufficient boiling water to cover the noodles in a bowl and mix. At the same time, the veggies are cooking, set aside for 5 mins.
2. Stir-fry the red pepper & ginger for ½ a min in 1 tbsp oil in a hot wok or big frying pan. Stir-fry for a minute with the sweetcorn, carrots, and asparagus, then add the sugar snaps & cook for another minute.
3. Combine the chili dipping sauce or hoisin sauce with 4 tbsp water, mix the red chili, beansprouts, pak choi, & spring onions, and heat for a few mins.
4. Drain the noodles and set them aside. Toss with coriander and mint. Serve with stir-fried veggies and a dash of soy sauce on top.

Nutritional Values

Calories 236kcal, Carbs 20g, Protein 10g, Fat 2.5g, Sodium 678mg

641. QUINOA AND BUTTERNUT SQUASH SALAD RECIPE

- Prep time: 10 mins, Cook time: 40 mins, Total time: 50 mins, Servings: 2

Ingredients

- 1 tbsp olive oil
- 150g quinoa
- ½ vegetable stock cube
- ½ red onion, finely sliced
- 1 butternut squash, peeled, deseeded, and diced
- 80g salad leaves

For The Dressing:
- 2 tbsp olive oil
- 1 tbsp red wine vinegar

Directions

1. Preheat the oven to 390°F. In a big ovenproof dish, spread out butternut

squash slices, sprinkle over the olive oil, and bake for 30 mins.
2. Meanwhile, rinse the quinoa in a colander under cold water to remove the bitter coating on the seeds. Cook the quinoa as per the package directions, using the cooking water to dissolve the veggie stock cube. The seeds will emit small white threads that coil around them when the quinoa is ripe. Drain any residual water, set it aside to cool, and then separate with a fork.
3. Combine the red onion, salad greens, quinoa, and butternut squash in a large mixing bowl. Combine the vinegar and oil in a mixing bowl and season with salt and pepper to make the dressing. Toss everything together after pouring the dressing over the salad.

Nutritional Values

Calories 261kcal, Carbohydrates-39g, Protein 5g, Fat 11g, Sodium 339mg

642. ROASTED MINTY BEETROOT AND GOAT'S CHEESE RECIPE

- Prep time: 5 mins, Cook time: 30 mins, Total time: 35 mins, Servings: 6

Ingredients

- 3 tbsp olive oil
- 100g soft goats'cheese, crumbled
- 2 tbsp mint sauce
- small bunch fresh mint, leaves only
- 400g beetroot, washed, trimmed, and unpeeled, cut into wedges
- 2 tsp balsamic vinegar

Directions

1. Preheat the oven to 425°F. Place the beets in a roasting pan, spray with olive oil, and roast for 20-25 mins, or until just soft.
2. Combine the mint sauce and vinegar in a mixing bowl and season with salt and black pepper. Sprinkle over the cooked beets, top with goats' cheese, and bake for another 5 mins. Before serving, scatter mint leaves on top.

Nutritional Values

Calories 129kcal, Carbohydrates-39g, Protein 15g, Fat 10g, Sodium 467mg

643. GRANOLA RECIPE

- Prep time: 10 mins, Cook time: 25 mins, Total time: 35 mins, Servings: 2

Ingredients

- 75ml sunflower oil
- 25g sunflower or pumpkin seeds
- 4tbsp honey
- 75g walnut or pecan halves
- 75g shelled almonds
- 100g dried fruits such as dried pineapple, mango, raisins
- 300g jumbo rolled oats
- 75g shelled hazelnuts

Directions

1. Preheat the oven to 375°F.
2. In a large mixing bowl, combine the oats, oil, and honey. Mix well before adding the other ingredients. Spread out on a big non-stick baking sheet and bake for 20–25 mins, flipping once or twice to ensure equal browning. Allow cooling fully before serving.
3. Add the dry fruits to the mix. Fill an airtight container halfway with the mixture and preserve for up to a month. Serve with fresh fruit and milk or yogurt.

Nutritional Values

Calories 140kcal, Carbohydrates-14g, Protein 3g, Fat 9g, Sodium 85mg

644. BEETROOT, POMEGRANATE, AND PARSNIP SOUP RECIPE

- Prep time: 10 mins, Cook time: 25 mins, Total time: 35 mins, Servings: 4

Ingredients

- 75g- 3oz onion, finely chopped
- 1 pomegranate
- 175g- 6oz carrots, diced
- 4tsp fresh dill, chopped
- 150g- 5oz parsnips, thinly sliced
- 350g- 12oz cooked beetroot- not in vinegar, sliced
- ½ tsp ground coriander
- 1tbsp light olive oil
- 800ml- 1⅓ pints light stock

To Garnish
- 2tbsp walnut pieces- optional

- 4tbsp soy yogurt

1. In a large saucepan, heat the oil & sweat the onion, carrot, and parsnip for 5 mins, or until they begin to soften. Cook for another 2 mins after adding the coriander.
2. Combine the stock & beetroot in a large mixing bowl. Bring to a boil, then reduce to low heat and cook for 20 mins, adding 2 tsp dill for the final 2 or 3 mins.
3. Using a lemon squeezer, cut the pomegranate in 2 and remove the juice. Toss the soup in a blender and season with lemon juice to taste.
4. Garnish with the remaining 2 tsp minced dill, yogurt, and walnut pieces.
5. Serve with walnut bread, granary rolls, or rye rolls.

Nutritional Values

Calories 158kcal, Carbohydrates-19g, Protein 6g, Fat 5.4g, Sodium 411mg

645. STIR-FRY PRAWNS WITH MUSHROOM AND BROCCOLI RECIPE

- Prep time: 30 mins, Cook time: 5 mins, Total time: 35 mins, Servings: 2

Ingredients

- 225g tiger prawns, uncooked
- 1 tbsp corn flour, a pinch of cayenne pepper
- 2 spring onions, diagonally sliced
- 2 tbsp soy sauce spray oil for frying
- 1 small piece of ginger root, finely chopped
- 25g unsalted cashew nuts
- 1 clove of garlic, crushed
- 120g shiitake mushrooms, halved
- 4 tbsp rice wine
- 200g broccoli, chopped into florets

Directions

1. In a bowl, combine the corn flour and cayenne, add the prawns and coat completely, add the soy sauce, and set aside for 30 mins.
2. Spray a wok with oil, set it over high heat, add the cashews & stir-fry for 30 secs or until brown, then transfer to a platter.
3. After that, add the mushrooms & cook for 1-2 mins, or until golden. Stir in the prawns

for approximately 1-2 mins, or until they become pink. Stir in the remaining ingredients for a further minute.
4. Return all nuts to the pan, reduce the heat to medium, stir in the rice wine & a splash of water, then cover and simmer for another minute. Serve with cooked rice or glass noodles.

Nutritional Values

Calories 271kcal, Carbohydrates-13g, Protein 8g, Fat 8g, Sodium 222mg

646. SEA BASS WITH SQUASH AND STIR-FRY RECIPE

- Prep time: 15 mins, Cook time: 20 mins, Total time: 35 mins, Servings: 2

Ingredients

- 2 tbsp olive oil
- 1 tbsp frozen chopped basil
- 220g pack of 2 frozen sea bass fillets
- 1 clove of garlic, peeled and thinly sliced
- 150g- 5oz frozen cauliflower florets
- 125g- 4oz frozen peas
- 250g- 8oz frozen butternut squash- from a 500g pack
- Salt and freshly ground black pepper

Directions

1. Microwave the butternut squash in a bowl on high for 5 mins.
2. Meanwhile, heat ½ the oil in a frying pan and cook the sea-bass slices for 3 mins on 1 side. Cook for another 1-2 mins, on the other side. Remove from the pan and place on a baking dish in a heated oven.
3. Cook for a few mins until the cauliflower is thawed and tinted brown in the hot oil remaining in the pan, then toss in the peas.
4. Sprinkle the mashed squash with salt and pepper, then divide it across 2 dishes. Combine the fish and stir-fried veggies in a large mixing bowl.
5. In the same pan, heat the remaining oil & add the garlic. Cook until the basil is just beginning to brown, then remove from the heat. Serve the sauce over the fish.

Nutritional Values

Calories 331kcal, Carbohydrates-54g, Protein 8g, Fat 15.5g, Sodium 654mg

647. Quinoa Lentil Salad

- Prep time: 30 mins, Cook time: 20 mins, Total time: 50 mins, Servings: 4

Ingredients

- ½ cup quinoa
- 2 tsp ground cumin
- 4 cloves garlic- minced
- 1 cup French lentils
- ¼ cup packed basil leaves- cut into thin ribbons
- 2 sweet potatoes- peeled & cut into small dice
- 1 green pepper- deseeded & finely diced
- Salt and ground black pepper to taste
- 1 tsp red pepper flakes or paprika
- 2 medium carrots- finely diced
- 1 medium onion- finely diced
- 2 stalks of celery- finely diced
- ½ tsp ground cinnamon
- 2 bay leaves
- 1 tsp extra virgin olive oil
- Juice of ½ lemon

Directions

1. Preheat the oven to 375°F. Combine the sweet potatoes & cinnamon on a baking sheet and arrange in a single layer. Sweet potatoes should be baked for 20-25 mins, or until fork-tender. Remove from the equation.
2. Rinse the lentils in a mixture of water and 1 tsp of salt. There should be around an inch of water covering the lentils. Allow 30 mins for preparation. It allows the lentils to keep their form while cooking.
3. Place the lentils in a saucepan after draining and washing them. 2 cups of water & bay leaves are added to the pot. Over medium heat, put the lentils to a boil, cover, and simmer until they are cooked but still maintain their form. It took me less than 5 mins, so keep an eye on your lentils, so they don't go mushy.
4. To cook the quinoa, rinse it completely before draining it. Roast the quinoa in a dry pan until it emits a nutty aroma.
5. Turn the heat off.
6. In a large saucepan, heat the olive oil or vegetable stock. With a sprinkle of salt and some ground black pepper, toss in the onions, carrots, and celery. Cook occasionally turns for approximately 8 mins, or until the onions have softened and the carrots have softened but retained their bite.
7. Garlic should be included now. Sauté for another minute with cumin and fresh chili flakes.
8. Continue to sauté the green peppers for another 2-3 mins, or until they are just tender.
9. Combine the roasted potatoes, quinoa, lentils, and lemon juice in a large mixing bowl and thoroughly combine. Add the basil and mix well.
10. Serve warm or hot.

Nutritional Values

Calories 295kcal, Carbohydrates-65g, Protein 16.4g, Fat 2g, Sodium 632mg

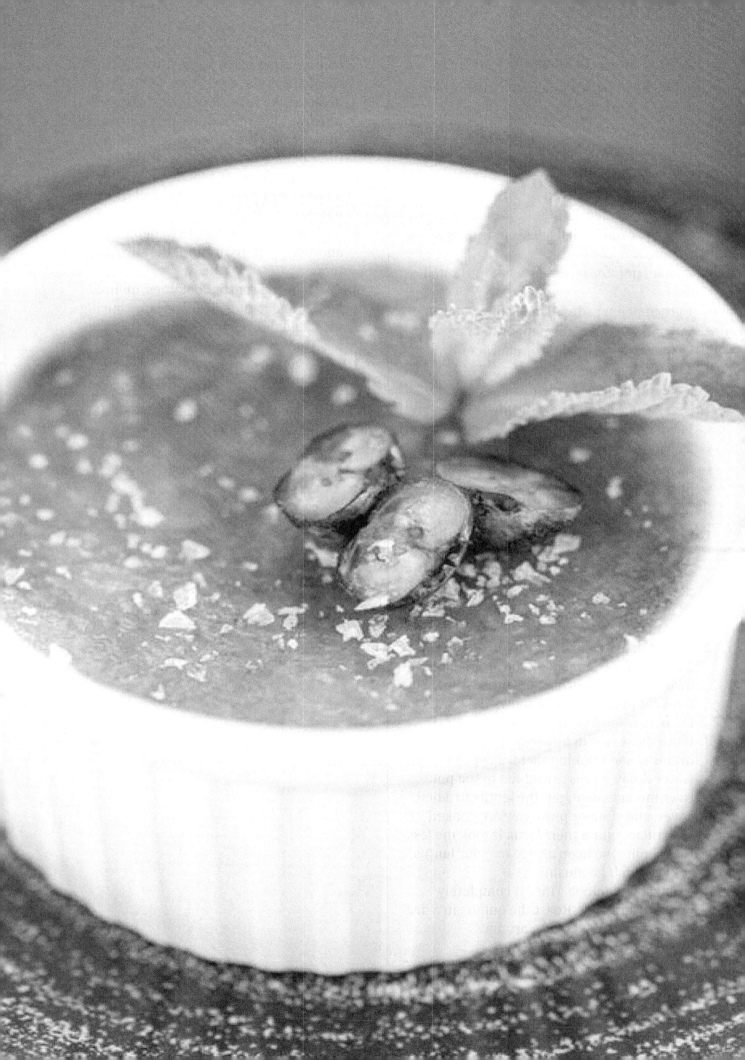

Chapter 17.

Sweet Dishes Recipes

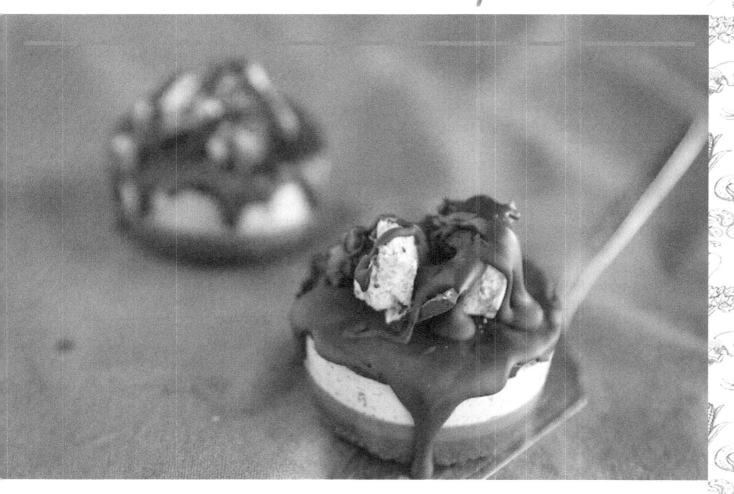

648. APRICOT-PEAR CAKE

- Dessert - Prep time: 5 mins, Cook time: 35 mins, Total time: 40 mins, Servings: 4 to 6, Grill temp: 300°F

Ingredients

- 1 ½ cups of water
- 1 cup of fresh chopped pears
- ½ cup of dried apricots
- 1 and ¼ cups of whole-wheat flour
- ½ tsp of baking soda
- ½ tsp of baking powder
- ½ tsp of ground nutmeg
- ⅛ tsp salt
- ½ cup of unsweetened coconut milk
- ¼ cup of pure maple syrup
- 2 tbsp of organic applesauce
- 2 tbsp of ground golden flax seeds

Directions

1. Grease a 7-inch bundt pan.
2. Mix dry ingredients in a bowl.
3. Mix wet ingredients in a separate bowl.
4. Mix wet into dry before folding in pears and cranberries.
5. Pour batter into pan and wrap in foil.
6. Pour water into your pressure cooker and lower it in a trivet or steamer basket.
7. Lower the pan in.
8. Close and seal the lid.
9. Cook on high pressure for 35 mins.
10. Turn down the heat and let the pressure come down on its own.
11. Take out the pan and throw away the foil.
12. Cool before serving.

Nutritional Values

Calories 163, Fat 2g, Chol 0mg, Sodium 71.4mg, Potassium 67.7mg, Carbs 35g, Protein 4g

649. APPLESAUCE CAKE

- Dessert - Prep time: ready in about: 35 mins, Servings: 8, Grill temp: Medium

Ingredients

- ½ cup of sugar
- 1 cup of applesauce
- ⅓ cup of avocado oil
- 3 eggs
- ¼ cup of almond milk
- 1 tsp vanilla extract
- ¾ cup of flour, all-purpose
- 1 tsp vinegar, apple cider
- ¾ cup of wheat flour
- 2 tsp Apple-Pie-Spice
- ½ cup of almond flour
- 2 tsp baking powder
- Cream Cheese for frosting
- ¼ tsp baking soda
- ½ tsp sea salt
- ½ cup of chopped walnuts

Directions

1. Preheat your oven to around 350°F.
2. Take a medium bowl, add applesauce, oil, sugar, almond milk, vanilla, eggs, and vinegar in it, and whisk well.
3. Take another bowl, and add the whole wheat, all-purpose, & almond flour, pie spice, salt, baking powder, & baking soda in it.
4. Combine dry ingredients with your, mix well, then add walnuts. Pour your batter into an already greased pan and bake for around 32-39 mins.
5. Let your cake cool for a while, then top with some cream cheese if required and enjoy the food.

Nutritional Values

Calories 202kcal, Carbs 30g, Protein 8g, Fat 11g, Sodium 886mg, Potassium 734mg, Chol 0mg

650. HOMEMADE BROWNIES

- Dessert - Prep time: ready in about: 40 mins, Servings: 16, Grill temp: Medium

Ingredients

- ¾ cup of flour, all-purpose
- 1 to ½ cups of granulated sugar
- 2/3 cup of cocoa powder
- ½ cup of chocolate chips
- ½ cup of powdered sugar
- ¾ tsp sea salt
- ½ cup of canola oil
- ½ tsp vanilla
- 2 eggs
- 2 tbsp water

Directions

1. Preheat your oven to around 325°F.
2. Take a bowl, add sugar, cocoa powder, flour, powdered sugar, salt & chocolate chips in it.
3. Take another bowl, combine eggs, water, olive oil, & vanilla in it, and whisk well. Add dry mix to your wet mix & stir well.
4. Pour your batter into an already greased pan and bake for around 40-48 mins
5. Serve hot.

Nutritional Values

Calories 272kcal, Carbs 30g, Protein 8g, Fat 15g, Sodium 186mg, Potassium 734mg, Chol 0mg

651. PALEO-BLACKBERRY-CASHEW-CHIA PUDDING

- Dessert - Prep time: ready in about: 30 mins, Servings: 4, Grill temp: Medium

Ingredients

- ½ cup of raw cashews
- 1 ½ cups of unsweetened cashew milk
- ½ cup blackberries
- 2 pitted dates
- 1/3 cup of chia seeds
- 1 tsp red-beet-powder
- 1/3 tsp ground cinnamon
- 1 tsp vanilla extract
- Salt
- Cocoa nibs
- - Toasted and unsweetened coconut flakes

Directions

1. Take a blender, add non-dairy milk, chia seeds, cashews, blackberries, vanilla, dates, cinnamon, and some salt to it, and blend well.
2. Divide this pudding mixture among cups and place them in a refrigerator; let them chill for around 4 hours.
3. Before serving, top each with cocoa nibs, coconut flakes, and some beet powder as well, then serve.

Nutritional Values

Calories 222kcal, Carbs 30g, Protein 8g, Fat 15g, Sodium 886mg, Potassium 634mg, Chol 0mg

652. APPLE-OATMEAL-COOKIES

- Dessert - Prep time: ready in about: 27 mins, Servings: 28, Grill temp: Medium

Ingredients

- 1½ cups of oat flour
- 2 tbsp ground flaxseed & 4 tbsp warm water
- 1 tsp baking soda
- ½ tsp sea salt
- 1 tsp cinnamon
- ½ cup of almond butter
- ¼ cup of applesauce
- ¼ cup of coconut oil
- 1 tsp of vanilla extract
- 1 cup rolled oats
- ½ cup brown sugar
- ¾ cup apple, chopped
- ¼ cup of raisins
- ½ cup of chopped walnuts

Directions

1. Preheat your oven to around 350°F. Take a bowl, add oat flour, cinnamon, salt, and baking soda in it, whisk well and fold apples, raisins, walnuts, and rolled oats into it.
2. Take another bowl, add almond butter, applesauce, coconut oil, vanilla, already thickened flaxseed mix, and brown sugar in it; stir to combine well.
3. Then mix the wet mix to your dry mix and mix well. Scoop your mix onto a lined baking sheet & flatten to the shape of cookies.
4. Bake them for around 12-15 mins, then serve by letting them cool for a while.

Nutritional Values

Calories 265kcal, Carbs 14g, Protein 14g, Fat 10g, Sodium 527mg, Potassium 834mg, Chol 0mg

653. JESSICA'S-PISTACHIO-OAT-SQUARES

- Dessert - Prep time: ready in about: 40 mins, Servings: 12, Grill temp: Medium

Ingredients

- 1 cup of rolled oats
- 1 cup of shelled pistachios
- ½ tsp sea salt
- 2 tbsp olive oil

- chopped pistachios, a handful
- ¼ cup of maple syrup
- ⅓ cup of coconut flakes, unsweetened

Directions

1. Preheat your oven to around 350°F.
2. Bring a food processor, put pistachios, maple syrup, oats, salt & some olive oil in it, and blend for around 30 seconds until the required dough-like consistency.
3. Put and flatten your dough smoothly into an already lined baking pan & sprinkle some coconut flakes as well as leftover pistachios on the top.
4. Bake for around 10-12 mins, and slice into squares.
5. Pour some maple syrup on them, if desired, and serve.

Nutritional Values

Calories 155kcal, Carbs 14g, Protein 8g, Fat 10g, Sodium 627mg, Potassium 834mg, Chol 0mg

654. OATMEAL COOKIES

- Dessert - Prep time: ready in about: 30 mins, Servings: 12, Grill temp: Medium

Ingredients

- 1 cup of oat flour
- 2 tbsp ground flaxseed & 5 tbsp warm water
- 1 cup of rolled oats
- zest from a lemon
- ½ cup of almond flour
- ½ tsp of baking powder
- ½ tsp of cinnamon
- ½ tsp of baking soda
- ½ tsp of sea salt
- ¼ cup of coconut oil
- ½ cup almond butter
- ½ cup of maple syrup
- ¾ cup of fresh blueberries
- ⅓ cup of walnuts

Directions

1. Preheat an oven to around 350°F.
2. Take a bowl, add oat flour, rolled oats, lemon zest, almond flour, baking powder, cinnamon, salt & baking soda in it, and stir well.

3. Take another bowl, add almond butter, maple syrup, coconut oil, and thickened flaxseed mixture in it, and stir well.
4. Combine your wet mix to dry mix also, and add blueberries & walnuts to it. Scoop your batter onto a lined baking sheet and flatten it to the shape of cookies.
5. Bake for around 20-24 mins, and enjoy after letting them cool for a while.

Nutritional Values

Calories 155kcal, Carbs 14g, Protein 7.4g, Fat 10g, Sodium 627mg, Potassium 834mg, Chol 0mg

655. VEGAN-ICE CREAM

- Dessert - Prep time: ready in about: 20 mins, Servings: 4, Grill temp: Medium

Ingredients

- ⅓ cup of pure maple syrup
- sesame seeds, chocolate, tart cherries- for topping
- 1 can of coconut milk
- ¼ cup of tahini

Directions

1. Take a bowl, add coconut milk, maple syrup & tahini, and whisk well.
2. Take the ice cream maker, pour your mixture into it & toss until thick for around 20 mins. Scoop it out & enjoy.
3. Before serving, you can also freeze for around 1-2 hours, if desired.

Nutritional Values

Calories 195kcal, Carbs 14g, Protein 18g, Fat 10g, Sodium 827mg, Potassium 834mg, Chol 0mg

656. TAHINI COOKIES

- Dessert - Prep time: ready in about: 25 mins, Servings: 10, Grill temp: Medium

Ingredients

- ½ cup of maple syrup
- ¾ cup of tahini
- ½ tsp vanilla extract
- ½ cup of pomegranate arils
- ½ tsp of cinnamon
- 2 cups of almond flour
- ¼ tsp of ground cardamom

- ½ tsp of baking powder
- ¼ tsp of ground ginger
- ½ tsp of sea salt

Directions

1. Preheat an oven to around 350°F.
2. Take a large bowl, combine tahini, almond extract, maple syrup, almond flour, cardamom, cinnamon, baking powder, salt, and ginger in it; stir well.
3. Then scoop your prepared dough on an already prepared baking sheet and flatten them in the shape of cookies.
4. Top with some pomegranates & bake for around 15-17 mins, then serve.

Nutritional Values

Calories 558 kcal, Carbs 76.3g, Protein 16.2g, Fat 23.5g, Sodium 607mg, Potassium 834mg, Chol 0mg

657. OATMEAL-WITH-PEANUT BUTTER & BANANA RECIPE

- Dessert - Prep time: ready in about: 40 mins, Servings: 4, Grill temp: Medium

Ingredients

- 2 cups of rolled oats
- 4 ½ cups of water
- 2 Tbsp of agave syrup
- Salt
- 2 Tbsp of peanut butter
- 2 sliced bananas
- ¼ cup of chopped almonds

Directions

1. Take a frying pan, add some water and bring it to a boil. Add salt & oatmeal to it and cook for around 5 mins while stirring.
2. Then put bananas, almonds, peanut butter, & agave syrup and whisk well with oatmeal.

Nutritional Values

Calories 320 kcal, Carbs 14g, Protein 16g, Fat 10g, Sodium 227mg, Potassium 334mg, Chol 0mg

658. HONEY PECAN GRANOLA WITH CHERRY RECIPE

- Dessert - Prep time: ready in about: 30 mins, Servings: 12, Grill temp: Medium

Ingredients

- 1 Tbsp of canola oil
- 1/4 cup of honey
- 1 tsp of vanilla extract
- 1/2 tsp of apple spice
- 1 tsp of orange zest
- 1/8 tsp of salt
- 1 cup of rolled oats
- 1 ½ cups of rice cereal
- 1/2 cup of chopped pecans
- 1/2 cup of dried cherries
- 1/4 cup of shredded coconut

Directions

1. Preheat your oven to around 350°F.
2. Take a bowl, add all of your ingredients except cherries, stir well, then layer your cereal batter in an already lined pan.
3. Bake for around 15 mins, then take off from the oven. Top with cherries, and then serve.

Nutritional Values

Calories 136kcal, Carbs 14g, Protein 6g, Fat 6g, Sodium 51mg, Potassium 434mg, Chol 0mg

659. CHOCOLATE-AVOCADO-PUDDING-POPS

- Dessert - Prep time: ready in about: 9 hr & 5 mins, Servings: 10, Grill temp: Medium

Ingredients

- ¼ cup of chocolate chips
- 2 ripe avocados
- 3 tbsp of cacao powder
- 3 tbsp of almond butter
- 3 tbsp of maple syrup
- 1 tsp of vanilla extract
- ¼ tsp of sea salt
- 2 cups of Vanilla Almond milk

Directions

1. Take a blender, add avocado pulp, chocolate chips, maple syrup, cacao powder, almond butter, almond milk, sea salt & vanilla in it, and blend well.
2. Transfer into ice-pop molds & freeze for about overnight and then serve with some delicious topping of your choice over them.

Nutritional Values

Calories 265kcal, Carbs 11g, Protein 7g, Fat 10g, Sodium 621mg, Potassium 834mg, Chol 0mg

660. VEGAN-BUTTERNUT-SQUASH-PUDDING

- Dessert - Prep time: ready in about: 40 mins, Servings: 6, Grill temp: Medium

Ingredients

- olive oil should be extra-virgin
- 1 butternut squash
- ½ cup of coconut cream
- 1 tbsp of coconut oil
- ¼ cup of maple syrup
- 1 tsp vanilla
- ¼ tsp nutmeg
- 1 tsp cinnamon
- ¼ tsp ginger
- 2 - 6 tbsp of almond milk
- ⅛ tsp sea salt

Directions

1. Preheat your oven to around 425°F.
2. Take squash cubes and place them on an already lined baking sheet, and brush with some olive oil. Roast them for around 30-35 mins.
3. Transfer this squash to your blender also, put coconut cream, coconut oil, maple syrup, vanilla, nutmeg, cinnamon, ginger, & salt in it, then blend until your desired consistency. Also, add almond milk, if required. Transfer this mixture to bowls & chill overnight. Later, serve with toppings of your choice.

Nutritional Values

Calories 325kcal, Carbs 14g, Protein 7g, Fat 10g, Sodium 627mg, Potassium 384mg, Chol 0mg

661. RASPBERRY-CHEESECAKE

- Dessert - Prep time: ready in about: 6 hr & 30 mins, Servings: 10, Grill temp: Medium-high

Ingredients

- 3 pitted Medjool dates
- 1 cup of walnuts
- ½ tbsp coconut oil
- 1½ cup cashews
- ¼ tsp sea salt
- ½ cup of coconut milk
- ¼ cup of lemon juice + 1 tbsp zest
- ¼ cup of maple syrup
- 2 tsp vanilla extract
- 1 bag of frozen raspberries
- ½ tsp sea salt
- ½ tsp lemon juice
- 2 tbsp chia seeds
- 2 tbsp maple syrup

Directions

1. Take a food processor, add walnuts, dates, salt & coconut oil to it and mix them well.
2. Transfer your crust material into your already lined pan and freeze it for around 15 mins.
3. Take a blender, put cashews, maple syrup, coconut milk, lemon juice, vanilla, salt, and lemon zest in it, and blend until smooth. Pour this filling over your crust and let it freeze for around 2 hours.
4. Take blender again, add raspberries, maple syrup, lemon juice, & chia seeds and blend well. Layer this mixture over frozen cheesecake, then again freeze for about 4 hours.
5. Before serving, remove your cheesecake from the freezer & slice it into 8-10 slices, then enjoy.

Nutritional Values

Calories 155kcal, Carbs 14g, Protein 16g, Fat 10g, Sodium 627mg, Potassium 544mg, Chol 0mg

662. TART-CHERRY AND MINT-SORBET

- Dessert - Prep time: ready in about: 10 mins, Servings: 2, Grill temp: 0

Ingredients

- ½ cup of maple syrup
- 2 cups of tart cherries, frozen
- ⅛ tsp salt
- 2 tsp of lemon juice
- ¼ cup of coconut milk
- ¼ cup of mint leaves
- ¼ cup of water

Directions

1. Take a blender, add tart cherries, lemon juice, maple syrup, mint, water, salt & coconut milk in it, and blend until smooth.

2. Serve fresh, or you can also chill it by keeping it in the freezer for some hours.

Calories 265kcal, Carbs 11g, Protein 7g, Fat 16g, Sodium 627mg, Potassium 534mg, Chol 0mg

663. PUMPKIN PUDDING

- Dessert - Prep time: ready in about: 5-6 hrs, Servings: 2-4, Grill temp: 0

Ingredients

- ½ cup of coconut solids
- 1 cup of pumpkin puree
- ¼ cup of maple syrup
- 1½ tsp cinnamon
- 2 tbsp almond butter
- 1½ tsp pure vanilla extract
- ½ cup of pecans, crushed & toasted
- ¼ tsp of sea salt
- Coconut-whip

Directions

1. Take a blender, put all of your ingredients except pecans & coconut whip in it, and blend until creamy.
2. Transfer this mixture to a bowl & let it chill for around 4-6 hours.
3. To combine the parfaits, put pecans equally among 4 dishes. Then put pumpkin pudding over it & a scoop of coconut whip in each dish and serve.

Nutritional Values

Calories 375kcal, Carbs 15g, Protein 7g, Fat 17g, Sodium 527mg, Potassium 834mg, Chol 0mg

664. OATMEAL-PANCAKES WITH APPLES-CINNAMON RECIPE

- Dessert - Prep time: ready in about: 45 mins, Servings: 4, Grill temp: Medium

Ingredients

- 3/4 cup of rolled oats
- 1 1/2 cups of buttermilk
- 3/4 cup of wheat flour
- 1 Tbsp of melted butter
- 2 Tbsp of milk
- 1 1/2 tsp of baking powder
- Cinnamon, a pinch
- 1/2 tsp of baking soda
- Nutmeg, a pinch
- 1/2 cup of apple juice
- 1 apple, chopped
- 2 Tbsp of brown sugar
- Confectioners' sugar
- Butter/cooking spray

Directions

1. Take a large bowl, add buttermilk, flour, oats, milk, baking powder, butter, baking soda, cinnamon, and nutmeg in it, and stir well.
2. Take a frying pan, add apple, brown sugar, apple juice, and leftover cinnamon in it, and cook for a while. Preheat your oven to around 200°F.
3. Scoop your batter into an already lined baking dish and flatten it into a circle shape.
4. Bake them for around 2-3 mins, flip and again bake for around 2 mins more.
5. Serve by topping with some sugar or warm apples, if desired.

Nutritional Values

Calories 280 kcal, Carbs 15g, Protein 7g, Fat 6g, Sodium 427mg, Potassium 834mg, Chol 0mg

665. PEACH COBBLER

- Dessert - Prep time: ready in about: 40 mins, Servings: 6, Grill temp: Medium

Ingredients

- 1 ½ tsp lemon juice
- 6 large peaches, sliced
- ¾ cup of flour, all-purpose
- ¼ tsp cinnamon
- ¼ cup of cane sugar
- ¼ tsp baking soda
- ¼ cup of coconut oil
- ice cream- for serving
- ¼ tsp salt
- 1 tsp vanilla extract

Directions

1. Preheat your oven to around 400°F.
2. Place peaches at the bottom of your already lined baking pan. Also, pour some lime juice over them.

3. Take a bowl, add flour, coconut oil, sugar, vanilla, cinnamon, salt, and baking soda in it, and mix well to form your dough.
4. Spread over layered peaches and bake for around 30 mins, then serve with some ice cream.

Nutritional Values

Calories 165kcal, Carbs 14g, Protein 7g, Fat 10g, Sodium 627mg, Potassium 445mg, Chol 0mg

666. SUMMER-STRAWBERRY-CRUMBLE

- Dessert - Prep time: ready in about: 30 mins, Servings: 4, Grill temp: Medium

Ingredients

- ½ tsp balsamic vinegar
- 2½ cups of chopped strawberries
- ⅓ cup of rolled oats
- ¼ cup of almond flour
- ⅓ cup of pistachios
- ¼ cup of coconut sugar, brown
- ⅛ tsp sea salt
- ½ tsp cinnamon
- 1 tbsp of coconut oil
- **For serving ice cream**
- 1 tbsp water

Directions

1. Preheat your oven to around 350°F.
2. Take a food processor, and add oats, coconut oil, pistachios, water, flour, cinnamon, salt, and coconut sugar to it. Blend until crumbly mixture.
3. Take a bowl, mix strawberries and balsamic vinegar in it, then transfer equally to lined small skillets.
4. Top each with prepared crumble and bake for around 15 mins.
5. Serve with the ice cream of your choice.

Nutritional Values

Calories 125kcal, Carbs 14g, Protein 78.g, Fat 10g, Sodium 427mg, Potassium 425mg, Chol 0mg

667. PEACH CRISP

- Dessert - Prep time: ready in about: 25 mins, Servings: 4-6, Grill temp: Medium-low

Ingredients

- 1 tbsp cornstarch
- 5 peaches, sliced
- 1 tbsp cane sugar
- 1 tsp of vanilla extract
- 1 tsp lemon juice
- ice cream- for serving
- ½ cup of almond flour
- ¼ cup of coconut oil
- ½ cup of rolled oats
- ⅓ cup of brown sugar
- ½ tsp cinnamon
- ¼ cup of crushed walnuts
- ¼ tsp sea salt

Directions

1. Preheat an oven to around 400°F.
2. Take a bowl, add peaches, sugar, cornstarch, lemon juice, & vanilla in it, stir well and your peach filling is prepared.
3. Take another bowl, add oats, brown sugar, almond flour, walnuts, salt, cinnamon, and coconut oil in it; mix until crumbly.
4. Put your peach filling into an already lined baking dish. Drizzle with some topping & bake for around 20-30 mins.
5. Serve with any ice cream of your choice.

Nutritional Values

Calories 245kcal, Carbs 18g, Protein 16g, Fat 10g, Sodium 427mg, Potassium 442mg, Chol 0mg

668. BEST-ZUCCHINI-BREAD

- Dessert/Breakfast - Prep time: ready in about: 60 mins, Servings: 16, Grill temp: Medium-high

Ingredients

- 2 cups of flour, all-purpose
- 2 cups of shredded zucchini
- 1 cup of almond flour
- 2 tsp baking powder
- 2 tsp cinnamon
- 1 tsp baking soda
- 4 cups flaxseed egg mixture
- 1 tsp sea salt
- 1 cup of cane sugar
- ½ cup of chocolate chips- optional
- ½ cup of almond milk
- ½ cup of olive oil, extra-virgin
- 2 tsp vanilla extract

Directions

1. Preheat your oven to around 350°F.
2. Take a bowl, and add flour, baking powder, cinnamon, baking soda, and salt. Mix well.
3. Take another bowl, and add your flaxseed egg mix, olive oil, sugar, almond milk, vanilla, and dried zucchini to it.
4. Combine your dry ingredients with wet ingredients and stir well.
5. Pour this batter into your lined pans also, add some chocolate chips on the top, as you want, and let them bake for around 45-50 mins, then serve.

Nutritional Values

Calories 155kcal, Carbs 14g, Protein 17g, Fat 10.1g, Sodium 427mg, Potassium 545mg, Chol 0mg

669. PUMPKIN BARS

- Dessert - Prep time: ready in about: 40 mins, Servings: 16, Grill temp: Medium

Ingredients

- ¼ cup of warm water
- ¼ cup flaxseed
- ¾ cup of flour, all-purpose
- 1 tbsp of pumpkin spice
- ¾ cup of almond flour
- 2 tsp of baking powder
- ½ tsp sea salt
- ½ tsp baking soda
- 1 cup of pumpkin puree
- ⅓ cup of maple syrup
- 2 tbsp coconut oil
- 1 tsp vanilla extract
- Cream-Cheese-Frosting
- chocolate chips- optional

Directions

1. Preheat your oven to around 350°F.
2. Take a bowl, add flours, pie spice, baking powder, salt, and baking soda in it; Stir well.
3. Take another bowl, add pumpkin, maple syrup, coconut oil, already thickened flaxseed mix, and vanilla in i. Mix well.
4. Combine your wet ingredients with dry ingredients mix.

5. Pour into your lined baking dish & bake for around 25-30. Serve with cream cheese frosting over it.

Nutritional Values

Calories 225kcal, Carbs 18g, Protein 10.6g, Fat 10g, Sodium 627mg, Potassium 405mg, Chol 0mg

670. HEALTHY-BANANA-BREAD

- Dessert - Prep time: ready in about: 55 mins, Servings: 8, Grill temp: Medium

Ingredients

- ½ cup of coconut sugar
- 2 bananas, mashed
- ¾ cup of almond milk
- 1 tsp of vanilla extract
- ⅓ cup of olive oil, extra-virgin
- 1 tsp apple-cider-vinegar
- ½ cup of almond flour
- 1½ cups of wheat-pastry-flour
- 2 tsp of baking powder
- 1 ½ tbsp rolled oats
- ½ tsp sea salt
- ¼ tsp baking soda
- ½ tsp cinnamon
- ½ cup walnuts, chopped
- ¼ tsp nutmeg
- 2 tbsp walnuts, additional

Directions

1. Preheat your oven to around 350°F.
2. Take a bowl, and add mashed bananas, sugar, olive oil, almond milk, vanilla, and apple cider vinegar in it. Stir well.
3. Take another bowl, add flour, baking soda, baking powder, salt, nutmeg, and cinnamon in it, and whisk well. Combine your dry ingredients to wet ingredients and stir, also. Add some walnuts.
4. Pour this batter into a lined pan & top with some oats and walnuts. Then, bake for around 42-50 mins, and serve hot.

Nutritional Values

Calories 265kcal, Carbs 12g, Protein 9.10g, Fat 10g, Sodium 647mg, Potassium 345mg, Chol 0mg

671. BLACK RICE PUDDING WITH COCONUT

- Dessert/Breakfast - Prep time: 5 mins, Cook time: 50 mins, Total time: 55 mins, Servings: 6 to 8, Grill temp: 300°F

Ingredients

- 6 ½ cups of water
- 2 cups of black rice
- ¾ cup sugar
- ½ cup of dried flaked coconut
- 2 cinnamon sticks snapped in ½
- 5 crushed cardamom pods
- 3 cloves
- ½ tsp of salt

Directions

1. Rinse the rice and pick out any stones.
2. Pour water into a deep-bottomed pot and add rice and salt.
3. Put the pot on heat and start heating it.
4. Add sugar and stir until it's dissolved and the bottom isn't gritty.
5. Wrap whole spices in a cheesecloth bag, tie them up, and put them in the pot.
6. Close and seal the lid.
7. Cook for about 40 mins on high pressure.
8. When time is up, let the pressure come down naturally.
9. Open the pot to stir the rice around.
10. Add coconut and turn your pot back to sauté until the rice liquid has become thick and syrupy.
11. When the consistency is the way you want it, take out the spice bag.
12. Serve warm or chill before eating.

Nutritional Values

Calories 135, Fat 3.2g, Chol 0mg, Sodium 71.4mg, Potassium 67.7mg, Carbs 26g, Protein 3.4g

672. BUCKWHEAT APPLE COBBLER

- Desserts - Prep time: 5 mins, Cook time: 15 mins, Total time: 20 mins, Servings: 4 to 6, Grill temp: 300°F

Ingredients

- 3 pounds of chopped apples
- 2 ½ cups of water
- ½ cup of chopped Medjool dates
- ½ cup of dry buckwheat
- 2 tsps of cinnamon

- ¼ tsp of ground nutmeg
- ¼ tsp of ground ginger

Directions

1. Mix everything in a deep-bottomed pot.
2. Cook for 12 mins on high pressure.
3. Turn down the heat and let it stand for some time.
4. Serve right away!

Nutritional Values

Calories 197, Fat 1g, Chol 0mg, Sodium 71.4mg, Potassium 67.7mg, Carbs 47g, Protein 3g

673. CHOCOLATE CHEESECAKE

- Desserts - Prep time: 5 mins, Cook time: 55 mins, Total time: 60 mins, Servings: 6 to 8, Grill temp: 300°F

Ingredients

- 1 ½ cups of almond flour
- ½ cup of sugar
- ¼ cup of melted coconut oil
- 1 ½ cups of soaked and drained cashews
- 1 cup of chocolate almond milk
- ⅔ cup of sugar
- ¼ cup of vegan chocolate chips
- 2 tbsp of coconut flour
- 2 tsps of vanilla
- ½ tsp of salt

Directions

1. Mix the ingredients in the first list together.
2. Press crust into the bottom of a 7-inch springform pan and 1-inch up the sides.
3. Put it in the fridge while you make the filling.
4. Mix the second ingredient list together-minus chocolate chips and flour in a food processor until smooth. Add coconut flour and mix. Add chocolate chips and mix with a spatula until evenly incorporated. Pour batter into the crust.
5. Pour 1 1/3 cups of water into your cooker and lower in the steamer basket or trivet.
6. Put the pan into the cooker and close and seal the lid.
7. Cook on high pressure for 55 mins.
8. Turn down the flame and wait for 10 mins before quick releasing pressure.

9. Carefully remove the pan and cool for 1 hour.
10. Cover the cheesecake and freeze for 4 hours before moving it to the fridge or serving.

Calories 493, Fat 29g, Chol 0mg, Sodium 71.4mg, Potassium 67.7mg, Carbs 42g, Protein 10g

674. CHOCOLATE FONDUE WITH COCONUT CREAM

- Desserts - Prep time: 5 mins, Cook time: 5 mins, Total time: 10 mins, Servings: 2 to 4, Grill temp: 300°F

Ingredients

- 2 cups of water
- 3 ½ ounces of 70% dark bittersweet chocolate
- 3 ½ ounces of coconut cream
- 1 tsp of sugar

Directions

1. Pour 2 cups of water into your pressure cooker and lower in a trivet.
2. In a heatproof bowl, add chocolate chunks.
3. Add coconut cream and sugar.
4. Put the bowl on top of the trivet.
5. Close and seal the lid.
6. Cook on high pressure for 2 mins.
7. Turn down the heat and let it stand for some time.
8. Carefully remove the bowl and whisk with a fork until it becomes smooth.
9. Serve!

Nutritional Values

Calories 216, Fat 20.3g, Chol 0mg, Sodium 71.4mg, Potassium 67.7mg, Carbs 11.7g, Protein 1.8g

675. CINNAMON-POACHED PEARS WITH CHOCOLATE SAUCE

- Desserts - Prep time: 5 mins, Cook time: 5 mins, Total time: 10 mins, Servings: 6, Grill temp: 300°F

Ingredients

- 6 ripe, firm pears
- 6 cinnamon sticks
- 3 cups of water
- 2 cups of sugar
- 2 cups of white wine
- 1 halved lemon
- 9 ounces of chopped bittersweet chocolate
- ½ cup of coconut milk
- ¼ cup of coconut oil
- 2 tbsp of maple syrup

Directions

1. Pour water, wine, sugar, and cinnamon into the deep-bottomed pot.
2. Stir until the sugar dissolves.
3. Peel pears, keeping the stems. Rub with the cut lemon.
4. Squeeze the juice into the pot and drop in the lemon.
5. Put pears in the pot. Close and seal the lid.
6. Cook for 3 mins on high pressure.
7. Turn down the heat and then quick-release pressure.
8. Take out the pears and let them cool before pouring on pressure cooker syrup.
9. For the chocolate sauce, put chocolate in a bowl. Heat coconut oil, coconut milk, and syrup in a saucepan until it just begins to boil.
10. Pour over chocolate and stir until smooth. 15. Pour over the pears.

Nutritional Values

Calories 210, Fat 2.8g, Chol 0mg, Sodium 71.4mg, Potassium 67.7mg, Carbs 50g, Protein 2.8g

676. ORANGE-GLAZED POACHED PEARS

- Desserts - Prep time: 5 mins, Cook time: 12 mins, Total time: 30 mins, Servings: 4, Grill temp: 300°F

Ingredients

- 4 ripe pears
- 1 cup of orange juice
- ⅓ cup of sugar
- 1 cinnamon stick
- 2 tsps of cinnamon
- 1 tsp nutmeg
- 1 tsp of ginger
- 1 tsp of ground clove

Directions

1. Peel the pears, leaving the stem alone.
2. Pour 1 cup of orange juice into a pot and add spices.
3. Arrange pears in the steamer basket and lower them into the pot.
4. Close and seal the lid.
5. Turn down the heat and cook for 7 mins on high pressure.
6. Turn down the heat and wait for 5 mins.
7. Carefully remove the trivet and pears.
8. Pick out the cinnamon stick.
9. Turn your pot to sauté and add sugar.
10. Stir until the liquid has reduced to a sauce.
11. Serve pears with sauce poured on top.

Nutritional Values

Calories 188, Fat 0g, Chol 0mg, Sodium 71.4mg, Potassium 67.7mg, Carbs 49g, Protein 1g

677. PINEAPPLE UPSIDE-DOWN CAKE

- Desserts - Prep time: 10 mins, Cook time: 25 mins, Total time: 35 mins, Servings: 6, Grill temp: 300°F

Ingredients

- 1 and ⅓ cups of whole-wheat flour
- 4 pineapple rings
- ⅓ cup of rapeseed oil
- ⅓ cup of unsweetened almond milk
- ¾ cup plus ¼ cup of white sugar
- 3 ½ cups of vegan butter
- 1 tsp of pure vanilla
- 1 tsp of apple cider vinegar
- ½ tsp of baking powder
- ¾ tsp of baking soda
- ¼ tsp of salt
- Pieces of fresh strawberry

Directions

1. Mix ¼ cup of sugar and butter together.
2. Spread on the bottom of your cooker-safe cake dish and up the sides, too.
3. Lay down pineapple slices in the dish.
4. Add in some pieces of strawberry.
5. In a bowl, mix flour, baking soda, baking powder, and salt.
6. Mix milk and apple cider vinegar together.
7. Into that mixture, add rapeseed oil, vanilla, and the rest of the sugar.

8. Mix wet into dry until just combined.
9. Pour the batter into your dish and cover with foil.
10. Pour 1 cup of water into a pressure cooker and lower in a trivet.
11. Set dish on trivet, and seal the lid.
12. Cook for 22 mins on high pressure.
13. Turn down the heat and wait for about 10 mins,
14. Unwrap the dish and let it cool for 30 mins before inverting.
15. Cool another 10 mins before slicing!

Nutritional Values

Calories 342, Fat 18g, Chol 0mg, Sodium 71.4mg, Potassium 67.7mg, Carbs 44g, Protein 4g

678. PUMPKIN-SPICE BROWN RICE PUDDING WITH DATES

- Desserts - Prep time: 10 mins, Cook time: 15 mins, Total time: 25 mins, Servings: 6, Grill temp: 300°F

Ingredients

- 3 cups of almond milk
- 1 cup of pumpkin puree
- 1 cup of brown rice
- 1 stick of cinnamon
- ½ cup of maple syrup
- ½ cup of water
- ½ cup of chopped pitted dates
- 1 tsp of vanilla extract
- 1 tsp of pumpkin spice
- ⅛ tsp of salt

Directions

1. Pour boiling water over your rice and wait at least 10 mins. Rinse.
2. Pour milk and water into a deep bottom med-pot.
3. Turn on the heat and when boiling, add rice, cinnamon, salt, and dates.
4. Close and seal the lid.
5. Cook on high pressure for 10 mins.
6. Wait for the pressure to descend naturally.
7. Add pumpkin puree, maple syrup, and pumpkin spice.
8. Stir for 3-5 mins, until thick. Turn off the heat.

9. Pick out the cinnamon stick and add vanilla.
10. Move pudding to a bowl and cover in plastic wrap so the plastic touches the top.
11. Wait 30 mins to cool.
12. Serve warm or chilled.

Calories 193, Fat 3g, Chol 0mg, Sodium 71.4mg, Potassium 67.7mg, Carbs 38g, Protein 1g

679. STUFFED PEARS WITH SALTED CARAMEL SAUCE

- Desserts - Prep time: 10 mins, Cook time: 20 mins, Total time: 30 mins, Servings: 4, Grill temp: 300°F

Ingredients

- 2 ripe, firm pears
- ½ cup of water plus 2 tbsp
- ¼ cup of raisins
- ¼ cup of rolled oats
- ¼ cup of walnuts
- ¼ cup of sugar
- 3 tbsp of vegan butter
- 1 tsp of vanilla extract
- ½ tsp of cinnamon
- ¼ tsp of sea salt

Directions

1. Cut pears in ½ and spoon out a well in the center.
2. Mix 1 tbsp of butter with oats, raisins, walnuts, vanilla, and cinnamon in your food processor.
3. When the mixture is like a crumble, stuff the pears.
4. Pour 2 tbsp of water and sugar into a pot.
5. Cook until the water has become dark amber.
6. Pour in the rest of the water.
7. Pour pears into the pot.
8. Cook for 9 mins on low pressure.
9. Turn down the heat and wait for 10 mins.
10. Turn the pot back to heat after removing the pears and reduce for 10 mins.
11. Whisk in 2 tbsp of butter and ¼ tsp salt.
12. Serve pears with caramel sauce on top.

Nutritional Values

Calories 244, Fat 12g, Chol 0mg, Sodium 71.4mg, Potassium 67.7mg, Carbs 35g, Protein 2g

680. TAPIOCA PUDDING

- Desserts/Breakfast - Prep time: 10 mins, Cook time: 10 mins, Total time: 20 mins, Servings: 4 to 6, Grill temp: 300°F

Ingredients

- 1 and ¼ cups of almond milk
- ½ cup of water
- ⅓ cup of sugar
- ½ split of vanilla bean
- ⅓ cup of seed tapioca pearls

Directions

1. Pour 1 cup of water into a deep-bottomed pot.
2. Rinse tapioca pearls.
3. In a 4l bowl- safe for a pressure cooker, add tapioca, water, milk, sugar, and vanilla and mix.
4. When the sugar has dissolved, lower it into a steamer basket and then into a cooker.
5. Cook on high pressure for 8 mins.
6. Turn down the heat and wait for the pressure to come down on its own.
7. When pressure is released, wait 5 mins before opening the lid. Stir.
8. Serve warm or cool in a fridge- covered with cling wrap for at least 3 hours.

Nutritional Values

Calories 187, Fat 2.5g, Chol 0mg, Sodium 71.4mg, Potassium 67.7mg, Carbs 39.6g, Protein 2.5g

681. VEGAN CHEESECAKE WITH RASPBERRIES

- Desserts - Prep time: 15 mins, Cook time: 10 mins, Total time: 25 mins, Servings: 6, Grill temp: 300°F

Ingredients

Crust
- 1 ½ cups of almonds
- ½ cup of soaked dates

Filling
- 1 ½ cups of soaked cashews
- ½ cup of firm silken tofu

- ¼ cup of pure maple syrup
- ¼ cup of unsweetened almond milk
- ½ lemon's worth of zest and juice
- 1 tsp of pure vanilla
- Pinch of salt
- Fresh raspberries

Directions

1. Grease 6 ramekins with a coconut oil-based spray.
2. To make the crust, pulse almonds until you get a crumb texture.
3. Add dates and pulse until sticky and together.
4. Press crust down into your ramekins and up the sides a little.
5. Stick in the fridge for now.
6. To make the filling, add the rest of the ingredients to a blender and pulse until smooth.
7. Divide among the ramekins and cover with foil.
8. Pour 1 ½ cups of water into a pressure cooker and add the trivet.
9. Set as many ramekins that fit on the trivet, and seal the lid.
10. Cook for just 4 mins.
11. Turn down the heat and wait 10 mins.
12. Repeat with any remaining ramekins.
13. Garnish with raspberries, and enjoy!

Nutritional Values

Calories 429, Fat 32g, Chol 0mg, Sodium 71.4mg, Potassium 67.7mg, Carbs 34g, Protein 13g

Chapter 18.

Staples & Seasonings

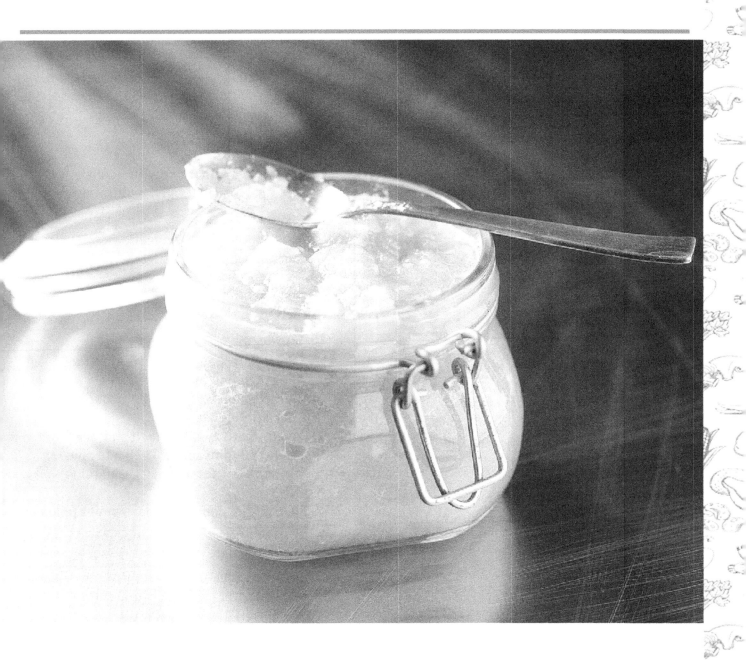

682. HONEY BUTTER

- Staple - Prep time: ready in about: 5 mins, Servings: 12, Grill temp: 0

Ingredients

- 3 tbsp honey
- ½ cup of unsalted butter
- ¾ tsp sea salt

Directions

1. Take a bowl, add honey, salt, and softened butter together and stir well.
2. Serve it with any bread or other snacks.

Nutritional Values

Calories 165kcal, Carbs 14g, Protein 7g, Fat 10g, Sodium 627mg, Potassium 445mg, Chol 0mg

683. APPLE-PIE-SPICE

- Staple - Prep time: ready in about: 5 mins, Servings: 8, Grill temp: 0

Ingredients

- 1 tsp ground ginger
- ½ tsp cardamom
- ¼ cup of cinnamon
- ½ tsp nutmeg

Directions

1. Take a bowl, add ginger, cinnamon, nutmeg, and cardamom. Stir well.

Nutritional Values

Calories 155kcal, Carbs 14g, Protein 17g, Fat 10.1g, Sodium 427mg, Potassium 545mg, Chol 0mg

684. CHILI POWDER

- Staple - Prep time: ready in about: 10 mins, Servings: 12, Grill temp: 0

Ingredients

- 3 tsp cumin seeds
- 6 dried chilies
- 1½ tsp of coriander seeds
- 1½ tsp garlic granules
- ¾ tsp fennel seeds
- ⅛ tsp sugar
- 1½ tsp of smoked paprika
- ¼ tsp all-spice
- ¾ tsp oregano

- ¼ tsp sea salt

Directions

1. Toast your chilies in a frying pan over low flame with coriander, fennel seeds, and cumin for around 30 seconds of time.
2. Cut them into pieces of small size, then transfer them to a grinder.
3. Put coriander seeds, cumin seeds, fennel seeds, paprika, garlic, oregano, salt, allspice & sugar.
4. Grind well until it becomes powdered form.

Nutritional Values

Calories 265kcal, Carbs 12g, Protein 9.10g, Fat 10g, Sodium 647mg, Potassium 345mg, Chol 0mg

685. HOMEMADE APPLESAUCE

- Staple - Prep time: ready in about: 45 mins, Servings: 8, Grill temp: Medium-low

Ingredients

- 2 tbsp apple-cider-vinegar
- 4 lb. apples, chopped
- ⅓ cup of water
- 1 tsp apple-pie-spice
- sea salt

Directions

1. Take a saucepan, and add apple cider vinegar, water, and apples to it.
2. Let it cook on low flame for around 4 mins while stirring well.
3. Cover it with a lid and let it simmer for around 10 mins more. Then add spice & salt, and cook for around 10-20 mins, again.
4. Turn off the flame and mash your apples to the required consistency.

Nutritional Values

Calories 195kcal, Carbs 14g, Protein 16g, Fat 12g, Sodium 547mg, Potassium 440mg, Chol 0mg

686. CHIPOTLE-RANCH-DRESSING

- Staple - Prep time: ready in about: 10 mins, Servings: 4, Grill temp: 0

Ingredients

- ¼ cup of mayonnaise

- ½ cup of Milk-Greek-yogurt
- 1 chipotle-pepper
- ½ tsp garlic powder
- 1 tsp apple-cider-vinegar
- ½ tsp onion powder
- ¼ tsp sea salt
- ½ tsp dried dill

Directions

1. Take a food processor, place all of your ingredients in it and blend well.

Nutritional Values

Calories 212kcal, Carbs 14g, Protein 14.2g, Fat 10g, Sodium 637mg, Potassium 425mg, Chol 0mg

687. OAT MILK

- Staple - Prep time: ready in about: 5 mins, Servings: 4, Grill temp: 0

Ingredients

- 3 cups of water
- ½ cup of rolled oats
- 2 tsp maple syrup
- ⅛ tsp sea salt
- ½ tsp vanilla extract

Directions

1. Take a blender, add all of your ingredients to it, and blend them for around 30 seconds.
2. Strain your milk without having any pulp remains as it'll give a creamy texture.
3. Add maple syrup for more taste, chill overnight and serve.

Nutritional Values

Calories 465kcal, Carbs 14g, Protein 19g, Fat 10g, Sodium 4327mg, Potassium 445mg, Chol 0mg

688. LENTILS

- Staple - Prep time: ready in about: 25 mins, Servings: 4-6, Grill temp: Low

Ingredients

- Water, a pot
- 1 cup of black lentils
- 3 tbsp lemon juice
- 1 tsp sea salt
- 1 tbsp olive oil, extra-virgin
- ¼ tsp Dijon mustard

- ½ cup of chopped parsley
- black pepper, ground
- red pepper flakes- optional

Directions

1. Take a medium frying pan, add lentils and water to it, bring it to a boil, and cook for around 20 mins, then drain and let them cool. You can use them in any of your recipes that include cooked lentils.
2. Transfer your cooked lentils to a bowl.
3. Combine olive oil, lemon juice, salt, red pepper flakes, mustard, parsley & pepper, stir them well to prepare your Lime-Herb dressing & serve with lentils.

Nutritional Values

Calories 365kcal, Carbs 10g, Protein 23g, Fat 10g, Sodium 427mg, Potassium 445mg, Chol 0mg

689. CASHEW CREAM

- Staple - Prep time: ready in about: 5 mins, Servings: 12, Grill temp: 0

Ingredients

- ½ cup of water
- 1 cup cashews
- 2 tbsp olive oil, extra-virgin
- 1 clove of garlic
- 2 tbsp lemon juice
- ½ tsp sea salt

Directions

1. Put all of the ingredients in a blender & blend them well until fully creamy.

Nutritional Values

Calories 158kcal, Carbs 12g, Protein 44g, Fat 10g, Sodium 427mg, Potassium 245mg, Chol 0mg

690. CHEESE SAUCE

- Staple - Prep time: ready in about: 15 mins, Servings: 4, Grill temp: Low

Ingredients

- ¾ cup of sweet potato
- ¾ cup of gold potato
- 2 cloves of garlic
- 1 tbsp apple-cider-vinegar
- ¼ cup of raw cashews

- 2 tbsp yeast
- ¼ cup of water
- ½ tsp sea salt
- ½ tsp onion powder
- ¼ cup of olive oil

Directions

1. Place potatoes in a frying pan, add salt and water to it and bring it to boil on low flame for around 8-12 mins.
2. Drain, then put it in a blender with all of the remaining ingredients and blend well. Serve with any snacks or over any pasta to enjoy food.

Nutritional Values

Calories 212kcal, Carbs 14g, Protein 18.25g, Fat 10g, Sodium 627mg, Potassium 435mg, Chol 0mg

691. PICO-DE-GALLO

- Staple - Prep time: ready in about: 10 mins, Servings: 6-8, Grill temp: 0

Ingredients

- ¾ cup of white onion
- 2 cups of tomato
- ½ cup cilantro
- 2 cloves of garlic
- ½ tsp sea salt
- ¼ cup of lime juice
- 1 jalapeño-pepper, diced well

Directions

1. Take a bowl, add all of the ingredients in it and stir well. Chill for some time.
2. Serve with any snacks & enjoy your food.

Nutritional Values

Calories 265kcal, Carbs 14g, Protein 18g, Fat 10g, Sodium 627mg, Potassium 245mg, Chol 0mg

692. ALMOND FLOUR

- Staple - Prep time: ready in about: 5 mins, Servings: 6, Grill temp: 0

Ingredients

- 1 ½ cups of slivered almonds

Directions

1. Put almonds in a blender and blend them well until smooth, for around 10 seconds.

2. Stir to avoid any almond pieces or large. Also, avoid over-blending. Otherwise, almonds will begin turning into a buttery consistency.
3. Later on, use it in any of your recipes that ask for almond meals or flour.

Nutritional Values

Calories 272kcal, Carbs 30g, Protein 8g, Fat 15g, Sodium 886mg, Potassium 734mg, Chol 0mg

693. CREAMY-CHIPOTLE-SAUCE

- Staple - Prep time: ready in about: 5 mins, Servings: 4, Grill temp: 0

Ingredients

- 1 chipotle-pepper
- ¾ cup of vegan mayo
- 1 clove of garlic
- 1 tsp olive oil, extra-virgin
- Sea salt & black pepper
- 1 tsp lime juice
- 1 tsp honey

Directions

1. Take a food processor, put all of your ingredients in it and blend well. Season with some extra pepper and salt, if required.

Nutritional Values

Calories 272kcal, Carbs 30.2g, Protein 8g, Fat 15g, Sodium 886mg, Potassium 714mg, Chol 0mg

694. OAT FLOUR

- Staple - Prep time: ready in about: 2 mins, Servings: 4, Grill temp: 0

Ingredients

- 2 cups of rolled oats

Directions

1. Take oats, put them in a food processor and blend for around 10 secs or until you will get a smooth flour.
2. Stir to avoid any lumps. Adopt any of your recipes that ask for oatmeal or flour.
3. Secure by using a container that should be airtight to avoid dampness.

Nutritional Values

Calories 262kcal, Carbs 20g, Protein 8g, Fat 15g, Sodium 886mg, Potassium 934mg, Chol 0mg

695. VEGAN MAYO

- Staple - Prep time: ready in about: 5 mins, Servings: 1 cup, Grill temp: 0

Ingredients

- 2 tsp of lemon juice
- ¼ cup of chickpea liquid
- ½ tsp Dijon mustard
- ½ tsp of sea salt
- ½ tsp cane sugar
- ¾ cup of sunflower oil

Directions

1. Take a blender, put all of your ingredients in it except sunflower oil and blend well. With the running blender, slowly pour in your sunflower oil & blend until saucy.

Nutritional Values

Calories 272kcal, Carbs 30g, Protein 8.4g, Fat 15g, Sodium 886mg, Potassium 634mg, Chol 0mg

696. RADISH-GREENS-PESTO

- Staple - Prep time: ready in about: 5 mins, Servings: 8, Grill temp: 0

Ingredients

- 1 garlic clove
- ½ cup of pine nuts
- ¼ tsp sea salt
- 2 tbsp lemon juice
- black pepper
- 1 cup of radish greens
- ¼ - 1/3 cup of olive oil, extra-virgin
- 1 cup of basil
- ¼ cup of Parmesan cheese

Directions

1. Take a food processor, garlic, pine nuts, salt, lemon juice, and pepper in it, and blend for a while.
2. Put basil, and radish greens, then blend again. While the blade is running, pour some olive oil in it also, add Parmesan cheese, and pulse again.
3. For a smooth consistency, put in some extra olive oil.

Nutritional Values

Calories 472kcal, Carbs 30g, Protein 8g, Fat 15.5g, Sodium 886mg, Potassium 734mg, Chol 0mg

697. EASY-VEGAN-CHILI

- Staple - Prep time: ready in about: 45 mins, Servings: 6-8, Grill temp: Low

Ingredients

- 1 yellow onion
- 2 tbsp olive oil, extra-virgin
- 2 cloves of garlic
- 1 can of roasted tomatoes
- 1 bell pepper- diced
- 1 can of red beans
- 1 cup of water
- 1 can of pinto beans
- 3 chipotle-peppers
- ½ tsp sea salt
- 1 tbsp lime juice
- 1 cup of corn kernels
- black pepper

Directions

1. Take a pan, add oil to it, and heat over medium flame.
2. Add pepper, salt and onion, stir and cook for around 5 mins.
3. Later put red pepper and garlic in it, stir and cook for around another 5-8 mins. Then add beans, tomatoes, water, adobo sauce, chipotle, corn, pepper, and some salt.
4. Cover and let it simmer for around 25 mins, on low flame, while stirring, until the consistency has thickened.
5. Also, add lime juice and some seasoning to it before serving any food.

Nutritional Values

Calories 222kcal, Carbs 30g, Protein 8g, Fat 15g, Sodium 886mg, Potassium 734mg, Chol 0mg

698. RANCH DRESSING

- Staple - Prep time: ready in about: 10 mins, Servings: 6, Grill temp: 0

Ingredients

- ½ cup of water
- 1 cup of cashews

- ⅓ cup of cucumber
- 1 tbsp yeast
- 2 tbsp of lemon juice
- ½ tsp garlic powder
- ½ tsp sea salt
- Chives
- ½ tsp of onion powder
- ¼ tsp dried dill

Directions

1. Bring a blender, put all of your ingredients in it except chives and blend them well until smooth.
2. Sprinkle with some extra salt if required. Also, add fresh chives, then serve.

Nutritional Values

Calories 272kcal, Carbs 30g, Protein 9.8g, Fat 15g, Sodium 886mg, Potassium 734mg, Chol 0mg

699. BEST HUMMUS

- Staple - Prep time: ready in about: 5 mins, Servings: 8, Grill temp: 0

Ingredients

- ⅓ cup of smooth tahini
- 1½ cups of cooked chickpeas
- 2 tbsp of olive oil, extra-virgin
- 1 clove of garlic
- 2 tbsp lemon juice
- ½ tsp of sea salt
- paprika, parsley, or red pepper flakes- used for garnishing
- 5 tbsp water

Directions

1. Take a blender, add tahini, chickpeas, olive oil, garlic, salt & lemon juice in it and blend well while adding water in batches to attain your required consistency.
2. Transfer it to your plate, garnish as you want, then serve with some warm food.

Nutritional Values

Calories 292kcal, Carbs 30g, Protein 8g, Fat 15g, Sodium 786mg, Potassium 734mg, Chol 0mg

Chapter 19.

Sauces, Dressing & Dips

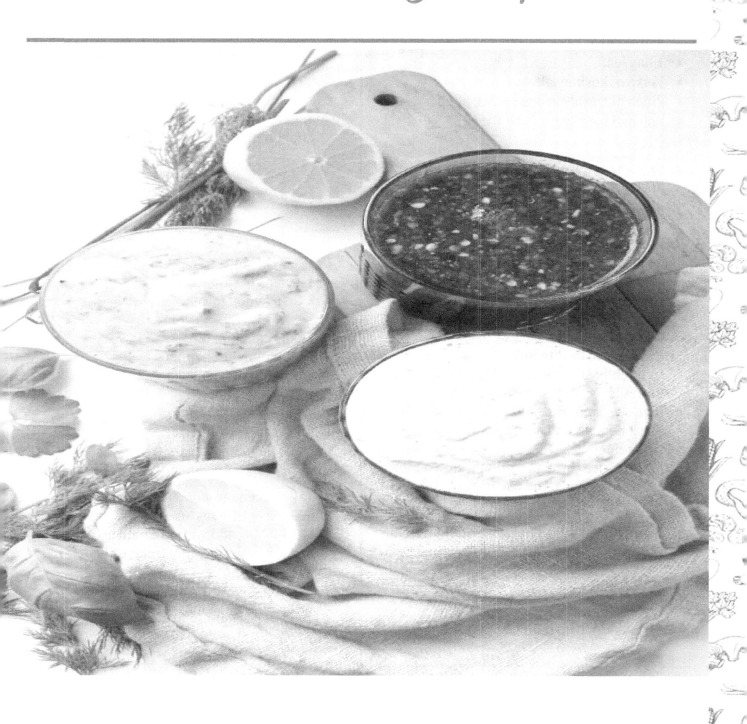

700. BÉCHAMEL SAUCE

- Sides - Prep time: 5 mins, Cook time: 15 mins, Total time: 20 mins, Servings: 2 cups, Grill temp: 300°F

Ingredients

- ¼ cup of grapeseed oil
- 3 tbsp of all-purpose flour
- 2 ½ cups of unflavored non-dairy milk, preferably soy or rice
- ¼ small yellow onion, studded with 1 whole clove
- 1 bay leaf
- ¼ tsp of kosher salt
- Pinch of freshly ground black pepper
- Pinch of freshly grated nutmeg

Directions

1. In a small saucepan over medium-high heat, heat grapeseed oil. Add all-purpose flour all at once, and stir vigorously with a whisk.
2. When the flour mixture is golden and begins to smell nutty- but before it browns about 2 mins, add non-dairy milk, continuing to whisk vigorously to prevent lumps.
3. Add clove-studded yellow onion and bay leaf, reduce heat to low, and cook, frequently stirring, for about 10 mins or until sauce is thickened.
4. Remove from heat, and stir in kosher salt, black pepper, and nutmeg. Taste and adjust seasonings.
5. Strain sauce through a fine-mesh strainer to remove solids, and use immediately.

Nutritional Values

Calories 73, Fat 1.8g, Chol 0mg, Sodium 64mg, Potassium 72mg, Carbs 12g, Protein 2.3g

701. WHITE-BEAN-DIP

- Staple - Prep time: ready in about: 5 mins, Servings: 4, Grill temp: 0

Ingredients

- 2 tbsp olive oil
- 1 ½ cups of cooked beans
- 2 tbsp lemon juice
- 1 garlic clove

- ½ tsp lemon zest
- ½ tsp sea salt
- 2 - 4 tbsp water
- 2 tsp rosemary leaves
- black pepper
- 2 tbsp basil leaves

Directions

1. Bring your food processor, add all of your ingredients in it except fresh herbs and blend them well while adding water in batches as per desired consistency.
2. Then add in fresh herbs, if required, and serve this dip with any food of your choice.

Nutritional Values

Calories 272kcal, Carbs 30g, Protein 10g, Fat 15g, Sodium 886mg, Potassium 734mg, Chol 0mg

702. VEGAN-PIMENTO-CHEESE-DIP

- Staple - Prep time: ready in about: 5 mins, Servings: 2 cups, Grill temp: 0

Ingredients

- ½ cup of water
- 1½ cups of raw cashews
- 3 tbsp lemon juice
- 1 tsp sriracha
- 2 tsp Dijon mustard
- 2 tbsp pimento peppers
- ½ tsp smoked paprika
- 1 clove of garlic
- ½ tsp salt
- 1 tsp chives- for garnish
- black pepper

Directions

1. Take a blender, put all of your ingredients in it except chives and blend them well.
2. Meanwhile, add water in batches according to your desired consistency. Chill before use.
3. Garnish your dip with sliced chives and serve with any food of your desire for dipping.

Nutritional Values

Calories 272kcal, Carbs 33g, Protein 8g, Fat 15g, Sodium 686mg, Potassium 734mg, Chol 0m

703. CARROT-TOMATO SAUCE

- Sides - Prep time: 5 mins, Cook time: 15 mins, Total time: 20 mins, Servings: 3 cups, Grill temp: 300°F

Ingredients

- 10 medium-sized, quartered tomatoes
- 8 medium-sized, diced carrots
- 8 minced garlic cloves
- ½ chopped white onion
- ½ cup of soaked cashews
- ¼ cup of water
- 1 tbsp of olive oil

Directions

1. Heat oil in a deep-bottomed saucepan and add garlic.
2. When fragrant, add onions and stir for 1-2 mins. Add carrots and tomatoes. Cook for another few mins. Pour in water and stir.
3. Close and seal the lid.
4. Cook on low pressure for 15 mins.
5. Turn down the heat and let it stand for some time.
6. Move to a blender and puree.
7. Pour the sauce back into the saucepan, leaving 1 cup in the blender.
8. Add your soaked cashews to the blender and puree.
9. Pour back into the pot and simmer without the lid for 10 mins, until thickened.
10. Season to taste.

Nutritional Values

Calories 284, Fat 14g, Chol 0mg, Sodium 71.4mg, Potassium 67.7mg, Carbs 35g, Protein 10g

704. CASHEW RICOTTA

- Sides - Prep time: 15 mins, Cook time: 0 mins, Total time: 15 mins, Servings: 2 cups, Grill temp: 300°F

Ingredients

- 2 cups of raw cashews
- ¼ cup of extra-virgin olive oil
- ¼ cup of warm water
- Juice of 1 ½ medium lemons
- 2 tbsp of nutritional yeast
- 1 tbsp of finely chopped fresh parsley
- 1 tbsp of finely chopped chives
- 1 tsp of white- Shiro miso
- ½ tsp of dried marjoram
- ½ tsp of kosher salt
- ½ tsp of freshly ground black pepper

Directions

1. Soak cashews in water overnight.
2. Discard soaking water, rinse cashews well, and drain.
3. In a food processor fitted with a metal blade, process cashews, extra-virgin olive oil, warm water, lemon juice, nutritional yeast, parsley, chives, white- Shiro miso, marjoram, kosher salt, and black pepper until smooth, scraping down the bowl several times with a spatula.
4. Use immediately, or store in the refrigerator for up to 5 days.

Nutritional Values

Calories 51, Fat 2g, Chol 0mg, Sodium 66mg, Potassium 42.7mg, Carbs 8g, Protein 0.3g

705. ENDO GUACAMOLE

- Prep time: 8 mins, Cook time: 0 mins, Total time: 8 mins, Servings: 2 cups, Grill temp: 0

Ingredients

- 2 ripe avocados (peeled)
- 1 garlic clove (minced)
- 1/3 medium cucumber (chopped)
- 1/3 medium red onion (chopped)
- 1 tbsp of lemon juice
- 1 tsp of cumin powder
- ½ tsp of salt
- Pepper to taste
- 1 tsp of chili flakes (optional)

Directions

1. Add all the ingredients to the blender and blend until it has reached a smooth consistency.
2. Serve chilled, and enjoy!

Nutritional Values

Calories 76, Carbs 4.70g, Fat 6.70g, Protein 1.00g

706. FAVA BEAN DIP

- Sides - Prep time: 5 mins, Cook time: 15 mins, Total time: 20 mins, Servings: 1 ½ cups, Grill temp: 300°F

Ingredients

- 3 cups of water
- 2 cups of soaked split fava beans
- 2 crushed garlic cloves
- 2 tbsp of vegetable oil
- 1 tbsp of olive oil
- 1 zested and juiced lemon
- 2 tsps of tahini
- 2 tsps of cumin
- 1 tsp of harissa
- 1 tsp of paprika
- Salt to taste

Directions

1. The night before, soak the fava beans and drain fava beans before beginning the recipe.
2. Heat oil in a deep-bottomed pot.
3. Add garlic when hot and cook until they become golden.
4. Add beans, veggie oil, and 3 cups of water.
5. Close and seal the lid.
6. Cook on high pressure for 12 mins.
7. Turn down the heat and wait 10 mins.
8. Drain the cooking liquid from the pot, leaving about 1 cup.
9. Toss in the tahini, cumin, harissa, and lemon zest.
10. Puree until smooth. Add the salt and blend again.
11. Serve with a drizzle of olive oil and a dash of paprika.

Nutritional Values

Calories 415, Fat 26g, Chol 0mg, Sodium 71.4mg, Potassium 67.7mg, Carbs 31g, Protein 15g

707. HOMEMADE KETCHUP

- Sides - Prep time: 5 mins, Cook time: 15 mins, Total time: 20 mins, Servings: 3 cups, Grill temp: 300°F

Ingredients

- 2 pounds of quartered plum tomatoes
- 1 tbsp of paprika
- 1 tbsp of agave syrup
- 1 tsp of salt
- 6 tbsp of apple cider vinegar
- ⅓ cup of raisins
- ⅛ wedged onion
- ½ tsp of Dijon mustard
- ¼ tsp of celery seeds
- ⅛ tsp of garlic powder
- ⅛ tsp of ground clove
- ⅛ tsp of cinnamon

Directions

1. Put everything in a deep-bottomed pot.
2. Mash down so the tomatoes release their juice, making sure you hit the 1 ½ cups minimum for the pot.
3. Close and seal the lid.
4. Cook for 5 mins on high pressure.
5. Turn down the heat and let it stand for some time.
6. Take the lid off and simmer for 10 mins, to reduce.
7. Puree in a blender before storing in a jar.
8. Wait until it's cooled down before putting it in the fridge.

Nutritional Values

Calories 20, Fat 0.3g, Chol 0mg, Sodium 71.4mg, Potassium 67.7mg, Carbs 1.7g, Protein 6g

708. LEMON AND THYME SAUCE

- Sides - Prep time: 5 mins, Cook time: o mins, Total time: 5 mins, Servings: 2 cups, Grill temp: 0

Ingredients

- 1 cup of low-Sodium vegetable broth
- ½ cup of freshly squeezed lemon juice
- ¼ cup of cooking oil
- ¼ cup of water
- 1 tbsp of finely minced fresh chives
- 1 tbsp of fresh thyme
- 1 tbsp of finely minced garlic

Directions

1. Put ingredients in a medium bowl and whisk until combined.
2. Use immediately or store refrigerated for up to 10 days.

Nutritional Values

Calories 20, Fat 0.3g, Chol 0mg, Sodium 71.4mg, Potassium 67.7mg, Carbs 1.7g, Protein 6g

709. LENTIL BOLOGNESE

- Sides - Prep time: 5 mins, Cook time: 15 mins, Total time: 20 mins, Servings: 4 to 6, Grill temp: 300°F

Ingredients

- 4 cups of water
- 1 cup of washed black lentils
- 1 28-ounce can of fire-roasted tomatoes
- 4 minced garlic cloves
- 3 diced carrots
- 1 diced yellow onion
- 1 can of tomato paste
- ¼ cup of balsamic vinegar
- 2 tbsp of Italian seasoning
- Red pepper flakes
- Salt and pepper

Directions

1. Add all your ingredients except the balsamic vinegar to a deep-bottomed saucepan. Stir. Close and seal the lid.
2. Cook for 15 mins on high pressure.
3. Turn down the heat and wait 10 mins.
4. Add the balsamic vinegar, salt, and pepper and stir.
5. Serve or pour in a jar that you let cool before storing in the fridge.

Nutritional Values

Calories 208, Fat 0g, Chol 0mg, Sodium 71.4mg, Potassium 67.7mg, Carbs 39g, Protein 12g

710. MANGO CHUTNEY

- Sides - Prep time: 5 mins, Cook time: 20 mins, Total time: 25 mins, Servings: 2 cups, Grill temp: 300°F

Ingredients

- 2 big, diced mangos
- 1 cored and diced apple
- 1 and ¼ cups of apple cider vinegar
- 1 and ¼ cups of raw sugar
- ¼ cup of raisins
- 1 chopped shallot
- 2 tbsp finely-diced ginger
- 1 tbsp of veggie oil
- 2 tsps of salt
- ½ tsp of red pepper flakes
- ¼ tsp of cardamom powder
- ⅛ tsp of cinnamon

Directions

1. Heat up a deep-bottomed saucepan.
2. When hot, add the oil and cook shallots and ginger until the shallot is soft.
3. Add cinnamon, chili powder, and cardamom, and cook for 1 minute.
4. Add the rest of the ingredients and mix.
5. When the sugar has melted, close and seal the lid.
6. Cook for 7 mins on high pressure.
7. Turn down the heat and wait for the pressure to come down on its own.
8. Turn on the heat and cook with the lid off until the chutney has a jam-like texture.
9. When you get the texture you want, move the chutney to glass jars and close them.
10. When the contents are cool, move to the fridge.

Nutritional Values

Calories 78.2, Fat 3g, Chol 0mg, Sodium 71.4mg, Potassium 67.7mg, Carbs 18.3g, Protein 0.9g

711. RASPBERRY VINAIGRETTE

- Sides - Prep time: 10 mins, Cook time: 8 mins, Total time: 18 mins, Servings: ¾ cup, Grill temp: 300°F

Ingredients

- ½ shallot
- ½ tsp of Dijon mustard
- ¼ cup of raspberry vinegar
- 6 drops of liquid stevia- plain
- ½ cup of olive oil
- Salt and ground black pepper to taste

Directions

1. Put the shallot and mustard in your food processor, and turn it on. As the shallots are reaching the minced stage, add the raspberry vinegar and liquid stevia. Now slowly pour in the olive oil. When it's well incorporated, turn off the processor.
2. Taste, add salt and pepper, then pulse just another second or 2 to mix, and it's ready to use.

Nutritional Values

Calories 121, Fat 14g, Chol 0mg, Sodium 71.4mg, Potassium 67.7mg, Carbs 1g, Protein 0.2g

712. MIXED-VEGGIE SAUCE

- Sides - Prep time: 10 mins, Cook time: 7 mins, Total time: 17 mins, Servings: 3, Grill temp: 300°F

Ingredients

- 4 chopped tomatoes
- 5 cubes of pumpkin
- 4 minced garlic cloves
- 2 chopped green chilies
- 2 chopped celery stalks
- 1 sliced leek
- 1 chopped onion
- 1 chopped red bell pepper
- 1 chopped carrot
- 1 tbsp of sugar
- 2 tsps of olive oil
- 1 tsp of red chili flakes
- Splash of vinegar
- Salt to taste

Directions

1. Prepare the vegetables.
2. Heat your oil in a pot
3. Add onion and garlic, and cook until the onion is clear.
4. Add pumpkin, carrots, green chilies, and bell pepper.
5. Stir before adding the leek, celery, and tomatoes.
6. After a minute or so, toss in salt and red chili flakes. Close and seal the lid of the pot.
7. Cook for 6 mins with the lid on.
8. Turn down the heat and let the pressure come down on its own. The veggies should be very soft.
9. Let the mixture cool a little before moving to a blender.
10. Puree until smooth.
11. Pour back into the pot and add vinegar and sugar.
12. Simmer on low for a few mins before serving.

Nutritional Values

Calories 126, Fat 3g, Chol 0mg, Sodium 71.4mg, Potassium 67.7mg, Carbs 22g, Protein 3g

713. SAGE-BUTTERNUT SQUASH SAUCE

- Sides - Prep time: 10 mins, Cook time: 10 mins, Total time: 20 mins, Servings: 4, Grill temp: 300°F

Ingredients

- 2 pounds of chopped butternut squash
- 1 cup of veggie broth
- 1 chopped yellow onion
- 2 chopped garlic cloves
- 2 tbsp of olive oil
- 1 tbsp of chopped sage
- ⅛ tsp of red pepper flakes
- Salt and black pepper to taste

Directions

1. Preheat your saucepan with oil.
2. Once the oil is hot, add the sage and stir so it becomes coated in oil.
3. When the sage crisps up, move it to a plate.
4. Add the onion to your cooker and cook until it begins to turn clear.
5. Add garlic and cook until fragrant.
6. Pour in 1 cup of broth and deglaze before adding squash.
7. Close and seal the lid.
8. Cook for straight 10 mins.
9. Turn down the heat and wait for 10 mins.
10. When a little cooler, add the pot's contents- and the sage to a blender and puree till smooth.
11. If it's too thick, add a little more veggie broth.
12. Serve right away or store in the fridge no longer than 3-4 days.

Nutritional Values

Calories 179, Fat 7g, Chol 0mg, Sodium 71.4mg, Potassium 67.7mg, Carbs 30g, Protein 3g

714. TANGY HONEY MUSTARD DRESSING

- Sides - Prep time: 10 mins, Cook time: 0 mins, Total time: 10 mins, Servings: 1 cup, Grill temp: 0

Ingredients

- ½ cup of light olive oil
- ¼ cup of cider vinegar
- ¼ cup of brown mustard
- 1/8 tsp of liquid stevia- plain
- ¼ tsp of ground black pepper
- ¼ tsp of salt

Directions

1. Just assemble everything in a clean jar, lid it tightly, and shake like mad.
2. Store in the fridge, right in the jar, and shake again before using.

Nutritional Values

Calories 7, Fat 0.1g, Chol 0mg, Sodium 2.4mg, Potassium 7.7mg, Carbs 1g, Protein 0.1g

715. WHITE WINE SHERRY SAUCE

- Sides - Prep time: 5 mins, Cook time: o mins, Total time: 5 mins, Servings: 2 cups, Grill temp: 0

Ingredients

- 1 cup of dry white wine
- ½ cup of water
- ¼ cup of cooking sherry
- ¼ cup of cooking oil
- 2 tbsp of finely minced shallots
- 1 tbsp of dried parsley
- 1 tbsp of finely minced garlic
- 1 tbsp of finely minced capers
- 1 tsp of salt
- 1 tsp of pepper

Directions

1. Put ingredients in a medium bowl and whisk until combined.
2. Use immediately or store refrigerated for up to 10 days.

Nutritional Values

Calories 32, Fat 2g, Chol 0mg, Sodium 11mg, Potassium 7.7mg, Carbs 2.3g, Protein 1g

716. VINEGAR HONEY SAUCE

- Sides - Prep time: 5 mins, Cook time: o mins, Total time: 5 mins, Servings: 2 cups, Grill temp: 0

Ingredients

- 1 and ¼ cups of balsamic vinegar
- ½ cup of water

- ¼ cup of honey
- ¼ cup of cooking oil
- 1 tbsp of Italian seasoning
- 1 tsp of salt
- 1 tsp of white pepper

Directions

1. Put ingredients in a medium bowl and whisk until combined.
2. Use immediately or store refrigerated for up to 10 days.

Nutritional Values

Calories 18.2, Fat 0.3g, Chol 0mg, Sodium 1.14mg, Potassium 6.3mg, Carbs 0.3g, Protein 0.2g

717. TERIYAKI SAUCE -ASIAN INSPIRED

- Sides - Prep time: 15 mins, Cook time: o mins, Total time: 15 mins, Servings: 2 cups, Grill temp: 0

Ingredients

- ½ cup of soy sauce
- 3 tbsp of honey
- 1 tbsp of rice wine or dry sherry
- 1 tbsp of rice vinegar
- 2 tsps of minced fresh ginger
- 2 smashed garlic cloves

Directions

1. Merge together all the ingredients in a small bowl.
2. Use immediately.

Nutritional Values

Calories 51, Fat 2g, Chol 0mg, Sodium 66mg, Potassium 42.7mg, Carbs 8g, Protein 0.3g

718. VEGAN "CHEESE" SAUCE

- Breakfast - Prep time: 5 mins, Cook time: 5 mins, Total time: 10 mins, Servings: 2 to 4, Grill temp: 300°F

Ingredients

- 2 cups of peeled and chopped white potatoes
- 2 cups of water
- 1 cup of chopped carrots
- 3 peeled, whole garlic cloves
- ½ cup of chopped onion
- ½ cup of nutritional yeast

- ½ cup of raw cashews
- 1 tsp of turmeric
- 1 tsp of salt

Directions

1. Put everything in a deep saucepan with a lid.
2. Close and seal the lid.
3. Cook for 5 mins on high pressure.
4. Turn down the heat and open the lid.
5. Let the sauce cool for 10-15 mins.
6. Blend until smooth and creamy.
7. Serve or store!

Nutritional Values

Calories 216, Fat 9g, Chol 0mg, Sodium 71.4mg, Potassium 67.7mg, Carbs 26g, Protein 13g

719. VEGAN ALFREDO SAUCE

- Sides - Prep time: 5 mins, Cook time: 5 mins, Total time: 10 mins, Servings: 2 to 4, Grill temp: 300°F

Ingredients

- Twelve ounces of cauliflower florets
- 2 minced garlic cloves
- ½ cup of water
- 1 tsp of coconut oil
- ½ tsp of sea salt
- Black pepper to taste

Directions

1. Heat the oil in a deep bottomed saucepan and add garlic.
2. When the garlic has become fragrant, pour ½ a cup of water into the pan.
3. Pour cauliflower into a steamer basket, and lower it into the pot.
4. Close and seal the lid.
5. Cook for 3 mins on high pressure.
6. Turn down the heat and wait for the pressure to come down on its own.
7. The cauliflower should be very soft. When a little cooler, add cauliflower and cooking liquid to a blender and process until smooth.
8. Season with salt and pepper before serving with pasta.

Nutritional Values

Calories 19, Fat 1g, Chol 0mg, Sodium 71.4mg, Potassium 67.7mg, Carbs 2g, Protein 1g

720. VINAIGRETTE

- Sides - Prep time: 10 mins, Cook time: 8 mins, Total time: 18 mins, Servings: 2 cups, Grill temp: 300°F

Ingredients

- ¾ cup of extra-virgin olive oil
- 1/3 cup of wine vinegar
- 1 tsp of Dijon mustard
- 1 clove of garlic, crushed
- ½ tsp of salt
- ¼ tsp of ground black pepper

Directions

1. Just put everything in a clean jar, lid it tightly, and shake vigorously.
2. You can store it in the jar and just shake it up again before use.

Nutritional Values

Calories 121, Fat 14g, Chol 0mg, Sodium 71.4mg, Potassium 67.7mg, Carbs 1g, Protein 0.3g

Chapter 20.

Smoothies & Fresh Juices

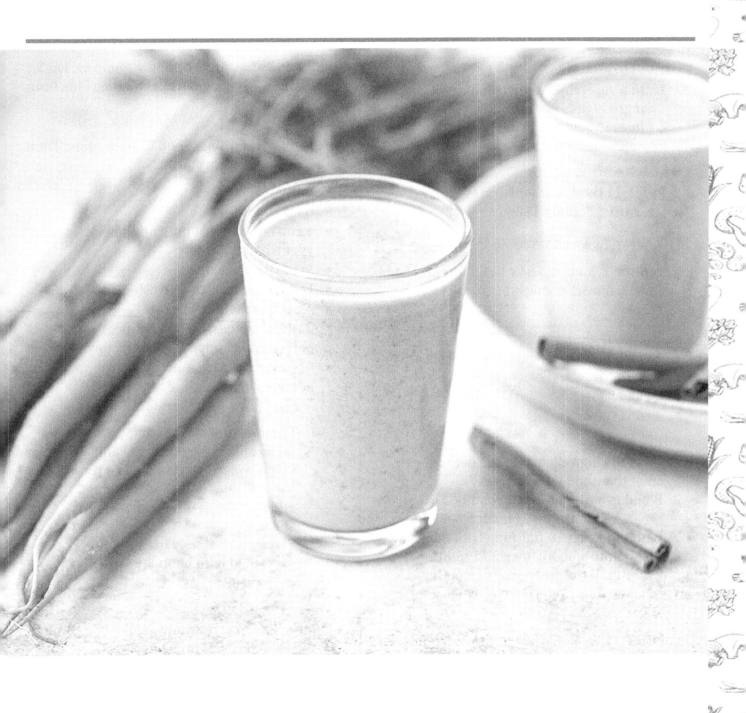

721. ANTI-INFLAMMATORY JUICE RECIPE

- Prep time: 5 mins, Cook time: 0 mins, Total time: 5 mins, Servings: 2

Ingredients

- 4 celery stalks
- ½ cucumber
- 1 cup pineapple
- ½ green apple
- 1 cup spinach
- 1 lemon
- 1 knob ginger

Directions

1. In a vegetable juicer, combine all of the ingredients.
2. Juice should be stirred gently and consumed right away.

Nutritional Values

Calories 114kcal, Carbohydrates-28g, Protein 2g, Fat 1g, Sodium 112mg

722. APPLE BERRY DETOX SMOOTHIE

- Prep time: 5 mins, Cook time: 0 mins, Total time: 5 mins, Servings: 1

Ingredients

- 1 large apple
- 1 cup mixed berries like raspberries, strawberries, and blueberries
- 1 cup water
- 2 cups spinach

Directions

1. All of the ingredients for the detox smoothie should be washed.
2. Blend in a weight-loss smoothie. Toss all of the ingredients into a blender, beginning with the greens & finishing with the fruit.
3. Blend until smooth, then add additional water until the green detox smoothie reaches your preferred consistency.

Nutritional Values

Calories 210kcal, Carbohydrates-50g, Protein 3.3g, Fat 1.1g, Sodium 234mg

723. APPLE-STRAWBERRY SMOOTHIE

- Drink/Breakfast - Prep time: ready in about: 2 mins, Servings: 1, Grill temp: 0

Ingredients

- 200 ml of almond milk
- 1 banana
- 160g of frozen strawberries
- 1 tbsp of peanut butter
- 60g of apple

Directions

1. Take a blender, add all of your ingredients to it, and blend until smooth.
2. Pour into a glass and serve fresh or chill, as you like.

Nutritional Values

Calories 281 kcal, Carbs 63g, Protein 6g, Fat 3g, Sodium 99mg, Potassium 521mg, Chol 0mg

724. APRICOT-MANGO MADNESS

- Prep time: 5 mins, Cook time: 0 mins, Total time: 5 mins, Servings: 2

Ingredients

- 8 ice cubes
- 1 cup reduced-Fat milk or plain low-fat yogurt
- ¼ tsp vanilla extract
- Lemon peel twists- garnish
- 4 tsp fresh lemon juice
- 2 ripe mangoes, 10 to 12 ounces each, peeled and chopped- about 2 cups
- 6 apricots, peeled, pitted, and chopped- about 2 cups

Directions

1. Combine the mangoes, apricots, lemon juice, milk or yogurt, and vanilla essence in a blender. For 8 seconds, process. Add the ice cubes and process for an additional 6 to 8 seconds, or until smooth.
2. Serve immediately in tall glasses garnished with lemon twists if preferred.

Nutritional Values

Calories 252kcal, Carbohydrates-53g, Protein 7g, Fat 3.5g, Sodium 57mg

725. AVOCADO DETOX SMOOTHIE

- Prep time: 5 mins, Cook time: 0 mins, Total time: 5 mins, Servings: 1

Ingredients

- 2 cups kale or spinach stemmed & chopped
- 1 ½ cups water
- ½ chopped avocado
- 1 apple unpeeled, cored & chopped

Directions

1. All of the detoxifying smoothie ingredients should be washed.
2. Toss all ingredients into a blender, beginning with the spinach and working your way to the fruit.
3. Blend until smooth, then add additional water until you have the green detox smoothie texture you want.

Nutritional Values

Calories 335kcal, Carbohydrates-41g, Protein 4.2g, Fat 20g, Sodium 484mg

726. BANANA GINGER SMOOTHIE

- Prep time: 5 mins, Cook time: 0 mins, Total time: 5 mins, Servings: 1

Ingredients

- 1 tbsp honey
- 1 banana, sliced
- ¾ cup- 6 oz. vanilla yogurt
- ½ tsp freshly grated ginger

Directions

1. Combine the yogurt, banana, ginger, and honey.
2. Blend until completely smooth.

Nutritional Values

Calories 157kcal, Carbohydrates-34g, Protein 5g, Fat 1g, Sodium 57mg

727. BANANA-BLUEBERRY-SOY SMOOTHIE

- Prep time: 5 mins, Cook time: 0 mins, Total time: 5 mins, Servings: 1

Ingredients

- ½ frozen banana, sliced
- 1¼ cup light soy milk
- 1 tsp pure vanilla extract
- ½ cup frozen loose-pack blueberries
- 2 tsp sugar

Directions

1. 1 cup milk, sugar or sweetener, banana, blueberries, and vanilla extract are

mixed. Blend for 20 - 30 secs or until the mixture is completely smooth.

2. If you want a thinner smoothie, add up to ¼ cup extra milk.

Nutritional Values

Calories 125kcal, Carbohydrates-25g, Protein 3g, Fat 1.5g, Sodium 60mg

728. BEET GREENS SMOOTHIE

- Breakfast/Snacks - Prep time: 10 mins, Cook time: 0 mins, Total time: 10 mins, Servings: 2, Grill temp: 0

Ingredients

- 1 cup of Beet Greens
- 2 tbsp of Pumpkin seeds butter
- 1 cup of Strawberry
- 1 tbsp of sesame seeds
- 1 tbsp of hemp seeds
- 1 cup of chamomile tea

Directions

1. Combine all the ingredients together in a food processor.
2. Pulse it 2 to 3 times.
3. Serve and enjoy.

Nutritional Values

Calories 51, Fat 2g, Chol 0mg, Sodium 71.4mg, Potassium 67.7mg, Carbs 8g, Protein 0.3g

729. BLACKBERRY SODA SYRUP

- Snacks - Prep time: 10 mins, Cook time: 15 mins, Total time: 25 mins, Servings: 2, Grill temp: 300°F

Ingredients

- Fourteen ounces of washed and dried blackberries
- 2 cups of white sugar
- 1 cup of water

Directions

1. Pour 1 cup of water into the pressure cooker.
2. Pour berries into your steamer basket and lower them into the cooker.
3. Close and seal the lid.
4. Cook on high pressure for 15 mins.
5. Turn off the heat. Wait for the pressure to come down.

6. Take out the steamer basket.
7. Pour juice-infused water into a measuring cup. Take note of how much it is.
8. Pour this cup into a saucepan and add twice the amount of sugar as there is juice water.
9. On medium heat, stir the pot until the sugar is fully dissolved.
10. Store in your fridge for 1-2 months.

Nutritional Values

Calories 167, Fat 0g, Chol 0mg, Sodium 71.4mg, Potassium 67.7mg, Carbs 46g, Protein 0g

730. BLUEBERRY DETOX SMOOTHIE

- Prep time: 10 mins, Cook time: 0 mins, Total time: 10 mins, Servings: 1

Ingredients

- 1 frozen banana, cut into pieces for easy blending
- 1 small handful of fresh cilantro leaves
- ½ cup orange juice
- ¼ cup water
- 1 cup frozen wild blueberries
- ¼ avocado

Directions

1. Mix the cilantro, orange juice, blueberries, avocado, banana, & water in a blender.
2. Blend until smooth.
3. Serve right away.

Nutritional Values

Calories 326kcal, Carbohydrates-65g, Protein 4g, Fat 8g, Sodium 11mg

731. BROCCOLI APPLE SMOOTHIE

- Breakfast/Snacks - Prep time: 10 mins, Cook time: 0 mins, Total time: 10 mins, Servings: 2, Grill temp: 0

Ingredients

- 1 Apple
- 1 cup of Broccoli
- 1 tbsp of Cilantro
- 1 Celery stalk
- 1 cup of crushed ice
- 1 tbsp of crushed Seaweed

Directions

1. Combine all the ingredients together in a food processor.
2. Pulse it 2 to 3 times.
3. Serve and enjoy.

Nutritional Values

Calories 89, Fat 2g, Chol 0mg, Sodium 31.4mg, Potassium 57.7mg, Carbs 7g, Protein 4g

732. CARROT AND APPLE JUICE

- Prep time: 10 mins, Cook time: 0 mins, Total time: 10 mins, Servings: 1

Ingredients

- 4 carrots, trimmed
- 2 apples, quartered
- 2 stalks celery
- 1- ½ inch piece of fresh ginger

Directions

1. Put apples, carrots, and celery in a juicer as per the manufacturer's Directions.
2. Add ginger to the juicer and blend.

Nutritional Values

Calories 277kcal, Carbohydrates-68.6g, Protein 4g, Fat 1.3g, Sodium 265mg

733. CARROT AND ORANGE JUICE

- Prep time: 10 mins, Cook time: 0 mins, Total time: 10 mins, Servings: 4

Ingredients

- 2 pounds organic carrots, trimmed and scrubbed
- 8 organic oranges, peeled

Directions

1. Add oranges and carrots to a juicer.
2. Pour into a big glass.

Nutritional Values

Calories 183kcal, Carbohydrates-44.3g, Protein 3.9g, Fat 0.8g, Sodium 156.6mg

734. CELERY CUCUMBER GREEN JUICE

- Prep time: 20 mins, Cook time: 5 mins, Total time: 25 mins, Servings: 4

Ingredients

- 1 head of celery broken into stalks
- 5 small Persian cucumbers, washed with the ends cut off

- 1 apple, red or green, sliced
- 1 lime, skin cut off
- 1 ½ " knob of fresh ginger, skin cut off

Directions

1. Blend the ingredients in a juicer, alternating the soft and hard pieces.
2. Serve as soon as possible.

Nutritional Values

Calories 323kcal, Carbohydrates-14g, Protein 1g, Fat 0.3g, Sodium 43mg

735. CHERRY BEET SMOOTHIE

- Prep time: 5 mins, Cook time: 0 mins, Total time: 5 mins, Servings: 1

Ingredients

- ¼ cup beet - peeled and diced
- 1 cup cherries
- ¼ banana - frozen
- ½ cup pomegranate juice
- ½ cup water
- fresh mint - for garnish
- 1 serving Protein Smoothie Boost - optional

Directions

1. Combine all ingredients in a blender and blend until smooth.
2. If desired, garnish with mint leaves.

Nutritional Values

Calories 195kcal, Carbohydrates-48g, Protein 3g, Fat 1g, Sodium 44mg

736. CHERRY MANGO ANTI-INFLAMMATORY SMOOTHIE

- Prep time: 10 mins, Cook time: 5 mins, Total time: 15 mins, Servings: 1

Ingredients

- 1 cup frozen sweet cherries
- ½ cup water
- 1 cup frozen mango
- ¾ cup water

Directions

1. Place the cherries & mangoes in 2 different dishes and set them aside for 10 mins to thaw.
2. Process the cherries first: in a blender, combine the cherries with ½ cup water

and mix on high until completely smooth. If it appears too thick, add the remaining ¼ cup water. Pour the mixture into a glass.

3. Fill the blender pitcher halfway with water and add the mango. Blend on high speed until completely smooth. If necessary, add extra water. Pour over the cherry layer in the glass.
4. Enjoy!

Nutritional Values

Calories 185kcal, Carbohydrates-46g, Protein 2g, Fat 1.5g, Sodium 17mg

737. COCONUT-WATER-SMOOTHIE

- Drink/Breakfast - Prep time: ready in about: 2 mins, Servings: 1, Grill temp: 0

Ingredients

- 100g of frozen mango
- 200 ml of coconut water
- 2 tsp of shredded coconut
- 1 tsp of peanut butter
- 60g of apple

Directions

1. Take a blender, add all of your ingredients to it, and blend until smooth.
2. Pour into a glass and serve fresh or chill, as you like.

Nutritional Values

Calories 281 kcal, Carbs 63g, Protein 6g, Fat 3g, Sodium 99mg, Potassium 521mg, Chol 0mg

738. CRANBERRY SIMPLE SYRUP

- Snacks - Prep time: 5 mins, Cook time: 5 mins, Total time: 10 mins, Servings: 2, Grill temp: 300°F

Ingredients

- 2 cups of dried cranberries
- 2 cups of water
- 2 cups of sugar

Directions

1. Pour water into the pressure cooker along with the fruit. Be sure it is no more than halfway full, or you'll have to reduce your measurements.
2. Close and seal the lid.
3. Cook for 5 mins, on high pressure.
4. Wait for the pressure to descend naturally.

5. Pour pot contents into a fine-mesh strainer and press down on the fruit to get all the juice out.
6. Pour pot contents back into the pressure cooker.
7. On the sauté setting, add sugar.
8. Bring to a boil and let it roll until liquid has reduced in ½.
9. Cool completely before pouring into glass jars.
10. Store in fridge and use for up to 2 weeks.

Calories 130, Fat 0g, Chol 0mg, Sodium 71.4mg, Potassium 67.7mg, Carbs 38g, Protein 0g

739. DAIRY, SUGAR & GLUTEN-FREE SMOOTHIE

- Prep time: 5 mins, Cook time: 0 mins, Total time: 5 mins, Servings: 1

Ingredients

- 1 cup spinach
- 1 apple cored [green preferred] or 1 green pear
- 1 ½ cup ice
- 1 stalk celery
- juice of 1 lemon
- ½ cucumber
- 2 droppers of liquid lemon stevia or plain
- ½ cup almond milk unsweetened
- 1 tbsp flax seed

Directions

1. In a high-powered blender, combine all ingredients until smooth.
2. Taste and, if necessary, adjust the sweetness.
3. Serve.

Nutritional Values

Calories 194kcal, Carbohydrates-34.1g, Protein 5.5g, Fat 6.2g, Sodium 171mg

740. DETOX GREEN SMOOTHIE WITH GRAPES

- Prep time: 5 mins, Cook time: 0 mins, Total time: 5 mins, Servings: 1

Ingredients

- 1 tbsp lime juice
- 1 tbsp apple cider vinegar
- ½ cup ice cubes
- 1 tbsp honey
- 1 pear, peeled & chopped
- 1 cup vanilla Greek yogurt
- 15 green grapes
- 1 medium ripe avocado, halved & pitted
- 2 cups fresh spinach

Directions

1. In a blender, combine all of the ingredients.
2. Blend until completely smooth.
3. Serve.

Nutritional Values

Calories 160kcal, Carbohydrates-24g, Protein 9g, Fat 5g, Sodium 35mg

741. DETOX SMOOTHIE

- Prep time: 5 mins, Cook time: 0 mins, Total time: 5 mins, Servings: 1

Ingredients

- 1 cucumber
- 1 ½ cups water- 375 ml
- 12 dates
- 1 cup chopped pineapple- 250 g
- 1 lemon

Directions

1. Add all the ingredients to a blender.
2. Blend until completely smooth.
3. Serve right away.

Nutritional Values

Calories 106kcal, Carbohydrates-28g, Protein 1.5g, Fat 0.3g, Sodium 237mg

742. DIGESTIVE AID GREEN JUICE

- Prep time: 10 mins, Cook time: 0 mins, Total time: 10 mins, Servings: 1

Ingredients

- 1 celery stick
- 2 handfuls of fresh kale- 40 g
- ¼ fennel
- ½ -inch piece of ginger root- about 1 cm
- 2 pears

Directions

1. Prepare the ingredients by chopping them up.
2. Everything should be put through the juicer.
3. For a smoother texture, strain the juice. It is an optional step.
4. It will be easy to clean the juicer after the juice is ready.
5. And now the juice is ready to drink! It's best to consume juice right away, but if you're making large amounts, you can keep it in an airtight jar in the fridge for 72 hrs.

Calories 237kcal, Carbohydrates-60.4g, Protein 3.3g, Fat 0.7g, Sodium 56mg

743. EASY DETOX SMOOTHIE

- Prep time: 5 mins, Cook time: 0 mins, Total time: 5 mins, Servings: 1

Ingredients

- ⅓ avocado, diced
- 1 cup spinach
- ½ cup mangos, diced
- ½ cup blueberries
- ½ cup soymilk or almond milk
- ½ lime
- ½ cup ice cubes

Directions

1. In a blender, combine all of the ingredients.
2. Lime juice should be squeezed in.
3. Blend well until smooth.
4. Serve and enjoy!

Nutritional Values

Calories 311kcal, Carbohydrates-50g, Protein 7.6g, Fat 16g, Sodium 96mg

744. ELDERBERRY SYRUP

- Snacks - Prep time: 10 mins, Cook time: 10 mins, Total time: 20 mins, Servings: 2 cups, Grill temp: 0

Ingredients

- 4 cups of water
- 1 cup of dried elderberries
- ¾-1 cup of agave syrup
- 1 split vanilla bean

Directions

1. Put all your ingredients- minus the agave in the pot and stir well.
2. Close and seal the lid.
3. Cook on high pressure for just 10 mins.
4. Turn off the heat and let it stand for a while.
5. Pour syrup into a fine-mesh strainer and throw away elderberries.
6. Let the syrup cool before whisking in agave.
7. Store in a fridge for up to 2 weeks, or freeze to make it last longer.

Nutritional Values

Calories 25, Fat 0g, Chol 0mg, Sodium 71.4mg, Potassium 67.7mg, Carbs 6g, Protein 0g

745. GLOWING GREEN DETOX SMOOTHIE

- Prep time: 5 mins, Cook time: 0 mins, Total time: 5 mins, Servings: 1

Ingredients

- ¼ cup pineapple
- 1 kiwi
- 1 cup water
- 1 banana
- 2 celery stalks
- 2 cups spinach

Directions

1. Clean all of the ingredients for the detox smoothie.
2. Add a weight-loss smoothie. Start with the greens & work your way to the fruit in the blender.
3. Blend until smooth, then add additional water until the green detox smoothie reaches the consistency you want.

Nutritional Values

Calories 191kcal, Carbohydrates-46.7g, Protein 4.3g, Fat 1.1g, Sodium 478mg

746. GOLDEN DETOX SMOOTHIE

- Prep time: 5 mins, Cook time: 0 mins, Total time: 5 mins, Servings: 1

Ingredients

- 2 tbsp honey Greek yogurt
- 1 banana
- ice cubes optional

- 1 carrot peeled and diced
- ½ cup water
- ½ cup fresh pineapple
- ½ cup orange juice fresh squeezed

Directions

1. In a blender, thoroughly combine all ingredients.
2. Before serving, pour into a glass.

Nutritional Values

Calories 472kcal, Carbohydrates-105g, Protein 13g, Fat 2g, Sodium 57mg

747. GRAPEFRUIT SMOOTHIE

- Prep time: 10 mins, Cook time: 0 mins, Total time: 10 mins, Servings: 2

Ingredients

- 1 Winter Sweets red grapefruit
- grapefruit segments, berries, and granola- for topping
- 1/3 cup Greek yogurt
- 2 cups frozen pineapple chunks
- 1 tbsp coconut oil
- ¼ inch knob of fresh ginger

Directions

1. Grapefruit should be segmented over a bowl so that all of the juice may be collected. Set aside 2-3 segments for topping.
2. Blend: In a high-powered blender, combine grapefruit juice, grapefruit segments, coconut oil, Greek yogurt, frozen pineapple, and fresh ginger until smooth.
3. If the smoothie is too thick, add a little bit of non-dairy milk.
4. Pour the mixture into 2 glasses and serve. Serve in a dish with a variety of toppings, such as granola, grapefruit segments, berries, and so on.

Nutritional Values

Calories 234kcal, Carbohydrates-37g, Protein 4g, Fat 7g, Sodium 256mg

748. GREEN DETOX SMOOTHIE

- Prep time: 10 mins, Cook time: 0 mins, Total time: 10 mins, Servings: 4

Ingredients

- 2 cups baby kale
- 2 cups baby spinach
- 1 tbsp chia seeds
- 2 ribs celery, chopped
- 1 tbsp grated fresh ginger
- 1 medium green apple, chopped
- 1 tbsp honey
- 1 cup frozen sliced banana
- 1 cup almond milk

Directions

1. Combine kale, spinach, apple, celery, almond milk, banana, chia seeds, ginger, and honey in a blender until completely smooth.
2. Serve right away.

Nutritional Values

Calories 136kcal, Carbohydrates-28g, Protein 1g, Fat 1g, Sodium 104mg

749. GREEN DRAGON VEGGIE JUICE

- Prep time: 5 mins, Cook time: 0 mins, Total time: 5 mins, Servings: 1

Ingredients

- ¼ large lemon
- 1 cup fresh spinach, or to taste
- 2 sprigs of fresh parsley, or more to taste
- 2 stalks celery
- ⅓ small jalapeno pepper- Optional
- 1 tomato, quartered
- 1 pinch salt
- 1 cup ice, or as desired

Directions

1. Add spinach, lemon, celery, parsley, tomato, and jalapeno pepper to a juicer.
2. Season with salt.
3. Add juice to a glass filled with ice.

Nutritional Values

Calories 74kcal, Carbohydrates-16.1g, Protein 4.8g, Fat 1.1g, Sodium 290mg

750. GREEN JUICE FOR BEGINNERS

- Prep time: 10 mins, Cook time: 0 mins, Total time: 10 mins, Servings: 2

Ingredients

- 2 pears

- 2 handfuls of fresh spinach- about 1.5 oz. or 40 g
- 1 stalk of celery
- ½ -inch piece of ginger root- about 1cm
- ¼ fennel bulb- or 2 stalks of celery

Directions

1. All of the ingredients should be washed and chopped. The pears and ginger root don't need to be peeled, but you should if they aren't organic.
2. Everything should be put through the juicer.
3. Because our juicer includes a strainer, we don't filter the juice. However, if your juicer doesn't have 1, you may want to sieve your juice for a nicer texture.
4. Although fresh green juice is preferable, it may be stored 72 hours in a jar or sealed container in the fridge. To avoid oxidation, fill your juice bottle to the top. It may be frozen for a week, but don't overfill the container, or it will explode.

Nutritional Values

Calories 139kcal, Carbohydrates-35.6g, Protein 1.8g, Fat 0.5g, Sodium 41mg

751. GREEN PROTEIN DETOX SMOOTHIE

- Prep time: 3 mins, Cook time: 0 mins, Total time: 3 mins, Servings: 1

Ingredients

- 1 tbsp almond butter
- 1 banana
- ½ cup unsweetened almond milk
- 2 cups baby spinach

Directions

1. Clean all of the ingredients for the detox smoothie.
2. Add a weight-loss smoothie. Start with the greens & work your way to the fruit in the blender.
3. Blend until smooth, then add additional water until the green detox smoothie reaches the consistency you want.

Nutritional Values

Calories 237kcal, Carbohydrates-33.1g, Protein 6.9g, Fat 1g, Sodium 439mg

752. GREEN TEA, BLUEBERRY, AND BANANA SMOOTHIE

- Prep time: 5 mins, Cook time: 0 mins, Total time: 5 mins, Servings: 1

Ingredients

- 1 green tea bag
- 1½ cups frozen blueberries
- 3 tbsp water
- 2 tsp honey
- ½ medium banana
- ¾ cups soy milk- vanilla

Directions

1. Fill a small bowl with boiling water. Allow 3 mins for the tea bag to brew. Take out the teabag. Honey should be stirred into the tea until it mixes.
2. In a blender, combine the berries, banana, and milk.
3. Blend the tea in a blender. Using an ice crush or the highest setting, blend the ingredients until smooth.- Depending on your blender, you may need to add more water to blend the mixture. Serve the smoothie in a large glass.

Nutritional Values

Calories 269kcal, Carbohydrates-63g, Protein 3.5g, Fat 2.5g, Sodium 52mg

753. HEALTHY GREEN JUICE

- Prep time: 10 mins, Cook time: 0 mins, Total time: 10 mins, Servings: 2

Ingredients

- 2 green apples, halved
- 4 stalks of celery, leaves removed
- 1 cucumber
- 6 leaves kale
- ½ lemon, peeled
- 1- 1 inch piece of fresh ginger

Directions

1. Process celery, green apples, kale, cucumber, ginger, and lemon through a juicer.
2. Pour in a glass and enjoy.

Nutritional Values

Calories 144kcal, Carbohydrates-36g, Protein 4.2g, Fat 1.1g, Sodium 95.2mg

754. HEALTHY GREEN JUICE WITH LEMON

- Prep time: 5 mins, Cook time: 0 mins, Total time: 5 mins, Servings: 2

Ingredients

- 1 bunch of kale
- 1 head of romaine lettuce
- 1 medium carrot optional
- 5 celery stalks
- 1 medium cucumber
- 1 green apple
- 2 lemons
- 1" piece of fresh ginger

Directions

1. All of your ingredients should be washed.
2. Ingredients for juice, as directed by your juicer's user manual. You can use a blender instead of a juicer if you don't have 1.
3. Slowly sip and enjoy!

Nutritional Values

Calories 184kcal, Carbohydrates-41g, Protein 9g, Fat 3g, Sodium 876mg

755. HOMEMADE GINGER-LEMON COUGH SYRUP

- Snacks - Prep time: 10 mins, Cook time: 20 mins, Total time: 30 mins, Servings: 2, Grill temp: 300°F

Ingredients

- 2 cups of water
- 1 cup of vegan honey
- 8 sprigs of fresh thyme
- ¼ cup of chopped ginger
- Juice of 1 lemon
- ⅛ tsp of cayenne pepper

Directions

1. Pour water into a pot, adding ginger and thyme.
2. Simmer until the water has reduced by ½.
3. Turn off the heat and wait until the liquid is warm, not hot.
4. Strain the herbs out, saving the infused water.
5. Pour water back into the pot.
6. Add lemon, honey, and pepper.
7. Pour into a jar.
8. Store in the cupboard for 1 week, and if there's still syrup left, move to the fridge.

Nutritional Values

Calories 31, Fat 0g, Chol 0mg, Sodium 71.4mg, Potassium 67.7mg, Carbs 8g, Protein 0g

756. HOMEMADE VANILLA EXTRACT

- Snacks - Prep time: 10 mins, Cook time: 30 mins, Total time: 40 mins, Servings: 10, Grill temp: 300°F

Ingredients

- 2 cups of 40% alcohol vodka
- 6-10 Madagascar vanilla beans

Directions

1. Slice the vanilla beans in ½.
2. Put the vanilla beans in a pint jar and pour in vodka, leaving 1-inch of space on top.
3. Put the ring and lid on, but only tighten a little.
4. Pour 1 cup of water into the pot.
5. Put the jar in the pot.
6. Close and seal the lid.
7. Cook on high pressure for 30 mins.
8. Turn down the heat and let it stand for 10 mins.
9. Take out the jar carefully, and cool overnight.
10. When cool, store in a cupboard.

Nutritional Values

Calories 12, Fat 0g, Chol 0mg, Sodium 71.4mg, Potassium 67.7mg, Carbs 1g, Protein 0g

757. JUMPING JACK SMOOTHIE RECIPE

- Prep time: 10 mins, Cook time: 0 mins, Total time: 10 mins, Servings: 2

Ingredients

- 100ml soya milk
- 1 pear, peeled
- 2tsp linseeds- also known as flaxseed
- 1 banana, peeled
- 75ml yogurt

Directions

1. Fill a smoothie maker halfway with peeled pears.
2. Chop the banana into bits and combine with the linseeds & yogurt in the pear.
3. Add the soya milk to the ingredients and mix until smooth.

Nutritional Values

Calories 149kcal, Carbohydrates-28g, Protein 4.1g, Fat 3.4g, Sodium 44.5mg

758. JUST PEACHY SMOOTHIE

- Prep time: 5 mins, Cook time: 0 mins, Total time: 5 mins, Servings: 1

Ingredients

- 1 cup milk
- 2 tbsp low-fat vanilla yogurt
- ½ cup frozen peaches
- ½ cup strawberries
- ⅛ tsp powdered ginger
- 2 tsp whey Protein powder- such as Source Organic Whey Protein
- 3 ice cubes

Directions

1. Any liquid ingredients- yogurt, milk, juice, etc. should be blended with the Protein powder to help break down the gritty powder and ensure it is equally distributed.
2. Add mushy ingredients first, such as pre-cooked oatmeal and bananas, and then ice last.
3. To make a thicker smoothie, add additional ice cubes; this will boost volume without adding calories.

Nutritional Values

Calories 150kcal, Carbohydrates-26.5g, Protein 9g, Fat 2g, Sodium 73mg

759. KALE AND APPLE GREEN DETOX SMOOTHIE

- Prep time: 5 mins, Cook time: 0 mins, Total time: 5 mins, Servings: 1

Ingredients

- ¾ cup ice
- ⅔ cup almond milk unsweetened
- 1 tbsp ground flax seed
- 1 ½ cups kale chopped
- 1 tsp honey optional
- 1 stalk celery chopped
- ½ red or green apple cored and chopped

Directions

1. All of the detox smoothie ingredients should be washed.

2. Smoothie for weight loss: Toss all ingredients into a blender, beginning with the greens & working your way to the fruit.
3. Blend until smooth, then add additional water until you have the green detox smoothie texture you want.

Nutritional Values

Calories 148kcal, Carbohydrates-17.5g, Protein 6g, Fat 0.3g, Sodium 154mg

760. KALE BANANA STRAWBERRY DETOX SMOOTHIE

- Prep time: 5 mins, Cook time: 0 mins, Total time: 5 mins, Servings: 1

Ingredients

- 1 cup fresh or frozen strawberries
- 1 banana
- 1 cup yogurt plain
- 1 cup kale chopped
- 1 cup ice

Directions

1. All of the detoxing smoothie ingredients should be washed.
2. Put all of the ingredients, including weight loss, into a blender, beginning with the veggies and working your way to the fruit.
3. Blend until smooth, then add additional water until you have the green detox smoothie texture you want.

Nutritional Values

Calories 358kcal, Carbohydrates-62g, Protein 18g, Fat 2.6g, Sodium 377mg

761. KALE COCONUT PINEAPPLE DETOX SMOOTHIE

- Prep time: 5 mins, Cook time: 0 mins, Total time: 5 mins, Servings: 1

Ingredients

- 1 cup coconut water
- 1 banana
- 2 cups chopped kale
- 1 cup pineapple

Directions

1. All of the ingredients should be washed.
2. In a blender, combine all ingredients, beginning with the kale and finishing with the fruit ingredient.

3. Blend until smooth, then add additional water until you have the green detox smoothie texture you want.

Nutritional Values

Calories 199kcal, Carbohydrates-71.5g, Protein 7.9g, Fat 1.1g, Sodium 344mg

762. KETO AVOCADO SMOOTHIE

- Prep time: 10 mins, Cook time: 0 mins, Total time: 10 mins, Servings: 1

Ingredients

- ¾ cup of full-Fat coconut milk- from a can
- ½ avocado- 3-4 oz
- ½ tsp turmeric
- ¼ cup almond milk
- 1 tsp lemon or lime juice- or more to taste
- 1 tsp fresh grated ginger- about ½ inch piece
- sugar-free sweetener to taste
- 1 cup crushed ice- or more for a thicker smoothie

Directions

1. In a blender, combine the first 6 ingredients and mix on low until smooth.
2. Mix in the crushed ice and the sweetener. Blend on high speed until completely smooth.
3. Taste and adjust the sweetness and tartness according to your taste. This recipe makes 2 avocado smoothies.

Nutritional Values

Calories 232kcal, Carbohydrates-6.9g, Protein 1.7g, Fat 22.4g, Sodium 25mg

763. MANGO-KALE SMOOTHIE

- Drink/Breakfast - Prep time: ready in about: 2 mins, Servings: 1, Grill temp: 0

Ingredients

- 15g of curly kale
- 1 banana
- 100g of frozen mango
- 1 tsp vanilla extract
- 200 ml of oat milk

Directions

1. Take a blender, add all of your ingredients to it, and blend until smooth.

2. Pour into a glass and serve fresh or chill, as you like.

Nutritional Values

Calories 281 kcal, Carbs 63g, Protein 6g, Fat 3g, Sodium 99mg, Potassium 521mg, Chol 0mg

764. MINT CHIP SMOOTHIE

- Prep time: 5 mins, Cook time: 5, Total time: 10 mins, Grill temp: 0, Servings: 1

Ingredients

- 4 ice cubes of coconut milk
- 1 & ½ cup spinach leaves frozen
- ¼ cup frozen mint leaves
- 3 soft dates Medjool
- 1 & ½ tbsp nibs' cacao
- 3 tbsp Protein Pea
- 1 & ½ cup milk almond

Directions

1. Combine the ingredients in a blender. Blend using the blender's baton to assist yourself.
2. Continue to add almond milk if you believe you need it.
3. Making a creamy smoothie is as easy as adding just enough liquid to get your blender blades spinning, but not so much that your smoothie becomes thin and watery.

Nutritional Values

Fat 4.3g, Chol 2.9mg, Sodium 27mg, Potassium 24mg, Carbs 42g, Calories 287, Protein 10 g

765. MIXED-FRUIT-SMOOTHIE

- Drink/Breakfast - Prep time: ready in about: 2 mins, Servings: 1, Grill temp: 0

Ingredients

- 40g of fresh raspberries
- 30 ml of grapefruit juice
- 45g of banana
- 100 ml of cold water
- 50g of frozen blueberries

Directions

1. Take a blender, add all of your ingredients to it, and blend until smooth.
2. Pour into a glass and serve fresh or chill, as you like.

Calories 281 kcal, Carbs 63g, Protein 6g, Fat 3g, Sodium 99mg, Potassium 521mg, Chol 0mg

766. MY FAVORITE GREEN JUICE

- Prep time: 10 mins, Cook time: 0 mins, Total time: 10 mins, Servings: 1

Ingredients

- 2 large kale leaves
- 1 head of romaine lettuce
- A handful of fresh parsley
- 1 large Granny Smith apple, chopped
- 2 lemons, peeled

Directions

1. All vegetables should be well washed.
2. Everything should be chopped into little bits that will fit down the juicer's funnel.
3. Place each ingredient in the juicer.
4. Pour the juice into a glass, mix well, and drink right away.

Nutritional Values

Calories 189kcal, Carbohydrates-38g, Protein 7g, Fat 1g, Sodium 490mg

767. ORANGE AND SPINACH JUICE

- Prep time: 10 mins, Cook time: 0 mins, Total time: 10 mins, Servings: 1

Ingredients

- 2 oranges, peeled
- 1 lemon, peeled
- 1 green apple, quartered
- 1 cup fresh spinach
- 1 leaf kale

Directions

1. Add lemon, oranges, spinach, green apple, and kale to a juicer.
2. Serve and enjoy.

Nutritional Values

Calories 44kcal, Carbohydrates-11g, Protein 0.9g, Fat 0.2g, Sodium 16.8mg

768. ORANGE DREAM CREAMSICLE

- Prep time: 5 mins, Cook time: 0 mins, Total time: 5 mins, Servings: 1

Ingredients

- ¼ tsp vanilla extract
- 1 navel orange, peeled
- 2 tbsp frozen orange juice concentrate
- ¼ cup Fat free ½-and-½ or Fat free yogurt
- 4 ice cubes

Directions

1. Mix the orange, orange juice concentrate, ½-and-½ or yogurt, ice cubes, and vanilla.
2. Blend until completely smooth.

Nutritional Values

Calories 160kcal, Carbohydrates-36g, Protein 3g, Fat 1g, Sodium 60mg

769. PEACH SIMPLE SYRUP

- Snacks - Prep time: 10 mins, Cook time: 40 mins, Total time: 50 mins, Servings: 4, Grill temp: 300°F

Ingredients

- 4 cups of fresh, chopped peaches
- 2 cups of water
- 2 cups of sugar

Directions

1. Pour peaches into a deep pot with water. Make sure it is no more than halfway full.
2. Close and seal the lid.
3. Cook on high pressure for 5 mins.
4. Turn down the heat and wait for the pressure to descend naturally.
5. Mash peaches before moving to a strainer.
6. Strain the contents back into the pot.
7. Bring to a boil, add sugar, and boil until the liquid has reduced by ½.
8. Cool before pouring into glass jars.
9. Store in fridge and use for up to 2 weeks.

Nutritional Values

Calories 97, Fat 0g, Chol 0mg, Sodium 71.4mg, Potassium 67.7mg, Carbs 28g, Protein 0g

770. PEACHES AND CREAM OATMEAL GREEN SMOOTHIE

- Prep time: 2 mins, Cook time: 0 mins, Total time: 2 mins, Servings: 1

Ingredients

- ¼ cup oatmeal
- 1 cup almond milk
- 1 cup frozen peach slices

- 1 cup baby spinach
- 1 cup Greek yogurt
- ¼ tsp vanilla extract

Directions

1. In a blender, mix all of the ingredients.
2. Blend until completely smooth.
3. Serve right away.
4. To prevent food from sticking to the blender, wash it right away.

Nutritional Values

Calories 331kcal, Carbohydrates-46g, Protein 29g, Fat 4g, Sodium 611mg

771. PEPPERMINT CRIO BRU

- Snacks - Prep time: 5 mins, Cook time: 5 mins, Total time: 10 mins, Servings: 8, Grill temp: 300°F

Ingredients

- 6 cups of water
- 2 cups of unsweetened vanilla almond milk
- ½ cup of Crio Bru ground cocoa beans-peppermint flavor
- ⅓ cup of agave syrup
- 1 tsp of pure vanilla
- 1 tsp of peppermint extract

Directions

1. Put beans, water, milk, puree, cinnamon, vanilla, and syrup in a deep-bottomed pot.
2. Close and seal the lid.
3. Cook for 5 mins, on high pressure.
4. Turn down the flame and let it wait for 10 mins.
5. Pour the drink through a fine-mesh strainer to filter out grounds.
6. Serve hot or chilled.

Nutritional Values

Calories 59, Fat 3g, Chol 0mg, Sodium 71.4mg, Potassium 67.7mg, Carbs 14g, Protein 3g

772. PINEAPPLE AND AVOCADO DETOX SMOOTHIE

- Prep time: 15 mins, Cook time: 0 mins, Total time: 15 mins, Servings: 1

Ingredients

- ¾ cup pineapple juice
- ½ cup fresh spinach leaves

- ¼ pear, chopped
- ¼ green apple, chopped
- ¼ avocado, chopped
- 3 broccoli florets

Directions

1. Blend spinach, pineapple juice, pear, avocado, broccoli florets, and apple in a blender until completely smooth.
2. Serve and Enjoy.

Nutritional Values

Calories 379kcal, Carbohydrates-70g, Protein 15g, Fat 9.4g, Sodium 169mg

773. PINEAPPLE BANANA DETOX SMOOTHIE

- Prep time: 5 mins, Cook time: 0 mins, Total time: 5 mins, Servings: 1

Ingredients

- 1 cup pineapple
- 1 banana
- 1 apple
- 2 cups spinach
- 1 cup water

Directions

1. All of the smoothie ingredients should be washed.
2. Toss all ingredients into a blender, beginning with the greens and then working your way to the fruit.
3. Blend until smooth, then add additional water until you have the green detox smoothie consistency you want.

Nutritional Values

Calories 310kcal, Carbohydrates-81.6g, Protein 4.5g, Fat 0.1g, Sodium 562mg

774. PINEAPPLE PASSION

- Prep time: 5 mins, Cook time: 0 mins, Total time: 5 mins, Servings: 1

Ingredients

- 1 cup pineapple chunks
- 1 cup low-fat or light vanilla yogurt
- 6 ice cubes

Directions

1. In a blender, combine all ingredients and add lemon juice to taste.
2. Puree until completely smooth.

3. Pour the mixture into 2 cold glasses.

Calories   283kcal,   Carbohydrates-53.5g, Protein 13g, Fat 3.5g, Sodium 167mg

775. PINEAPPLE SUNRISE

- Prep time: 10 mins, Cook time: 0 mins, Total time: 10 mins, Servings: 2

Ingredients

- 1 lime, halved
- 1 pound of carrots, chopped
- 2 cups fresh pineapple chunks
- ice, as desired

Directions

1. Using a juicer, mix the lime, carrots, and pineapple.
2. Serve over ice.

Nutritional Values

Calories   186kcal,   Carbohydrates-46.9g, Protein 3.2g, Fat 0.8g, Sodium 159mg

776. POMEGRANATE, RASPBERRY, AND BANANA SMOOTHIE

Prep Time: 10 min, Cook time: 5 min, Total time: 15 min, Servings: 2

Ingredients

- 125g raspberry and vanilla soy yogurt alternative
- 100g/4oz raspberries
- 1 banana, sliced
- 300ml/½ pint pomegranate juice

Directions

1. In a blender, combine the raspberry, banana, raspberries, vanilla yogurt, and pomegranate juice to produce this superfood dish.
2. Blend until smooth and blended, then divide between 2 glasses & serve.

Nutritional Values

Calories: 169kcal, Carbs: 32g, Protein: | Fat: 1.7g, Sodium: 456mg

777. POMEGRANATE SMOOTHIE

- Drink/Breakfast - Prep time: ready in about: 2 mins, Servings: 1, Grill temp: 0

Ingredients

- 50g of pomegranate seeds
- 1 banana
- 200 ml of almond milk
- 1 apple
- 100g of frozen raspberries
- 2 tsp of agave syrup

Directions

1. Take a blender, add all of your ingredients to it, and blend until smooth.
2. Pour into a glass and serve fresh or chill, as you like.

Nutritional Values

Calories 281 kcal, Carbs 63g, Protein 6g, Fat 3g, Sodium 99mg, Potassium 521mg, Chol 0mg

778. PRESSURE-COOKER CHAI TEA

- Breakfast/Snacks - Prep time: 5 mins, Cook time: 5 mins, Total time: 10 mins, Servings: 4, Grill temp: 300°F

Ingredients

- 1 cup of water plus a ½ cup of water
- 1 cup of almond milk
- 1 ½ tsps of black loose-leaf tea powder
- 2 crushed cardamom pods
- 2 crushed cloves
- 2 tsps of sugar
- 1 tsp of crushed ginger

Directions

1. Pour 1 cup of water into the pressure cooker.
2. Put a bowl in the cooker on top of a trivet, and add all the ingredients.
3. Close and seal the cooker.
4. Cook on low pressure for 3 mins.
5. When time is up, turn down the heat and quick-release.
6. Strain the tea into a favorite mug, and enjoy!

Nutritional Values

Calories 93, Fat 4g, Chol 0mg, Sodium 71.4mg, Potassium 67.7mg, Carbs 10g, Protein 1g

779. RASPBERRY & BLUEBERRY SMOOTHIE

- Drink/Breakfast - Prep time: ready in about: 2 mins, Servings: 1, Grill temp: 0

Ingredients

- 75g of frozen raspberries

- 1 apple
- 75g of frozen raspberries
- ½ tsp of agave syrup
- 200 ml of oat milk

1. Take a blender, add all of your ingredients to it, and blend until smooth.
2. Pour into a glass and serve fresh or chill, as you like.

Nutritional Values

Calories 281 kcal, Carbs 63g, Protein 6g, Fat 3g, Sodium 99mg, Potassium 521mg, Chol 0mg

780. STRAWBERRY-BANANA SMOOTHIE

- Drink/Breakfast - Prep time: ready in about: 5 mins, Servings: 2-3, Grill temp: 0

Ingredients

- 1 cup of strawberries
- 1-½ cup of raspberries
- ½ banana
- 1 tbsp maple syrup
- basil or mint, optional
- 1 cup of almond milk
- 1-½ cups of ice

Directions

1. Take a blender, add all of your ingredients to it and blend them well until smooth.
2. Chill for a while, then serve.

Nutritional Values

Calories 282kcal, Carbs 30g, Protein 16g, Fat 15g, Sodium 886mg, Potassium 734mg, Chol 0mg

781. STRAWBERRY-KIWI SMOOTHIE

- Prep time: 10 mins, Cook time: 0 mins, Total time: 10 mins, Servings: 4

Ingredients

- 1 ripe banana, sliced
- 1¼ cups cold apple juice
- 1½ tsp honey
- 1 kiwi fruit, sliced
- 5 frozen strawberries

Directions

1. Combine the banana, juice, strawberries, kiwifruit, and honey.
2. Keep blending until smooth.

Nutritional Values

Calories 87kcal, Carbohydrates-22g, Protein 0.5g, Fat 0.3g, Sodium 3.5mg

782. SUNRISE DETOX SMOOTHIE

- Prep time: 5 mins, Cook time: 0 mins, Total time: 5 mins, Servings: 1

Ingredients

- ½ cup pineapple- fresh or frozen
- 1 medium banana- frozen
- 1 juice of a lemon- optional
- ½ cup strawberries- frozen
- ½ cup mango- frozen
- 1 cup coconut water- or filtered water

Directions

1. In a high-powered blender, mix all of the ingredients & blend for 2 mins, or until totally smooth.
2. Serve right away.

Nutritional Values

Calories 296kcal, Carbohydrates-75g, Protein 6g, Fat 2g, Sodium 258mg

783. SUNRISE SMOOTHIE

- Prep time: 10 mins, Cook time: 0 mins, Total time: 10 mins, Servings: 4

Ingredients

- 1 cup apricot nectar, chilled
- 1 banana
- ½ cup club soda, chilled
- 1 container- 8 oz. low-Fat peach yogurt
- 1 tbsp frozen lemonade concentrate

Directions

1. Combine the apricot nectar, banana, lemonade concentrate, and yogurt. Process for almost 30 secs, or until creamy and smooth.
2. Serve immediately after stirring in the club soda.

Nutritional Values

Calories 130kcal, Carbohydrates-29g, Protein 2.5g, Fat 0.5g, Sodium 43.5mg

784. TOMATO-KALE GAZPACHO SMOOTHIE

- Prep time: 5 mins, Cook time: 0 mins, Total time: 5 mins, Servings: 2

Ingredients

- ¼ cup water
- 2 tbsp lime juice
- ½ cup plain Greek yogurt
- ¼ tsp ground cumin
- 2 large kale leaves, stems removed
- 1 cup fresh or canned diced tomatoes
- 1 small carrot, chopped
- 1 small English cucumber, chopped
- ½ rib celery, chopped
- ½ cup ice

Directions

1. Toss in a pinch of spicy sauce and mix until smooth.
2. Divide the mixture between 2 glasses.
3. Serve and enjoy.

Nutritional Values

Calories 112kcal, Carbohydrates-16g, Protein 8g, Fat 2.5g, Sodium 79mg

785. TROPICAL PAPAYA PERFECTION

- Prep time: 5 mins, Cook time: 0 mins, Total time: 5 mins, Servings: 1

Ingredients

- 1 papaya, cut into chunks
- 1 cup Fat free plain yogurt
- ½ cup fresh pineapple chunks
- ½ cup crushed ice
- 1 tsp coconut extract
- 1 tsp ground flaxseed

Directions

1. Combine the yogurt, papaya, ice, pineapple, flaxseed, and coconut extract.
2. Process for 30 seconds or until completely frosty and smooth.

Nutritional Values

Calories 299kcal, Carbohydrates-64g, Protein 13g, Fat 1.5g, Sodium 149mg

786. TURMERIC GINGER C BOOST LIFE JUICE

- Prep time: 5 mins, Cook time: 0 mins, Total time: 5 mins, Servings: 1

Ingredients

- 2 Fuji apples, cored and sliced
- 1 orange, peeled and sectioned
- ½ lemon, peeled

- 1- 1 inch piece of fresh ginger
- ½ tsp ground turmeric

Directions

1. Add orange, apples, ginger, and lemon to a juicer, and stir in the turmeric until completely mixed.
2. Serve and enjoy.

Nutritional Values

Calories 163kcal, Carbohydrates-45.8g, Protein 1.6g, Fat 0.8g, Sodium 5.6mg

787. VANILLA-GINGER SYRUP

- Snacks - Prep time: 10 mins, Cook time: 25 mins, Total time: 35 mins, Servings: 4 to 6, Grill temp: 300°F

Ingredients

- 2 cups of water
- 2 cups of sugar
- 1 split vanilla bean
- The 8-ounce thumb of fresh ginger
- Pinch of salt

Directions

1. Rinse the ginger before slicing and then chopping up.
2. Pour water, chopped ginger, salt, sugar, and vanilla bean into a deep pot.
3. Close and seal the pot.
4. Cook for 25 mins on high pressure.
5. When time is up, turn down the heat and let the pressure come down on its own.
6. Pour through a strainer into a glass container.
7. Store in the fridge for up to 3 weeks.

Nutritional Values

Calories 104, Fat 0g, Chol 0mg, Sodium 71.4mg, Potassium 67.7mg, Carbs 26g, Protein 0g

788. VERY BERRY BREAKFAST

- Prep time: 5 mins, Cook time: 0 mins, Total time: 5 mins, Servings: 1

Ingredients

- 1½ tbsp honey
- 1 cup frozen unsweetened raspberries
- 2 tsp fresh lemon juice
- 1 tsp ground flaxseed

- ¼ cup frozen pitted cherries or raspberries, unsweetened
- ¾ cup chilled unsweetened almond or rice milk
- 2 tsp fresh ginger, finely grated

Directions

1. In a blender, combine all ingredients and add lemon juice to taste.
2. Puree until completely smooth.
3. Pour the mixture into 2 cold glasses.

Nutritional Values

Calories 112kcal, Carbohydrates-25g, Protein 1g, Fat 1.5g, Sodium 56mg

789. WASSAIL- HOT MULLED CIDER

- Snacks - Prep time: 10 mins, Cook time: 10 mins, Total time: 20 mins, Servings: 10, Grill temp: 300°F

Ingredients

- 8 cups of apple cider
- 4 cups of orange juice
- 10 cloves
- 2 split vanilla beans
- 5 cinnamon sticks, a 1-inch piece of peeled ginger
- Juice and zest of 2 lemons
- ½ tsp of nutmeg

Directions

1. Pour juice and cider into a pot.
2. Add the lemon, cinnamon, cloves, nutmeg, ginger, and vanilla beans to your steamer basket, and lower them into the pot.
3. Close and seal the lid.
4. Cook on high for 10 mins.
5. Turn down the heat and let the pressure come down naturally.
6. Take out the steamer basket and throw away stuff.

Nutritional Values

Calories 83, Fat 0g, Chol 0mg, Sodium 71.4mg, Potassium 67.7mg, Carbs 9g, Protein 1g

790. WATERMELON WONDER

- Prep time: 5 mins, Cook time: 0 mins, Total time: 5 mins, Servings: 1

Ingredients

- 2 cups ice
- 2 cups chopped watermelon
- ¼ cup Fat free milk

Directions

1. Blend the watermelon and milk for 15 seconds, or until completely smooth.
2. Add the ice and mix for another 20 seconds, or until you reach your desired consistency. If necessary, add additional ice and combine for another 10 seconds.

Nutritional Values

Calories 56kcal, Carbohydrates-13g, Protein 2g, Fat 0.3g, Sodium 19.5mg

791. WORLD'S BEST SMOOTHIE

- Prep time: 5 mins, Cook time: 0 mins, Total time: 5 mins, Servings: 1

Ingredients

- ½ cup orange juice
- 1 cup plain nonFat yogurt
- 1 banana
- 6 frozen strawberries

Directions

1. Combine the banana, yogurt, strawberries, and juice for 20 secs.
2. Scrape down the edges and mix for another 15 secs.

Nutritional Values

Calories 300kcal, Carbohydrates-63g, Protein 14g, Fat 0.5g, Sodium 180mg

792. YUMMY MANGO CITRUS DRINK

- Prep time: 10 mins, Cook time: 0 mins, Total time: 10 mins, Servings: 2

Ingredients

- 1 banana, peeled
- ½ lemon, peeled
- 1 mango - peeled, seeded, and cut into wedges
- ½ orange, peeled
- 2 apples, cut into chunks
- 2 slices of fresh ginger root

Directions

1. Process lemon, banana, orange, mango, ginger, and apples through a juicer.
2. Serve.

Nutritional Values

Calories 180kcal, Carbohydrates-48.5g, Protein 1.7g, Fat 0.7g, Sodium 4.5mg

793. Avocado Pesto Pasta Salad

- Prep time: 10 mins, Cook time: 10 mins, Total time: 20 mins, Servings: 4 cups, Grill temp: 0

Ingredients

- 15 oz. of dry whole wheat fusilli
- 1 cup of spinach
- 2 finely chopped cloves garlic cloves
- 1 ripe avocado
- 1 handful of fresh basil
- 3 tsps of fresh lemon juice
- 1 tsp of extra-virgin olive oil
- Salt and pepper to taste
- ½ cup of halved baby plum tomatoes

Directions

1. Cook the fusilli pasta according to the instructions on the package. Once cooked, drain, then rinse with cold water until the pasta is no longer warm. Set aside.
2. In a blender, add spinach, garlic, avocado, basil leaves, lemon juice, olive oil, and purée. If the sauce is too thick, you may add water. Add salt and pepper to taste and blend some more.
3. Combine the pasta and avocado pesto in a dish and top with the plum tomatoes.

Nutritional Values

Calories 259, Carbs 36.9g, Protein 6g, Fat 9.8g

794. Endo Parm Asparagus

- Prep time: 3 mins, Cook time: 10 mins, Total time: 23 mins, Servings: 4 cups, Grill temp: 0

Ingredients

- ¼ cup of parmesan cheese (grated)
- 3–4 cups of fresh asparagus
- 1 tbsp of extra virgin olive oil
- Salt and pepper to taste

Directions

1. Preheat the oven to 400°F.
2. Place the asparagus on an oven or baking tray.

3. Glaze with extra virgin olive oil and coat with parmesan cheese.
4. Add some salt and pepper.
5. Bake for 10 minutes and enjoy.

Nutritional Values

Calories 259, Carbs 36.9g, Protein: 6g, Fat 9.8g, Protein 3.90g

795. Green Quinoa Salad

- Prep time: 10 mins, Cook time: 25 mins, Total time: 35 mins, Servings: 1 cup, Grill temp: 0

Ingredients

- ⅓ cup of dried quinoa
- ½ medium zucchini, diced
- ½ cup of asparagus, diced
- ½ cup of kale washed with water left on the leaves
- ¼ cup of dried cranberries

Directions

1. Rinse the quinoa well. Cover with 1 inch of water, then cook it over medium heat. Stir the quinoa while cooking. Once there is only a little bit of water left, turn off the heat and cover the pan with a cloth.
2. Stir-fry the zucchini and asparagus for 3 minutes over medium heat. Then add the kale, cover the pan, and cook for a few minutes.
3. Mix the asparagus, zucchini, kale, and quinoa together and top with the dried cranberries.

Nutritional Values

Calories 264, Carbs 53.8g, Protein 8.7g, Fat 3.4g

796. Vegetable Fried Rice

- Prep time: 20 mins, Cook time: 20 mins, Total time: 40 mins, Servings: 6 cups, Grill temp: 0

Ingredients

- 1 tbsp olive oil.
- ½ sweet onion (chopped)
- 1 tbsp grated fresh ginger
- 2 tsp minced garlic
- 1 cup sliced carrots
- ½ cup chopped eggplant

- ½ cup peas
- ½ cup green beans, cut into 1-inch pieces
- 2 tbsp chopped fresh cilantro
- 3 cups cooked rice

Directions

1. Heat the olive oil in a skillet.
2. Sauté the ginger, onion, and garlic for 3 minutes or until softened.
3. Stir in carrot, eggplant, green beans, and peas and sauté for 3 minutes more.
4. Add cilantro and rice.
5. Sauté, constantly stirring, for about 10 minutes or until the rice is heated through.
6. Serve.

Nutritional Values

Calories 189, Fat 7g, Carbs 28g, Phosphorus-89mg, Potassium 172mg, Sodium 13mg, Protein 6g

797. TOFU STIR-FRY

- Prep time: 20 mins, Cook time: 20 mins, Total time: 40 mins, Servings: 4 cups, Grill temp: 0

Ingredients

For the tofu
- 1 tbsp lemon juice
- 1 tsp minced garlic
- 1 tsp grated fresh ginger
- Pinch red pepper flakes
- 5 ounces extra-firm tofu, pressed well and cubed

For the stir-fry
- 1 tbsp olive oil.
- ½ cup cauliflower florets
- ½ cup thinly sliced carrots
- ½ cup julienned red pepper
- ½ cup fresh green beans
- 2 cups cooked white rice

Directions

1. In a bowl, mix the lemon juice, garlic, ginger, and red pepper flakes.
2. Add the tofu and toss to coat.
3. Place the bowl in the refrigerator and marinate for 2 hours.
4. To make the stir-fry, heat the oil in a skillet.
5. Sauté the tofu for 8 minutes or until it is lightly browned and heated through.

6. Add the carrots and cauliflower, and sauté for 5 minutes. Stirring and tossing constantly.
7. Add the red pepper and green beans, and sauté for 3 minutes more.
8. Serve over white rice.

Nutritional Values

Calories 190, Fat 6g, Carb-30g, Phosphorus-90mg, Potassium 199mg, Sodium 22mg, Protein 6g

798. ALMONDS & BLUEBERRIES SMOOTHIE

- Prep time: 5 mins, Cook time: 0 mins, Total time: 5 mins, Servings: 2 cups, Grill temp: 0

Ingredients

- ¼ cup of ground almonds, unsalted
- 1 cup of fresh blueberries
- Fresh juice of 1 lemon
- 1 cup of fresh Kale leaves
- ½ cup of coconut water
- 1 cup of water
- 2 tbsp of plain yogurt (optional)

Directions

1. Put all the ingredients in your high-speed blender, and blend until your smoothie is smooth.
2. Pour the mixture into a chilled glass.
3. Serve and enjoy!

Nutritional Values

Calories 110, Carbs 8g, Proteins-2g, Fat 7g, Fiber-2g

799. ALMONDS AND ZUCCHINI SMOOTHIE

- Prep time: 5 mins, Cook time: 0 mins, Total time: 5 mins, Servings: 2 cups, Grill temp: 0

Ingredients

- 1 cup of zucchini, cooked and mashed - unsalted
- 1 ½ cup of almond milk
- 1 tbsp of almond butter (plain, unsalted)
- 1 tsp of pure almond extract
- 2 tbsp of ground almonds or Macadamia almonds
- ½ cup of water
- 1 cup of Ice cubes crushed (optional for serving)

Directions

1. Put all the ingredients from the list above in your fast-speed blender; blend for 45 - 60 seconds or to taste.
2. Serve with crushed ice.

Nutritional Values

Calories 322, Carbs 6g, Proteins-6g, Fat 30g, Fiber-3.5g

800. AVOCADO WITH WALNUT BUTTER SMOOTHIE

- Prep time: 5 mins, Cook time: 0 mins, Total time: 5 mins, Servings: 2 cups, Grill temp: 0

Ingredients

- 1 avocado (diced)
- 1 cup of baby spinach
- 1 cup of coconut milk (canned)
- 1 tbsp of walnut butter, unsalted
- 2 tbsp of natural sweeteners, such as Stevia, Erythritol, Truvia...etc.

Directions

1. Place all the ingredients into a food processor or a blender; blend until smooth or to taste.
2. Add more or less walnut butter.
3. Drink and enjoy!

Nutritional Values

Calories 364, Carbs 7g, Proteins-8g, Fat 35g, Fiber-5.5g

801. BABY SPINACH AND DILL SMOOTHIE

- Prep time: 5 mins, Cook time: 0 mins, Total time: 5 mins, Servings: 2 cups, Grill temp: 0

Ingredients

- 1 cup of fresh baby spinach leaves
- 2 tbsp of fresh dill, chopped
- 1 ½ cup of water
- ½ avocado, chopped into cubes
- 1 tbsp of chia seeds
- 2 tbsp of natural sweetener Stevia

Directions

1. Place all the ingredients into a fast-speed blender. Beat until smooth and all ingredients united well.
2. Serve and enjoy!

Nutritional Values

Calories 136, Carbs 8g, Proteins-7g, Fat 10g, Fiber-9g

802. BLUEBERRIES AND COCONUT SMOOTHIE

- Prep time: 5 mins, Cook time: 0 mins, Total time: 5 mins, Servings: 5 cups, Grill temp: 0

Ingredients

- 1 cup of frozen blueberries, unsweetened
- 1 cup of Stevia or Erythritol sweetener
- 2 cups of coconut milk (canned)
- 1 cup of fresh spinach leaves
- 2 tbsp of shredded coconut (unsweetened)
- 3/4 cup of water

Directions

1. Place all the ingredients from the list in the food processor or in your strong blender.
2. Blend for 45 - 60 seconds or to taste. Ready for a drink!
3. Serve!

Nutritional Values

Calories 190, Carbs 8g, Proteins-3g, Fat 18g, Fiber-2g

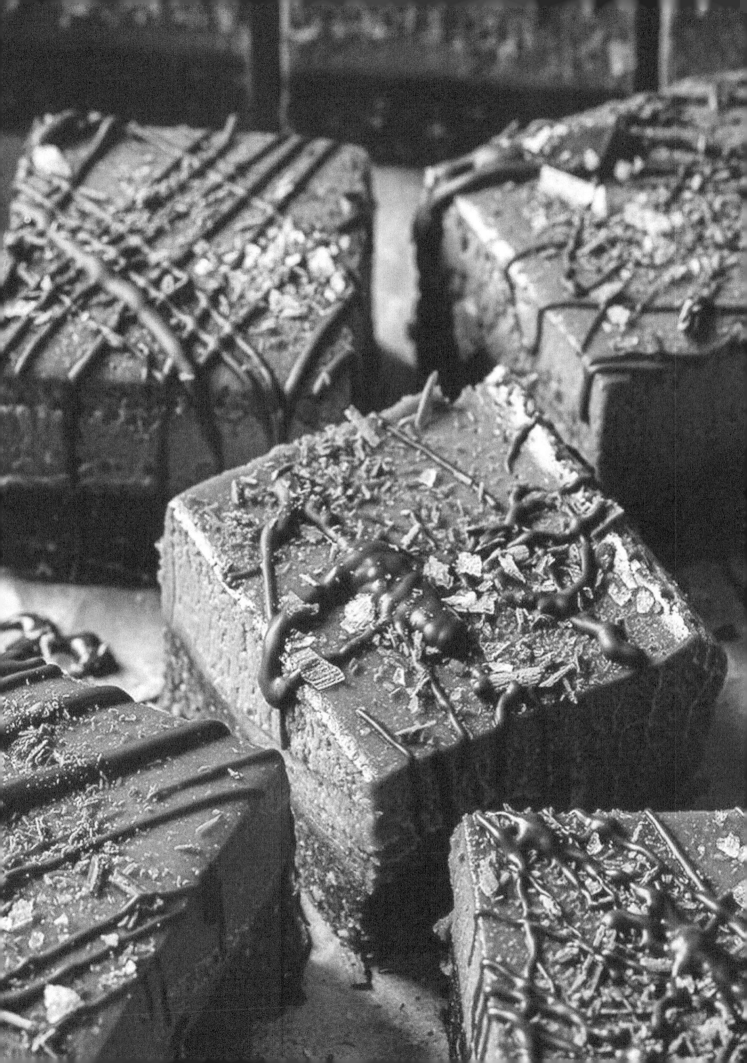

Chapter 21.

Measurement Conversion Chart

COOKING CONVERSION CHART

Measurement

CUP	ONCES	MILLILITERS	TABLESPOONS
8 cup	64 oz	1895 ml	128
6 cup	48 oz	1420 ml	96
5 cup	40 oz	1180 ml	80
4 cup	32 oz	960 ml	64
2 cup	16 oz	480 ml	32
1 cup	8 oz	240 ml	16
3/4 cup	6 oz	177 ml	12
2/3 cup	5 oz	158 ml	11
1/2 cup	4 oz	118 ml	8
3/8 cup	3 oz	90 ml	6
1/3 cup	2.5 oz	79 ml	5.5
1/4 cup	2 oz	59 ml	4
1/8 cup	1 oz	30 ml	3
1/16 cup	1/2 oz	15 ml	1

Temperature

FAHRENHEIT	CELSIUS
100 °F	37 °C
150 °F	65 °C
200 °F	93 °C
250 °F	121 °C
300 °F	150 °C
325 °F	160 °C
350 °F	180 °C
375 °F	190 °C
400 °F	200 °C
425 °F	220 °C
450 °F	230 °C
500 °F	260 °C
525 °F	274 °C
550 °F	288 °C

Weight

IMPERIAL	METRIC
1/2 oz	15 g
1 oz	29 g
2 oz	57 g
3 oz	85 g
4 oz	113 g
5 oz	141 g
6 oz	170 g
8 oz	227 g
10 oz	283 g
12 oz	340 g
13 oz	369 g
14 oz	397 g
15 oz	425 g
1 lb	453 g

The measurement conversion charts are given below for a variety of parameters. In addition, here are some conversion tables to help you measure recipes accurately.

WEIGHTS

SOLIDS

g	kg	oz	lb.
30g	0.03kg	1oz	
90g	0.09kg	3oz	
125g	0.125kg	4oz	¼ lb.
250g	0.25kg	8oz	½ lb.
500g	0.5kg	16oz	1 lb.
1,000g	1kg	32oz	2 lb.
1,500g	1.5kg	48oz	3 lb.
2,000g	2 kg	64 oz	4 lb.

LIQUIDS

Imperial measures	ml	fl oz
¼ tsp	1.25ml	
½ tsp	2.5ml	
1 tsp	5ml	⅛ fl oz
1 tsp	10ml	¼ fl oz
½ tbs	10ml	¼ fl oz
1 tbs	20ml	½ fl oz
¼ cup	60ml	2 fl oz
⅓ cup	80ml	
½ cup	125ml	4 fl oz
1 cup	250ml	8 fl oz

Ingredient	Amount	g
Almond meal	1 cup	120g
Almonds	1 cup	140g
Barley, pearled uncooked	1 cup	200g
Black beans, dry	1 cup	190g
Breadcrumbs, dry	1 cup	90g
Buckwheat, uncooked	1 cup	190g
Cashews	1 cup	140g
Chia seeds	1 tps	5g
Chia seeds	¼ cup	50g
Chickpea dry	1 cup	190g
Chickpea flour	½ cup	60g
Cocoa powder	1 cup	100g
Coconut, desiccated	1 cup	85g
Couscous, uncooked	1 cup	180g
Dates. pitted	1 cup	155g
Flour, buckwheat	1 cup	140g
Flour, plain	1 cup	150g
Flour, rice	1 cup	180g
Freekeh, uncooked	1 cup	200g
honey	½ cup	160g
Kidney beans, red, dry	1 cup	190g
Lentils, brown, dry	1 cup	210g
Lentils, puy, dry	1 cup	200g
Lentils, red, split, dry	1 cup	190g
Linseeds, whole	1 tbs	5g
Linseeds, whole	¼ cup	45g
Milk	1 cup	250g
Millet, hulled, uncooked	1 cup	190g
Olive oil	1 tbs	20g
Peanut butter	1 tbs	20g
Peanut butter	¼ cup	70g

Ingredient	Amount	g
Pepitas	¼ cup	40g
Popcorn kernels	1 cup	225g
Quinoa, uncooked	1 cup	190g
Rice, arborio rice, uncooked	1 cup	220g
Rice, long-grain, basmati, uncooked	1 cup	210g
Rice, long-grain, brown, uncooked	1 cup	210g
Rice, sushi rice, uncooked	1 cup	225g
Rolled oats, traditional	1 cup	105g
Sugar, raw	1 cup	205g
Sugar, caster	1 cup	215g
Sugar, brown	1 cup	200g
Sultanas	1 cup	170g
Sunflower seeds	¼ cup	40g
Yogurt	1 cup	250g
Tahini	1 tbs	20g
Tahini	¼ cup	65g
Walnuts, whole pieces	1 cup	110g

BAKING MEASUREMENTS

If a recipe calls for this amount	You can also measure it this way
Dash	2 or 3 drops (liquid) or less than 1/8 teaspoon of (dry)
One tablespoon of	3 teaspoons or Half ounce
Two tablespoons of	1 ounce
A quarter cup of	4 tablespoons or 2 ounces
1/3 cup	5 tablespoons plus one teaspoon
Half cup of	8 tablespoons or 4 ounces
3/4 cup	1Two tablespoons of or 6 ounces
One cup of	16 tablespoons or 8 ounces
1 pint	2 cups or 16 ounces or 1 pound
1 quart	Four cups of or 2 pints
1 gallon	4 quarts
1 pound	16 ounces

VOLUME MEASUREMENTS

US Units	Canadian Units	Australian Units
A quarter teaspoon of	1 ml	1 ml
Half teaspoon of	2 ml	2 ml
One teaspoon of	5 ml	5 ml
One tablespoon of	15 ml	20 ml
A quarter cup of	50 ml	60 ml
1/3 cup	75 ml	80 ml
Half cup of	125 ml	125 ml
2/3 cup	150 ml	170 ml
3/4 cup	175 ml	190 ml
One cup of	250 ml	250 ml
1 quart	1 liter	1 liter
1 and a half quarts	One and a half liters	One and a half liters
2 quarts	2 liters	2 liters
2 and a half quarts	2.5 liters	2.5 liters
3 quarts	3 liters	3 liters
4 quarts	4 liters	4 liters

WEIGHT MEASUREMENTS

US Units	Canadian Metric	Australian Metric
1 ounce	30 grams	30 grams
2 ounces	55 grams	60 grams
3 ounces	85 grams	90 grams
4 ounces (1/4 pound)	115 grams	125 grams
8 ounces (half a pound)	225 grams	225 grams
16 ounces (1 pound)	455 grams	500 grams (half a Kg)

Fahrenheit (F)	Celsius (C) Approximate
212	100
250	120
275	140
300	150
325	160
350	180
375	190
400	200
425	220
450	230
475	240
500	260

TEMPERATURES

C	F	
110°	225°	very cool
120°	250°	
140°	275°	cool
150°	300°	
160°	325°	warm
180°	350°	moderate
190°	375°	moderately hot
200°	400°	
220°	425°	
230°	450°	hot
240°	475°	very hot
250°	500°	

CONVERSION CHART

Liquid Measure

8 ounces =	1 cup
2 cups =	1 pint
16 ounces =	1 pint
4 cups =	1 quart
1 gill =	1/2 cup or 1/4 pint
2 pints =	1 quart
4 quarts =	1 gallon
31.5 gal. =	1 barrel

3 tsp =	1 tbsp
2 tbsp =	1/8 cup or 1 fluid ounce
4 tbsp =	1/4 cup
8 tbsp =	1/2 cup
1 pinch =	1/8 tsp or less
1 tsp =	60 drops

Conversion of US Liquid Measure to Metric System

1 fluid oz. =	29.573 milliliters
1 cup =	230 milliliters
1 quart =	.94635 liters
1 gallon =	3.7854 liters
.033814 fluid ounce =	1 milliliter
3.3814 fluid ounces =	1 deciliter
33.814 fluid oz. or 1.0567 qt.=	1 liter

Dry Measure

2 pints =	1 quart
4 quarts =	1 gallon
8 quarts =	2 gallons or 1 peck
4 pecks =	8 gallons or 1 bushel
16 ounces =	1 pound
2000 lbs. =	1 ton

Conversion of US Weight and Mass Measure to Metric System

.0353 ounces =	1 gram
1/4 ounce =	7 grams
1 ounce =	28.35 grams
4 ounces =	113.4 grams
8 ounces =	226.8 grams
1 pound =	454 grams
2.2046 pounds =	1 kilogram
.98421 long ton or 1.1023 short tons =	1 metric ton

Linear Measure

12 inches =	1 foot
3 feet =	1 yard
5.5 yards =	1 rod
40 rods =	1 furlong
8 furlongs (5280 feet) =	1 mile
6080 feet =	1 nautical mile

Conversion of US Linear Measure to Metric System

1 inch =	2.54 centimeters
1 foot =	.3048 meters
1 yard =	.9144 meters
1 mile =	1609.3 meters or 1.6093 kilometers
.03937 in. =	1 millimeter
.3937 in.=	1 centimeter
3.937 in.=	1 decimeter
39.37 in.=	1 meter
3280.8 ft. or .62137 miles =	1 kilometer

To convert a Fahrenheit temperature to Centigrade, do the following:
a. Subtract 32   b. Multiply by 5   c. Divide by 9

To convert Centigrade to Fahrenheit, do the following:
a. Multiply by 9   b. Divide by 5   c. Add 32

CUPS	TBSP	TSP	ML
1	16	48	250
3/4	12	36	175
2/3	11	32	150
1/2	8	24	125
1/3	5	16	70
1/4	4	12	60
1/8	2	6	30
1/16	1	3	15

Conclusion

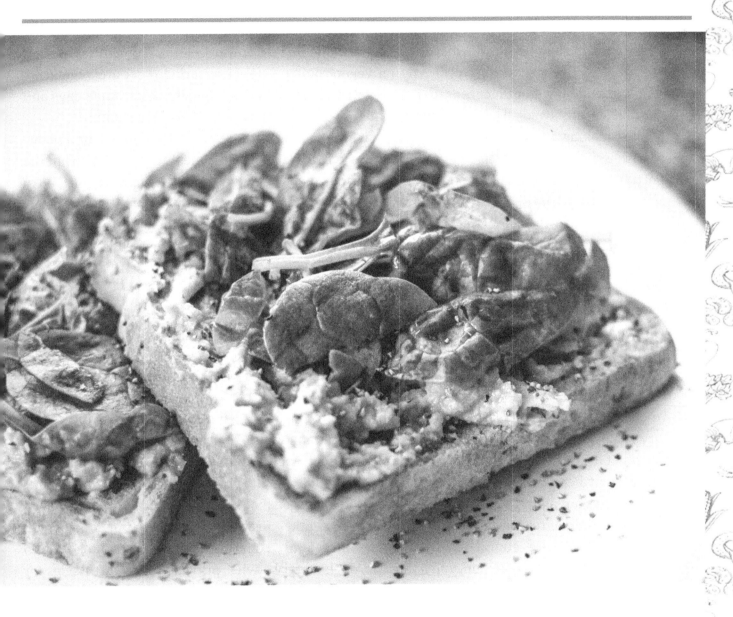

A plant-based diet is a group of diets, and all have one thing in common: they reduce animal-derived meals in favor of plant-based meals. Rather than a meat-and-dairy-centered diet, fruits, vegetables, & whole grains take center stage. It is a light, tasty way of eating that's been linked to various health advantages, including weight reduction and illness prevention. Plant-based meals exclude meat, milk, and eggs and comprise only plant foods such as fruits, veggies, legumes, and grains. Plant-based meals are high in fiber, vitamins & minerals, are cholesterol-free, and have a low calorie & saturated fat content. Consuming a mix of these meals will offer your body all of the calcium, protein, and other critical nutrients it requires. It's critical to get enough vitamin B12 from a reputable source. A regular dose of protected foods, such as vitamin B12-enriched plant milk, morning cereals, and nutritional yeast, may easily satisfy your vitamin-B12 requirements.

Eaters of plant-based food have a decreased risk of cardiovascular disease, obesity, type 2 diabetes, and other diseases. According to research, a plant-based meal is not as costly as an omnivorous one. It's worth emphasizing, though, that the plant-based does not always imply healthy, especially when it is packaged and processed foods. Although goods like white flour, refined sugar, and some vegetable fats are essentially plant-based, this doesn't imply that they must make up the majority of a balanced diet. People frequently have various ideas about what it means to eat a "plant-based" diet.

A flexitarian or semi-vegetarian diet allows some individuals to consume limited quantities of meat and seafood while concentrating primarily on vegetarian cuisine. Pescatarian diets are vegetarian diets that exclude meat but incorporate fish. Vegetarians avoid fish and meat but consume eggs and dairy, while vegans avoid all animal-derived foods, including honey, eggs, dairy, and gelatin.

If you're making a substantial dietary change, it's a good idea to ease into it by adding 2 or 3 plant-based dishes a day or each week. This enables the body to adjust to new meals and variations in the proportions of specific nutrients, such as fiber, in your diet. It also gives you the opportunity to try new items and stock up on store-cupboard favorites over time.

Whole foods plant-based eating promotes plant foods while avoiding unhealthy foods such as refined grains and added sugars. It has long been known that eating a plant-based diet may help prevent heart disease, cancer, obesity, diabetes, and cognitive decline. Plant-based eating is also beneficial to the environment. You will see a big improvement in your health regardless of what kind of whole-foods, plant-based diet you follow. Veganism is both a way of life and philosophy. Diet has no bearing on it at all. In addition to health and environmental considerations, those who follow plant-based diets do so for several other reasons. Various levels of animal product exclusion are permissible. There are three types of plant-based diets: veganism, flexitarians, and pescatarians. For both humans and the ecosystem, eating a plant-based diet is beneficial.

To prevent nutritional deficiency, those who desire to consume a plant-based diet must meet their dietary requirements. Many people are reducing or eliminating their use of animal products. Some people don't describe themselves as vegan or plant-based, whereas others do. The term "plant-based" is often used in diets, mostly plant-based meals, and excludes animal products. The whole foods, plant-based diet does not allow the use of oils or processed packaged foods.

For a multitude of reasons, vegans eat this way. One of the most important factors of good health. Additionally, there are ethical, environmental, and moral concerns that must be taken into consideration. In this introduction, you'll find thorough dietary advice, purchasing tips, strategies for altering eating habits, and information and thoughts on the issue. However, the recipes are what pique the interest of the audience. In the end, it's a cookbook! Everyone who wants to eat tasty, nutritious, and pleasant cuisine may find it at our establishment. What you put in your mouth is more important than what you don't put in your mouth to keep yourself in good health via your vegan lifestyle. When it comes to veganism, it's not about deprivation; it's about enjoyment.

A precise definition of what constitutes a plant-based diet is missing (WFPB diet). The WFPB diet is more of a way of life than a strict diet plan. It's because plant-based diets may vary substantially depending on how many animal items are included in a person's diet.

Nonetheless, the following are the essential concepts of a plant-based diet:
- Whole, less processed meals are emphasized.

- Animal products are limited or avoided.
- Plants, such as fruits, vegetables, legumes, whole grains, seeds, and nuts, should make up the bulk of your diet.
- Refined foods, such as added sugars, white flour, and processed oils, are excluded.
- Food quality is prioritized, with many supporters of the WFPB diet advocating for locally produced, organic foods wherever feasible.

This diet is often mistaken for vegetarian or vegan diets as a result of these factors. However, although comparable in some aspects, these diets are not the same. Vegans avoid eating animal products, including poultry, dairy, meat, eggs, fish, and honey. Vegetarians avoid all meat and poultry. However, some vegetarians consume eggs, shellfish, or dairy products. On the other side, the WFPB diet is more adaptable. For example, animal items are not forbidden to followers, mostly consuming vegetables. Moreover, while one WFPB dieter may avoid all animal products, others may have limited quantities of eggs, poultry, fish, meat, or dairy. Plant-based foods are prioritized in the whole-foods, plant-based diet, limiting animal products and processed meals. It Has the Potential to Assist You in Losing Weight and Improving Your Health.

Obesity has become a global problem. Over 69 percent of people in the United States are obese or overweight. Fortunately, implementing dietary and lifestyle adjustments may help you lose weight and improve your health in the long run. Plant-based diets have been found to help people lose weight in several studies.

The WFPB diet's high fiber content, along with its avoidance of processed foods, is a good combo for losing weight. Plant-based diets resulted in considerable weight loss — around 4.5 pounds (2 kilograms) over an average of Eighteen weeks —compared to non-vegetarian diets, according to a study of 12 trials involving over 1,100 participants. Adopting a plant-based eating pattern may also help you maintain your weight loss over time.

A study of 65 overweight and obese people revealed that those on a WFPB diet dropped much more weight than those on a control diet and that the weight reduction of 9.25 pounds (4.2kg) was maintained throughout a 1-year follow-up period. Furthermore, eliminating processed items that aren't permitted on the WFPB diet, such as soda, sweets, fast food, and refined grains, is a potent weight reduction technique in and of itself.

If you're looking to lose weight and improve your health, you'll want to focus on eating primarily plant-based food instead of animal-based food. This is because animal products and synthetic chemicals are absent from plant-based foods, including those above (such as fruits, vegetables, grains, seeds, nuts, legumes, and other grains and legume products). In contrast to a vegan diet, a plant-based diet may not always exclude or limit the consumption of animals. Pregnancy, childhood, lactation, and adulthood, as well as athletes, can all benefit from properly-planned plant-based diets, according to the Academy of Nutritional facts per servings and Dietetics.

Dietary patterns that emphasize plant-based foods like fruits, vegetables, whole grains, nuts, legumes, and seeds are called "plant-based diets." There is a wide range of definitions for "plant-based diet," including vegan diets (consisting entirely of plant-based foods), vegetarian diets (which may include dairy or eggs but no meat), and real Mediterranean diets (which contain some meat).

Due to crop, freshwater, and energy resource limitations, around four billion people are expected to subsist on a plant-based diet, either by choice or necessity. As a result of worries about health, food security, and animal welfare, the European market for plant-based meat substitutes accounted for

40% of the global market in 2019. Foods made from plants grew at an eight-fold rate quicker than food from other sources in 2019.

This book focuses on the recipes that help you lose weight and the meal plan specifically designed for beginners. Hope you like the book and acknowledge the vitality and importance of a plant-based diet.

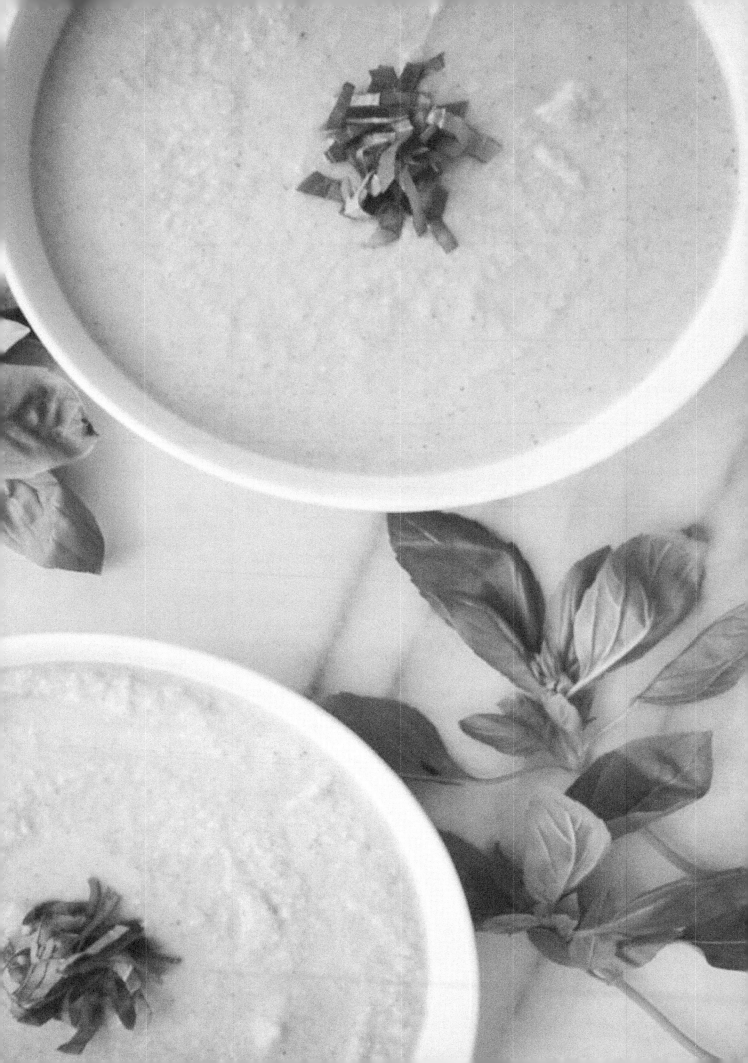

Recipes Index

2

2-Minute Steamed Asparagus 135

6

6 Ingredients Mexican Quinoa 286

A

Acai-Bowl Recipe 56
Adzuki-Bean-Bowls 158
Air Fryer-French- Fries 149
Air-Fryer Onion-Rings 143
Alanna's Pumpkin Cranberry Nut & Seed Loaf 87
Almond and breadcrumb–stuffed piquillo peppers 106
Almond Butter Brown Rice Crispy Treats 78
Almond Flour 376
Almost-Raw Carrot Balls 87
American Goulash 317
Anna's Avocado & Lemon Zest Spaghetti...................252
Anthony Worrall Thompson's herby fruit salad recipe 354
Anti-Inflammatory Juice Recipe 388
Apple Berry Detox Smoothie 388
Apple Chicken Stew 212
Apple-Oatmeal-Cookies 361
Apple-Pie-Spice 374
Applesauce Cake 360
Apple-Strawberry-Smoothie 388
Apricot-Mango Madness.....................................388
Apricot-Pear Cake..360
Arancini (Risotto balls) 214
Arugula-Salad with Lemon-Vinaigrette 153
Asparagus Avocado Soup 111
Autumn Wheat Berry Salad.................................302
Avocado and White-Bean-Salad Wraps....................93
Avocado couscous salad recipe 352

Avocado Cucumber Sushi Roll...............................298
Avocado Detox Smoothie....................................388
Avocado Fries 144
Avocado-Crispbreads w/ Everything-Bagel-Seasoning.....167
Avocado-Cucumber-Sushi-Roll..............................162
Avocado-Sweet-Potato-Tacos...............................156

B

Baba Ganoush 130
Baby Bok Choy Salad with Sesame Dressing 302
Baby Lima Bean and Quinoa Salad........................302
Baked Apples...55
Baked Bean Toast (3-Ingredient)...........................264
Baked Potato-Wedges 145
Baked-Sweet-Potato-Fries...................................149
Balela Salad 277
Banana Ginger Smoothie 389
Banana-Amaranth Porridge..................................54
Banana-Blueberry-Soy Smoothie 389
Banana-Buckwheat Porridge.................................58
Banh-Mi-Sandwich 125
Barley Bowl 274
Barley with Winter Vegetable Soup 184
Bean Chili 273
Béchamel sauce 380
Beefless Stew 212
Beefy Cabbage Bean Stew..................................207
Beet Greens Smoothie 389
Beetroot, pomegranate, and parsnip soup recipe 355
Best Ever Sauteed Kale......................................347
Best Hummus 378
Best Lentil Soup...80
Best Roasted Vegetables (Perfectly Seasoned 338
Best-Zucchini-Bread 366
Bibim-bap 166
Bisteeya (Moroccan phyllo pie).............................214
Black Bean + Quinoa Burritos...............................277
Black Bean + Sweet Potato Hash...........................58
Black Bean Breakfast Burritos 265

Black Bean Chili 267
Black Bean Soup 184
Black Bean, Corn & Avocado Salad 270
Black Beans 279
Black beans and rice 330
Black Rice Pudding with Coconut 367
Black-Bean-Chili 152
Blackberry Soda Syrup 389
Blistered Shishito Peppers 70
BLT Pasta Salad 234
BLT Sandwich 126
Blueberry Detox Smoothie 390
Blueberry Muffins 59
Blueberry overnight oats 333
Blueberry Pancakes 55
Blueberry-Banana-Wraps 91
Box-Buddha-Bowls 154
Braised brussels sprouts with chestnuts 107
Braised Pork Stew 205
Breakfast Bowl with Amaranth Granola 64
Breakfast burritos 59
Breakfast Scramble 60
Breakfast Tofu Scramble 60
Breakfast-Veggie-Burger Recipe 58
Broccoli and Arugula Soup 203
Broccoli Apple Smoothie 390
Broccoli Basil Cream Soup 197
Broccoli Tahini Pasta Salad 248
Brown Rice 154
Buckwheat Apple Cobbler 368
Buffalo-Cauliflower-Pita-Pockets 129
Bulgur, Cucumber and Tomato Salad 303
Burrata 70
Burrito 263
Burrito with Tofu Scramble 262
Butternut Squash Black Bean Enchiladas with Jalapeño Cashew
    Crema 266
Butternut Squash Burrito Bowls 299
Butternut Squash Noodle Pasta 245
Butternut Squash Soup with Apple Grilled Cheese Sandwiches 312
Butternut squash tagine 215
Butternut-Squash-Risotto 153
Butternut-Squash-Soup 172
Buttery Garlic Green Beans 303

C

Cabbage Roll Casserole 318
Cabbage Soup 181
Caesar Salad 269
California Burritos 91
Carrot and Apple Juice 390
Carrot and ginger soup recipe 313
Carrot and Orange Juice 390
Carrot Muffins 288
Carrot Smorrebrod Crisps 68
Carrot-Coconut-Soup 177
Carrot-Smorrebrod-Crisps 126
Carrot-Soup-Recipe w/ Ginger 176
Carrot-Tomato Sauce 380
Cashew Broccoli Soba Noodles 238
Cashew Cream 375
Cashew Cream for Two 87
Cashew ricotta 381
Cassoulet 215
Cauliflower Mac & Cheese 251
Cauliflower Rice Kimchi Bowls 293
Cauliflower Soup 176
Cauliflower-Rice-Kimchi-Bowls 160
Celery Cucumber Green Juice 390
Chai-Spiced Oatmeal with Mango 61
Chana Masala 295
Cheese Sauce 375
Cheesy Ground Beef & Cauliflower Casserole 314
Cherry Beet Smoothie 391
Cherry Mango Anti-Inflammatory Smoothie 391
Chia Overnight Oats 2 Ways! 300
Chicken Cutlets with Sun-Dried Tomato Cream Sauce 316
Chicken Detox Soup 194
Chicken Mushroom Stew 207
Chicken(less) Soup 112
Chickpea Noodle Soup 279
Chickpea Tikka Masala 272
Chickpea-Salad Sandwich 125
Chickpea-Salad-Sandwiches 100
Chickpea-Salad-Wraps with Avocado-Dill-Sauce 96
Chili Powder 374
Chipotle Black Bean Avocado Toast 264
Chipotle-Ranch-Dressing 374
Chocolate Avocado Pudding Pops 81
Chocolate Cheesecake 368
Chocolate Chip, Apricot, And Orange Scones 287
Chocolate Cups 71
Chocolate Fondue with Coconut Cream 369
Chocolate peanut butter oatmeal 335
Chocolate-Avocado-Pudding-Pops 363
Chunky English garden salad recipe 352
Cilantro Lime Rice 72
Cinnamon-Poached Pears with Chocolate Sauce 369
Cinnamon-Roasted-Sweet-Potato-Salad with Wild-Rice 155
Citrus Green Beans with Pine Nuts 303
Classic (Vegan) Chili 184
Classic Hummus 123
Classic vegetable soup 112
Clean Vegan Pad Thai 216
Cleanse & Detox Smoothie: Dairy, Sugar & Gluten-Free 392
Cleansing carrot autumn squash soup 195
Cleansing detox soup 193
Coconut Bacon 156
Coconut Curry 166
Coconut lemongrass noodle soup 350

Coconut-Almond Risotto 61
Coconut-Water-Smoothie 391
Cold Cucumber Soba 237
Cold Sesame Noodles with Kale & Shiitakes 244
Cold Tomato Summer Vegetable Soup 113
Collard Greens 274
Cooked Brown Rice 294
Corn "Ceviche" Crostini 85
Corn Pakora, baked, no oil 342
Cowboy Caviar 148
Cranberry Simple Syrup 391
Cranberry-Walnut Quinoa 61
Cream of mushroom soup 113
Cream of Mushroom Soup 68
Cream of Thyme Tomato Soup 113
Creamy Broccoli Soup with "Chicken" and Rice 185
Creamy Butternut Squash Pasta 242
Creamy Butternut Squash Soup 196
Creamy Cauliflower Soup 114
Creamy corn chowder 114
Creamy Dill Potato Salad 276
Creamy Nutmeg Broccoli Soup 202
Creamy Pasta Pomodoro 256
Creamy pasta with Swiss chard and tomatoes 216
Creamy pea and watercress soup recipe 353
Creamy Potato Soup 268
Creamy Pumpkin Pasta Sauce 248
Creamy tomato, basil & rice soup 291
Creamy Vegan Pasta 249
Creamy Vegan Pasta Bake with Brussels Sprouts 259
Creamy Vegan Shiitake & Kale Pasta 247
Creamy-Chipotle-Sauce 376
Creamy-Mushroom-Soup 173
Creamy-Potato-Soup 182
Cremini Mushroom Soup 198
Crispy Chickpeas 279
Crispy quinoa cakes 217
Crispy-Roasted-Chickpeas 146
Crunchy-Egg-Salad 57
Cucumber and prawn stir-fry recipe 351
Cucumber Mango Miso Noodle Bowl...........................239
Curried Beef Stew 210
Curried cauliflower coconut soup 115
Curried Chickpea Salad 270
Curried Rice Salad 304
Curried Tempeh Quinoa Breakfast Hash 339
Curried-Lentil-Salad 154
Curry Roasted Cauliflower 105

D

Detox Deliciously: Ginger-Carrot Soup 203
Detox Green Smoothie with Grapes.............................392
Detox Smoothie...392
Detox Turmeric Ginger Miso Soup 340

Deviled-Potato Sandwiches...89
Digestive Aid Green Juice 392

E

Easiest Chia Pudding 66
Easy Detox Smoothie 393
Easy Garlic-Roasted Potatoes......................................106
Easy guacamole 323
Easy Italian Wedding Soup 315
Easy low fodmap shakshuka 292
Easy Oil-Free Granola (with lots of crunchy clusters!) 290
Easy Peanut Noodles...237
Easy Pesto Pasta 258
Easy Sauteed Cabbage 346
Easy-Vegan-Chili 377
Edible Cookie Dough 75
Eggplant and roasted tomato polenta lasagna 217
Eggplant chickpea curry 326
Elderberry Syrup 393
Enchilada Rice 287

F

Falafel..79
Falafel Flatbread 157
Farro risotto with roasted fennel and mushrooms 218
Fat-Free Crock Pot Chili...339
Fava Bean Dip..381
Fettuccine & Sweet Corn Cream 255
Flush the Fat Away Vegetable Soup 199
Four ingredient cookies...324
Fragrant Cauliflower Rice 138
French-Onion-Dip...148
French-Onion-Soup 178
Fresh Spring Rolls 88
Fresh Spring-Rolls 95
Fruited Millet Salad 304

G

Garlic Sautéed Spinach..138
Giambotta (Italian summer vegetable stew)...............115
Ginger kale soup 116
Ginger Miso Noodles with Eggplant 246
Ginger Noodles with Kale & Shiitakes 238
Ginger-Miso-Soup 180
Glowing Green Detox Smoothie...................................393
Gluten-free, vegan breakfast cookies 334
Golden Detox Smoothie...393
Golden Turmeric Noodle Miso Soup 247
Grandma's chicken-y noodle soup 116
Granola recipe...355

Grapefruit Smoothie..394
Greek Broccoli Salad..305
Greek Quinoa Salad...270
Green Beans Almondine (Amandine) 271
Green curry vegetable stew 117
Green detox smoothie..394
Green Dragon Veggie Juice....................................394
Green Juice for Beginners......................................394
Green Pea, Lettuce and Tomato Sandwich............100
Green Protein Detox Smoothie 395
Green Tea, Blueberry, and banana 395
Greens & Things Sandwiches................................127
Grilled Tartines 84
Grilled tofu caprese 219
Grilled-Ratatouille-Tartines 131
Grilled-Vegetable-Wrap W/ Balsamic-Mayo 168
Guacamole Soup...117
Gumbo filé 118

H

Hazelnut tahini pasta...252
Healthy Baked Beans..278
Healthy Banana-Muffins...133
Healthy Carrot Cake Cookies 288
Healthy Chai-Spiced Carrot Banana Bread with Cream Cheese
    Frosting 289
Healthy Green Juice..395
Healthy Green Juice with Lemon 396
Healthy Huevos Rancheros Tacos 286
Healthy Loaded Vegan Nachos 81
Healthy-Banana-Bread 367
Hearty Lentil Soup 272
Hearty seitan roast 219
Herb Compound Butter 89
Herbed zucchini 123
Homemade Applesauce..374
Homemade Brownies 360
Homemade Ginger-Lemon Cough Syrup 396
Homemade Granola 145
Homemade Ketchup 382
Homemade Marinated Mushrooms 124
Homemade Salsa 147
Homemade Soft-Pretzels...98
Homemade Taquitos 146
Homemade Vanilla Extract 396
Honey Butter 374
Honey Pecan Granola with Cherry Recipe 363
How to Make Veggie Noodles 235
Huevos Rancheros Casserole 263

I

Imam bayildi (Turkish stuffed eggplant) 108

Instant Pot Black Beans 268
Instant Pot Buckwheat Porridge............................291
Instant-Pot Mashed-Potatoes 145
Instant-Pot-Black-Beans 152
Instant-Pot-Lentil-Soup 183
Israeli Quinoa Salad...305

J

Jackfruit-Barbecue-Sandwiches and Broccoli-Slaw 128
Jackfruit-BBQ-Sandwiches 126
Jalapeño Cornbread..54
Jamaican Jerk Vegan Tacos......................................82
Japanese-Pumpkin Rice 54
Jessica's-Pistachio-Oat-Squares............................361
Jumping Jack smoothie recipe...............................396
Just Peachy 397

K

Kale + Black Bean Burrito Bowl..............................275
Kale and Apple Green Detox Smoothie 397
Kale Banana Strawberry Detox Smoothie 397
Kale Coconut Pineapple Detox Smoothie 397
Kale Pesto...74
Kale-Salad w/ Carrot-Ginger-Dressing...................164
Keto Avocado Smoothie with Coconut Milk, Ginger, and Turmeric
   398
Kimchi Brown Rice Bliss Bowls 295
Kimchi-Brown-Rice-Bliss-Bowls 154

L

Latkes 105
Lemon and Thyme Sauce..382
Lemon Chickpea Orzo Soup....................................282
Lemon pepper cauliflower steaks...........................329
Lemon Rosemary White Bean Soup 271
Lemon Thyme oil & Burrata 67
Lentil and Kale Soup 196
Lentil and vegetable dal 185
Lentil Bolognese...383
Lentil Soup with Cumin and Coriander 186
Lentils 375
Lime-Mint Soup..118
Loaded-Potato-Skins..131

M

Macro-Veggie-Bowl 156
Maki-Sushi-Recipe 134
Manchester Stew 208

Mango Chutney 383
Mango Coconut Muffins 70
Mango Ginger Oats Recipe 56
Mango Ginger Rice Bowl 298
Mango Salsa 147
Mango-Coconut-Muffins 133
Mango-Ginger-Rice-Bowl 159
Mango-Kale-Smoothie 398
Many-Veggie Vegetable Soup 83
Maple Cashew Apple Toast 56
Marinated Baked Tempeh 82
Match chia pudding 334
Matcha Milkshakes 71
Mean Green Detox Vegetable Soup 192
Meaty mushroom stew 119
Meaty Seitan Stew 187
Mediterranean quinoa salad 322
Mexican Baked Potato Soup 187
Mexican Cauliflower Rice 136
Mexican-style stuffed zucchini boats 325
Millet medley nourish bowl 349
Minestrone 187
Mint Chip Smoothie 398
Minted peas and baby potatoes 136
Miso Soup 67
Miso udon bowl 120
Mixed Beans Bowl with Sweet Potatoes & Turmeric Rice........341
Mixed spice muesli recipe 350
Mixed vegetable cottage pie 220
Mixed-Fruit-Smoothie 398
Mixed-Greens-Salad w/ Pumpkin-Vinaigrette 168
Mixed-Veggie Sauce 384
Moroccan couscous 221
Moroccan Vegetarian Stew 206
Mushroom & Jalapeño Stew 188
Mushroom and cabbage borscht 120
Mushroom barley soup 121
Mushroom bun sliders 124
Mushroom lasagna 221
Mushroom Risotto 137
Mushroom-Cheesesteak Recipe 169
My Favorite Green Juice 399

N

No-Bake Cookies 57
No-Bake-Energy-Balls 57
No-Boil Vegetable Lasagna 234
Nori Wraps 96
No-Tuna-Salad-Sandwich 127
Nutrient Packed-Simmered-Lentils Recipe............169
Nutty granola 61

O

Oat Flour 376
Oat Milk 375
Oatmeal Cookies 362
Oatmeal-Pancakes with Apples-Cinnamon Recipe...365
Oatmeal-With-Peanut Butter & Banana Recipe 363
One Pot Chili Mac 273
One Pot Vegetable Penne Pasta 258
One-pan pasta primavera 222
One-Pot Beef & Pepper Stew 208
One-Pot Chicken & Cabbage Soup 317
One-Pot Vegan Turmeric Cauliflower Chickpea Stew 193
Orange and Spinach Juice 399
Orange Dream Creamsicle 399
Orange-Glazed Poached Pears 369
Orange-Scented Green Beans with Toasted Almond 109
Orecchiette with Broccoli Rabe 257
Original Baba Ganoush 74
Oyster-Mushroom-Soup 178

P

Paleo-Blackberry-Cashew-Chia Pudding 361
Peach Cobbler 365
Peach Crisp 366
Peach Simple Syrup 399
Peaches and Cream Oatmeal Green Smoothie 399
Peanut Butter Cinnamon Toast 289
Peanut Butter plus Rice Crispy Cacao Nibs Treats....280
Pear Oats with Walnuts 62
Peppermint Crio Bru 400
Perfect Sauteed Carrots 346
Perfect Sauteed Green Beans 348
Perfect Sauteed Zucchini 346
Pesto Pasta Salad 235
Pesto White Bean Soup 201
Pico-De-Gallo 376
Pina Colada Granola (vegan & can be GF) 292
Pineapple and Avocado Detox Smoothie 400
Pineapple Banana Detox Smoothie 400
Pineapple Passion 400
Pineapple Sunrise 401
Pineapple Upside-Down Cake 370
Plant-Based Burrito Breakfast 56
Polenta with Herbs 54
Pomegranate Potato Crostini 76
Pomegranate Rice Salad 295
Pomegranate Smoothie 401
Porcini Mushroom Pate 103
Pork and Green Chile Stew 205
Portobello Mushroom Burger 64
Portobello steaks 327
Portobello-Mushroom-Burger 134
Potato-Leek-Soup 174

Pozole (Posole Verde).. 271
Pressure-Cooker Chai Tea....................................... 401
Protein-Packed Black Bean and Lentil Soup 198
Protein-packed chia pudding................................... 333
Puffed Rice Balls 101
Pumpkin Bars... 367
Pumpkin Pudding.. 365
Pumpkin Spice Oatmeal with Brown Sugar Topping 62
Pumpkin Spice Overnight Oats Recipe 288
Pumpkin Spiced Corn Muffins 79
Pumpkin-Spice Brown Rice Pudding with Dates........ 370
Pumpkin-Tortilla-Soup.. 174

Q

Quick Sauteed Peppers and Onions.......................... 344
Quinoa & Chia Oatmeal Mix 290
Quinoa and butternut squash salad recipe 354
Quinoa Arugula Salad 305
Quinoa Lentil Salad 357
Quinoa Salad 348
Quinoa Tabbouleh 306
Quinoa vegetable salad 222
Quinoa, Corn and Black Bean Salad 306
Quinoa-Pilaf-Recipe 163

R

Radish-Greens-Pesto 377
Radish-Salad w/ Radish-Top-Pesto 164
Rainbow-Veggie-Slaw Wrap 92
Ranch Dressing 377
Raspberry & Blueberry Smoothie 401
Raspberry vinaigrette 383
Raspberry-Cheesecake 364
Raw carrot cake bites 331
Raw chocolate chia pudding................................... 330
Raw chocolate peanut butter cups.......................... 333
Raw chunky monkey ice cream 332
Raw Red Pepper Soup 197
Red Beans & Rice.. 280
Red cabbage with apples and pecans...................... 137
Red Curry-Coconut Milk Soup 188
Red pepper hummus in cucumber cups 103
Red-Curry-Lemongrass-Soup................................... 177
Refried Beans... 278
Rhubarb Chia Strawberry Overnight Oat Parfaits...... 78
Ribollita Tuscan Bean Soup..................................... 181
Rice Salad with Fennel, Chickpeas, and Orange 306
Risotto milanese 223
Roast tomato and orange soup recipe 352
Roasted Brussels Sprouts 66
Roasted Cauliflower & Lemon Zest 147
Roasted cauliflower hummus 101

Roasted Cauliflower Pasta......................................240
Roasted Cauliflower Soup 196
Roasted Chickpeas..66
Roasted corn with poblano-cilantro butter 102
Roasted garlic hummus 324
Roasted minty beetroot and goat's cheese recipe 355
Roasted Poblano Tacos...276
Roasted Pumpkin-Seeds..144
Roasted Radishes and Carrots with a Lemon Butter Dill Sauce.106
Roasted root vegetable medley 109
Roasted Tomato Brown Rice Pasta...........................241
Roasted Tomato Soup 121
Roasted tomatoes 139
Roasted Veggie Brown Rice Buddha Bowl 294
Roasted-Cauliflower-Salad......................................165
Roasted-Golden-Beets...152
Roasted-Kabocha Squash 144
Roasted-Red-Pepper-Soup.......................................176
Roasted-Veggie-Grain-Bowl.....................................158
Root Bowl with Meyer Garlic Sauce Recipe..............350
Root Stew 210
Root Veggie Soup 189
Rosemary Bread 283
Rosemary Garlic Popcorn..123
Rosemary lemon pasta 249
Rosemary-Focaccia-Bread..99
Rustic Cabbage, Potato & White Bean Soup 274

S

Sage-Butternut Squash Sauce 384
Santa Fe Black Bean Burger.....................................269
Sautéed broccoli rabe...139
Sautéed Brussels-Sprouts..130
Sauteed Mushrooms...347
Sauteed Rainbow Chard..346
Sauteed Spinach (That Tastes Amazing)...................345
Sautéed Zucchini and Cherry Tomatoes 139
Savory stuffed cabbage 223
Savory Vegan Breakfast Bowl..................................290
Sea bass with squash and stir-fry recipe 356
Seitan and dumplings 224
Seitan satay 225
Sesame asparagus 140
Sesame ginger broccoli 140
Sesame Noodle Bowl 246
Sesame noodles..225
Sesame Soba Noodles 236
Sesame tofu cutlets 226
Sesame-Soba-Noodles...159
Seven-veg stir-fry recipe...354
Sheet Pan Nachos...73
Sheet-Pan-Nachos..146
Shells & Roasted Cauliflower...................................253
Shiitake Bacon 155

Simple Sauteed Broccoli 345
Simple Sauteed Onions 348
Skinny Detox Soup 201
Slimming Detox Soup 194
Slow Cooker Black Bean & Veggie Soup 200
Slow Cooker Butternut Squash & Kale Stew 200
Slow Cooker Butternut Squash Dal 342
Slow Cooker Chana Masala 343
Slow Cooker Chicken Enchilada Stew 200
Slow Cooker Savory Superfood Soup 199
Slow roasted tomato pasta 250
Slow-Cooked Lentil Stew 209
Slow-Cooker Chicken & Chickpea Soup 312
Slow-Cooker Chicken & White Bean Stew 315
Smokey Tempeh Bacon 262
Smoky Lima Beans 140
Smoky Roasted Eggplant Soup with Za'atar (Fat-Free) ... 340
Smoky Sweet Potatoes with Black Beans & Corn 268
Smoky white bean and tomato soup 122
Soba noodles with shishitos & avocado 243
Socca Recipe 131
Southern sweet potatoes with pecan streusel 141
Southern-style braised greens 141
Southwest quinoa salad 322
Soy Yogurt 62
Soy-cured tuna noodles recipe 351
Spaghetti Aglio e Olio 259
Spaghetti and Meatballs 236
Spaghetti Bolognese 254
Spaghetti Squash 161
Spanish Vegan Paella 281
Spanish-Rice & Black-Beans with Burrito 92
Spicy Asian Quinoa Salad 307
Spicy Beef Vegetable Stew 211
Spicy Chicken Stew 211
Spicy Chili with Red Lentils 189
Spicy kohlrabi noodles 244
Spicy Weight-Loss Cabbage Soup 316
Spicy-Mango AND Avocado-Rice-Bowl 163
Spicy-Tempeh-Mango-Spring Rolls 90
Spinach & Artichoke Casserole with Chicken and Cauliflower Rice
.... 315
Spinach & Chickpeas with 5 Ingredient Ziti Baked 232
Spinach and rice–stuffed tomatoes 109
Spinach Parmesan Zucchini Noodles 234
Spinach, Feta & Rice Casserole 294
Spinach-Tomatillo-Wraps with Hearty-Tahini-Spread ... 93
Spiralized Daikon "Rice Noodle" Bowl 243
Spiralized-Zucchini-Vegetable-Noodle Soup 180
Split-Pea Soup 189
Spring Asparagus Salad with Lemon Vinaigrette 307
Spring Detox: Asparagus, Spinach, and Quinoa Soup ... 204
Spring Green Lemon & Basil Pasta 254
Stacked-Vegetable-Sandwiches & Cilantro-Chutney 128
Steamed Artichokes 142
Steamed Bao-Buns 97

Steamed Dumplings 97
Stir-fried Chinese cress with fermented black beans ... 103
Stir-fry prawns with mushroom and broccoli recipe ... 356
Strawberry Basil Avocado Toast 76
Strawberry muffins 63
Strawberry Rhubarb Bars 77
Strawberry-Banana-Smoothie 402
Strawberry-Kiwi Smoothie 402
Stuffed artichokes 104
Stuffed mushrooms 104
Stuffed Pears with Salted Caramel Sauce 371
Stuffed Poblano Peppers 296
Stuffed Yellow Peppers 293
Stuffed-Acorn Squash 161
Stuffed-Poblano-Peppers 162
Summer Rolls 95
Summer Squash & Corn Orzo 258
Summer squash and onion bake 226
Summer-Strawberry-Crumble 366
Sun-Dried-Tomato & Chickpea Sliders 136
Sunrise Detox Smoothie 402
Sunrise Smoothie 402
Super crunch salad 348
Superfoods Detox Soup 202
Super-Sloppy-Joes 129
Sweet & Spicy Popcorn 69
Sweet Potato & Black Bean Chili 342
Sweet potato (vegan) alfredo 250
Sweet Potato Appetizer Bites 102
Sweet Potato Lentil Stew 210
Sweet Potato Stew 211
Sweet Potato Surprise 256
Sweet Thai Coconut Rice 142
Sweet Vegan Nachos 75
Sweet-Potato & Veggie-Roll-Ups 90
Sweet-Potato-Appetizer-Bites 108
Sweet-Potato-Quinoa-Bowl 159
Sweet-Potato-Soup 183
Swiss chard ravioli 227

T

Taco Salad 165
Tagliatelle with Tomatoes and Greens 253
Tahini Cookies 362
Tahini Noodle Salad with Roasted Carrots & Chickpeas ... 239
Tahini Zucchini Noodles 241
Tamago-Kake-Gohan 167
Tamale casserole 227
Tangy honey mustard dressing 384
Tapioca Pudding 371
Tart-Cherry and Mint-Sorbet 364
Tempeh milanese 228
Teriyaki Beef Stew 208
Teriyaki Sauce -Asian Inspired 385

Teriyaki Tofu-Tempeh Casserole 281
Thai Chickpeas 101
Thai Quinoa Salad 353
Thai Roasted Sweet Potato Soup 198
Thai salad with ginger peanut sauce 320
The Best Guacamole 72
The ultimate detox salad with lemon ginger dressing 320
Toast with Radishes & Dandelion Greens 65
Toasted Oats Cereal (Camping Breakfast) 299
Tofu and veggie stir-fry 229
Tofu Scramble Stuffed Breakfast Sweet Potatoes 265
Tofu Stir Fry with Asparagus Stew 190
Tofu stir fry with broccoli and bell peppers 329
Tofu Stir-Fry 232
Tofu summer rolls 229
Tom yum soup 122
Tomatillo-Salsa-Verde 148
Tomato Basil Soup 195
Tomato- Basil Soup 173
Tomato Bruschetta 130
Tomato rice soup 190
Tomato-Basil-Soup 175
Tomato-Kale Gazpacho Smoothie 402
Tortellini Soup 179
Tortilla-Roll-Ups & Lentils-Spinach 92
Tropical Papaya Perfection 403
Turkish Soup 190
Turmeric Ginger C Boost Life Juice 403
Turmeric Ginger Spiced Cauliflower 110
Turmeric noodle soup 349
Tuscan Portobello Stew 205
Twice Baked Sweet Potatoes 84
Tzatziki Sauce 76

U

Ultimate Sauteed Vegetables 338

V

Vanilla Vegan Buckwheat Pancakes 286
Vanilla-Ginger Syrup 403
Vegan "Cheese" Sauce 385
Vegan Alfredo Sauce 386
Vegan Almond Flour Shortbread Cookies 318
Vegan Apple Cinnamon Oatmeal 339
Vegan Bacon 75
Vegan Black Bean Soup 204
Vegan bolognese sauce with mushrooms. 327
Vegan Burrito Bowl 297
Vegan Carrot Almond Breakfast Pudding 319
Vegan Cashews Dip 73
Vegan cheddar cheese with jalapeño 323
Vegan Cheesecake with Raspberries 371

Vegan chocolate banana cream pie 332
Vegan chocolate cheesecake bars 330
Vegan coconut rice pudding 291
Vegan Collard Greens 264
Vegan enchiladas skillet 326
Vegan Gumbo 344
Vegan Lemon Muffins 80
Vegan Lentil Tacos 343
Vegan Mayo 377
Vegan Pasta Salad 71
Vegan Pimento Dip 72
Vegan Portobello-Pizzas 132
Vegan queso 324
Vegan quinoa salad 321
Vegan Seven Layer Dip 73
Vegan spring rolls with sweet potato noodles 323
Vegan Stuffed Eggplant Provençal 110
Vegan Sushi 296
Vegan sushi bowl 328
Vegan taco salad 321
Vegan zucchini noodle lasagna 327
Vegan-7-Layer-Dip 135
Vegan-Broccoli-Soup 172
Vegan-Burrito-Bowl 160
Vegan-Butternut-Squash-Pudding 364
Vegan-Egg-Salad 157
Vegan-Ice Cream 362
Vegan-Lemon-Muffins 132
Vegan-Miso Soup 119
Vegan-Pecan-Apple-Chickpea-Salad Wraps 99
Vegan-Pimento-Cheese-Dip 380
Vegan-Poke-Bowl 167
Vegan-Pumpkin Bars 77
Vegan-Snack-Wrap 95
Vegan-Spring-Rolls 94
Vegan-Welsh-Rarebit & Mushrooms 142
Vegetable Chili 283
Vegetable detox soup 192
Vegetable enchiladas with roasted tomato sauce 230
Vegetable Stock 182
Vegetarian Chili 267
Vegetarian Pho 179
Vegetarian Tacos with Avocado Sauce 69
Veggie Soup 181
Veggie-Quinoa Soup 191
Veggie-Rice-Bowl Recipe 168
Verde Avocado Salsa 67
Very Berry Breakfast 403
Vinaigrette 386
Vinegar Honey Sauce 385

W

Warm broccoli and chicken salad recipe 314
Warm Caper with Beet Salad 107

Warm Rice and Bean Salad 307
Wasabi-Ginger-Beet & Avocado with Tartines.........................143
Wassail (Hot Mulled Cider).......................................404
Watermelon Wonder 404
Weeknight Three-Bean Chili.......................................191
Weight Loss Soup 202
West African Chicken Stew 209
Wheat Berry Salad with Roasted Beets & Curry Cashew Dressing
....313
White Wine Sherry Sauce.......................................385
White-Bean-Dip.......................................380
Whole-wheat banana pecan pancakes 63
Whole-wheat Pasta e Ceci (Pasta with chickpeas) 230
Wild Rice 174
Wild rice Mason jar salad with basil pesto 319
Wild Rice Soup 65
Winter Greens Salad with Pomegranate & Kumquats 308
Winter vegetable pot pie 231

Wintertime Braised Beef Stew...............................206
World's Best Smoothie.......................................404

Y

Yellow Split Pea Soup 83
Yummy Mango Citrus Drink 404

Z

Zucchini and Avocado Salad with Garlic Herb Dressing 308
Zucchini coconut noodles.......................................245
Zucchini Noodles 242
Zucchini Noodles & Avocado-Miso Sauce 238
Zucchini noodles & lemon /ricotta.......................................236
Zucchini noodles with pesto.......................................320

Made in the USA
Las Vegas, NV
04 January 2024

83820866R00236